Rehabilitation Techniques

in Sports Medicine

Third Edition

Rehabilitation Techniques

in Sports Medicine

William E. Prentice, Ph.D., P.T., A.T.C.

Professor, Coordinator of Sports Medicine Program
Department of Physical Education, Exercise, and Sport Science
Clinical Professor, Division of Physical Therapy
Department of Medical Allied Professions
Associate Professor, Department of Orthopaedics
School of Medicine
The University of North Carolina
Chapel Hill, North Carolina

Director, Sports Medicine Education and Fellowship Programs
HEALTHSOUTH Corporation
Birmingham, Alabama

With 400 illustrations

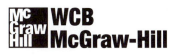

WCB McGraw-Hill

Boston Burr Ridge, IL Dubuque, IA Madison, WI New York San Francisco St. Louis
Bangkok Bogotá Caracas Lisbon London Madrid
Mexico City Milan New Delhi Seoul Singapore Sydney Taipei Toronto

WCB/McGraw-Hill

A Division of The **McGraw·Hill** Companies

REHABILITATION TECHNIQUES IN SPORTS MEDICINE, THIRD EDITION

This book is printed on acid-free paper.

1 2 3 4 5 6 7 8 9 0 QPF/QPF 9 3 2 1 0 9 8

ISBN 0-07-289470-9

Vice president and editorial director: *Kevin T. Kane*
Publisher: *Edward G. Bartell*
Executive editor: *Vicki Malinee*
Developmental editor: *Sarah Reed*
Marketing manager: *Pamela S. Cooper*
Project manager: *Cathy Ford Smith*
Production supervisor: *Deborah Donner*
Coordinator of freelance design: *Michelle D. Whitaker*
Photo research coordinator: *Lori Hancock*
Compositor: *Shepherd, Inc.*
Typeface: *9/11 Photina*
Printer: *Quebecor Printing Book Group/Fairfield, PA*

Freelance cover and interior designer: *David Zielinski*

Library of Congress Cataloging-in-Publication Data

Rehabilitation techniques in sports medicine / [edited by] William E. Prentice. — 3rd ed.
    p. cm.
  Includes bibliographical references and index.
  ISBN 0-07-289470-9
  1. Sports—Accidents and injuries—Patients—Rehabilitation.
2. Sports physical therapy. I. Prentice, William E.
  [DNLM: 1. Athletic Injuries—rehabilitation. 2. Athletic
Injuries—therapy. 3. Physical Therapy—methods. QT 261 R345 1999]
RD97.R44   1999
617.1'027—dc21
DNLM/DLC
for Library of Congress   98-6338
                                  CIP

Preface

As the art and science of sports medicine becomes more sophisticated and specialized, the need has arisen for textbooks that deal with specific aspects of sports injury management. Rehabilitation is certainly one of the major areas of responsibility for the sports therapist. For the classroom instructor, there are a number of texts available that present a general overview of the various aspects of sports medicine. This third edition of *Rehabilitation Techniques in Sports Medicine* is for the student of sports medicine who is interested in gaining more in-depth exposure to the theory and practical application of rehabilitation techniques used in a sports medicine environment.

The purpose of this text is to provide the sports therapist with a comprehensive guide to the design, implementation, and supervision of rehabilitation programs for sport-related injuries. It is intended for use in advanced courses in sports medicine that deal with the practical application of theory in a clinical setting. The contributing authors have collectively attempted to combine their expertise and knowledge to produce a single text that encompasses all aspects of sports medicine rehabilitation.

ORGANIZATION

The text is essentially divided into three sections. The first section deals with achieving the goals of rehabilitation. It begins by discussing the important considerations in designing a rehabilitation program for the injured athlete and provides a basic overview of the rehabilitative process (Chapter 1). It is critical for the sports therapist to understand the importance of the *healing process* and how it should dictate the course of rehabilitation (Chapter 2). It is also essential to be aware of the *psychological* aspects of rehabilitation that the injured athlete must deal with (Chapter 3). The goals of any sports medicine rehabilitation program, including *Restoring Range of Motion and Improving Flexibility* (Chapter 4), *Regaining Muscular Strength, Endurance, and Power* (Chapter 5), *Reestablishing Neuromuscular Control* (Chapter 6), *Regaining Balance and*

Stability (Chapter 7), and *Maintaining Cardiorespiratory Fitness* (Chapter 8), are also discussed in this first section.

The sports therapist has many rehabilitation "tools" with which they can choose to treat an injured athlete. How they choose to use these "tools" is often a matter of personal preference. The second section provides a detailed discussion concerning how these tools may best be incorporated into a rehabilitation program to achieve the goals identified in the first section. The tools of rehabilitation included in this section are: *Isokinetics* (Chapter 9), *Plyometric Exercise* (Chapter 10), *Open- versus Closed-Chain Exercise* (Chapter 11), *Joint Mobilization and Traction Techniques* (Chapter 12), *Proprioceptive Neuromuscular Facilitation Techniques* (Chapter 13), *Aquatic Therapy* (Chapter 14), *Using Therapeutic Modalities* (Chapter 15), *Using Pharmacologic Agents* (Chapter 16), and *Functional Progressions and Functional Testing* (Chapter 17).

The third section of this text goes into great detail on specific rehabilitation techniques that are used in treating a variety of injuries. This section begins by discussing the importance of the *Evaluation process* in first determining the exact nature of an existing injury and then designing a rehabilitation program based on the findings of that evaluation (Chapter 18). Specific rehabilitation techniques are included for the *Shoulder* (Chapter 19), the *Elbow* (Chapter 20), the *Hand and Wrist* (Chapter 21), the *Groin, Hip, and Thigh* (Chapter 22), the *Knee* (Chapter 23), the *Lower Leg* (Chapter 24), the *Ankle and Foot* (Chapter 25), and the *Spine* (Chapter 26). Each chapter begins with a discussion of the pertinent functional anatomy and biomechanics of the region. An extensive series of photographs illustrating a wide variety of rehabilitative exercises is presented in each chapter. The last portion of each chapter involves in-depth discussion of the pathomechanics, injury mechanism, rehabilitation concerns, rehabilitation progressions, and finally, criteria for return to activity for specific injuries.

As will become readily apparent, the third edition of *Rehabilitation Techniques in Sports Medicine* has been significantly expanded and updated to offer a comprehensive reference and guide on sports injury rehabilitation to the sports therapist overseeing programs of rehabilitation. There are a total of eight chapters that are new to this edition.

Comprehensive Coverage of Research-Based Material

Relative to some of the other health-care specializations, sports medicine is still in its infancy. Growth dictates the necessity for expanding our research efforts to identify new and more effective methods and techniques for dealing with sport-related injury. Any sports therapist charged with the responsibility of supervising a rehabilitation program knows that the most currently accepted and up-to-date rehabilitation protocols tend to change rapidly. A sincere effort has been made by the contributing authors to present the most recent information on the various aspects of injury rehabilitation currently available from the literature.

Additionally, this manuscript has been critically reviewed by selected athletic trainers and physical therapists who are well respected clinicians, educators, and researchers in this field to further ensure than the material presented is accurate and current.

Pertinent to Sports Medicine

There are many texts currently available that deal with the subject of rehabilitation of injury in various patient populations. However, the third edition of this text concentrates exclusively on the application of rehabilitation techniques in a sport-related setting. The emphasis on sports medicine makes this text somewhat unique.

Pedagogical Aids

The aids provided in this text to assist the student in its use include the following:

Objectives. These are listed at the beginning of each individual chapter to identify the concepts to be presented.

Figures and Tables. The number of figures and tables included throughout the text has been significantly increased in an effort to provide as much visual and graphic demonstration of specific rehabilitation techniques and exercises as possible.

Summary. Each chapter has a summary that outlines the major points discussed.

References. A comprehensive list of up-to-date references is presented at the end of each chapter to provide additional information relative to chapter content.

Acknowledgments

The preparation of the manuscript for a textbook is a long term commitment and extremely demanding of everyone involved. It demands input, effort, and cooperation on the part of many different individuals. I would like to personally thank each of the contributing authors. They were asked to contribute to this text because I have tremendous respect for them both personally and professionally. These individuals have distinguished themselves as educators and clinicians dedicated to the field of Sports Medicine. I am exceedingly grateful for their input.

Sarah Reed, my developmental editor at WCB/McGraw-Hill, has been persistent and diligent in the completion of this text. She has patiently encouraged me along and I have certainly appreciated her support.

The following individuals have invested a significant amount of time and energy as reviewers for this manuscript and I appreciate their efforts:

Thomas Kaminski, Ph.D., A.T.C.
University of Florida

Dan Brown, M.S., L.A.T., A.T.C.
Midwestern State University

Robert Moss, Ph.D., A.T.C.
Western Michigan University

Finally, and most importantly, this is for my family—Tena, Brian, and Zachary, who make an effort such as this worthwhile.

—Bill Prentice

Contributors

John Marc Davis, P.T., A.T.C.

Physical Therapist/Athletic Trainer
Division of Sports Medicine
The University of North Carolina
Chapel Hill, North Carolina

Bernard DePalma, M.Ed., P.T., A.T.C.

Head Athletic Trainer
Cornell University
Ithaca, New York

Freddie Fu, M.D.

Blue Shield/Blue Cross Professor of Orthopaedic Surgery
Department of Orthopaedic Surgery
Director, Center for Sports Medicine
University of Pittsburgh Medical Center
Pittsburgh, Pennsylvania

Joe Gieck, Ed.D., P.T., A.T.C.

Professor, Department of Human Services, Curry School
  of Education
Assistant Clinical Professor, Department of Orthopaedics
  and Rehabilitation
Head Athletic Trainer
The University of Virginia
Charlottesville, Virginia

Kevin Guskiewicz, Ph.D., A.T.C.

Assistant Professor, Department of Physical Education,
  Exercise, and Sport Science
Director, Undergraduate Athletic Training Program
The University of North Carolina
Chapel Hill, North Carolina

Elizabeth Hedgepath, Ed.D.

Sport Psychology Consultant
Durham, North Carolina

Chris Hirth, M.S., P.T., A.T.C.

Athletic Trainer/Physical Therapist
Division of Sports Medicine
The University of North Carolina
Chapel Hill, North Carolina

Daniel N. Hooker, Ph.D., P.T., SCS, A.T.C.

Coordinator of Athletic Training and Physical Therapy
Division of Sports Medicine
The University of North Carolina
Chapel Hill, North Carolina

Patsy Huff, Pharm.D., F.A.S.H.P.

Director of the Pharmacy, Student Health Service
Professor, School of Pharmacy
The University of North Carolina
Chapel Hill, North Carolina

Stuart L. (Skip) Hunter, P.T., A.T.C.

Director, Clemson Physical Therapy
Clemson, South Carolina

Scott M. Lephart, Ph.D., A.T.C.

Associate Professor, Education
Assistant Professor of Orthopaedic Surgery
Director, Neuromuscular Research Laboratory
Sports Medicine Program
University of Pittsburgh
Pittsburgh, Pennsylvania

Michael McGee, M.A., A.T.C.

Director of Sports Medicine
Instructor, Department of Physical Education
Lenori Rhyne
Hickory, North Carolina

Janine Oman, M.S., P.T., A.T.C.

Athletic Trainer/Physical Therapist
The Ohio State University
Columbus, Ohio

David H. Perrin, Ph.D., A.T.C.

Director, Graduate Athletic Training Program
Professor, Curry School of Education
The University of Virginia
Charlottesville, Virginia

William E. Prentice, Ph.D., P.T., A.T.C.

Professor, Coordinator of the Sports Medicine Program
Department of Physical Education, Exercise, and Sport
  Science
Clinical Professor, Division of Physical Therapy
Department of Medical Allied Professions
Associate Professor, Department of Orthopaedics
School of Medicine
The University of North Carolina
Chapel Hill, North Carolina
Director, Sports Medicine Education and Fellowship
  Programs
HEALTHSOUTH Corporation
Birmingham, Alabama

Gina Selepak, M.A., A.T.C.

Head Athletic Trainer
Lake Highland Preparatory School
Orlando, Florida

Ann Marie Schneider, O.T.R., C.H.T.

Coordinator, Hand Center
Raleigh Orthopaedic and Rehabilitation Specialists
Raleigh, North Carolina

Rob Schneider, M.S., P.T., A.T.C.

Athletic Trainer/Physical Therapist
Division of Sports Medicine
The University of North Carolina
Chapel Hill, North Carolina

C. Buz Swanik, M.S., A.T.C.

Neuromuscular Research Laboratory
Sports Medicine Program
University of Pittsburgh
Pittsburgh, Pennsylvania

Steve Tippett, M.S., P.T., SCS, A.T.C.

Assistant Professor, Department of Physical Therapy
Director, Great Plains Sports Medicine and Rehabilitation
  Center
Peoria, Illinois

Michael L. Voight, D.P.T., P.T., SCS, OCS, A.T.C.

Associate Professor
Department of Physical Therapy
Belmont University
Nashville, Tennessee

Pete Zulia, P.T., A.T.C.

Director, Oxford Physical Therapy
Instructor, Athletic Training Curriculum
Miami University of Ohio
Oxford, Ohio

Brief Contents

Contents

PART TWO   The Tools of Rehabilitation

PART THREE Rehabilitation Techniques for Specific Injuries

PART ONE

Achieving the Goals of Rehabilitation

CHAPTER 1

Considerations in Designing a Rehabilitation Program for the Injured Athlete

William E. Prentice

After completion of this chapter, the student should be able to do the following:

- Discuss the philosophy of the rehabilitative process in a sports medicine environment.

- Realize the importance of understanding the healing process, the biomechanics, and the psychological aspects of a rehabilitation program.

- Identify the individual short-term and long-term goals of a rehabilitation program.

- Discuss the criteria and the decision-making process for determining when the injured athlete may return to full activity.

One of the primary goals of every sports medicine professional is to create a playing environment for the athlete that is as safe as it can possibly be. Regardless of that effort, the nature of athletic participation dictates that injuries will eventually occur. Fortunately, few of the injuries that occur in an athletic setting are life-threatening. The majority of the injuries are not serious and lend themselves to rapid rehabilitation. When injuries do occur, the focus of the sports therapist shifts from injury prevention to injury treatment and rehabilitation. In a sports medicine setting, the sports therapist generally assumes primary responsibility for the design, implementation, and supervision of the rehabilitation program for the injured athlete.

The sports therapist responsible for overseeing an exercise rehabilitation program must have as complete an understanding of the injury as possible, including knowledge of how the injury was sustained, the major anatomical structures affected, the degree or grade of trauma, and the stage or phase of the injury's healing.[7]

THE PHILOSOPHY OF SPORTS MEDICINE REHABILITATION

The approach to rehabilitation is considerably different in a sports medicine environment than in most other rehabilitation settings.[2] The competitive nature of athletics necessitates an aggressive approach to rehabilitation. Because the competitive season in most sports is relatively short, the athlete does not have the luxury of being able to sit around and do nothing until the injury heals. The goal is to return to activity as soon as is safely possible. Consequently, the sports therapist tends to play games with the healing process, never really allowing enough time for an injury to completely heal. The sports therapist who is supervising the rehabilitation program usually performs a "balancing act"—walking along a thin line between not pushing the athlete hard enough or fast enough and being overly aggressive. In either case, a mistake in judgment on the part of the sports therapist can hinder the athlete's return to activity.

Understanding the Healing Process

Decisions as to when and how to alter or progress a rehabilitation program should be based primarily on the process of injury healing. The sports therapist must possess a sound understanding of both the sequence and the time frames for the various phases of healing, realizing that certain physiological events must occur during each of the phases. Anything that is done during a rehabilitation program that interferes with this healing process will likely increase the length of time required for rehabilitation and slow return to full activity. The healing process must have an opportunity to accomplish what it is supposed to. At best the sports therapist can only try to create an environment that is conducive to the healing process. Little can be done to speed up the process physiologically, but many things can impede healing (see Chapter 2).

Exercise Intensity. The **SAID Principle** (an acronym for *specific adaptation to imposed demand*) states that when an injured structure is subjected to stresses and overloads of varying intensities, it will gradually adapt over time to whatever demands are placed upon it.[9] During the rehabilitation process, the stresses of reconditioning exercises must not be so great as to exacerbate the injury before the injured structure has had a chance to adapt specifically to the increased demands. Engaging in exercise that is too intense or too prolonged can be detrimental to the progress of rehabilitation. Indications that the intensity of the exercises being incorporated into the rehabilitation program exceed the limits of the healing process include an increase in the amount of swelling, an increase in pain, a loss or a plateau in strength, a loss or a plateau in range of motion, or an increase in the laxity of a healing ligament.[16] If an exercise or activity causes any of these signs, the sports therapist must back off and become less aggressive in the rehabilitation program.

In most injury situations, early exercise rehabilitation involves submaximal exercise performed in short bouts that are repeated several times daily. Exercise intensity must be commensurate with healing. As recovery increases, the intensity of exercise also increases, with the exercise performed less often. Finally, the athlete returns to a conditioning mode of exercise, which often includes high-intensity exercise three to four times per week.

Understanding the Pathomechanics of Injury

When a joint or other anatomic structure is damaged by injury, normal biomechanical function is compromised. Adaptive changes occur that alter the manner in which various forces collectively act upon that joint to produce motion. Thus the biomechanics of joint motion are changed as a result of that injury.

It is critical that the sports therapist supervising a rehabilitation program has a solid foundation in biomechanics and functional human anatomy, to be effective in designing a rehabilitation program. A sports therapist who does not understand the biomechanics of normal motion will find it very difficult to identify existing adaptive or compensatory changes in motion and then to know what must be done in a rehabilitation program to correct the pathomechanics.

Understanding the Psychological Aspects of Rehabilitation

The psychological aspects of how the individual athlete deals with an injury are a critical yet often neglected factor in the rehabilitation process. Injury and illness produce a wide range of emotional reactions; therefore the sports therapist needs to develop an understanding of the psyche of each athlete. Athletes vary in terms of pain threshold, cooperation and compliance, competitiveness, denial of disability, depression, intrinsic and extrinsic motivation, anger, fear, guilt, and the ability to adjust to injury. Besides dealing with the mental aspect of the injury, sports psychology can also be used to improve total athletic performance through the use of visualization, self-hypnosis, and relaxation techniques (see Chapter 3).

The Tools of Rehabilitation

Sports therapists have many tools at their disposal—such as manual therapy techniques, therapeutic modalities, aquatic therapy, and the use of physician-prescribed medications—that can individually or collectively facilitate the rehabilitative process. How different sports therapists choose to utilize those tools is often a matter of individual preference and experience.

Additionally, patients differ in their responses to various treatment techniques. Thus the sports therapist should avoid "cookbook" rehabilitation protocols that can be followed like a recipe. In fact, use of rehabilitation "recipes" should be strongly discouraged. Instead the sports therapist must develop a broad theoretical knowledge base from which specific techniques or tools of rehabilitation can be selected and practically applied to each individual case.

Therapeutic Exercise versus Conditioning Exercise

Exercise is an essential factor in fitness conditioning, injury prevention, and injury rehabilitation. To compete successfully at a high level, the athlete must be fit. An athlete who is not fit is more likely to sustain an injury. Coaches and athletic trainers both recognize that improper conditioning is one of the major causes of sport injuries. It is essential that the athlete engage in training and conditioning exercises that minimize the possibility of injury while maximizing performance.[12]

The basic principles of training and conditioning exercises also apply to techniques of therapeutic, rehabilitative, or reconditioning exercises that are specifically concerned with restoring normal body function following injury. The term **therapeutic exercise** is perhaps most widely used to indicate exercises that are used in a rehabilitation program.[6]

GOALS OF A REHABILITATION PROGRAM

Designing an effective rehabilitation program is relatively simple if the sports therapist routinely addresses several basic components. These basic components can also be considered the short-term goals of a rehabilitation program. They should include (1) providing correct immediate first aid and management following injury to limit or control swelling; (2) reducing or minimizing pain; (3) restoring full range of motion; (4) restoring or increasing muscular strength, endurance, and power; (5) reestablishing neuromuscular control; (6) improving balance; (7) maintaining cardiorespiratory fitness, and; (8) incorporating appropriate functional progressions. The long-term goal is almost invariably to return the injured athlete to practice or competition as quickly and safely as possible.

Establishing reasonable, attainable goals and including specific exercises or activities to address these goals is the easy part of overseeing a rehabilitation program. The difficult part comes in knowing exactly when and how to progress, change, or alter the rehabilitation program to most effectively accomplish both long- and short-term goals.

Athletes tend to be goal-oriented individuals. Thus, the sports therapist should design a goal-oriented rehabilitation program in which the athlete can have a series of progressive "successes" in achieving attainable short-term goals throughout the rehabilitation process. Injured

athletes are almost always most concerned to know precisely how long they will be out and when exactly they can return to full activity. The sports therapist should not make the mistake of giving an injured athlete an exact time frame or date. Instead, the athlete should be given a series of sequenced challenges, involving increasing skill and ability, that must be met before progressing to the next level in their rehabilitation program. It is critical that the athlete be actively involved in planning the process of rehabilitating their injury.

The Importance of Controlling Swelling

The process of rehabilitation begins immediately after injury. Thus, in addition to understanding exactly how the injury occurred, the sports therapist must be competent in providing correct and appropriate initial care. Initial first aid and management techniques are perhaps the most critical part of any rehabilitation program. The manner in which the injury is initially managed unquestionably has a significant impact on the course of the rehabilitative process.[10]

The one problem all injuries have in common is swelling. Swelling can be caused by any number of factors, including bleeding, production of synovial fluid, an accumulation of inflammatory by-products, edema, or a combination of several factors. No matter which mechanism is involved, swelling produces an increased pressure in the injured area, and increased pressure causes pain.[17] Swelling can also cause neuromuscular inhibition, which results in weak muscle contraction. Swelling is most likely during the first 72 hours after an injury.

Once swelling has occurred, the healing process is significantly retarded. The injured area cannot return to normal until all the swelling is gone. Therefore everything that is done in first aid management of any of these conditions should be directed toward controlling the swelling.[1] If the swelling can be controlled initially in the acute stage of injury, the time required for rehabilitation is likely to be significantly reduced.

To control and significantly limit the amount of swelling, the PRICE principle—*protection, restricted activity, ice, compression, and elevation*—should be applied (Figure 1-1). Each factor plays a critical role in limiting swelling, and all of these elements should be used simultaneously.

Protection. The injured area should be protected from additional injury by applying appropriate splints, braces, pads, or other immobilization devices. If the injury involves the lower extremity, it is recommended that the athlete go non-weight-bearing on crutches at least until the acute inflammatory response has subsided.

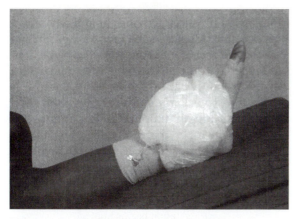

Figure 1-1 The PRICE technique should be used immediately following injury to limit swelling.

Restricted Activity (Rest). The period of restricted activity following any type of injury is absolutely critical in any treatment program. Once an anatomical structure is injured, it immediately begins the healing process. In an injured structure that is not rested and is subjected to unnecessary external stress and strains, the healing process never really gets a chance to begin. Consequently, the injury does not get well, and the time required for rehabilitation is markedly increased. This is not to minimize the importance of early mobility. Controlled mobility has been shown to be superior to immobilization for scar formation, revascularization, muscle regeneration, and reorientation of muscle fibers and tensile properties.[12] The amount of time necessary for resting varies with the severity of the injury, but most minor injuries should rest for approximately 24 to 48 hours before an active rehabilitation program is begun.

It must be emphasized that rest does not mean that the athlete does nothing. The term *rest* applies only to the injured body part. During this period, the athlete should continue to work on cardiovascular fitness and strengthening and flexibility exercises for the other parts of the body not affected by the injury.[18]

Ice. The use of cold is the initial treatment of choice for virtually all conditions involving injuries to the musculoskeletal system.[14] It is most commonly used immediately after injury to decrease pain and promote local vasoconstriction, thus controlling hemorrhage and edema. Cold applied to an acute injury will lower metabolism in the injured area, and thus the tissue demands for oxygen, thus reducing hypoxia. This benefit extends to uninjured tissue, preventing injury-related tissue death from spreading to adjacent normal cellular structures. It is also used in the acute phase of inflammatory conditions, such as bursitis, tenosynovitis, and tendinitis, in which heat can cause additional pain and swelling. Cold is also used to reduce the reflex muscle guarding and spastic conditions that accompany pain. Its analgesic effect is probably one of its greatest benefits. One explanation of the analgesic effect is that cold decreases the velocity of nerve conduction, although it does not entirely eliminate it. Cold can also bombard cutaneous sensory nerve receptor areas with so many cold impulses that pain impulses are lost. With ice treatments, the athlete reports an uncomfortable sensation of cold, followed by burning, an aching sensation, and finally complete numbness.[8,14]

Because of the low thermal conductivity of underlying subcutaneous fat tissues, applications of cold for short periods are ineffective in cooling deeper tissues. For this reason longer treatments of 20 to 30 minutes are recommended. Cold treatments are generally believed to be more effective in reaching deeper tissues than most forms of heat. Cold applied to the skin is capable of significantly lowering the temperature of tissues at a considerable depth. The extent of this lowered tissue temperature depends on the type of cold applied to the skin, the duration of its application, the thickness of the subcutaneous fat, and the region of the body to which it is applied. Ice should be applied to the injured area until the signs and symptoms of inflammation have disappeared and there is little or no chance that swelling will be increased by using some form of heat. Ice should be used for at least 72 hours after an acute injury.[8,14]

Compression. Compression is likely the single most important technique for controlling initial swelling. The purpose of compression is to mechanically reduce the amount of space available for swelling by applying pressure around an injured area. The best way of applying pressure is to use an elastic wrap, such as an Ace bandage, to apply firm but even pressure around the injury.

Because of the pressure buildup in the tissues, having a compression wrap in place for a long time can become painful. However, the wrap must be kept in place despite significant pain because it is so important in the control of swelling. The compression wrap should be left in place continuously for at least 72 hours after an acute injury. In many overuse problems, such as tendinitis, tenosynovitis, and particularly bursitis, which involve ongoing inflammation, the compression wrap should be worn until the swelling is almost entirely gone.

Elevation. The fifth factor that assists in controlling swelling is elevation. The injured part, particularly an extremity, should be elevated to eliminate the effects of gravity on blood pooling in the extremities. Elevation assists venous and lymphatic drainage of blood and other fluids from the injured area back to the central circulatory system. The greater the degree of elevation, the more effective the reduction in swelling. For example, in an ankle sprain, the leg should be placed in such a position that the ankle is virtually straight up in the air. The injured part should be elevated as much as possible during the first 72 hours.

The appropriate technique for initial management of the acute injuries discussed in this chapter, regardless of where they occur, would be the following:

1. Apply a compression wrap directly over the injury. Wrapping should be from distal to proximal. Tension should be firm and consistent. Wetting the elastic wrap to facilitate the passage of cold from ice packs might be helpful.
2. Surround the injured area entirely with ice bags, and secure them in place. Ice bags should be left on for 45 minutes initially and then 1 hour off and 30 minutes on as much as possible over the next 24 hours. During the following 48-hour period, ice should be applied as often as possible.
3. The injured part should be elevated as much as possible during the initial 72-hour period after injury. Keeping the injured part elevated while sleeping is particularly important.
4. Allow the injured part to rest for approximately 24 hours after the injury.

Controlling Pain

When an injury occurs, the sports therapist must realize that the athlete will experience some degree of pain. The extent of the pain will be determined in part by the severity of the injury, by the athlete's individual response to and perception of pain, and by the circumstances in which the injury occurred. The athlete's pain is real. The sports therapist can effectively modulate acute pain by using the PRICE technique immediately after injury.[12] A physician can also make use of various medications to help ease pain.

Persistent pain can make strengthening or flexibility exercises more difficult, thus interfering with the rehabilitation process. The sports therapist should routinely address pain during each individual treatment session. Making use of appropriate therapeutic modalities—including various techniques of cryotherapy, thermotherapy, and electrical stimulating currents—will help modulate pain throughout the rehabilitation process[14] (Figure 1-2).

To a great extent, pain will dictate the rate of progression. With initial injury, pain is intense and tends to decrease and eventually subside altogether as healing progresses. Any exacerbation of either pain, swelling, or other clinical symptoms during or following a particular

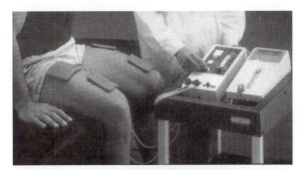

Figure 1-2 Several modalities, including electrical stimulating currents, may be used to modulate pain.

exercise or activity indicates that the load is too great for the level of tissue repair or remodeling.

Restoring Range of Motion

Following injury to a joint, there will always be some associated loss of motion. That loss of movement can be attributed to a number of pathological factors, including resistance of the musculotendinous unit (i.e., muscle, tendon, fascia) to stretch; contracture of connective tissue (i.e., ligaments, joint capsule); or some combination of the two.

It is critical for the sports therapist to closely evaluate the injured joint to determine whether motion is limited due to physiological movement constraints involving musculotendinous units or due to limitation in accessory motion (joint arthrokinematics) involving the joint capsule and ligaments. If physiological movement is restricted, the athlete should engage in stretching activities designed to improve flexibility (Figure 1-3). Stretching exercises should be used whenever there is musculotendinous resistance to stretch. If accessory motion is limited due to some restriction of the joint capsule or the ligaments, the sports therapist should incorporate joint mobilization and traction techniques into the treatment program (Figure 1-4). Mobilization techniques should be used whenever there are tight articular structures.[11] Traditionally, rehabilitation programs tend to concentrate more on passive physiological movements without paying much attention to accessory motions.

Restoring Muscular Strength, Endurance, and Power

Muscular strength, endurance and power are among the most essential factors in restoring the function of a body part to preinjury status. Isometric, progressive resistive (isotonic), isokinetic, and plyometric exercises can bene-

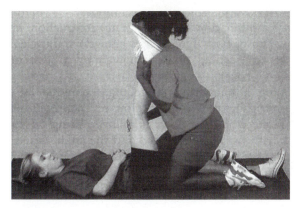

Figure 1-3   Stretching techniques are used with tight musculotendinous structures to improve physiological range of motion.

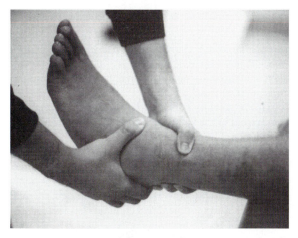

Figure 1-4   Joint mobilization techniques are used with tight ligamentous or capsular structures to improve accessory motion.

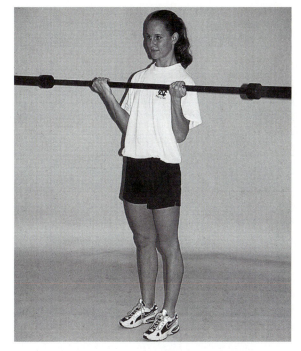

Figure 1-5   Progressive resistive exercise using isotonic contractions is the most widely used rehabilitative strengthening technique.

ing (Figure 1-5). Progressive resistive exercise uses isotonic contractions in which force is generated while the muscle is changing in length. Isotonic contractions may be either concentric or eccentric. In a rehabilitation program the sports therapist should incorporate both eccentric and concentric strengthening exercises. Traditionally, progressive resistive exercise has concentrated primarily on the concentric component and has to some extent minimized the importance of the eccentric component.

Isokinetic Exercise.   Isokinetic exercise is commonly used in the rehabilitative process.[13] It is most often incorporated during the later phases of a rehabilitation program. Isokinetics uses a fixed speed with accommodating resistance to provide maximal resistance throughout the range of motion (Figure 1-6). The speed of movement can be altered in isokinetic exercise. Isokinetic measures are commonly used as a criteria for return of the athlete to functional activity following injury.

Plyometric Exercise.   Plyometric exercises are most often incorporated into the later stages of a rehabilitation program. Plyometrics use a quick eccentric stretch to facilitate a subsequent concentric contraction. Plyometric exercises are useful in restoring or developing the athlete's ability to produce dynamic movements associated with muscular power (Figure 1-7). The ability to

fit rehabilitation. A major goal in performing strengthening exercises is to work through a full pain-free range of motion.

Isometric Exercise.   Isometric exercises are commonly performed in the early phase of rehabilitation when a joint is immobilized for a period of time. They are useful when using resistance training through a full range of motion might make the injury worse. Isometrics increase static strength and assist in decreasing the amount of atrophy. Isometrics also can lessen swelling by causing a muscle pumping action to remove fluid and edema.

Progressive Resistive Exercise.   Progressive resistive exercise (PRE) is the most commonly used strengthening technique in a rehabilitation program. PRE may be done using free weights, exercise machines, or rubber tub-

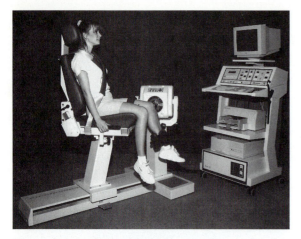

Figure 1-6 Isokinetic exercise is most often used in the later stages of rehabilitation.

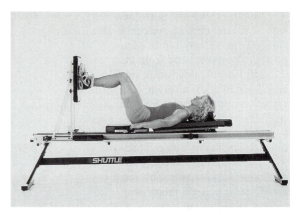

Figure 1-8 Closed-kinetic-chain exercises are widely used in rehabilitation.

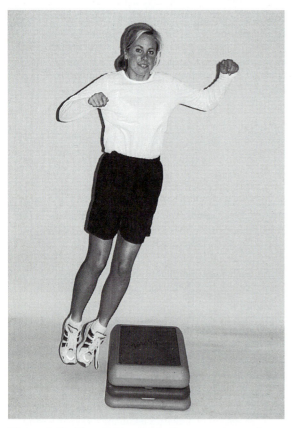

Figure 1-7 Plyometric exercise focuses on improving dynamic, power movements.

generate force very rapidly is a key to successful performance in many sport activities. It is critical to address the element of muscular power in rehabilitation programs for the injured athlete.

Open- versus Closed-Kinetic-Chain Exercise. The concept of the kinetic chain deals with the anatomical functional relationships that exist in the upper and lower extremities. An open kinetic chain exists when the foot or hand is not in contact with the ground or some other surface.[4] In a closed kinetic chain, the foot or hand is weight-bearing (Figure 1-8). In rehabilitation, the use of closed-chain strengthening techniques has become the treatment of choice for many sports therapists. Closed-kinetic-chain exercises use varying combinations of isometric, concentric, and eccentric contractions that must occur simultaneously in different muscle groups within the chain.

Reestablishing Neuromuscular Control

Reestablishing neuromuscular control should be of prime concern to the sports therapist in all rehabilitation programs.[5] The ability to sense the position of a joint in space is mediated by mechanoreceptors found in both muscles and joints, in addition to cutaneous, visual, and vestibular input. Neuromuscular control relies on the central nervous system to interpret and integrate proprioceptive and kinesthetic information and then to control individual muscles and joints to produce coordinated movement.[16]

Following injury and subsequent rest and immobilization, the central nervous system "forgets" how to put together information coming from muscle and joint mechanoreceptors, and from cutaneous, visual, and vestibular input. Regaining neuromuscular control means regaining the ability to follow some previously established sensory pattern. Neuromuscular control is the mind's attempt to teach the body conscious control of a specific movement. Successful repetition of a patterned movement makes its performance progressively less difficult, thus requiring less concentration, until the movement becomes automatic. This requires many repetitions of the same movement, progressing step-by-step from simple to more complex movements. Strengthening exercises, particularly those that tend to be more functional, such as closed-kinetic-chain exercises, are essential for reestablishing neuromuscular control.[16] Addressing neuromuscular control is critical throughout the recovery process, but it is perhaps most critical during the early stages of rehabilitation to avoid reinjury.[16]

Balance

Balance involves the complex integration of muscular forces, neurological sensory information received from the mechanoreceptors, and biomechanical information.[3,5] The ability to balance and maintain postural stability is essential to acquiring or reacquiring complex motor skills.[16] Athletes who show a decreased sense of balance or a lack of postural stability following injury might lack sufficient proprioceptive and kinesthetic information and/or might have muscular weakness, either of which can limit the ability to generate an effective correction response when there is not equilibrium. A rehabilitation program must include functional exercises that incorporate balance and proprioceptive training that prepares the athlete for return to activity (Figure 1-9). Failure to address balance problems can predispose the athlete to reinjury.

Maintaining Cardiorespiratory Fitness

Maintaining cardiorespiratory fitness is perhaps the single most neglected component of a rehabilitation program. An athlete spends a considerable amount of time preparing the cardiorespiratory system to be able to handle the increased demands made upon it during a competitive season. When injury occurs and the athlete is forced to miss training time, cardiorespiratory fitness can decrease rapidly. Thus the sports therapist must design or substi-

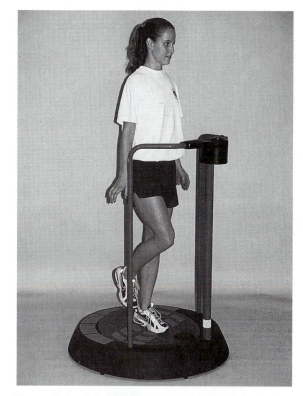

Figure 1-9   Reestablishing neuromuscular control and balance is critical to regaining functional performance capabilities.

tute alternative activities that allow the athlete to maintain existing levels of cardiorespiratory fitness as early as possible in the rehabilitation period[11] (Figure 1-10).

Depending on the nature of the injury, there are a number of possible activities that can help the athlete maintain fitness levels. When there is a lower-extremity injury, non-weight-bearing activities should be incorporated. Pool activities provide an excellent means for injury rehabilitation. Cycling also can positively stress the cardiorespiratory system.

Functional Progressions

The purpose of any program of rehabilitation is to restore normal function following injury. Functional progressions involve a series of gradually progressive activities designed to prepare the individual for return to a specific sport.[15] Those skills necessary for successful participation in a given sport are broken down into component parts, and the athlete gradually reacquires those skills within the limitations

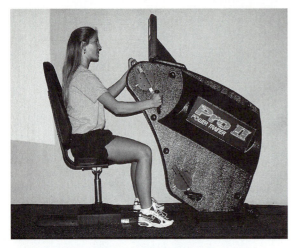

Figure 1-10 Every rehabilitation program must include some exercise designed to maintain cardiorespiratory fitness.

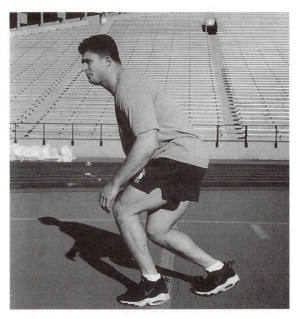

Figure 1-11 Performance on functional tests can determine the athlete's capability to return to full activity.

of his or her own individual progress.[16] Every new activity introduced must be carefully monitored by the sports therapist to determine the athlete's ability to perform and her or his physical tolerance. If an activity does not produce additional pain or swelling, the level should be advanced; new activities should be introduced as quickly as possible.

Functional progressions will gradually help the injured athlete achieve normal pain-free range of motion, restore adequate strength levels, and regain neuromuscular control throughout the rehabilitation program.

Functional Testing

Functional testing uses functional progression drills to assess the athlete's ability to perform a specific activity (Figure 1-11). Functional testing involves a single maximal effort performed to indicate how close the athlete is to a full return to activity. For years sports therapists have assessed athletes' progress with a variety of functional tests, including agility runs (Figure eights, shuttle run, carioca), sidestepping, vertical jump, hopping for time or distance, and co-contraction tests.[16]

Criteria for Full Recovery

All exercise rehabilitation plans must determine what is meant by complete recovery from an injury. Often it means that the athlete is fully reconditioned and has achieved full range of movement, strength, neuromuscular control, car-

diovascular fitness, and sport-specific functional skills. Besides physical well-being, the athlete must also have regained full confidence to return to his or her sport.

Specific criteria for a return to full activity after rehabilitation of the injured knee is largely determined by the nature and severity of the specific injury, but it also depends on the philosophy and judgment of both the physician and the sports therapist. Traditionally, return to activity has been dictated through both objective and subjective evaluations. Objective evaluation techniques have made use primarily of isokinetic testing and arthrometry. The advantage of testing with an isokinetic device that indicates levels of strength and an arthrometer that measures joint laxity is that the sports therapist is provided with some hard, quantifiable data relative to the athlete's progress in the rehabilitation program. Recently, however, considerable debate has taken place in the sports medicine community on the functional application of isokinetic testing. The question has been raised whether the ability to generate torque at a fixed speed is indicative of the athlete's capability of returning to an activity in which success more often depends on the ability to generate force at a high velocity.

For the athlete, it might be more practical to base criteria for return on functional capabilities as indicated by performance on specific functional tests that are more closely related to the demands of a particular sport. Performance on functional tests, such as those described in Chapter 17 (hop test, co-contraction test), should serve as primary determinants of the athlete's capability to return to full activity. Currently data on the majority of these tests are limited. Thus at present they remain as purely subjective evaluations until research data become available to objectively quantify performance on various functional tests. Once results are objectively quantified, these functional tests will be extremely useful and valuable tools for determining readiness to return to full activity.

The decision to release an athlete recovering from injury to a full return to athletic activity is the final stage of the rehabilitation/recovery process. The decision should be carefully considered by each member of the sports medicine team involved in the rehabilitation process. The team physician should be ultimately responsible for deciding that the athlete is ready to return to practice and/or competition. That decision should be based on collective input from the sports therapist, the coach, and the athlete.

In considering the athlete's return to activity, the following concerns should be addressed:

- *Physiological healing constraints.* Has rehabilitation progressed to the later stages of the healing process?
- *Pain status.* Has pain disappeared, or is the athlete able to play within her or his own levels of pain tolerance?
- *Swelling.* Is there still a chance that swelling could be exacerbated by return to activity?
- *ROM.* Is ROM adequate to allow the athlete to perform both effectively and with minimized risk of reinjury?
- *Strength.* Is strength, endurance, or power great enough to protect the injured structure from reinjury?
- *Neuromuscular control/proprioception/ kinesthesia.* Has the athlete "relearned" how to use the injured body part?
- *Cardiorespiratory fitness.* Has the athlete been able to maintain cardiorespiratory fitness at or near the level necessary for competition?
- *Sport-specific demands.* Are the demands of the sport or a specific position such that the athlete will not be at risk of reinjury?
- *Functional testing.* Does performance on appropriate functional tests indicate that the extent of recovery is sufficient to allow successful performance?
- *Prophylactic strapping, bracing, padding.* Are any additional supports necessary for the injured athlete to return to activity?
- *Responsibility of the athlete.* Is the athlete capable of listening to his or her body and recognizing situations that present a potential for reinjury?
- *Predisposition to injury.* Is this athlete prone to reinjury or a new injury when she or he is not 100 percent?
- *Psychological factors.* Is the athlete capable of returning to activity and competing at a high level without fear of reinjury?
- *Athlete education and preventive maintenance program.* Does the athlete understand the importance of continuing to engage in conditioning exercises that can greatly reduce the chances of reinjury?

THE RELATIONSHIP OF THE SPORTS THERAPIST AND THE PHYSICIAN

Certainly, the sports therapist has an obligation to the injured athlete to understand the nature of the injury, the function of the structures damaged, and the different tools available to safely rehabilitate the athlete. Additionally, the sports therapist must understand the treatment philosophy of the athlete's physician and be careful in applying different treatment regimens, because what might be a safe but outdated technique in the opinion of one physician might be the treatment of choice to another. Communication is crucial to prevent misunderstandings and a subsequent loss of rapport with the athlete or the physician. Successful sports therapists are flexible in their approach to rehabilitation, incorporating techniques that are sound and effective but somewhat variable from athlete to athlete and physician to physician.

Under ideal conditions, the physician, the sports therapist, the athlete, and the athlete's family will communicate freely and function as a team. This group is intimately involved with the rehabilitative process, beginning with patient assessment, treatment selection, and implementation and ending with functional exercises and return to activity. The sports therapist directs the postacute phase of the rehabilitation, and it is crucial that the athlete understand that this part of the recovery is just as crucial as surgical technique to the return of normal joint function and the subsequent return to athletic competition. This is the area of the sports therapist's specialization where he or she can provide a strong link in the treatment chain.

Summary

1. The sports therapist is responsible for the design, implementation, and supervision of the rehabilitation program for the injured athlete.
2. The rehabilitation philosophy in sports medicine is aggressive, with the ultimate goal being to return the injured athlete to full activity as quickly and safely as possible.
3. To be effective in overseeing a rehabilitation program, the sports therapist must have a sound understanding of the healing process, the biomechanics of normal movement, and the psychological aspects of the rehabilitative process.
4. The sports therapist must develop a broad theoretical knowledge base from which specific techniques or tools of rehabilitation can be selected and practically applied to each individual case without relying on "recipe" rehabilitation protocols.
5. Therapeutic exercises are rehabilitative, or reconditioning, exercises that are specifically concerned with restoring normal body function following injury.
6. Short-term goals of a rehabilitation program: (1) providing correct immediate first aid and management following injury to limit or control swelling; (2) reducing or minimizing pain; (3) restoring full range of motion; (4) restoring or increasing muscular strength, endurance, and power; (5) reestablishing neuromuscular control; (6) improving balance; (7) maintaining cardiorespiratory fitness, and; (8) incorporating appropriate functional progressions.
7. Controlling swelling immediately following injury is perhaps the single most important aspect of injury rehabilitation in a sports medicine setting. If the swelling can be controlled initially in the acute stage of injury, the time required for rehabilitation is likely to be significantly reduced.

References

1. Arnheim, D. and W. Prentice. 1997. *Principles of athletic training.* 9th ed. Madison, WI: Brown & Benchmark.
2. Buschbacher, R., and R. Braddom. 1994. *Sports medicine and rehabilitation: A sport specific approach.* Philadelphia: Hanley & Belfus.
3. Guskiewicz, K. and D. Perrin. 1996. Research and clinical applications of assessing balance. *Journal of Sport Rehabilitation* 5(1): 45–63.
4. Hillman, S. 1994. Principles and techniques of open kinetic chain rehabilitation. *Journal of Sport Rehabilitation* 3(4): 319–30.
5. Irrgang, J., S. Whitney, and E. Cox. 1994. Balance and proprioceptive training for rehabilitation of the lower extremity. *Journal or Sport Rehabilitation* 3(1): 68–83. 1994.
6. Kisner C. and A. Colby. 1996. *Therapeutic exercise: Foundations and techniques.* Philadelphia: F.A. Davis.
7. Knight, K. J. 1985. Guidelines for rehabilitation of sports injuries. In *Rehabilitation of the injured athlete: Clinics in sports medicine,* vol. 4, no. 3, edited by J. S. Harvey. Philadelphia: W. B. Saunders.
8. Knight, K. L. 1995. *Cryotherapy in sport injury management.* Champaign, IL: Human Kinetics.
9. Logan, G. A., and E. L. Wallis. 1960. *Recent findings in learning and performance.* Paper presented at the Southern Section Meeting, California Association for Health, Physical Education and Recreation, Pasadena, CA.
10. MacMaster, J. H. 1982. *The ABC's of sports medicine.* Melbourne, FL: R. E. Kreiger.
11. Magnusson, P., and M. McHugh. 1995. Current concepts on rehabilitation in sports medicine. In *The lower extremity and spine in sports medicine,* edited by J. Nicholas and E. Hirschman. St. Louis: Mosby.
12. Malone, T., ed. 1996. *Orthopedic and sports physical therapy.* St Louis: Mosby/Yearbook.
13. Perrin, D. 1993. *Isokinetic exercise and assessment.* Champaign, IL: Human Kinetics.
14. Prentice, W. 1998. *Therapeutic modalities in sports medicine.* Dubuque, IA: WCB/McGraw-Hill.
15. Tippett, S. 1990. Sports rehabilitation concepts. In *Sports physical therapy,* edited by B. Sanders. Norwalk, CT: Appleton & Lange.
16. Tippett, S., and M. Voight. 1995. *Functional progressions for sport rehabilitation.* Champaign, IL: Human Kinetics.
17. Wells, P. E., V. Frampton, and D. Bowsher. 1988. *Pain management in physical therapy.* Norwalk, CT: Appleton & Lange.
18. Zachazewski, J., D. Magee, and S. Quillen. 1996. *Athletic injuries and rehabilitation.* Philadelphia: W. B. Saunders.

CHAPTER 2

Understanding and Managing the Healing Process through Rehabilitation

William E. Prentice

After completion of this chapter, the student should be able to do the following:

• Describe the pathophysiology of the healing process.

• Identify the factors that can impede the healing process.

• Identify the four types of tissue in the human body.

• Discuss the etiology and pathology of various musculoskeletal injuries associated with various types of tissue.

• Discuss the healing process relative to specific musculoskeletal structures.

• Explain the importance of initial first aid and injury management of these injuries and their impact on the rehabilitation process.

Rehabilitation of sport-related injuries requires sound knowledge and understanding of the etiology and pathology involved in various musculoskeletal injuries that might occur.[6,38,63] When injury occurs, the sports therapist is charged with designing, implementing, and supervising the rehabilitation program. Rehabilitation protocols and progressions must be based primarily on the physiological responses of the tissues to injury and on an understanding of how various tissues heal.[34,35] Thus the sports therapist must understand the healing process to effectively supervise the rehabilitative process. This chapter discusses the healing process relative to the various musculoskeletal injuries that might be encountered in a sports medicine setting.

UNDERSTANDING THE HEALING PROCESS

Rehabilitation programs must be based on the framework of the healing process (Figure 2-1). The sports therapist must have a sound understanding of the sequence of the various phases of the healing process. The physiological responses of the tissues to trauma follow a predictable sequence and time frame.[35] Decisions on how and when to alter and progress a rehabilitation program should be primarily based on recognition of signs and symptoms, as well as on an awareness of the time frames associated with the various phases of healing.[2,45]

The healing process consists of the inflammatory response phase, the fibroblastic-repair phase, and the maturation-remodeling phase. It must be stressed that although the phases of healing are presented as three separate entities, the healing process is a continuum.

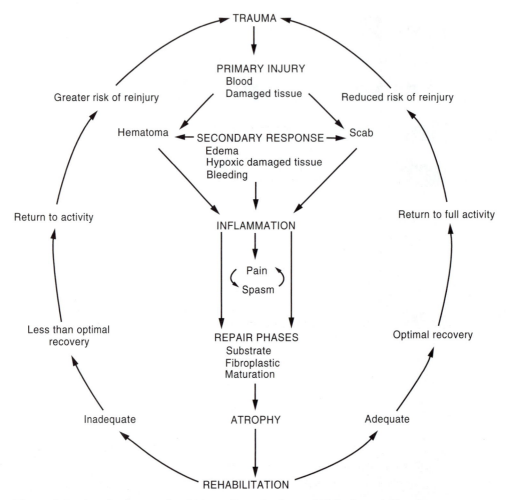

Figure 2-1 A cycle of sport-related injury. (From Booher and Thibadeau, *Athletic Injury Assessment,* Mosby, 1994.)

Phases of the healing process overlap one another and have no definitive beginning or end points.[21]

The Primary Injury

In the athletic population, injuries most often involve the musculoskeletal system and in fewer instances the nervous system. In sports medicine, **primary injuries** are almost always described as being either chronic or acute in nature resulting from **macrotraumatic** or **microtraumatic** forces. Injuries classified as macrotraumatic occur as a result of acute trauma and produce immediate pain and disability. Macrotraumatic injuries include fractures, dislocations, subluxations, sprains, strains, and contusions. Microtraumatic injuries are most often called overuse injuries and result from repetitive overloading or

incorrect mechanics associated with continuous training or competition.[47] Microtraumatic injuries include tendinitis, tenosynovitis, bursitis, etc. A **secondary injury** is essentially the inflammatory or hypoxia response that occurs with the primary injury.

Inflammatory Response Phase

Once a tissue is injured, the process of healing begins immediately[1,8] (Figure 2-2A). The destruction of tissue produces direct injury to the cells of the various soft tissues.[27] Cellular injury results in altered metabolism and the liberation of materials that initiate the inflammatory response. It is characterized symptomatically by redness, swelling, tenderness, and increased temperature.[11,42] *This initial inflammatory response is critical to the entire*

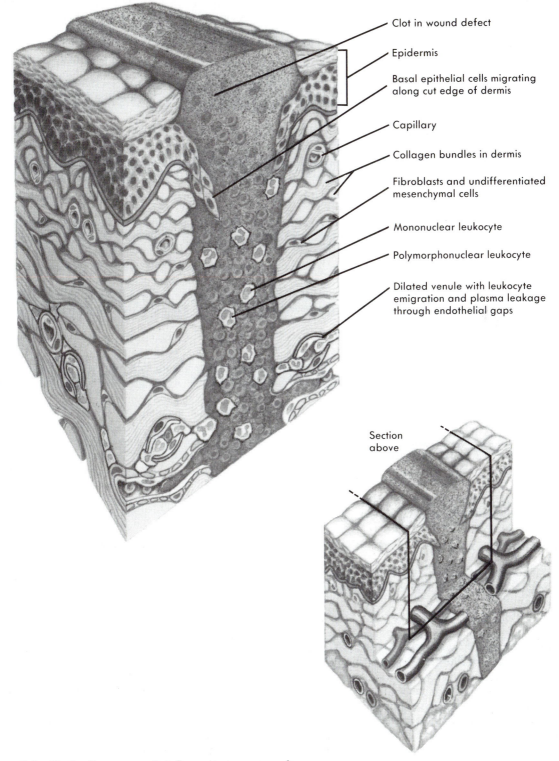

Clot in wound defect

Epidermis

Basal epithelial cells migrating along cut edge of dermis

Capillary

Collagen bundles in dermis

Fibroblasts and undifferentiated mesenchymal cells

Mononuclear leukocyte

Polymorphonuclear leukocyte

Dilated venule with leukocyte emigration and plasma leakage through endothelial gaps

A

Section above

Figure 2-2   The healing process. **A,** Inflammatory response phase.

healing process. If this response does not accomplish what it is supposed to or if it does not subside, normal healing cannot take place.

Inflammation is a process through which **leukocytes** and other **phagocytic cells** and exudate are delivered to the injured tissue. This cellular reaction is generally protective, tending to localize or dispose of injury by-products (e.g., blood and damaged cells) through phagocytosis and thus setting the stage for repair. Local vascular effects, disturbances of fluid exchange, and migration of leukocytes from the blood to the tissues occur.

Vascular Reaction. The vascular reaction involves vascular spasm, formation of a platelet plug, blood coagulation, and growth of fibrous tissue.[61] The immediate response to tissue damage is a vasoconstriction of the vascular walls that lasts for approximately 5 to 10 minutes. This spasm presses the opposing endothelial linings together to produce a local anemia that is rapidly replaced by hyperemia of the area due to dilation. This increase in blood flow is transitory and gives way to a slowing of the flow in the dilated vessels, which then progresses to stagnation and stasis. The initial effusion of blood and plasma lasts for 24 to 36 hours.

Chemical mediators. Three chemical mediators, histamine, leukotaxin, and necrosin, are important in limiting the amount of exudate and thus swelling after injury. Histamine released from the injured mast cells causes vasodilation and increased cell permeability, owing to swelling of endothelial cells and then separation between the cells. Leukotaxin is responsible for **margination,** in which leukocytes line up along the cell walls. It also increases cell permeability locally, thus affecting passage of the fluid and white blood cells through cell walls via diapedesis to form exudate. Therefore vasodilation and active hyperemia are important in exudate (plasma) formation and supplying leukocytes to the injured area. Necrosin is responsible for phagocytic activity. The amount of swelling that occurs is directly related to the extent of vessel damage.

Formation of a Clot. Platelets do not normally adhere to the vascular wall. However, injury to a vessel disrupts the endothelium and exposes the collagen fibers. Platelets adhere to the collagen fibers to create a sticky matrix on the vascular wall, to which additional platelets and leukocytes adhere and eventually form a plug. These plugs obstruct local lymphatic fluid drainage and thus localize the injury response.

The initial event that precipitates clot formation is the conversion of **fibrinogen** to **fibrin.** This transformation occurs because of a cascading effect beginning with the release of a protein molecule called **thromboplastin** from the damaged cell. Thromboplastin causes **prothrombin** to be changed into **thrombin,** which in turn causes the conversion of fibrinogen into a very sticky fibrin clot that shuts off blood supply to the injured area. Clot formation begins around 12 hours after injury and is completed within 48 hours.

As a result of a combination of these factors, the injured area becomes walled off during the inflammatory stage of healing. The leukocytes phagocytize most of the foreign debris toward the end of the inflammatory phase, setting the stage for the fibroblastic phase. This initial inflammatory response lasts for approximately 2 to 4 days after initial injury.

Chronic Inflammation. A distinction must be made between the acute inflammatory response as described above and chronic inflammation. **Chronic inflammation** occurs when the acute inflammatory response does not eliminate the injuring agent and restore tissue to its normal physiological state. Chronic inflammation involves the replacement of leukocytes with **macrophages,** lymphocytes, and **plasma cells.** These cells accumulate in a highly vascularized and innervated loose connective tissue matrix in the area of injury.[41]

The specific mechanisms that convert an acute inflammatory response to a chronic inflammatory response are to date unknown; however, they seem to be associated with situations that involve overuse or overload with cumulative microtrauma to a particular structure.[20,41] Likewise, there is no specific time frame in which a classification of acute inflammation is changed to chronic inflammation.

It does appear that chronic inflammation is resistant to both physical and pharmacological treatments.[35]

The Use of Anti-inflammatory Medications. A sports medicine physician will routinely prescribe nonsteroidal anti-inflammatory drugs (NSAID) for an athlete who has sustained an injury. These medications are certainly effective in minimizing pain and swelling associated with inflammation and can enhance return to full activity. However, there are some concerns that use of NSAID acutely following injury might actually interfere with inflammation, thus delaying the healing process. The use of NSAID will be further discussed in Chapter 16.

Fibroblastic-Repair Phase

During the fibroblastic phase of healing, proliferative and regenerative activity leading to scar formation and repair of the injured tissue follows the vascular and exudative phenomena of inflammation[32] (Figure 2-2 *B*, p. 17). The period of scar formation referred to as **fibroplasia** begins within the first few hours after injury and can last as long as 4 to 6 weeks. During this period, many of the signs and symptoms associated with the inflammatory response subside. The athlete might still indicate some tenderness

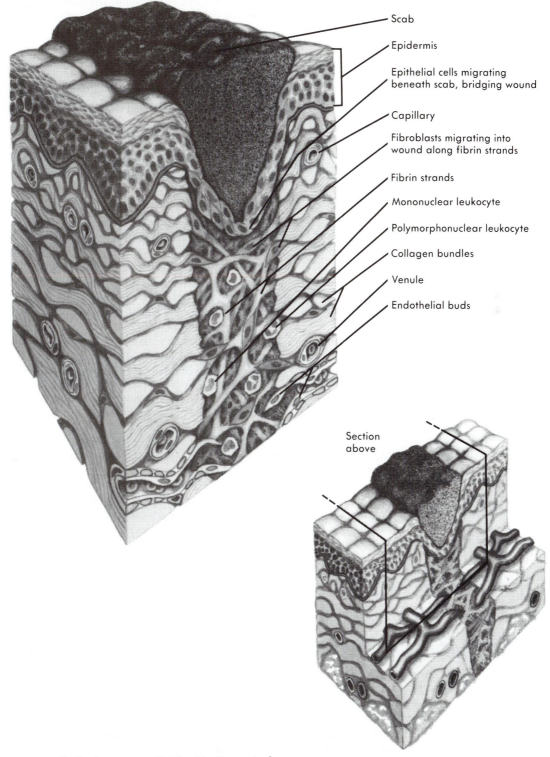

Scab

Epidermis

Epithelial cells migrating
beneath scab, bridging wound

Capillary

Fibroblasts migrating into
wound along fibrin strands

Fibrin strands

Mononuclear leukocyte

Polymorphonuclear leukocyte

Collagen bundles

Venule

Endothelial buds

B

Section
above

Figure 2-2   The healing process. **B,** Fibroblastic-repair phase.

to touch and will usually complain of pain when particular movements stress the injured structure. As scar formation progresses, complaints of tenderness or pain gradually disappear.[59]

During this phase, growth of endothelial capillary buds into the wound is stimulated by a lack of oxygen, after which the wound is capable of healing aerobically.[15] Along with increased oxygen delivery comes an increase in blood flow, which delivers nutrients essential for tissue regeneration in the area.[12]

The formation of a delicate connective tissue called **granulation tissue** occurs with the breakdown of the fibrin clot. Granulation tissue consists of **fibroblasts,** collagen, and capillaries. It appears as a reddish granular mass of connective tissue that fills in the gaps during the healing process.

As the capillaries continue to grow into the area, fibroblasts accumulate at the wound site, arranging themselves parallel to the capillaries. Fibroblastic cells begin to synthesize an extracellular matrix that contains protein fibers of **collagen** and **elastin,** a ground substance that consists of nonfibrous proteins called proteoglycans, glycosaminoglycans, and fluid. On about day 6 or 7, fibroblasts also begin producing collagen fibers that are deposited in a random fashion throughout the forming scar. As the collagen continues to proliferate, the tensile strength of the wound rapidly increases in proportion to the rate of collagen synthesis. As the tensile strength increases, the number of fibroblasts diminishes, signaling the beginning of the maturation phase.

This normal sequence of events in the repair phase leads to the formation of minimal scar tissue. Occasionally, a persistent inflammatory response and continued release of inflammatory products can promote extended fibroplasia and excessive fibrogenesis, which can lead to irreversible tissue damage.[69] Fibrosis can occur in synovial structures, as with adhesive capsulitis in the shoulder, in extra-articular tissues including tendons and ligaments, in bursa, or in muscle.

Maturation-Remodeling Phase

The maturation-remodeling phase of healing is a long-term process (Figure 2-2C, p. 19). This phase features a realignment or remodeling of the collagen fibers that make up scar tissue according to the tensile forces to which that scar is subjected. Ongoing breakdown and synthesis of collagen occur with a steady increase in the tensile strength of the scar matrix. With increased stress and strain, the collagen fibers realign in a position of maximum efficiency parallel to the lines of tension. The tissue gradually assumes normal appearance and func-

tion, although a scar is rarely as strong as the normal injured tissue. Usually by the end of approximately 3 weeks, a firm, strong, contracted, nonvascular scar exists. The maturation phase of healing might require several years to be totally complete.

The Role of Progressive Controlled Mobility During the Healing Process

Wolff's law states that bone and soft tissue will respond to the physical demands placed on them, causing them to remodel or realign along lines of tensile force.[72] Therefore it is critical that injured structures be exposed to progressively increasing loads throughout the rehabilitative process.[55]

In animal models, controlled mobilization is superior to immobilization for scar formation, revascularization, muscle regeneration, and reorientation of muscle fibers and tensile properties.[75] However, a brief period of immobilization of the injured tissue during the inflammatory response phase is recommended and will likely facilitate the process of healing by controlling inflammation, thus reducing clinical symptoms. As healing progresses to the repair phase, controlled activity directed toward return to normal flexibility and strength should be combined with protective support or bracing.[37] Generally, clinical signs and symptoms disappear at the end of this phase.

As the remodeling phase begins, aggressive active range-of-motion and strengthening exercises should be incorporated to facilitate tissue remodeling and realignment. To a great extent, pain will dictate rate of progression. With initial injury, pain is intense; it tends to decrease and eventually subside altogether as healing progresses. Any exacerbation of pain, swelling, or other clinical symptoms during or after a particular exercise or activity indicates that the load is too great for the level of tissue repair or remodeling. The sports therapist must be aware of the time required for the healing process and realize that being overly aggressive can interfere with that process.

Factors That Impede Healing

Extent of Injury. The nature of the inflammatory response is determined by the extent of the tissue injury. **Microtears** of soft tissue involve only minor damage and are most often associated with overuse. **Macrotears** involve significantly greater destruction of soft tissue and result in clinical symptoms and functional alterations. Macrotears are generally caused by acute trauma.[37]

Edema. The increased pressure caused by swelling retards the healing process, causes separation of tissues, inhibits neuromuscular control, produces reflexive neurological changes, and impedes nutrition in

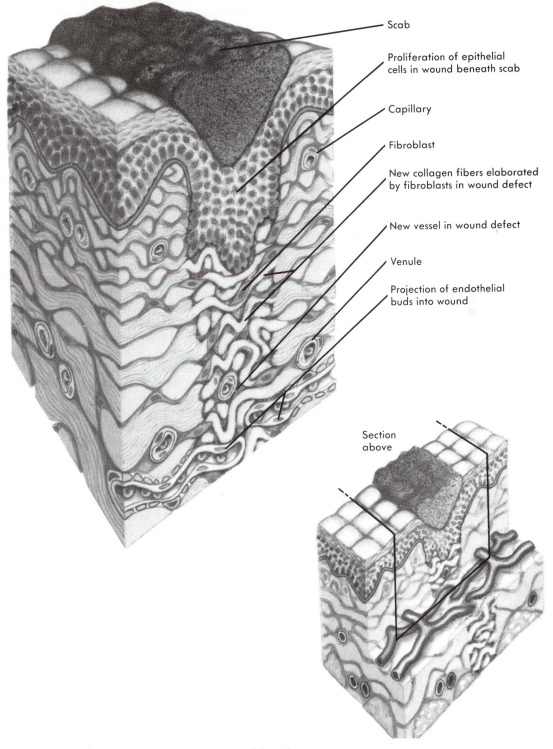

Scab

Proliferation of epithelial cells in wound beneath scab

Capillary

Fibroblast

New collagen fibers elaborated by fibroblasts in wound defect

New vessel in wound defect

Venule

Projection of endothelial buds into wound

C

Section above

Figure 2-2   The healing process. **C,** Maturation-remodeling phase.

the injured part. Edema is best controlled and managed during the initial first-aid management period as described previously.[10]

Hemorrhage.   Bleeding occurs with even the smallest amount of damage to the capillaries. Bleeding produces the same negative effects on healing as does the accumulation of edema, and its presence produces additional tissue damage and thus exacerbation of the injury.[54]

Poor Vascular Supply.   Injuries to tissues with a poor vascular supply heal poorly and at a slow rate. This response is likely related to a failure in the initial delivery of phagocytic cells and fibroblasts necessary for scar formation.[54]

Separation of Tissue.   Mechanical separation of tissue can significantly impact the course of healing. A wound that has smooth edges in good apposition will tend to heal by primary intention with minimal scarring. Conversely, a wound that has jagged, separated edges must heal by secondary intention, with granulation tissue filling the defect and excessive scarring.[60]

Muscle Spasm.   Muscle spasm causes traction on the torn tissue, separates the two ends, and prevents approximation. Local and generalized ischemia can result from spasm.

Atrophy.   Wasting away of muscle tissue begins immediately with injury. Strengthening and early mobilization of the injured structure retard atrophy.

Corticosteroids.   Use of corticosteroids in the treatment of inflammation is controversial. Steroid use in the early stages of healing has been demonstrated to inhibit fibroplasia, capillary proliferation, collagen synthesis, and increases in tensile strength of the healing scar. Their use in the later stages of healing and with chronic inflammation is debatable.

Keloids and Hypertrophic Scars.   Keloids occur when the rate of collagen production exceeds the rate of collagen breakdown during the maturation phase of healing. This process leads to hypertrophy of scar tissue, particularly around the periphery of the wound.

Infection.   The presence of bacteria in the wound can delay healing, causes excessive granulation tissue, and frequently causes large, deformed scars.[29]

Humidity, Climate, and Oxygen Tension. Humidity significantly influences the process of epithelization. Occlusive dressings stimulate the epithelium to migrate twice as fast without crust or scab formation. The formation of a scab occurs with dehydration of the wound and traps wound drainage, which promotes infection. Keeping the wound moist provides an advantage for the necrotic debris to go to the surface and be shed.

Oxygen tension relates to the neovascularization of the wound, which translates into optimal saturation and maximal tensile strength development. Circulation to the wound can be affected by ischemia, venous stasis, hematomas, and vessel trauma.

Health, Age, and Nutrition.   The elastic qualities of the skin decrease with aging. Degenerative diseases, such as diabetes and arteriosclerosis, also become a concern of the older athlete and can affect wound healing. Nutrition is important for wound healing—in particular, vitamins C (for collagen synthesis and immune system), K (for clotting), and A (for the immune system); zinc (for the enzyme systems) and amino acids play critical roles in the healing process.

PATHOPHYSIOLOGY OF INJURY TO VARIOUS BODY TISSUES

Classification of Body Tissues

There are four types of fundamental tissues in the human body: epithelial, connective, muscular, and nervous[66] (Table 2-1). According to Guyton, all tissues of the body except bone can be defined as soft tissue.[30] Cailliet, however, more technically defines **soft tissue** as the matrix of the human body comprised of cellular elements within a ground substance. Furthermore, Cailliet believes that soft tissue is the most common site of functional impairment of the musculoskeletal system.[9] Most sport-related injuries occur to the soft tissues.

Epithelial Tissue

The first fundamental tissue is epithelial tissue (Figure 2-3). This specific tissue covers all internal and external body surfaces and therefore encompasses structures such as the skin, the outer layer of the internal organs, and the inner lining of the blood vessels and glands. A basic purpose of epithelial tissue, as presented by Fahey, is to protect and form structure for other tissues and organs.[19] In addition, this tissue functions in absorption (e.g., in the digestive tract) and secretion (as in glands). A principal physiological characteristic of epithelial tissue is that it contains no blood supply per se, so it must depend on the process of diffusion for nutrition, oxygenation, and elimination of waste products. Most sport-related injuries to this type of tissue are traumatic, including abrasions, lacerations, punctures, and avulsions. Other injuries to this tissue can include infection, inflammation, or disease.

■ **TABLE 2-1** Tissues

Tissue	Location	Function
Epithelial		
Simple squamous	Alveoli of lungs	Absorption by diffusion of respiratory gases between alveolar air and blood
	Lining of blood and lymphatic vessels	Absorption by diffusion, filtration, and osmosis
Stratified squamous	Surface of lining of mouth and esophagus	Protection
	Surface of skin (epidermis)	
Simple columnar	Surface layer of lining of stomach, intestines, and parts of respiratory tract	Protection; secretion; absorption
Stratified transitional	Urinary bladder	Protection
Connective (most widely distributed of all tissues)		
Areolar	Between other tissues and organs	Connection
Adipose (fat)	Under skin	Protection
	Padding at various points	Insulation; support; reserve food
Dense fibrous	Tendons; ligaments	Flexible but strong connection
Bone	Skeleton	Support; protection
Cartilage	Part of nasal septum; covering articular surfaces of bones; larynx; rings in trachea and bronchi	Firm but flexible support
	Disks between vertebrae	
	External ear	
Blood	Blood vessels	Transportation
Muscle		
Skeletal (striated voluntary)	Muscles that attach to bones	Movement of bones
	Eyeball muscles	Eye movements
	Upper third of esophagus	First part of swallowing
Cardiac (striated involuntary)	Wall of heart	Contraction of heart
Visceral (nonstriated involuntary or smooth)	In walls of tubular viscera of digestive, respiratory, and genitourinary tracts	Movement of substances along respective tracts
	In walls of blood vessels and large lymphatic vessels	Changing of diameter of blood vessels
	In ducts of glands	Movement of substances along ducts
	Intrinsic eye muscles (iris and ciliary body)	Changing of diameter of pupils and shape of lens
	Arrector muscles of hairs	Erection of hairs (gooseflesh)
Nervous		
	Brain; spinal cord; nerves	Irritability; conduction

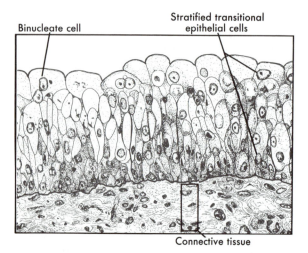
Binucleate cell

Stratified transitional
epithelial cells

Connective tissue

Figure 2-3 Epithelial cells exist in several layers.

Connective Tissue

The functions of connective tissue in the body are to support, provide a framework, fill space, store fat, help repair tissues, produce blood cells, and protect against infection. Connective tissue consists of various types of cells separated from one another by some type of extracellular matrix. This matrix consists of fibers and ground substance and can be solid, semisolid, or fluid. The primary types of connective tissue cells are macrophages, which function as phagocytes to clean up debris; mast cells, which release chemicals (histamine and heparin) associated with inflammation; and the fibroblasts, which are the principal cells of the connective tissue.

Collagen. Fibroblasts produce collagen and elastin found in varying proportions in different connective tissues. Collagen is a major structural protein that forms strong, flexible, inelastic structures that hold connective tissue together. Collagen enables a tissue to resist mechanical forces and deformation. Elastin, however, produces highly elastic tissues that assist in recovery from deformation. Collagen fibrils are the load-bearing elements of connective tissue. They are arranged to accommodate tensile stress but are not as capable of resisting shear or compressive stress. Consequently the direction of orientation of collagen fibers is along lines of tensile stress.

Collagen has several mechanical and physical properties that allow it to respond to loading and deformation, permitting it to withstand high tensile stress. The mechanical properties of collagen include *elasticity,* which is the capability to recover normal length after elongation; *viscoelasticity,* which allows for a slow return to normal length and shape after deformation; and *plasticity,* which

allows for permanent change or deformation. The physical properties include *force-relaxation,* which indicates the decrease in the amount of force needed to maintain a tissue at a set amount of displacement or deformation over time; the *creep response,* which is the ability of a tissue to deform over time while a constant load is imposed; and *hysteresis,* which is the amount of relaxation a tissue has undergone during deformation and displacement. If the mechanical and physical limitations of connective tissue are exceeded, injury results.

Types of Connective Tissue. There are several types of connective tissue.[5,33,62] **Fibrous connective tissue** is composed of strong collagenous fibers that bind tissues together. There are two types of fibrous connective tissue. **Dense connective tissue** is composed primarily of collagen and is found in tendons, fascia, aponeurosis, ligaments, and joint capsule. **Tendons** connect muscles to bone. An **aponeurosis** is a thin, sheet-like tendon. A **fascia** is a thin membrane of connective tissue that surrounds individual muscles and tendons or muscle groups. **Ligaments** connect bone to bone. All synovial joints are surrounded by a **joint capsule,** which is a type of connective tissue similar to a ligament. The orientations of collagen fibers in ligaments and joint capsules are less parallel than in tendons. **Loose connective tissue** forms many types of thin membranes found beneath the skin, between muscles, and between organs. **Adipose tissue** is a specialized form of loose connective tissue that stores fat, insulates, and acts as a shock absorber. The blood supply to fibrous connective tissue is relatively poor, so healing and repair are slow processes.

Cartilage is a type of rigid connective tissue that provides support and acts as a framework in many structures. It is composed of chondrocyte cells contained in small chambers called lacunae surrounded completely by an intracellular matrix. The matrix consists of varying ratios of collagen and elastin and a ground substance made of proteoglycans and glycosaminoglycans, which are nonfibrous protein molecules. These proteoglycans act as sponges and trap large quantities of water, which allows cartilage to spring back after being compressed. Cartilage has a poor blood supply, thus healing after injury is very slow. There are three types of cartilage. **Hyaline cartilage** is found on the articulating surfaces of bone and in the soft part of the nose. It contains large quantities of collagen and proteoglycan. **Fibrocartilage** forms the intervertebral disks and menisci located in several joint spaces. It has greater amounts of collagen than proteoglycan and is capable of withstanding a great deal of pressure. **Elastic cartilage** is found in the auricle of the ear and the larynx. It is more flexible than the other types of cartilage and consists of collagen, proteoglycan, and elastin.

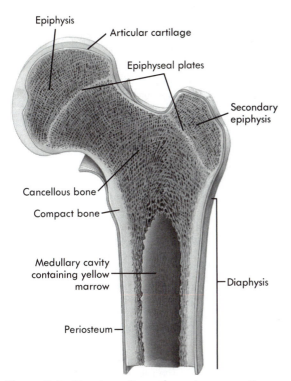

Epiphysis

Articular cartilage

Epiphyseal plates

Secondary epiphysis

Cancellous bone

Compact bone

Medullary cavity containing yellow marrow

Diaphysis

Periosteum

Figure 2-4   Structure of bone shown in cross section.

Reticular connective tissue is also composed primarily of collagen. It provides the support structure of the walls of various internal organs, including the liver and kidneys.

Elastic connective tissue is composed primarily of elastic fibers. It is found primarily in the walls of blood vessels, airways, and hollow internal organs.

Bone is a type of connective tissue consisting of both living cells and minerals deposited in a matrix (Figure 2-4). Each bone consists of three major components. The **epiphysis** is an expanded portion at each end of the bone that articulates with another bone. Each articulating surface is covered by an articular, or hyaline, cartilage. The diaphysis is the shaft of the bone. The **epiphyseal** or **growth plate** is the major site of bone growth and elongation. Once bone growth ceases, the plate ossifies and forms the epiphyseal line. With the exception of the articulating surfaces, the bone is completely enclosed by the **periosteum,** a tough, highly vascularized and innervated fibrous tissue.[43]

The two types of bone material are **cancellous,** or spongy, bone and cortical, or compact, bone. Cancellous bone contains a series of air spaces referred to as trabeculae, whereas cortical bone is relatively solid. Cortical bone

in the diaphysis forms a hollow medullary canal in long bone, which is lined with **endosteum** and filled with bone **marrow.** Bone has a rich blood supply that certainly facilitates the healing process after injury. Bone has the functions of support, movement, and protection. Furthermore, bone stores and releases calcium into the bloodstream and manufactures red blood cells.

One additional type of connective tissue in the body is **blood.** Blood is composed of various cells suspended in a fluid intracellular matrix referred to as plasma. Plasma contains red blood cells, white blood cells, and platelets. Although this component does not function in structure, it is essential for the nutrition, cleansing, and physiology of the body.

With connective tissue playing such a major role throughout the human body, it is not surprising that many sport-related injuries involve structures composed of connective tissue. Although tendons are classified as connective tissue, injuries to tendons and tendon healing will be incorporated into the discussion of the musculotendinous unit.

LIGAMENT SPRAINS

A sprain involves damage to a ligament that provides support to a joint. A ligament is a tough, relatively inelastic band of tissue that connects one bone to another. A ligament's primary function is threefold: to provide stability to a joint, to provide control of the position of one articulating bone to another during normal joint motion, and to provide proprioceptive input or a sense of joint position through the function of free nerve endings or mechanoreceptors located within the ligament.

Before discussing injuries to ligaments, a review of joint structure is in order[53] (Figure 2-5). All **synovial joints** are composed of two or more bones that articulate with one another to allow motion in one or more places. The articulating surfaces of the bone are lined with a very thin, smooth, cartilaginous covering called a hyaline cartilage. All joints are entirely surrounded by a thick, ligamentous **joint capsule.** The inner surface of this joint capsule is lined by a very thin **synovial membrane** that is highly vascularized and innervated. The synovial membrane produces **synovial fluid,** the functions of which include lubrication, shock absorption, and nutrition of the joint.

Some joints contain a thick fibrocartilage called a **meniscus.** The knee joint, for example, contains two wedge-shaped menisci that deepen the articulation and provide shock absorption in that joint. Finally, the main structural support and joint stability is provided by the ligaments, which may be either thickened portions of a

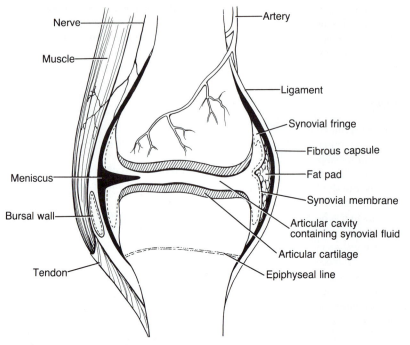

Figure 2-5 Structure of a synovial joint.

joint capsule or totally separate bands. Ligaments are composed of dense connective tissue arranged in parallel bundles of collagen composed of rows of fibroblasts. Although bundles are arranged in parallel, not all collagen fibers are arranged in parallel.

Ligaments and tendons are very similar in structure. However, ligaments are usually more flattened than tendons, and collagen fibers in ligaments are more compact. The anatomical positioning of the ligaments determines in part what motions a joint can make.

If stress is applied to a joint that forces motion beyond its normal limits or planes of movement, injury to the ligament is likely[23] (Figure 2-6). The severity of damage to the ligament is classified in many different ways; however, the most commonly used system involves three grades (degrees) of ligamentous sprain:

Grade 1 sprain: There is some stretching or perhaps tearing of the ligamentous fibers, with little or no joint instability. Mild pain, little swelling, and joint stiffness might be apparent.

Grade 2 sprain: There is some tearing and separation of the ligamentous fibers and moderate instability of the joint. Moderate to severe pain, swelling, and joint stiffness should be expected.

Grade 3 sprain: There is total rupture of the ligament, manifested primarily by gross instability of the joint.

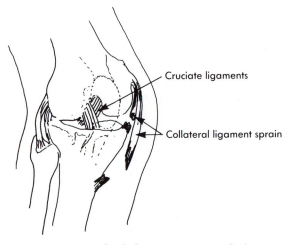

Figure 2-6 Example of a ligament sprain in the knee joint.

Severe pain might be present initially, followed by little or no pain due to total disruption of nerve fibers. Swelling might be profuse, and thus the joint tends to become very stiff some hours after the injury. A third-degree sprain with marked instability usually requires some form of immobilization lasting several weeks. Frequently the force producing the ligament injury is so great that other ligaments or structures surrounding the joint are also injured. With cases in which there is injury to multiple joint structures, surgical repair or reconstruction may be necessary to correct an instability.

Ligament Healing

The healing process in the sprained ligament follows the same course of repair as with other vascular tissues. Immediately after injury and for approximately 72 hours there is a loss of blood from damaged vessels and attraction of inflammatory cells into the injured area. If a ligament is sprained outside of a joint capsule (extra-articular ligament), bleeding occurs in a subcutaneous space. If an intra-articular ligament is injured, bleeding occurs inside of the joint capsule until either clotting occurs or the pressure becomes so great that bleeding ceases.

During the next 6 weeks, vascular proliferation with new capillary growth begins to occur along with fibroblastic activity, resulting in the formation of a fibrin clot. It is essential that the torn ends of the ligament be reconnected by bridging of this clot. Synthesis of collagen and ground substance of proteoglycan as constituents of an intracellular matrix contributes to the proliferation of the scar that bridges between the torn ends of the ligament. This scar initially is soft and viscous but eventually becomes more elastic. Collagen fibers are arranged in a random woven pattern with little organization. Gradually there is a decrease in fibroblastic activity, a decrease in vascularity, and an increase to a maximum in collagen density of the scar.[3] Failure to produce enough scar and failure to reconnect the ligament to the appropriate location on a bone are the two reasons why ligaments are likely to fail.

Over the next several months the scar continues to mature, with the realignment of collagen occurring in response to progressive stresses and strains. The maturation of the scar may require as long as 12 months to complete.[3] The exact length of time required for maturation depends on mechanical factors such as apposition of torn ends and length of the period of immobilization.

Factors Affecting Ligament Healing

Surgically repaired extra-articular ligaments have healed with decreased scar formation and are generally stronger than unrepaired ligaments initially, although this strength advantage might not be maintained as time progresses. Nonrepaired ligaments heal by fibrous scarring effectively lengthening the ligament and producing some degree of joint instability. With intra-articular ligament

tears, the presence of synovial fluid dilutes the hematoma, thus preventing formation of a fibrin clot and spontaneous healing.[33]

Several studies have shown that actively exercised ligaments are stronger than those that are immobilized. Ligaments that are immobilized for periods of several weeks after injury tend to decrease in tensile strength and also exhibit weakening of the insertion of the ligament to bone.[44] Thus it is important to minimize periods of immobilization and progressively stress the injured ligaments while exercising caution relative to biomechanical considerations for specific ligaments.[3,52]

It is not likely that the inherent stability of the joint provided by the ligament before injury will be regained. Thus, to restore stability to the joint, the other structures that surround that joint, primarily muscles and their tendons, must be strengthened. The increased muscle tension provided by strength training can improve stability of the injured joint.[64,65]

FRACTURES OF BONE

Fractures are extremely common injuries among the athletic population. They can be generally classified as being either open or closed. A closed fracture involves little or no displacement of bones and thus little or no soft-tissue disruption. An open fracture involves enough displacement of the fractured ends that the bone actually disrupts the cutaneous layers and breaks through the skin. Both fractures can be relatively serious if not managed properly, but an increased possibility of infection exists in an open fracture. Fractures may also be considered complete, in which the bone is broken into at least two fragments, or incomplete, where the fracture does not extend completely across the bone.

The varieties of fractures that can occur include greenstick, transverse, oblique, spiral, comminuted, impacted, avulsive, and stress. A **greenstick** fracture (Figure 2-7A) occurs most often in children whose bones are still growing and have not yet had a chance to calcify and harden. It is called a greenstick fracture because of the resemblance to the splintering that occurs to a tree twig that is bent to the point of breaking. Because the twig is green, it splinters but can be bent without causing an actual break.

A **transverse fracture** (Figure 2-7B) involves a crack perpendicular to the longitudinal axis of the bone that goes all the way through the bone. Displacement might occur; however, because of the shape of the fractured ends, the surrounding soft tissue (for example, muscles, tendons, and fat) sustains relatively little damage. A **linear fracture** runs parallel to the long axis of a bone and is similar in severity to a transverse fracture.

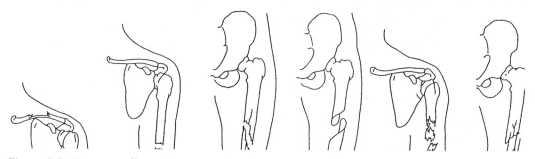

Figure 2-7 Fractures of bone. **A,** Greenstick; **B,** transverse; **C,** oblique; **D,** spiral; **E,** comminuted; **F,** impacted; **G,** avulsion.

An **oblique fracture** (Figure 2-7C) results in a diagonal crack across the bone and two very jagged, pointed ends that, if displaced, can potentially cause a good bit of soft-tissue damage. Oblique and spiral fractures are the two types most likely to result in compound fractures.

A **spiral fracture** (Figure 2-7D) is similar to an oblique fracture in that the angle of the fracture is diagonal across the bone. In addition, an element of twisting or rotation causes the fracture to spiral along the longitudinal axis of the bone. Spiral fractures used to be fairly common in ski injuries occurring just above the top of the boot when the bindings on the ski failed to release when the foot was rotated. These injuries are now less common due to improvements in equipment design.

A **comminuted fracture** (Figure 2-7E) is a serious problem that can require an extremely long time for rehabilitation. In the comminuted fracture, multiple fragments of bone must be surgically repaired and fixed with screws and wires. If a fracture of this type occurs to a weight-bearing bone in the leg, a permanent discrepancy in leg length can develop.

In an **impacted fracture** (Figure 2-7F), one end of the fractured bone is driven up into the other end. As with the comminuted fracture, correcting discrepancies in the length of the extremity can require long periods of intensive rehabilitation.

An **avulsion fracture** (Figure 2-7G) occurs when a fragment of bone is pulled away at the bony attachment of a muscle, tendon, or ligament. Avulsion fractures are common in the fingers and some of the smaller bones but can also occur in larger bones whose tendinous or ligamentous attachments are subjected to a large amount of force.

Perhaps the most common fracture resulting from physical activity is the **stress fracture.** Unlike the other types of fractures that have been discussed, the stress fracture results from overuse or fatigue rather than acute trauma.[40,50] Common sites for stress fractures include the weight-bearing bones of the leg and foot. In either case, repetitive forces transmitted through the bones produce irritations and microfractures at a specific area in the bone. The pain usually begins as a dull ache that becomes progressively more painful day after day. Initially, pain is most severe during activity. However, when a stress fracture actually develops, pain tends to become worse after the activity is stopped.

The biggest problem with a stress fracture is that often it does not show up on an X-ray film until the osteoblasts begin laying down subperiosteal callus or bone, at which point a small white line, or a callus, appears. However, a bone scan might reveal a potential stress fracture in as little as 2 days after onset of symptoms. If a stress fracture is suspected, the athlete should, for a minimum of 14 days, stop any activity that produces added stress or fatigue to the area. Stress fractures do not usually require casting but might become normal fractures that must be immobilized if handled incorrectly. If a fracture occurs, it should be managed and rehabilitated by a qualified orthopedist and sports therapist.

Bone Healing

Healing of injured bone tissue is similar to soft-tissue healing in that all phases of the healing process can be identified, although bone regeneration capabilities are somewhat limited. However, the functional elements of healing differ significantly from those of soft tissue. Tensile strength of the scar is the single most critical factor in soft-tissue healing, whereas bone has to contend with a number of additional forces, including torsion, bending, and compression.[22] Trauma to bone can vary from contusions of the periosteum to closed, nondisplaced fractures to severely displaced open fractures that also involve significant soft-tissue damage. When a fracture occurs, blood vessels in the bone and the periosteum are damaged, resulting in bleeding and subsequent clot formation. Hemorrhaging from the marrow is contained by the periosteum and the surrounding soft tissue in the region of the fracture. In about 1 week, fibroblasts have begun laying down a fibrous collagen network. The fibrin strands within the clot serve as the framework for proliferating vessels. **Chondroblast** cells begin producing fibrocartilage, creating a **callus** between the broken bones. At first, the callus is soft and firm because it is composed primarily of collagenous fibrin. The callus becomes firm and more rubbery as cartilage begins to predominate. Bone-producing cells called **osteoblasts** begin to proliferate and enter the callus, forming cancellous bone trabeculae, which eventually replace the cartilage. Finally the callus crystalizes into bone, at which point remodeling of the bone begins. The callus can be divided into two portions, the external callus located around the periosteum on the outside of the fracture and the internal callus found between the bone fragments. The size of the callus is proportional both to the damage and to the amount of irritation to the fracture site during the healing process. Also during this time, **osteoclasts** begin to appear in the area to resorb bone fragments and clean up debris.[33,62]

The remodeling process is similar to the growth process of bone in that the fibrous cartilage is gradually replaced by fibrous bone and then by more structurally efficient lamellar bone. Remodeling involves an ongoing process during which osteoblasts lay down new bone and osteoclasts remove and break down bone according to the forces placed upon the healing bone.[71] Wolff's law maintains that a bone will adapt to mechanical stresses and strains by changing size, shape, and structure. Therefore, once the cast is removed, the bone must be subjected to normal stresses and strains so that tensile strength can be regained before the healing process is complete.[28,67]

The time required for bone healing is variable and based on a number of factors, such as severity of the fracture, site of the fracture, extensiveness of the trauma, and age of the patient. Normal periods of immobilization range from as short as 3 weeks for the small bones in the hands and feet to as long as 8 weeks for the long bones of the upper and lower extremities. In some instances, such as fractures in the four small toes, immobilization might not be required for healing. The healing process is certainly not complete when the splint or cast is removed. Osteoblastic and osteoclastic activity might continue for 2 to 3 years after severe fractures.

CARTILAGE DAMAGE

Osteoarthrosis is a degenerative condition of bone and cartilage in and about the joint. **Arthritis** should be defined as primarily an inflammatory condition with possible secondary destruction. **Arthrosis** is primarily a degenerative process with destruction of cartilage, remodeling of bone, and possible secondary inflammatory components.

Cartilage fibrillates—that is, releases fibers or groups of fibers and ground substance into the joint. Peripheral cartilage that is not exposed to weight-bearing or compression-decompression mechanisms is particularly likely to fibrillate. Fibrillation is typically found in the degenerative process associated with poor nutrition or disuse. This process can then extend even to weight-bearing areas, with progressive destruction of cartilage proportional to stresses applied on it. When forces are increased, thus increasing stress, osteochondral or subchondral fractures can occur. Concentration of stress on small areas can produce pressures that overwhelm the tissue's capabilities. Typically, lower-limb joints have to handle greater stresses, but their surface area is usually larger than the surface area of upper limbs. The articular cartilage is protected to some extent by the synovial fluid, which acts as a lubricant. It is also protected by the subchondral bone, which responds to stresses in an elastic fashion. It is more compliant than compact bone, and microfractures can be a means of force absorption. Trabeculae might fracture or might be displaced due to pressures applied on the subchondral bone. In compact bone, fracture can be a means of defense to dissipate force. In the joint, forces might be absorbed by joint movement and eccentric contraction of muscles.

In the majority of joints where the surfaces are not congruent, the applied forces tend to concentrate in certain areas, which increases joint degeneration. **Osteophytosis** occurs as a bone attempts to increase its surface area to decrease contact forces. Typically people describe this growth as "bone spurs." **Chondromalacia** is the nonprogressive transformation of cartilage with irregular surfaces and areas of softening. Typically it occurs first in non-weight-bearing areas and may progress to areas of excessive stress.

In athletes, certain joints may be more susceptible to a response resembling osteoarthrosis.[57] The proportion of body weight resting on the joint, the pull of musculotendinous unit, and any significant external force applied to the joint are predisposing factors. Altered joint mechanics caused by laxity or previous trauma are also factors that come into play. The intensity of forces can be great, as in the hip, where the above-mentioned factors can produce pressures or forces four times that of body weight and up to ten times that of body weight on the knee.

Typically, muscle forces generate more stress than body weight itself. Particular injuries are conducive to osteoarthritic changes such as subluxation and dislocation of the patella, osteochondritis dissecans, recurrent synovial effusion, and hemarthrosis. Also, ligamentous injuries can bring about a disruption of proprioceptive mechanisms, loss of adequate joint alignment, and meniscal damage in the knees with removal of the injured meniscus.[31] Other factors that have an impact are loss of full range of motion, poor muscular power and strength, and altered biomechanics on the joint. In sport participation, spurring and spiking of bone are not synonymous with osteoarthrosis if the joint space is maintained and the cartilage lining is intact. It may simply be an adaptation to the increased stress of physical activity.

Cartilage Healing

Cartilage has a relatively limited healing capacity. When chondrocytes are destroyed and the matrix is disrupted, the course of healing is variable, depending on whether damage is to cartilage alone or also to subchondral bone. Injuries to articular cartilage alone fail to elicit clot formation or a cellular response. For the most part the chondrocytes adjacent to the injury are the only cells that show any signs of proliferation and synthesis of matrix. Thus the defect fails to heal, although the extent of the damage tends to remain the same.[25,46]

If subchondral bone is also affected, inflammatory cells enter the damaged area and formulate granulation tissue. In this case, the healing process proceeds normally, with differentiation of granulation tissue cells into chondrocytes occurring in about 2 weeks. At approximately 2 months normal collagen has been formed.

INJURIES TO MUSCULOTENDINOUS STRUCTURES

Muscle is often considered to be a type of connective tissue, but here it is treated as the third of the fundamental tissues. The three types of muscles are smooth (involuntary), cardiac, and skeletal (voluntary). **Smooth muscle** is found within the viscera, where it forms the walls of the internal organs, and within many hollow chambers. **Cardiac muscle** is found only in the heart and is responsible for its contraction. A significant characteristic of the car-

diac muscle is that it contracts as a single fiber, unlike smooth and skeletal muscles, which contract as separate units. This characteristic forces the heart to work as a single unit continuously; therefore, if one portion of the muscle should die (as in myocardial infarction), contraction of the heart does not cease.

Skeletal muscle is the striated muscle within the body responsible for the movement of bony levers (Figure 2-8). Skeletal muscle consists of two portions: (1) the muscle belly and (2) its tendons, which are collectively referred to as a musculotendinous unit. The muscle belly is composed of separate, parallel elastic fibers called myofibrils. Myofibrils are composed of thousands of small sarcomeres, which are the functional units of the muscle. Sarcomeres contain the contractile elements of the muscle, as well as a substantial amount of connective tissue that holds the fibers together. Myofilaments are small contractile elements of protein within the sarcomere. There are two distinct types of myofilaments: thin actin myofilaments and thicker myosin myofilaments. Finger-like projections, or crossbridges, connect the actin and myosin myofilaments. When a muscle is stimulated to contract, the crossbridges pull the myofilaments closer together, thus shortening the muscle and producing movement at the joint that the muscle crosses.[20]

The **muscle tendon** attaches muscle directly to bone. The muscle tendon is composed primarily of collagen fibers and a matrix of proteoglycan, which is produced by the tenocyte cell. The collagen fibers are grouped together into **primary bundles.** Groups of primary bundles join together to form hexagonal shaped **secondary bundles.** Secondary bundles are held together by intertwined loose connective tissue containing elastin called the **endotenon.** The entire tendon is surrounded by a connective tissue layer called the **epitenon.** The outermost layer of the tendon is the **paratenon,** which is a double-layer connective tissue sheath lined on the inside with synovial membrane (Figure 2-9).

All skeletal muscles exhibit four characteristics: (1) elasticity, the ability to change in length or stretch; (2) extensibility, the ability to shorten and return to normal length; (3) excitability, the ability to respond to stimulation from the nervous system; and (4) contractility, the ability to shorten and contract in response to some neural command.[75]

Skeletal muscles show considerable variation in size and shape. Large muscles generally produce gross motor movements at large joints, such as knee flexion produced by contraction of the large, bulky hamstring muscles. Smaller skeletal muscles, such as the long flexors of the fingers, produce fine motor movements. Muscles producing

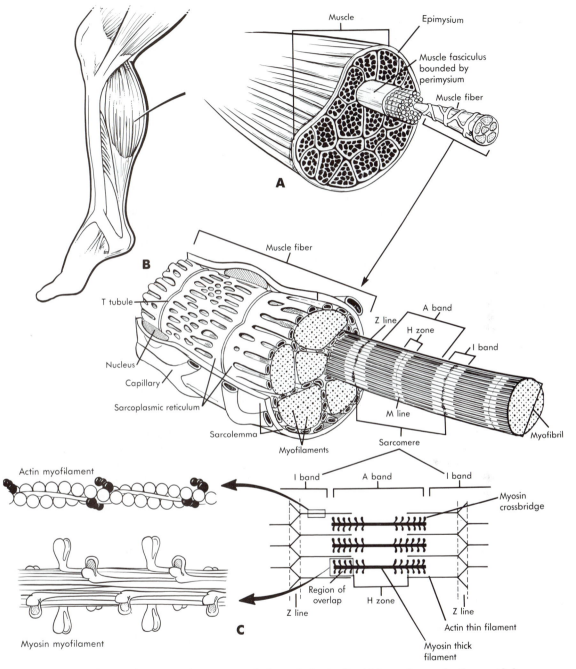

Figure 2-8 Parts of a muscle. **A,** Muscle is composed of muscle fasciculi, which can be seen by the unaided eye as striations in the muscle. The fasciculi are composed of bundles of individual muscle fibers (muscle cells). **B,** Each muscle fiber contains myofibrils in which the banding patterns of the sarcomeres are seen. **C,** The myofibrils are composed of actin myofilament and myosin myofilaments, which are formed from thousands of individual actin and myosin molecules.

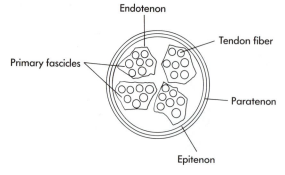

Figure 2-9 Structure of a tendon.

movements that are powerful in nature are usually thicker and longer, whereas those producing finer movements requiring coordination are thin and relatively shorter. Other muscles may be flat, round, or fan-shaped.[33,62] Muscles may be connected to bone by a single tendon or by two or three separate tendons at either end. Muscles that have two separate muscle and tendon attachments are called *biceps,* and muscles with three separate muscle and tendon attachments are called *triceps.*

Muscles contract in response to stimulation by the central nervous system. An electrical impulse transmitted from the central nervous system through a single motor nerve to a group of muscle fibers causes a depolarization of those fibers. The motor nerve and the group of muscle fibers that it innervates are referred to collectively as a **motor unit.** An impulse coming from the central nervous system and traveling to a group of fibers through a particular motor nerve causes all the muscle fibers in that motor unit to depolarize and contract. This is referred to as the **all-or-none** response and applies to all skeletal muscles in the body.[33]

Muscle Strains

If a musculotendinous unit is overstretched or forced to contract against too much resistance, exceeding the extensibility limits or the tensile capabilities of the weakest component within the unit, damage can occur to the muscle fibers, at the musculotendinous juncture, in the tendon, or at the tendinous attachment to the bone.[26,36] Any of these injuries may be referred to as a **strain** (Figure 2-10). Muscles strains, like ligament sprains, are subject to various classification systems. The following is a simple system of classification of muscle strains:

Grade 1 strain: Some muscle or tendon fibers have been stretched or actually torn. Active motion produces some tenderness and pain. Movement is painful, but full range of motion is usually possible.

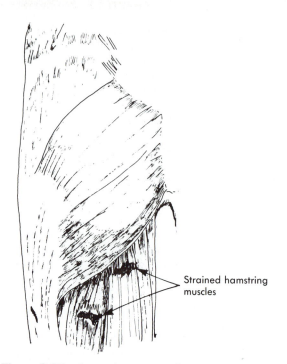

Figure 2-10 A muscle strain results in tearing or separation of fibers.

Grade 2 strain: Some muscle or tendon fibers have been torn, and active contraction of the muscle is extremely painful. Usually a palpable depression or divot exists somewhere in the muscle belly at the spot where the muscle fibers have been torn. Some swelling might occur because of capillary bleeding.

Grade 3 strain: There is a complete rupture of muscle fibers in the muscle belly, in the area where the muscle becomes tendon, or at the tendinous attachment to the bone. The athlete has significant impairment to, or perhaps total loss of, movement. Pain is intense initially but diminishes quickly because of complete separation of the nerve fibers. Musculotendinous ruptures are most common in the biceps tendon of the upper arm or in the Achilles heelcord in the back of the calf. When either of these tendons ruptures, the muscle tends to bunch toward its proximal attachment. With the exception of an Achilles rupture, which is frequently surgically repaired, the majority of third-degree strains are treated conservatively with some period of immobilization.

Muscle Healing

Injuries to muscle tissue involve similar processes of healing and repair as discussed with other tissues. Initially there will be hemorrhage and edema followed almost immediately by phagocytosis to clear debris. Within a few days there is a proliferation of ground substance, and fibroblasts begin producing a gel-type matrix that surrounds the connective tissue, leading to fibrosis and scarring. At the same time, myoblastic cells form in the area of injury, which will eventually lead to regeneration of new myofibrils. Thus regeneration of both connective tissue and muscle tissue has begun.[73]

Collagen fibers undergo maturation and orient themselves along lines of tensile force according to Wolff's law. Active contraction of the muscle is critical in regaining normal tensile strength.[4,48]

Regardless of the severity of the strain, the time required for rehabilitation is fairly lengthy. In many instances, rehabilitation time for a muscle strain is longer than for a ligament sprain. These incapacitating muscle strains occur most frequently in the large, force-producing hamstring and quadriceps muscles of the lower extremity. The treatment of hamstring strains requires a healing period of at least 6 to 8 weeks and a considerable amount of patience. Attempts to return to activity too soon frequently cause reinjury to the area of the musculotendinous unit that has been strained, and the healing process must begin again.

Tendinitis

Of all the overuse problems associated with physical activity, tendinitis is among the most common. **Tendinitis** is a catchall term that can describe many different pathological conditions of a tendon. It essentially describes any inflammatory response within the tendon without inflammation of the paratenon. **Paratenonitis** involves inflammation of the outer layer of the tendon only and usually occurs when the tendon rubs over a bony prominence. **Tendinosis** describes a tendon that has significant degenerative changes with no clinical or histological signs of an inflammatory response.[14]

In cases of what is most often called **chronic tendinitis,** there is evidence of significant tendon degeneration, loss of normal collagen structure, loss of cellularity in the area, but absolutely no inflammatory cellular response in the tendon. The inflammatory process is an essential part of healing. Inflammation is supposed to be a brief process with an end point after its function in the healing process has been fulfilled. The point or the cause in the pathological process where the acute inflammatory cellular response terminates and the chronic degeneration begins is difficult to determine. As mentioned previously, with chronic tendinitis the cellular response involves a replacement of leukocytes with macrophages and plasma cells.

During muscle activity a tendon must move or slide on other structures around it whenever the muscle contracts. If a particular movement is performed repeatedly, the tendon becomes irritated and inflamed. This inflammation is manifested by pain on movement, swelling, possibly some warmth, and usually crepitus. Crepitus is a crackling sound similar to the sound produced by rolling hair between the fingers by the ear. Crepitus is usually caused by the adherence of the paratenon to the surrounding structures while it slides back and forth. This adhesion is caused primarily by the chemical products of inflammation that accumulate on the irritated tendon.[14]

The key to treating tendinitis is rest. If the repetitive motion causing irritation to the tendon is eliminated, chances are the inflammatory process will allow the tendon to heal. Unfortunately, an athlete who is seriously involved with some physical activity might have difficulty in resting for 2 weeks or more while the tendinitis subsides. Anti-inflammatory medications and therapeutic modalities are also helpful in reducing the inflammatory response. An alternative activity, such as bicycling or swimming, is necessary to maintain fitness levels to a certain degree while allowing the tendon a chance to heal.

Tendinitis most commonly occurs in the Achilles tendon in the back of the lower leg in runners or in the rotator cuff tendons of the shoulder joint in swimmers or throwers, although it can certainly flare up in any tendon in which overuse and repetitive movements occur.

Tenosynovitis

Tenosynovitis is very similar to tendinitis in that the muscle tendons are involved in inflammation. However, many tendons are subject to an increased amount of friction due to the tightness of the space through which they must move. In these areas of high friction, tendons are usually surrounded by synovial sheaths that reduce friction on movement. If the tendon sliding through a synovial sheath is subjected to overuse, inflammation is likely to occur. The inflammatory process produces by-products that are "sticky" and tend to cause the sliding tendon to adhere to the synovial sheath surrounding it.

Symptomatically, tenosynovitis is very similar to tendinitis, with pain on movement, tenderness, swelling, and crepitus. Movement may be more limited with tenosynovitis because the space provided for the tendon and its synovial covering is more limited. Tenosynovitis occurs most commonly in the long flexor tendons of the fingers as they cross over the wrist joint and in the biceps tendon around the shoulder joint. Treatment for tenosynovitis is the same as for tendinitis. Because both conditions involve inflammation, mild anti-inflammatory drugs, such as aspirin, might be helpful in chronic cases.

Tendon Healing

Unlike most soft-tissue healing, tendon injuries pose a particular problem in rehabilitation.[34] The injured tendon requires dense fibrous union of the separated ends and both extensibility and flexibility at the site of attachment. Thus an abundance of collagen is required to achieve good tensile strength. Unfortunately, collagen synthesis can become excessive, resulting in fibrosis, in which adhesions form in surrounding tissues and interfere with the gliding that is essential for smooth motion. Fortunately, over a period of time the scar tissue of the surrounding tissues becomes elongated in its structure because of a breakdown in the cross-links between fibrin units and thus allows the necessary gliding motion. A tendon injury that occurs where the tendon is surrounded by a synovial sheath can be potentially devastating.

A typical time frame for tendon healing would be that during the second week the healing tendon adheres to the surrounding tissue to form a single mass, and during the third week the tendon separates to varying degrees from the surrounding tissues. However, the tensile strength is not sufficient to permit a strong pull on the tendon for at least 4 to 5 weeks, the danger being that a strong contraction can pull the tendon ends apart.

INJURY TO NERVE TISSUE

The final fundamental tissue is nerve tissue (Figure 2-11). This tissue provides sensitivity and communication from the central nervous system (brain and spinal cord) to the muscles, sensory organs, various systems, and the periphery. The basic nerve cell is the neuron. The neuron cell body contains a large **nucleus** and branched extensions called **dendrites,** which respond to neurotransmitter substances released from other nerve cells. From each nerve cell arises a single **axon,** which conducts the nerve impulses. Large axons found in peripheral nerves are enclosed in sheaths composed of **Schwann cells,** which are tightly wound around the axon. A nerve is a bundle of nerve cells held together by some connective tissue, usually a lipid-protein layer called the **myelin sheath** on the outside of the axon. Neurology is an extremely complex science, and only a brief presentation of its relevance to sport-related injuries is covered here.[7]

In a sports medicine setting, nerve injuries usually involve either contusions or inflammations. More serious injuries involve the crushing of a nerve or complete division (severing). This type of injury can produce a lifelong physical disability, such as paraplegia or quadriplegia, and should therefore not be overlooked in any circumstance.

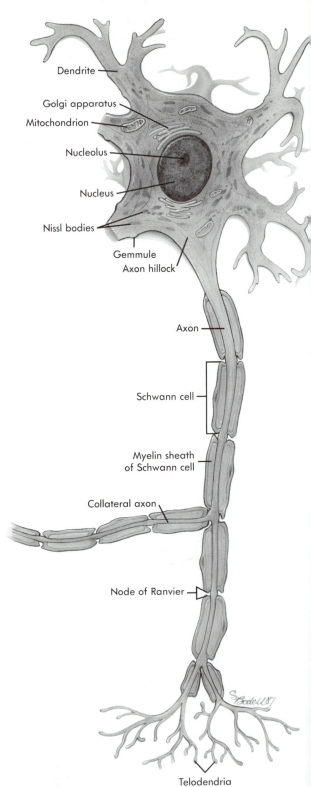

Figure 2-11 Structural features of a nerve cell.

Of critical concern to the sports therapist is the importance of the nervous system in proprioception and neuromuscular control of movement as an integral part of a rehabilitation program. This will be discussed in great detail in Chapter 6.

Nerve Healing

Nerve cell tissue is specialized and cannot regenerate once the nerve cell dies. In an injured peripheral nerve, however, the nerve fiber can regenerate significantly if the injury does not affect the cell body. The proximity of the axonal injury to the cell body can significantly affect the time required for healing. The closer an injury is to the cell body, the more difficult the regenerative process. In the case of a severed nerve, surgical intervention can markedly enhance regeneration.

For regeneration to occur, an optimal environment for healing must exist. When a nerve is cut, several degenerative changes occur that interfere with the neural pathways. Within the first 3 to 5 days the portion of the axon distal to the cut begins to degenerate and breaks into irregular segments. There is also a concomitant increase in metabolism and protein production by the nerve cell body to facilitate the regenerative process. The neuron in the cell body contains the genetic material and produces chemicals necessary for maintenance of the axon. These substances cannot be transmitted to the distal part of the axon, and eventually there will be complete degeneration.

In addition, the myelin portion of the Schwann cells around the degenerating axon also degenerates, and the myelin is phagocytized. The Schwann cells divide, forming a column of cells in place of the axon. If the cut ends of the axon contact this column of Schwann cells, the chances are good that an axon may eventually reinnervate distal structures. If the proximal end of the axon does not make contact with the column of Schwann cells, reinnervation will not occur.

The axon proximal to the cut has minimal degeneration initially and then begins the regenerative process with growth from the proximal axon. Bulbous enlargements and several axon sprouts form at the end of the proximal axon. Within about 2 weeks, these sprouts grow across the scar that has developed in the area of the cut and enter the column of Schwann cells. Only one of these sprouts will form the new axon, while the others will degenerate. Once the axon grows through the Schwann cell columns, remaining Schwann cells proliferate along the length of the degenerating fiber and form new myelin around the growing axon, which will eventually reinnervate distal structures.

Regeneration is slow, at a rate of only 3 to 4 millimeters per day. Axon regeneration can be obstructed by scar formation due to excessive fibroplasia. Damaged nerves within the central nervous system regenerate very poorly compared to nerves in the peripheral nervous system. Central nervous system axons lack connective tissue sheaths, and the myelin-producing Schwann cells fail to proliferate.[33,62]

ADDITIONAL MUSCULOSKELETAL INJURIES

Dislocations and Subluxations

A dislocation occurs when at least one bone in an articulation is forced out of its normal and proper alignment and stays out until it is either manually or surgically put back into place or reduced.[51] Dislocations most commonly occur in the shoulder joint, elbow, and fingers, but they can occur wherever two bones articulate.

A subluxation is like a dislocation except that in this situation a bone pops out of its normal articulation but then goes right back into place. Subluxations most commonly occur in the shoulder joint, as well as in the kneecap in females.

Dislocations should never be reduced immediately, regardless of where they occur. The sports therapist should take the athlete to an X-ray facility and rule out fractures or other problems before reduction. Inappropriate techniques of reduction might only exacerbate the problem. Return to activity after dislocation or subluxation is largely dependent on the degree of soft-tissue damage.

Bursitis

In many areas, particularly around joints, friction occurs between tendons and bones, skin and bone, or two muscles. Without some mechanism of protection in these high-friction areas, chronic irritation would be likely.

Bursae are essentially pieces of synovial membrane that contain small amounts of synovial fluid. This presence of synovium permits motion of surrounding structures without friction. If excessive movement or perhaps some acute trauma occurs around these bursae, they become irritated and inflamed and begin producing large amounts of synovial fluid. The longer the irritation continues or the more severe the acute trauma, the more fluid is produced. As the fluid continues to accumulate in a limited space, pressure tends to increase and causes irritation of the pain receptors in the area.

Bursitis can be extremely painful and can severely restrict movement, especially if it occurs around a joint. Synovial fluid continues to be produced until the movement or trauma producing the irritation is eliminated.

A bursa that occasionally completely surrounds a tendon to allow more freedom of movement in a tight area is referred to as a **synovial sheath.** Irritation of this synovial sheath may restrict tendon motion.

All joints have many bursae surrounding them. Perhaps the three bursae most commonly irritated as a result of various types of physical activity are the subacromial bursa in the shoulder joint, the olecranon bursa on the tip of the elbow, and the prepatellar bursa on the front surface of the patella. All three of these bursae have produced large amounts of synovial fluid, affecting motion at their respective joints.

Muscle Soreness

Overexertion in strenuous muscular exercise often results in muscular pain. At one time or another most everyone has experienced muscle soreness, usually resulting from some physical activity to which we are unaccustomed.

There are two types of muscle soreness. The first type of muscle pain is acute and accompanies fatigue. It is transient and occurs during and immediately after exercise. The second type of soreness involves delayed muscle pain that appears approximately 12 hours after injury. It becomes most intense after 24 to 48 hours and then gradually subsides so that the muscle becomes symptom-free after 3 or 4 days. This second type of pain may best be described as a syndrome of delayed muscle pain, leading to increased muscle tension, edema formation, increased stiffness, and resistance to stretching.[49]

The cause of **delayed-onset muscle soreness (DOMS)** has been debated. Initially it was hypothesized that soreness was due to an excessive buildup of lactic acid in exercised muscles. However, recent evidence has essentially ruled out this theory.[18]

It has also been hypothesized that DOMS is caused by the tonic, localized spasm of motor units, varying in number with the severity of pain. This theory maintains that exercise causes varying degrees of ischemia in the working muscles. This ischemia causes pain, which results in reflex tonic muscle contraction that increases and prolongs the ischemia. Consequently a cycle of increasing severity is begun.[17] As with the lactic acid theory, the spasm theory has also been discounted.

Currently there are two schools of thought relative to the cause of DOMS. DOMS seems to occur from very small tears in the muscle tissue, which seem to be more likely with eccentric or isometric contractions.[18] It is generally believed that the initial damage caused by eccentric exercise is mechanical damage to either the muscular or the connective tissue. Edema accumulation and delays in the rate of glycogen repletion are secondary reactions to mechanical damage.[56]

DOMS might be caused by structural damage to the elastic components of connective tissue at the musculotendinous junction. This damage results in the presence of hydroxyproline, a protein by-product of collagen breakdown, in blood and urine.[13] It has also been documented that structural damage to the muscle fibers results in an increase in blood serum levels of various protein/enzymes, including creatine kinase. This increase indicates that there is likely some damage to the muscle fiber as a result of strenuous exercise.[18]

Muscle soreness can best be prevented by beginning at a moderate level of activity and gradually progressing the intensity of the exercise over time. Treatment of muscle soreness usually also involves some type of stretching activity. As for other conditions discussed in this chapter, ice is important as a treatment for muscle soreness, particularly within the first 48 to 72 hours.

Contusions

Contusion is synonymous with *bruise*. The mechanism that produces a contusion is a blow from some external object that causes soft tissues (e.g., skin, fat, muscle, ligaments, joint capsule) to be compressed against the hard bone underneath. If the blow is hard enough, capillaries rupture and allow bleeding into the tissues. The bleeding, if superficial enough, causes a bluish-purple discoloration to the skin that persists for several days. The contusion may be very sore to the touch. If damage has occurred to muscle, pain may be elicited on active movement. In most cases the pain ceases within a few days, and discoloration disappears in usually 2 to 3 weeks.

The major problem with contusions occurs where an area is subjected to repeated blows. If the same area, or more specifically the same muscle, is bruised over and over again, small calcium deposits might begin to accumulate in the injured area. These pieces of calcium might be found between several fibers in the muscle belly, or calcium might form a spur that projects from the underlying bone. These calcium formations, which can significantly impair movement, are referred to as **myositis ossificans.** In some cases myositis ossificans develops from a single trauma.

The key to preventing myositis ossificans from occurring from repeated contusions is protection of the injured area by padding. If the area is properly protected after the first contusion, myositis ossificans might never develop. Protection, along with rest, might allow the calcium to be reabsorbed and eliminate any need for surgical intervention. The two areas that seem to be the most vulnerable to repeated contusions during physical activity are the quadriceps muscle group on the front of the thigh and the biceps muscle on the front of the upper arm. The formation of myositis ossificans in either of these or any other areas can be detected on X-ray films.

MANAGING THE HEALING PROCESS THROUGH REHABILITATION

Rehabilitation exercise progressions in sports medicine can generally be subdivided into three phases based primarily on the three stages of the healing process: phase 1, the acute phase; phase 2, the repair phase; and phase 3, the remodeling phase. Depending on the type and extent of injury and the individual response to healing, phases will usually overlap. Each phase must include carefully considered goals and a criteria for progressing from one phase to another.

Presurgical Exercise Phase

This phase would apply only to those athletes who sustain injuries that require surgery. If surgery can be postponed, exercise may be used as a means to improve its outcome. By allowing the initial inflammatory response phase to resolve, by maintaining or, in some cases, increasing muscle strength and flexibility, levels of cardiorespiratory fitness, and improving neuromuscular control, the athlete may be better prepared to continue the exercise rehabilitative program after surgery.

Phase 1, the Acute Injury Phase

Phase 1 begins immediately when injury occurs and can last as long as day 4 following injury. During this phase, the inflammatory stage of the healing process is attempting to "clean up the mess," thus creating an environment that is conducive to the fibroblastic stage. As indicated in Chapter 1, the primary focus of rehabilitation during this stage is to control swelling and to modulate pain by using the PRICE technique immediately following injury. Ice, compression, and elevation should be used as much as possible during this phase[58] (Figure 2-12).

Rest of the injured part is critical during this phase. It is widely accepted that early mobility during rehabilitation is essential. However, if the sports therapist becomes overly aggressive during the first 48 hours following injury, and does not allow the injured part to be rested during the inflammatory stage of healing, the inflammatory process never really gets a chance to accomplish what it

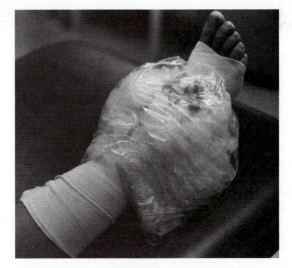

Figure 2-12 Musculoskeletal injuries should be treated initially with protection, restricted activity, ice, compression, and elevation.

is supposed to. Consequently, the length of time required for inflammation might be extended. Therefore, immobility during the first 24 to 48 hours following injury is necessary to control inflammation.

By day 3 or 4, swelling begins to subside and eventually stops altogether. The injured area may feel warm to the touch, and some discoloration is usually apparent. The injury is still painful to the touch, and some pain is elicited on movement of the injured part.[70] At this point the athlete should have already begun active mobility exercises, working through a pain-free range of motion. If the injury involves the lower extremity, the athlete should be encouraged to progressively bear more weight.

The team physician may choose to have the athlete take nonsteroidal anti-inflammatory drugs (NSAIDs) to help control swelling and inflammation. It is usually helpful to continue this medication throughout the rehabilitative process.

Phase 2, the Repair Phase

Once the inflammatory response has subsided, the repair phase begins. During this stage of the healing process, fibroblastic cells are laying down a matrix of collagen fibers and forming scar tissue. This stage might begin as early as 2 days after the injury and can last for several weeks. At this point, swelling has stopped completely. The injury is still tender to the touch but is not as painful as during the previous stage. Pain is also less on active and passive motion.[58]

As soon as inflammation is controlled, the sports therapist should immediately begin to incorporate into the rehabilitation program activities that can maintain levels of cardiorespiratory fitness, restore full range of motion, restore or increase strength, and reestablish neuromuscular control as discussed in Chapter 1.

As in the acute phase, modalities should be used to control pain and swelling. Cryotherapy should still be used during the early portion of this phase to reduce the likelihood of swelling. Electrical stimulating currents can help with controlling pain and improving strength and range of motion.[58]

Phase 3, the Remodeling Phase

The remodeling phase is the longest of the three phases and can last for several years, depending on the severity of the injury. The ultimate goal during this maturation stage of the healing process is return to activity. The injury is no longer painful to the touch, although some progressively decreasing pain might still be felt on motion. The collagen fibers must be realigned according to tensile stresses and strains placed upon them during functional sport specific exercises.

The focus during this phase should be on regaining sport-specific skills. Dynamic functional activities related to individual sport performance should be incorporated into the rehabilitation program. Functional training involves the repeated performance of an athletic skill for the purpose of perfecting that skill. Strengthening exercises should progressively place on the injured structures stresses and strains that would normally be encountered during that sport. Plyometric strengthening exercises can be used to improve muscle power and explosiveness.[31] Functional testing should be done to determine specific skill weaknesses that need to be addressed prior to full return.

At this point some type of heating modality is beneficial to the healing process. The deep-heating modalities, ultrasound, or the diathermies should be used to increase circulation to the deeper tissues. Massage and gentle mobilization may also be used to reduce guarding, increase circulation, and reduce pain. Increased blood flow delivers the essential nutrients to the injured area to promote healing, and increased lymphatic flow assists in breakdown and removal of waste products.[58]

THE SPORTS MEDICINE APPROACH TO THE HEALING PROCESS

In sports medicine, the rehabilitation philosophy relative to inflammation and healing after injury is to assist the natural processes of the body while doing no harm.[41] The chosen course of rehabilitation must focus on the sports therapist's knowledge of the healing process and its therapeutic modifiers to guide, direct, and stimulate the structural function and integrity of the injured part. The primary goal should be to have a positive influence on the inflammation and repair process to expedite recovery of function in terms of range of motion, muscular strength and endurance, neuromuscular control, and cardiorespiratory endurance.[22] The sports therapist must try to minimize the early effects of excessive inflammatory processes, including pain modulation, edema control, and reduction of associated muscle spasm, which can produce loss of joint motion and contracture. Finally, the sports therapist should concentrate on preventing the recurrence of injury by influencing the structural ability of the injured tissue to resist future overloads by incorporating various training techniques.[41] The subsequent chapters throughout this text can serve as a guide for the sports therapist in using the many different rehabilitation tools available.

Summary

1. The three phases of the healing process are the inflammatory response phase, the fibroblastic-repair phase, and the maturation-remodeling phase. These occur in sequence but overlap one another in a continuum.

2. Factors that can impede the healing process include edema, hemorrhage, lack of vascular supply, separation of tissue, muscle spasm, atrophy, corticosteroids, hypertrophic scars, infection, climate and humidity, age, health, and nutrition.

3. The four fundamental types of tissue in the human body are epithelial, connective, muscle, and nerve.

4. Ligament sprains involve stretching or tearing the fibers that provide stability at the joint.

5. Fractures can be classified as greenstick, transverse, oblique, spiral, comminuted, impacted, avulsive, or stress.

6. Osteoarthritis involves degeneration of the articular cartilage or subchondral bone.

7. Muscle strains involve a stretching or tearing of muscle fibers and their tendons and cause impairment to active movement.

8. Tendinitis, an inflammation of a muscle tendon that causes pain on movement, usually occurs because of overuse.

9. Tenosynovitis is an inflammation of the synovial sheath through which a tendon must slide during motion.

10. Dislocations and subluxations involve disruption of the joint capsule and ligamentous structures surrounding the joint.

11. Bursitis is an inflammation of the synovial membranes located in areas where friction occurs between various anatomic structures.

12. Muscle soreness can be caused by spasm, connective tissue damage, muscle tissue damage, or some combination of these.

13. Repeated contusions can lead to the development of myositis ossificans.

14. All injuries should be initially managed with rest, ice, compression, and elevation to control swelling and thus reduce the time required for rehabilitation.

References

1. Anonymous. 1994. The healing process. *Nursing Times* 90(16): 95.

2. Arnheim D., and W. Prentice. 1997. *Principles of athletic training.* 9th ed. Madison, WI: Brown & Benchmark.

3. Arnoczky, S. P. 1991. Physiologic principles of ligament injuries and healing. In *Ligament and extensor mechanism injuries of the knee,* edited by W. N. Scott. St Louis: Mosby.

4. Bandy, W., and K. Dunleavy. 1996. Adaptability of skeletal muscle: Response to increased and decreased use. In *Athletic injuries and rehabilitation,* edited by J. Zachazewski, D. Magee, and W. Quillen. Philadelphia: W. B. Saunders.

5. Beck, E. W. 1982. *Mosby's atlas of functional human anatomy.* St Louis: Mosby.

6. Booher, J. M., and G. A. Thibodeau. 1994. *Athletic injury assessment.* 2d ed. St Louis: Mosby.

7. Butler, D. 1996. Nerve structure, function, and physiology. In *Athletic injuries and rehabilitation,* edited by J. Zachazewski, D. Magee, and W. Quillen. Philadelphia: W. B. Saunders.

8. Bryant, M. W. 1997. Wound healing. *CIBA Clinical Symposia* 29(3): 2–36.

9. Cailliet, R. 1988. *Soft tissue pain and disability.* 2d ed. Philadelphia: F. A. Davis.

10. Carley, P. J., and S. F. Wainapel. 1985. Electrotherapy for acceleration of sound healing: Low intensity direct current. *Archives of Physical Medicine and Rehabilitation* 66:443–46.

11. Carrico, T. J., A. I. Mehrhof, and I. K. Cohen. 1984. Biology and wound healing. *Surg Clin North Am* 64(4): 721–34.

12. Cheng, N. 1982 The effects of electrocurrents on A.T.P. generation, protein synthesis and membrane transport. *Journal of Orthopaedic Research* 171:264–72.

13. Clancy, W. 1990. Tendon trauma and overuse injuries. In *Sports-induced inflammation,* edited by W. Leadbetter, J. Buckwalter, and S. Gordon. Park Ridge, IL: American Academy of Orthopaedic Surgeons.

14. Clarkson, P. M., and I. Tremblay. 1988. Exercise-induced muscle damage, repair and adaptation in humans. *Journal of Applied Physiology* 65:1–6.

15. Cox, D. 1993. Growth factors in wound healing. *Journal of Wound Care* 2(6): 339–42.

16. Curwin, S. 1996. Tendon injuries, pathophysiology and treatment. In *Athletic injuries and rehabilitation,* edited by J. Zachazewski, D. Magee, and W. Quillen. Philadelphia: W. B. Saunders.

17. deVries, H. A. 1996. Quantitative EMG investigation of spasm theory of muscle pain, *American Journal of Physical Medicine* 45:119–34.

18. Evans, W. J. 1987. Exercise induced skeletal muscle damage. *Physician and Sports Medicine* 15:189–200.

19. Fahey, T. D. 1986. *Athletic training: Principles and practice.* Palo Alto, CA: Mayfield.

20. Fantone, J. 1990. Basic concepts in inflammation. In *Sports-induced inflammation,* edited by W. Leadbetter, J. Buckwalter, and S. Gordon. Park Ridge, IL: American Academy of Orthopaedic Surgeons.

21. Fernandez, A., and J. M. Finlew. 1983. Wound healing: Helping a natural process. *Postgraduate Medical Journal* 74(4): 311–18.

22. Flynn, M., and D. Rovee. 1982. Influencing repair and recovery. American Journal of Nursing 82:1550–58.

23. Frank, C. 1986. Ligament injuries: Pathophysiology and healing. In *Athletic injuries and rehabilitation,* edited by J. Zachazewski, D. Magee, and W. Quillen, Philadelphia: W. B. Saunders.

24. Frankel. V. H., and M. Nordin. 1980. *Basic biomechanics of the skeletal system.* Philadelphia: Lea & Febiger.

25. Gelberman, R., V. Goldberg, K.-N. An, et al. 1988. Soft tissue healing. In *Injury and repair of musculoskeletal soft tissues,* edited by S.L.-Y. Woo, and J. Buckwalter. Park Ridge, IL: American Academy of Orthopaedic Surgeons.

26. Glick, J. M. 1980. Muscle strains: Prevention and treatment. *Physician and Sports Medicine* 8(11): 73–77.

27. Goldenberg, M. 1996. Wound care management: Proper protocol differs from athletic trainers' perceptions. *Journal of Athletic Training* 31(1): 12–16.

28. Gradisar, I. A. 1985. Fracture stabilization and healing. In *Orthopaedic and sports physical medicine,* edited by J. A. Gould, and G. J. Davies. St Louis: Mosby.

29. Gross, A., D. Cutright, and S. Bhaskar, et al. 1972. Effectiveness of pulsating water jet lavage in treatment of contaminated crush wounds. *American Journal of Surgery* 124:373–75.

30. Guyton, A. C. 1986. *Textbook of medical physiology,* Philadelphia: W. B. Saunders.

31. Henning, C. E. 1988. Semilunar cartilage of the knee: function and pathology. In *Exercise and sport science review,* edited by K. B. Pandolf. New York: Macmillan.

32. Hettinga, D. L. 1985. Inflammatory response of synovial joint structures. In *Orthopaedic and sports physical therapy,* edited by J. A. Gould, and G. J. Davies. St Louis: Mosby.

33. Hole, J. 1984. *Human anatomy and physiology.* Dubuque, IA: Wm. C. Brown.

34. Houglum, P. 1992. Soft tissue healing and its impact on rehabilitation. *Journal of Sport Rehabilitation* 1(1): 19–39.

35. Hubbel, S., and R. Buschbacher. 1994. Tissue injury and healing: Using medications, modalities, and exercise to maximize recovery. In *Sports medicine and rehabilitation: A sport specific approach,* edited by R. Bushbacher, and R. Branddom. Philadelphia: Hanley & Belfus.

36. Keene, J. S. 1985. Ligament and muscle tendon unit injuries. In *Orthopaedic and sports physical therapy,* edited by J. A. Gould, and G. J. Davies. St Louis: Mosby.

37. Kibler, W. B. 1990. Concepts in exercise rehabilitation of athletic injury. In *Sports-induced inflammation,* edited by W. Leadbetter, J. Buckwalter, and S. Gordon. Park Ridge, IL: American Academy of Orthopaedic Surgeons.

38. Kissane, J. M. 1985. *Anderson's pathology.* 8th ed. St Louis: Mosby.

39. Knight, K. L. 1995. *Cryotherapy in sport injury management.* Champaign, IL: Human Kinetics.

40. Lane, N. E., D. Bloch, P. Wood, et al. 1987. Aging, long-distance running, and the development of musculoskeletal disability. *American Journal of Medicine* 82:772–80.

41. Leadbetter, W. 1990. Introduction to sports-induced soft-tissue inflammation. In *Sports-induced inflammation,* edited by W. Leadbetter, J. Buckwalter, and S. Gordon. Park Ridge, IL: American Academy of Orthopaedic Surgeons.

42. Leadbetter, W., J. Buckwalter, and S. Gordon. 1990. *Sports-induced inflammation.* Park Ridge, IL: American Academy of Orthopaedic Surgeons.

43. Loitz-Ramage, B., and R. Zernicke. 1996. Bone biology and mechanics. In *Athletic injuries and rehabilitation,* edited by J. Zachazewski, D. Magee, and W. Quillen. Philadelphia: W. B. Saunders.

44. MacMaster, J. H. 1982. *The ABC's of sports medicine,* Melbourne, FL: Kreiger.

45. Marchesi, V. T. 1985. Inflammation and healing. In *Anderson's pathology,* edited by J. M. Kissane. 8th ed., St Louis: Mosby.

46. Martinez-Hernandez, A., and P. Amenta. 1990. Basic concepts in wound healing. In *Sports-induced inflammation,* edited by W. Leadbetter, J. Buckwalter, and S. Gordon. Park Ridge, IL: American Academy of Orthopaedic Surgeons.

47. Matheson, G., J. MacIntyre, and J. Taunton. 1989. Musculoskeletal injuries associated with physical activity in older adults. *Medicine and Science in Sports and Exercise* 21:379–85.

48. Malone, T., W. Garrett, and J. Zachewski. 1996. Muscle: Deformation, injury and repair. In *Athletic injuries and rehabilitation,* edited by J. Zachazewski, D. Magee, and W. Quillen. Philadelphia: W. B. Saunders.

49. Malone, T., and T. McPhoil, eds. *Orthopaedic and sports physical therapy.* St Louis: Mosby.

50. Messier, S. P., and K. A. Pittala. 1988. Etiologic factors associated with selected running injuries. *Medicine and Science in Sports and Exercise* 20(5): 501–5.

51. Muckle, D. S. 1985. *Outline of fractures and dislocations.* Bristol, England: Wright.

52. Musacchia, X. J. 1988. Disuse atrophy of skeletal muscle: Animal models. In *Exercise and sport sciences review,* edited by K. B. Pandolf. New York: Macmillan.

53. Norkin, C., and P. Levangie. 1983. *Joint structure and function: A comprehensive analysis.* Philadelphia: F. A. Davis.

54. Norris, S., B. Provo, and N. Stotts. 1990. Physiology of wound healing and risk factors that impede the healing process. *AACN Clinical Issues in Critical Care Nursing* 1(3): 545–52.

55. Noyes, F. R. 1977. Functional properties of knee ligaments and alterations induced by immobilization. *Clin Orthop* 123:210–42.

56. O'Reilly, K., M. Warhol, R. Fielding, et al. 1987. Eccentric exercise induced muscle damage impairs muscle glycogen depletion. *Journal of Applied Physiology* 63:252–56.

57. Panush, R. S., and D. G. Brown. 1987. Exercise and arthritis. *Sports Medicine* 4:54–64.

58. Prentice, W. E., ed. 1988. *Therapeutic modalities in sports medicine.* St Louis: Mosby.

59. Riley, W. B. 1981. Wound healing. *American Family Physician* 24:5.

60. Robbins, S. L., R. S. Cotran, and V. Kumar. 1984. *Pathologic basis of disease.* 3d ed. Philadelphia: W. B. Saunders.

61. Rywlin, A. M. 1985. Hemopoietic system. In *Anderson's pathology,* 8th ed., edited by J. M. Kissane. St. Louis: Mosby.

62. Seeley, R., T. Stephens, and P. Tate. 1995. *Anatomy and physiology.* St. Louis: Mosby.

63. Seller, R. H. 1986. *Differential diagnosis of common complaints.* Philadelphia: W. B. Saunders.

64. Stanish, W. D., and B. Gunnlaugson. 1988. Electrical energy and soft tissue injury healing. *Sportcare and Fitness* 9:12.

65. Stanish, W. D., M. Rubinovich, J. Kozey, et al. 1985. The use of electricity in ligament and tendon repair. *Physician and Sports Medicine* 13:8.

66. Stewart, J. 1986. *Clinical anatomy and physiology.* Miami: Medmaster.

67. Stone, M. H. 1988. Implications for connective tissue and bone alterations resulting from rest and exercise training. *Medicine and Science in Sports and Exercise* 20(5): S162–68.

68. Walker, J. 1996. Cartilage of human joints and related structures. In *Athletic injuries and rehabilitation,* edited by J. Zachazewski, D. Magee, and W. Quillen, Philadelphia: W. B. Saunders.

69. Wahl, S., and P. Renstrom. 1990. Fibrosis in soft-tissue injuries. In *Sports-induced inflammation,* edited by W. Leadbetter, J. Buckwalter, and S. Gordon. Park Ridge, IL: American Academy of Orthopaedic Surgeons.

70. Wells, P. E, V. Frampton, and D. Bowsher. 1988. *Pain management in physical therapy.* Norwalk, CT: Appleton & Lange.

71. Whiteside, J. A., S. B. Fleagle, and A. Kalenak. 1981. Fractures and refractures in intercollegiate athletes: An eleven year experience. *American Journal of Sports Medicine* 9(6): 369–77.

72. Woo, S.L.-Y., and J. Buckwalter, eds. *Injury and repair of musculoskeletal soft tissues.* Park Ridge, IL: American Academy of Orthopaedic Surgeons.

73. Woodman, R., and L. Pare. 1982. Evaluation and treatment of soft tissue lesions of the ankle and foot using the Cyriax approach. *Phys Ther* 62:1144–47.

74. Zachezewski, J. 1990. Flexibility for sports. In *Sports physical therapy,* edited by B. Sanders. Norwalk, CT: Appleton & Lange.

CHAPTER 3

Psychological Considerations for Rehabilitation of the Injured Athlete

Joe Gieck
Elizabeth G. Hedgpeth

After completion of this chapter, the student should be able to do the following:

- Discuss various predictors of injury and interventions.

- Identify stressors in the athlete's life.

- Discuss the concept of buffers for stress management.

- Describe the progressive reactions to injury, dependent on length of rehabilitation.

- Describe interventions for the four time periods of rehabilitation.

- Recognize irrational thinking and its resolution.

- Explain the importance of athletes' taking responsibility for their actions in regard to injury.

- Define compliance and adherence.

- Explain the importance of rehabilitation compliance and its deviations.

- Discuss one strategy for the management of pain.

- Discuss goal setting and rehabilitation compliance.

- Describe the coping skills necessary for successful rehabilitation.

- Recognize the importance of the relationship between the sports therapist and the athlete.

A thletic injuries are considered to be one of the major health hazards of sport.[47] The fear of injury might cause a negative view of participation in an activity that has a positive impact on the health and well-being of millions of participants.[38] Sports medicine and athletic training are still inexact sciences. Nowhere is this more evident than in the psychological process of responding to injury in a rational and productive manner and completing the rehabilitation process to the best of the athlete's ability. Early writings often mention that one should never attempt to cure the body without curing the soul.

Most athletes have the self-confidence to adapt to a mild or moderate injury, and most have the support, understanding, and proper encouragement to adapt to more severe injury, but even the most self-confident athletes have their doubts. One athlete put it this way, expressing the positive aspects of return to competition but also some of the doubts involved: "The best competitors like to compete, and to me this is just a game—an inner game. It's an inner soul game. Can I beat my knee back?" But he also expressed doubts about the real test when a tackler "takes a whack at the knee": "I haven't thought about it, but I've had nightmares about it. My buddy told me he broke his ankle. He said once you get that real good hit and you pop up and it pops up with you, then everything is going to fall into place and you're going to be rolling. You're going to go out there like it's never been hurt and just play."

With the emergence of sport psychology, more attention is being paid to getting the mind ready to return to competition to match the adjustment of the body. Athletes have begun to describe the nightmares, fears, and anxiety of returning to competition. Also, in the current trend of professional athletes receiving extremely high salaries, some athletes describe their injuries and surgery as the most important things in their lives because the ability to play will either make or break them. Surgery and subsequent rehabilitation can determine whether athletes make either millions of dollars in a sports career or only thousands in a regular job if the injury career ends.

Athletes don't all deal with injury in the same manner. Rotella[49] describes how one might view the injury as disastrous, another might view it as an opportunity to show courage, whereas another athlete might relish the injury as a means to avoid embarrassment over poor performance, to escape from a losing team, or to discourage a domineering parent. When injuries are career-threatening, athletes whose lives have revolved around a sport may have to make major adjustments in how they perceive themselves as well as how they are perceived within their society. Olympic and other top-caliber athletes are often emotionally and socially years behind their chronological peers because they have spent so much time in their sport that their social interactions have suffered. Therefore many top or single-minded athletes have difficulty with emotional control when they sustain a serious injury. Figure 3-1 demonstrates the physical and emotional aspects of return to performance. The return to performance is either enhanced or negated by the physiological results of both elements.

PREDICTORS OF INJURY

The Injury-Prone Athlete

Some athletes seem to have a pattern of injury, whereas others in exactly the same position with the same physical makeup are injury-free. Certain researchers suggest that some psychological traits might predispose the ath-

lete to a repeated injury cycle.[43,45,55,58,64] No one particular personality type has been recognized as injury-prone. However, the individual who likes to take risks seems to represent the injury-prone athlete.[24] Other factors that are seen as predisposing an athlete to risk of injury are being reserved, detached, tender-minded,[30] apprehensive, overprotective, or easily distracted.[48] These individuals usually also lack the ability to cope with the stress associated with the risks and their consequences. Sanderson[50] suggests some other factors leading to a propensity for injury, such as attempts to reduce anxiety by being more aggressive, fear of failure, or guilt over unobtainable or unrealistic goals.

Stress and Risk of Injury

Much has been written about life stress events and the likelihood of illness.[2,12,28,34] Stressors are both positive (e.g., making All-American) and negative (e.g., not making the starting lineup, or failing a drug test). Stressors that seem to predispose an athlete to injury are the negative stressors.[60]

Andersen and Williams[2] suggest that negative stressors lead to a lack of attentional focus and to muscle tension, which in turn lead to the stress-injury connection. Loss of attentional focus can cause the athlete to miss cues during a play, setting the stage for a possible injury. Muscle tension (bracing or guarding) leads to reduced flexibility, reduced motor coordination, and reduced muscle efficiency, which set the athlete up for a variety of injuries (e.g., getting hit by a golf ball or missing an obstacle during a run).

Attentional focusing is perceived on two planes (width and directional). A major component is the ability to change focus when the situation demands it. Width of focus ranges from broad (attending to a number of cues) to narrow (attending to one cue), and direction of focus is internal (attending to feelings or thoughts) or external (attending to events outside of the body). The trick is not only to be able to change focus, but to know the optimal time to make the change in order to minimize the possibility of injury or reinjury. For instance, a football player can be blindsided and take an unanticipated hit, or the gymnast can be distracted and miss a landing.

Life stress is a more global assessment, taking into account events that cause stress over the past year to 18 months. The Life Events Survey for Collegiate Athletes (LESCA) asks collegiate-athlete-specific questions, eliciting a negative or positive response on a Likert-type 8-point scale.[45] Typical events asked about are "major change in playing status" and "pressure to gain or lose weight for sport participation." Another life events

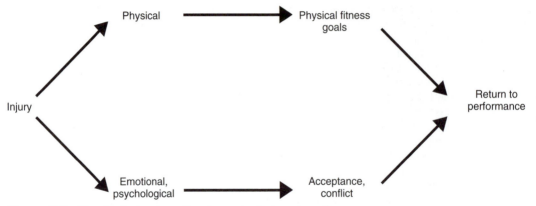

Figure: 3-1 The physical and emotional aspects of return to performance.

assessment is the Social and Athletic Readjustment Rating Scale[6] (SARRS). The events most likely to elicit a negative stress response are listed in Table 3-1.

Profiles of Mood States[39] (POMS) is a more immediate response inventory assessing moods within the last few days or at the most the last few weeks. The POMS identifies six mood states. Five are negative, and one (vigor) is positive. The six mood states are (1) tension-anxiety, (2) depression-dejection, (3) anger-hostility, (4) vigor-activity, (5) fatigue-inertia, and (6) confusion-bewilderment. When the POMS results were compared using elite athletes and the general population, a visual "iceberg profile" was noted for the elite athletes by Morgan.[42] The elite athletes' scores on the five negative scales fall below the 50th percentile, and their scores on the sixth, positive scale (vigor) peak considerably above the 50th percentile, indeed resembling the silhouette of an "iceberg."

The POMS has been used to measure the mood states of athletes at the time of injury as well as at 2-week intervals during the rehabilitation process.[54] When the POMS was used within 2 days of injury, the injured athletes showed significant elevations in depression and anger, no change in tension and vigor, but less fatigue and confusion as compared to the college norms. When the athletes were divided into groups according to severity of injury based on length of rehabilitation, the data is more explicit concerning reactions to injury and rehabilitation. Group 1 consists of athletes with less than 1 week of rehabilitation; they had less tension, depression, fatigue, and confusion. Group 2 consists of athletes in rehabilitation for more than 2 weeks but less than 4 weeks; they had more anger but less fatigue and confusion. Group 3 consists of athletes in rehabilitation more than 4 weeks; they had more tension, depression, and anger and less vigor. This finding is important in that it sends a wake-up call to the

■ **TABLE 3-1** Examples of Events in the Lives of Athletes Most Likely to Elicit a Stress Response

Life Stress Events

Death of family member
Detention or jail
Injury
Death of close friend
Playing for a new coach
Playing on a new team
Personal achievements
Change in living habits
Social readjustments
Change to new school
Change in social activities

sports medicine team to be aware of the ramifications of severe injury that entails a long rehabilitation period.

Interventions for Stress Reduction

Not all athletes need or want counseling, and the close relationship between the athlete and the sports therapist is invaluable in making this decision (Figure 3-2). Few athletes react to stress events by verbalizing their feelings of stress, yet most handle them very well by themselves. James Michener[41] makes the following point:

For many athletes physical activity, rather than talking things out, appears to offer a means of expressing feelings and aggressions. Perhaps this substitution of actions for words contributes to the seeming reluctance of athletes to come to a service that requires that they articulate their feelings.

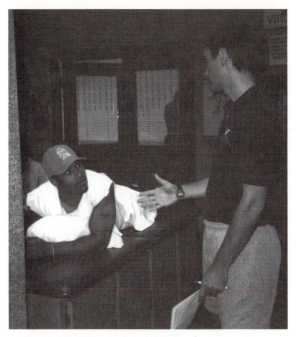

Figure 3-2 A close relationship between the athlete and the sports therapist is invaluable.

Unfortunately, many coaches do not have the interest or ability to work with athletes who need help. Some sort of screening device should be used to identify athletes who are experiencing life situations that they are unprepared to handle. Obviously the staff of a smaller team is more familiar with the athletes and their problems and can more effectively deal with them, but larger teams' staffs should attempt to deal with the athlete through the position coach or other available support personnel (e.g., counseling centers, sport psychologists, grief support groups).

Using Buffers In many instances athletes feel that their sport is the one positive thing in life that helps them get through times of extreme stress. Areas outside of sports are often stressful, and athletes tend to respond to interventions that are within their framework of emotional comfort. The use of buffers might be all the athlete needs to handle the stress of injury and rehabilitation. Buffers are techniques that allay the symptom of stress but do not address the problem that originally caused the stressors. Several buffers that can be beneficial in reducing the stress of injury and rehabilitation are progressive relaxation with or without imagery, aerobic exercise, diet modifications (e.g., reduction of caffeine), treatment of sleep disorders, and time management programs.

Progressive Relaxation Techniques. Progressive relaxation techniques[31] are most effective for ath-

letes who tend to be stressed regarding an injury and who have problems sleeping, tension headaches, or general muscle bracing or tightness. Relaxation training, with or without imagery, allows athletes to control their feelings of stress and anxiety with a series of deep breathing, voluntary muscular contraction, and relaxation exercise.[4] Relaxation and imagery are used by athletes to reduce the symptoms of anxiety associated with the reaction to injury and rehabilitation. Athletes who are coping well on their own should not be forced to spend extra time on relaxation training.

Jacobsen's[32] progressive relaxation technique is thought to be effective because of the assumption that it is impossible to be nervous or tense when the muscles are relaxed. The tenseness of the involuntary muscles and organs can be reduced when the contiguous skeletal muscles are relaxed. The muscles are tensed and relaxed in order for the athlete to become familiar with how the muscle feels in a relaxed state and in a tense state. The relaxation method involves the tensing and relaxing of muscles in a predetermined order. The arm and hand are done first because the difference in tense and relaxed muscles is more apparent in these muscle groups. The repetitions should last approximately 10 to 15 seconds for the tension segment and 15 to 20 seconds for the relaxation segment, with about three repetitions for each muscle group. After the athlete is comfortable with the relaxation training, then imagery can be introduced.

Imagery. Imagery is the use of one's senses to create or recreate an experience in the mind.[5] Visual images used in the rehabilitation process include *visual rehearsal, emotive imagery rehearsal,* and *body rehearsal.* Visual rehearsal uses both coping and mastery rehearsal. *Coping rehearsal* has athletes visually rehearsing problems they feel might stand in the way of a return to competition. They then rehearse how they will overcome these problems. *Mastery rehearsal* aids in gaining confidence and motivational skills. Athletes visualize their successful return to competition, beginning with early practice drills and continuing on to the game situation.

In emotive rehearsal, the athlete gains confidence and security by visualizing scenes relating to positive feelings of enthusiasm, confidence, and pride—in other words, the emotional rewards of praise and success from participating well in competition. Body rehearsal empirically helps athletes in the healing process. It is suggested that athletes visualize their bodies healing internally both during the rehabilitation procedures as well as throughout their daily activities.[23] To do this, the athletes have to have a good understanding of the injury and of the type of healing occurring during the

Length of rehabilitation	Reaction to injury	Reaction to rehabilitation	Reaction to return
Short (< 4 weeks)	Shock Relief	Impatience Optimism	Eagerness Anticipation
Long (> 4 weeks)	Fear Anger	Loss of vigor Irrational thoughts Alienation	Acknowledgment
Chronic (recurring)	Anger Frustration	Dependence or independence Apprehension	Confident or skeptical
Termination (career-ending)	Isolation Grief process	Loss of athletic identify	Closure and renewal

Figure 3-3   Progressive reactions of injured athletes based on severity of injury and length of rehabilitation.

rehabilitation process. Ievleva and Orlick[29] had athletes use imagery during physiotherapy by imagining that the ultrasound was increasing blood flow and thus promoting recovery.

Care should be taken to explain the healing and rehabilitative process clearly but not to overwhelm athletes with so much information that they become intimidated and fearful. This mistake is often made by the inexperienced sports therapist who wants to impress the athletes. Educate athletes only to the amount of knowledge required. By the same token, don't hold back information athletes require for this imagery.

PROGRESSIVE REACTIONS DEPEND ON LENGTH OF REHABILITATION

The literature on reactions to injury has dispelled the stage theory of reaction to injury, according to an extensive literature review by Wortman and Silver.[66] However, there are factors that are commonly seen among athletes going through adjustment to injury and rehabilitation in the athletic training room. Severity of injury usually determines length of rehabilitation. Regardless of length of rehabilitation, the injured athlete has to deal with three reactive phases of the injury and rehabilitation process (Figure 3-3). These phases are reaction to injury, reaction to rehabilitation, and reaction to return

to competition or career termination. These reactions can be cumulative in nature depending on the length of rehabilitation. Other factors that influence reactions to injury and rehabilitation are the athlete's coping skills, past history of injury, social support, and personality traits. These reactions fall into four time frames: short-term (less than 4 weeks), long-term (more than 4 weeks), chronic (recurring), and termination (career-ending). Reactions are primary and secondary, but athletes do not all have all reactions, nor do all reactions fall into the suggested sequence.

DEALING WITH SHORT-TERM INJURY

Short-term injuries are usually of less than 4 weeks but may be a few days over depending on how the length is measured in terms of the end of rehabilitation. For practical purposes the rehabilitation is complete when the athlete and the sports medicine team feel it is safe for the athlete to return, when an appropriate level of competitive fitness has been reached, and the athlete feels ready physically and psychologically to return to competition. Short-term injuries can include, but are not limited to, first- or second-degree sprains/strains, bruises, and simple dislocations. These are the type of injury that are fairly common and are part of playing the game.

Reactions to Short-Term Injury

The primary reaction to these injuries is the **shock** of surprise—the shock that the injury cannot be just "walked off" or "shaken off." At the time of the injury, the athlete tries to walk it off or shake it off on the court or playing field. Athletes have probably experienced this type of injury before with no residual complaint and need time to accept that, this time, it is not immediately going away. Rehabilitation compliance is often compromised when athletes envision themselves returning in a couple of days without treatment. The sport therapist assesses the athlete's injury and explains the process of rehabilitation to the athlete.

The secondary reaction is **relief**—relief that it is not something really major, given that it couldn't be discounted as just a "nick" or "ding." The sense of relief is contingent on the athlete's trust of the sports therapist. At this point the relationship between the sports therapist and the athlete is forged and trust is established. This sets the tone for the success or failure of the rehabilitation process.

Reactions to Rehabilitation of Short-Term Injury

Once short-term injury rehabilitation begins, the primary reaction the athlete displays is **impatience**—an impatience to get started, to do something, to get on with the program as quickly as possible. During this time the athlete is often experiencing peaks and valleys in the recovery process. The athlete is accustomed to two speeds: no speed and full speed. Athletes often express the belief that they should heal faster because they are in better shape, and they are not happy to spend time in the sequential phases of rehabilitation. If it is a sprained ankle, the athlete does not react with exhilaration to the crutch phase, then the walking phase, then the walk-jog phase, then the jog-run phase, then the run phase, and then finally the full-speed activity phase. The sport therapist can reassure the athlete that the phases are necessary and that to push it could set back the rehabilitation time.

The secondary reaction is one of **optimism.** This optimism is due to the confidence and trust established between the sports therapist and the athlete. The athlete is able to believe the sports therapist's assessment that because the injury turned out to be less serious than originally thought, it stands to reason that the rehabilitation will work out as well. It is important that compliance be consistent with the sport therapist's treatment plan and that the athlete does not try to return to practice or play

too soon. This level of injury has a good track record for excellent recovery.

Intervention for Short-Term Injury

Intervention should include allowing the athlete to vent frustrations and reiterating that there is a light at the end of the tunnel. At the collegiate level, athletes have frequently had this type of injury and consider it to be part and parcel of playing the game. The athlete should be encouraged to remain involved with the team, attending practices while performing rehabilitation, attending team meetings, and interacting with teammates after hours. At this stage the sports therapist and the athlete will have to conduct some reality checks to ascertain that the concerns that come up are in the realm of the athlete's control. Losing their spot on the team, losing their speed, or losing their best shot is not within athletes' control. Doing effective rehabilitation on a consistent basis is within their control. Staying current with the team will keep them current with plays and coaching changes. Effective rehabilitation is the only way to return to their sport. Compliance is not usually a factor for short-term injuries.

Reactions to Return to Competition after Short-Term Injury

The primary reaction to returning to competition is **eagerness** and the secondary reaction is **anticipation.** At the time of return to competition, the athletes with short-term injuries are usually eager to begin to practice and play. They anticipate that they will return to their preinjury competence the first day back. By the time the sports therapist feels the athlete is ready to return, it is assumed that a level of trust has been established. The athlete and the sports therapist must agree on a realistic plan for return to activity so that the transition will be safe and satisfactory for all concerned.

DEALING WITH LONG-TERM INJURY

Long-term injuries are considered to have a rehabilitation time of more than 4 weeks and can be anywhere from 4 weeks to 6 months to a year. These injuries are the most severe and tend to be the most difficult for the athlete to handle because of the length of inactivity and the lack of rapid progress during rehabilitation. Long-term injuries include, but are not limited to, fractures, orthopedic surgery, general surgery, second- and third-degree sprains/strains, and debilitating illness.

Reaction to Long-Term Injury

The primary reaction to long-term injury is **fear**—fear that they will never get better, fear that they can never play again, fear that they cannot handle a long rehabilitation period, fear of pain, and fear of the unknown (Figure 3-4). Most athletes have heard the horror stories of the athlete who had this same injury and never came back for a multitude of reasons. They hear stories of athletes who came back but were never again as fast or as talented or as fearless . . . the list goes on. At this point the sports therapist must allay the fear with pertinent information in terms that are easy to understand. It is not helpful to overload the athlete with all the latest information on that particular injury. The rule of thumb is to present the truth in appropriate doses that the athlete can handle. Again, establishing a trusting relationship with the sports therapist is a vital component of this long-term process.

The secondary reaction to a long-term injury is **anger**—anger that the injury happened, that it happened to them, that it happened at the time it did, and so on. Anger cannot be reasoned with, and the sports medicine team must understand and not react to the athlete's anger. An angry, hostile, or surly attitude toward the personnel or program should not offend the sports therapist. Whoever happens to be around the athlete often bears the brunt of the anger. This response is merely an emotional release. With anger the athlete is usually reacting to the situation and not necessarily to the individual.

Reaction to Long-Term Rehabilitation

The primary reaction to long-term rehabilitation is twofold: *loss of vigor* and *irrational thoughts.* At this point the sports therapist needs to be aware that a loss of vigor can be masked as depression, although depression can also be a possible reaction. The athlete appears to be lacking the usual vim, vigor, and vitality but does not have the common signs and symptoms of a true depression (loss of appetite, sleep disruption, withdrawal, change in mood state, thoughts of or plans for attempting suicide, etc.). Understanding this phenomenon will enable the sports therapist to understand the athlete's change in temperament and disposition. The athlete should understand that it is reasonable to feel somewhat discouraged concerning the injury, as long there are no other presenting symptoms of clinical depression.

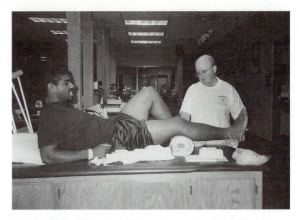

Figure 3-4 The sports therapist assists the athlete to quell the fear associated with long-term injuries.

In one study, it was found that clinical depression occurs in only 4.8 percent of the injured athletic population.[7] The possibility of attempted suicide by the clinically depressed athlete warrants the vigilance of the sports medicine team. If signs of clinical depression (loss of appetite, sleep disruption, withdrawal, change in mood state, thoughts of or plans for attempting suicide, etc.) are present, then the possibility of attempted suicide must be addressed. According to Smith and Milliner,[53] the incidence of attempted suicide is high among the age group of 15 to 24 years. In Smith and Milliner's study of five athletes who had attempted suicide, the common factors were a serious injury that required surgical intervention, rehabilitation of 6 weeks to a year while not participating in sport, diminished athletic skill upon return after successful rehabilitation, and being replaced in their position on the team. Adaptation to the physical, mental, and emotional frustration is hard work during the rehabilitative process. The work the athlete is doing is not producing the same rewards as participation in the sport; plus the athlete is becoming anxious about falling farther behind in the sport. At this point it is prudent to ask the athlete if psychological intervention is needed or desired, since not all athletes require or desire psychological intervention.

The other primary reaction to long-term rehabilitation is **irrational thoughts** (Figure 3-5). If irrational thoughts are persistent, interfere with the normal routine of daily life, and disrupt the rehabilitation process, then psychological intervention is recommended and is frequently effective. Irrational thoughts can be negative perceptions of pain, reinjury, social support, performance, and so on. These athletes might harbor thoughts of not being to return to play or not being able to return

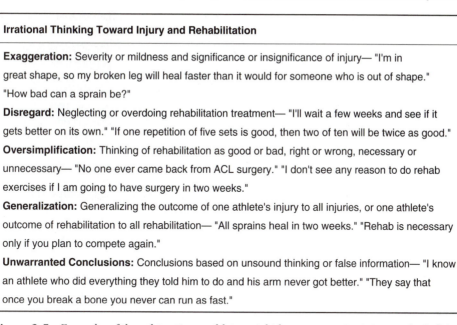

Irrational Thinking Toward Injury and Rehabilitation

Exaggeration: Severity or mildness and significance or insignificance of injury— "I'm in great shape, so my broken leg will heal faster than it would for someone who is out of shape." "How bad can a sprain be?"

Disregard: Neglecting or overdoing rehabilitation treatment— "I'll wait a few weeks and see if it gets better on its own." "If one repetition of five sets is good, then two of ten will be twice as good."

Oversimplification: Thinking of rehabilitation as good or bad, right or wrong, necessary or unnecessary— "No one ever came back from ACL surgery." "I don't see any reason to do rehab exercises if I am going to have surgery in two weeks."

Generalization: Generalizing the outcome of one athlete's injury to all injuries, or one athlete's outcome of rehabilitation to all rehabilitation— "All sprains heal in two weeks." "Rehab is necessary only if you plan to compete again."

Unwarranted Conclusions: Conclusions based on unsound thinking or false information— "I know an athlete who did everything they told him to do and his arm never got better." "They say that once you break a bone you never can run as fast."

Figure 3-5   Examples of thought patterns athletes might have concerning injury and rehabilitation.

to their previous level of play. Previously rational and positive perceptions of situations now become negative and irrational as self-destructive emotions color the thought process. Emotional reaction is exacerbated when the athlete fails to heal or return faster than the nonathlete. Frequently, athletes feel that because they are in better shape at the time of injury, they should heal faster than nonathletes who are out of shape at the time of injury. The athlete has often put in years of training and imposes pressures to heal faster and return quicker. The athlete's common sense and judgment become altered. This mood change might occur daily or weekly, so continual interaction between the sports therapist and the athlete is necessary to restore rationality and change negative thoughts.

The secondary reaction to long-term rehabilitation is a feeling of **alienation.** With an injury that requires weeks or months of rehabilitation before the athlete's return to competition, the athlete often feels that the coaches have ceased to care, teammates have no time to spend with them, friends are no longer around, and their social life consists of time put into rehabilitation. The athletes may have had little support from coaches and teammates, since the coaches are concerned with the results of the team. Injured athletes feel neglected if their daily activities have revolved around the sport and they are no longer part of the sport.

The athlete must understand that the coach cares but has no expertise in injury management and must be concerned with getting the rest of the team ready. The sports therapist has no expertise in coaching but is primarily interested in getting the athlete back to optimal fitness. Coaches work with players on playing their sport, sports therapist work with athletes on rehabilitating injuries: two different fields, two different abilities, two different areas of expertise. Some coaches, unfortunately, might also want the injured athlete kept away from other players to remove the reminder that injury is a possibility.[17]

The injured athlete may feel unable to maintain or regain normal relationships with teammates. The injured athlete is a reminder that injury can happen, and teammates might pull away from that constant reminder. Friendships based on athletic identification are now compromised, because the athletic identification is gone, and they can be related to in athletic terms only by what they did yesterday or as injured teammates and not as individuals. Injured athletes no longer have the camaraderie of the dressing room, the practice bashing, the travel to away events, and the other interactions mired in tradition that give athletes a sense of belonging, a sense of being important. When injured athletes can remain involved with the team, however, they feel less isolated and less guilty for not putting it on the line to help the team.

Intervention for Long-Term Rehabilitation

Whenever possible, anger should not be challenged, since no one can reason with anger. Instead, the sports therapist should wait until the individual is in control of the anger and then discuss the inappropriate behavior that cannot be tolerated in the rehabilitation setting. Then the sports therapist and the athlete can work out the cause of the anger and together arrive at a solution. The sports therapist must act as an emotional blotter and, if possible, not further aggravate the situation by attempting to exert power to calm down the athlete. It is as important to listen to what the athlete is feeling in addition to what the athlete is saying. At this point the athlete has a need to vent the anger, and the sports therapist must simply listen to the athlete's reaction.

At this time active listening by the sports therapist is a move toward developing a supportive and trusting relationship with the athlete. Having a trusting relationship between the athlete and the sports therapist can make all the difference in getting the athlete into the proper frame of mind for successful completion of the rehabilitation process.

One of the more difficult aspects of adjusting to injury is stopping negative thoughts, which are devastating to a successful rehabilitation process. These thoughts have to be recognized by the athlete and then controlled. Controlling inner thoughts determines future behavior. This process is one of awareness, education, and encouragement for ultimate positive change.

Negative thoughts have a detrimental effect on both mental and physical performance.[49] It is helpful to keep a daily record of when these thoughts take place, as well as the correlated physical progress and the time and circumstances in which they occur. Then athletes are helped to stop these negative thoughts and instill a positive regimen. This step is followed by an evaluation of the whole negative thought-stopping program on a regular basis. In this manner, athletes have the practice and feedback to begin their own positive outlook in terms of constructive thoughts, concentration, cues, images, and calming responses to change inappropriate attitudes. This positive outlook, plus seeing physical progress, can help athletes return more quickly to competition with better abilities to perform. The reinforcement of sayings such as "You will get better" and "This too will pass" aid in the blockage of the negative thoughts. Negative thoughts block the athlete's road to recovery by increasing pain, anxiety, and anger. Athletes should be encouraged to put their efforts into recovery rather than into the downward spiral of self-pity. Thoughts create emotions, therefore these negative thoughts have to be recognized and dealt with for a more rapid recovery. The athlete should never be allowed to say "I can't" but rather substitute "I'll try."

The technique of restructuring perceptions helps the athlete become aware of these destructive, self-defeating behaviors. The athlete, however, might fall into the mode of "I can't do it, I'll never get well." This irrational thinking produces anxiety, fear, and possibly depression, which are detrimental to progress in rehabilitation. The athlete might be illogical, distort perceptions of events, or reach unrealistic decisions and conclusions. The athlete has replaced the old set of worries about simply playing well and helping the team win with the set of "Woe is me," with its resultant anxiety. Obviously, these thought patterns are detrimental to the positive attitude necessary in the rehabilitation process.

The sports therapist must recognize and challenge irrational thinking. Examination of these thoughts with athletes reassures them that it is normal to feel unhappy, frustrated, angry, or insecure, but that the injury is not hopeless, they do not lack courage, and all is not lost and life is not over. The athlete should be challenged to replace irrational thoughts with positive and rational ones. In short, the injury is aggravating and unfortunate, but it can be handled and overcome. The injury is placed in perspective and viewed in the same way as the athlete would consider preparation for the next athletic contest. The athlete must identify faulty thinking, gain understanding of it, and actively work for its change. Research[63] indicates that the self-thoughts, images, and attitudes during the recovery period impact the length and quality of the rehabilitation.

Lost social support can be replaced by organizing support groups or similar injury groups or mentoring by athletes who have completed rehabilitation successfully.[20] A supporting relationship between the athlete and the sports therapist can be the mainstay in attainment of successful rehabilitation (Figure 3-6). Establishing this relationship may be difficult for athletes who have been catered to when healthy and are now in a reversed role. At this time athletes question many aspects of the rehabilitation procedure. They question the doctor's diagnosis, the sports therapist for working them possibly too much, and the coach for not paying attention to them. They question whether they are thought of as malingerers. They question whether the rehabilitation personnel know how important competition is to them.

Toward the end of rehabilitation, the athlete should begin sport-specific drills during practice time with the team. The athlete then begins to re-enter the team culture and is not isolated from the team environment. Thus more effort is put into functional sport-specific situations that are generally less boring to the athlete. In so doing, the athlete gains a more realistic appreciation of the skills

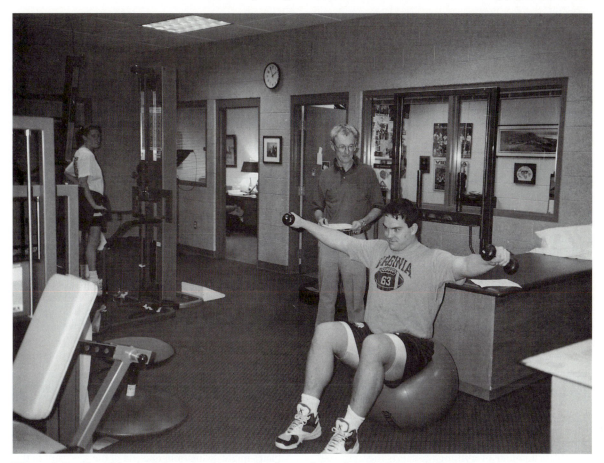

Figure 3-6   The athlete and the sports therapist develop a relationship of respect and trust.

needed to attain preinjury performance levels. The rehabilitation routine is more easily tolerated by athletes if they can see some carryover to their particular sport.

After injury, athletes need the support of teammates. To prevent possible feelings of negative self-worth and problems of loss of identity for athletes, their support groups need to stress that they are interested in the athlete as a person as well as a team member. If the rehabilitation personnel have established prior personal contact with the athlete as a worthwhile person, this transition can be easier.

Reaction to Return to Competition for Long-Term Injury

The primary reaction to return to competition from a long-term injury is an **acknowledgment** that the rehabilitation process is completed. This is a feeling of "I have done my best and all that I can do in the area of rehabili-

tation." The athlete might go down a checklist of performance abilities. The team physician who has the final vote on medically clearing an athlete to return to competition has given the OK to return. The sports therapist has set functional criteria to be followed before returning to play. The sports therapist and the athlete have discussed the use of additional padding, the wearing of a brace, or other equipment adjustments to minimize reinjury. The physician, the sports therapist, the sports psychologist, and the coach have determined that the athlete is ready to play at 100 percent, the athlete fits back into the chemistry of the current lineup, the athlete is knowledgeable about recent changes in coaching strategy, and the athlete feels psychologically ready. The athlete and the sports medicine team have discussed feelings of confidence about returning, willingness to play with pain or soreness, and willingness to risk reinjury or permanent damage. The athlete has gained the emotional self-control to think rationally about the injury and cope successfully with the return to competition. It is now up to the athlete to make the decision to return to play.

After going through the checklist of concerns that the athlete feels are important, the secondary reaction is **trust**—trust that everything has been done to be as prepared as possible to return to play. Trust at this time is trust that everything has been done, not that the injury is healed—this won't come until it has been tested and proven. When the athlete has been cleared to return, everything has been completed that is within the athlete's control. It is now time to "put it to the test—to step up to the plate and give it a shot." Acceptance that the rehabilitation process is successful will not come until the athlete makes the first move, takes the first hit or runs the first race. Then, and only then, will the athlete play with the freedom and confidence she or he had prior to the injury.

DEALING WITH CHRONIC INJURY

Chronic injury can be defined as an injury having a slow, insidious onset, most often starting with pain and/or signs of inflammation that might last for months or years and giving the impression of recurring over time.[1] These injuries are usually overuse injuries and can include tendinitis, stress fractures (shin splints), compartment syndrome, and other second- or third-degree injuries.

Reaction to Chronic Injury

The primary reaction to a chronic injury is **anger.** Often the athlete has done everything the sports therapist suggested as far as rehabilitation and even maintenance rehabilitation, and still the injury recurred. The athlete desperately wants to return to previous form and remembers that rehabilitation is going to be another long, drawn-out process. The sports therapist often has to explain over and over that setbacks occur even without provocation. Such repetition is necessary because an angry athlete has selective hearing and a short attention span. It might take several meetings for the athlete to cool down enough to hear what is being said. Because many chronic injuries are overuse injuries, rest and inactivity are frequently the treatment of choice. Athletes often describe this inactivity during injury as being harder than playing. When they are playing, all their energy is directed toward the goal of running, throwing, jumping, or whatever other activity is part of their sport. When they are doing rehabilitation for a chronic injury, most physical activity screeches to a halt.

Inactivity leads to **frustration,** the secondary reaction to chronic injury. The fact that many of these injuries are overuse injuries increases the frustration brought on by a sense of somehow having caused the recurrence or at least done something to increase the chance of it. "If I hadn't run the extra mile." "If I hadn't played the second set." If the athlete has used sport as a buffer to control stress, that outlet is gone for the time being. Stress then accelerates. Often these athletes are used to being very active and the forced inactivity is frustrating. These athletes are well acquainted with the rehabilitation process to come, the emotional ups and downs, the time commitment, the expense, and the hard work that goes into successful rehabilitation. The thoughts of going through the process again with no real expectation of a permanent solution is indeed frustrating.

Reaction to Rehabilitation of Chronic Injury

The primary reactions to rehabilitation of a chronic injury are **dependence** and **independence.** These reactions are manifested by athletes' reacting to the rehabilitation process as if they have no control or as if they have complete control. The stance in either reactive or proactive and is seen in the athlete's either not taking control or responsibility for getting better or assuming total control over the rehabilitation process.

There is very little middle ground for these athletes in the treatment protocol: they either try everything new or they are unwilling to try anything new. They either question every treatment the sports therapist recommends or accept every treatment the sports therapist recommends. Athletes might swing from one end of the spectrum to the other, depending on factors such as how well the last rehabilitation worked, how fast the last rehabilitation moved, how well they liked the last sports therapist, where they are in their season, and any other situation they perceived as warranting a change.

Dependent athletes don't take part in the decisions of rehabilitation, they don't give their input concerning what worked before or what didn't, and they often leave all decisions up to the sports therapist or team physician. Often these athletes become dependent on the sports therapist and relinquish all power regarding rehabilitation decisions. These athletes want someone else to be responsible for their welfare and to meet their every need at their whim and command. They demand that more time be spent on them. Failure of one staff member to meet their demands results in their selecting a staff member who will meet their demands. Staff members with the greatest need to help others will be easily taken advantage of, at the sacrifice of time needed for other athletes.

The independent reaction is just the opposite. These athletes want to call all the shots and are up-to-date on the latest fads. They are likely to change the treatment plan—or the therapist—if progress is not as fast or as productive as they expect or want. They have a strong urge to find the perfect treatment by trying new techniques, changing physicians and therapists, or shopping around for any solution that might work better and faster. The sports therapist must not take this personally. It is important to accept that shopping around is not a rejection of the therapist but a reaction to the chronic injury rehabilitation.

The secondary reaction to chronic injury rehabilitation is **apprehension.** Athletes with chronic injuries know that although they might get through this flareup, there is a strong possibility that the injury will return, for in fact it never completely heals. They approach rehabilitation with trepidation, not knowing what will work this time and what will last. They tend to feel stress over every sign and symptom that the rehabilitation is not going as well or as rapidly as expected. Dependent athletes react to this apprehension by being overcompliant, thinking that they just need to work harder at what the sports therapist suggests. Independent athletes, reacting to apprehension, tend to make more changes if rehabilitation is not going well—trying new and different things, looking for the perfect treatment.

Interventions for Chronic Injury

If athletes become dependent and they no longer receive the special attention they feel they deserve, they often lash out in anger or frustration. The sports therapist needs to head off this response by firmly explaining the restrictions on time and what is required of the athlete in terms of rehabilitation. This response should be pointed out to the athlete as inappropriate, and it should be examined by the sports therapist and the athlete if it becomes a continual problem, because it is only a detriment to recovery. At this time the athlete is encouraged to transfer the time and energy formerly given to the sport into the rehabilitation process. The athlete has to become an active, not a passive, participant. The injury is now the competitor, rather than next week's opponent. Care should be taken to prevent the athlete from becoming a dependent patient.

In order to be more proactive rather than reactive, the dependent athlete is encouraged to take part in the rehabilitation. This does not mean that the athlete assumes the role of the sports therapist, but it does mean that they work as a team. This is where the trust and respect between the sports therapist and the athlete is of paramount importance. It is a two-way street where the sports therapist provides the expertise concerning the injury and the athlete has the expertise concerning his or her body.

The independent athlete is encouraged to develop a relationship with the sports therapist that is one of respect and trust. At this point the sports therapist can facilitate this trust by being current with the latest literature on the athlete's particular injury. Knowledge of the injury, its healing mechanism, and the rehabilitation progression gives athletes an orderly timetable within which to proceed. It will help if the sports therapist and the athlete have a plan that is mutually acceptable. The sports therapist can make an effort to be particularly flexible when working with these athletes; thus will go a long way in strengthening the relationship of trust and respect so necessary to a smooth rehabilitation.

All athletes are participants in the rehabilitation process, but they must be active participants and become engaged in the process. Athletes have to be encouraged and believe in future success. All efforts should point toward a positive result, with the athletes working with what is available and not with wishful thinking.

Reaction to Chronic Injury Recovery

Recovery from chronic injury is in some ways a misnomer, because the very nature of the injury assumes it will recur if the athlete continues to play. The single level reaction is twofold—either skeptical or confident.

The *skeptical* reaction is not necessarily a negative reaction but one born of multiple experiences with rehabilitation. Skeptical athletes are realistic in their options and have usually made peace with the nature of a chronic injury. This is not to say defeat is accepted but that reality is acknowledged. They have not given up hope, but the hope is tempered with acceptance of factors that they have no power to control. These athletes rehabilitate to the best of their ability but accept that some things are not within their control.

The *confident* reaction to recovery from chronic injury is not necessarily an unrealistic or unenlightened reaction regarding the course of this injury. These athletes have an unyielding faith that is untarnished by repeated experiences with recurrence of a chronic injury. Often confidence is more global for these athletes and is not necessarily an injury-specific reaction. This may be a personality trait and is not tied into the injury or lack of participation in their sport. Identity for these athletes is not contingent upon sport. This does not mean these athletes do not care, but just that they do not allow the injury to design and mandate their disposition or to define and outline their life.

It is unclear whether one reaction comes before the other. It can be assumed that athletes are not relegated to one or the other reaction but can move between the two.

The mitigating factors for moving between the two could be maturity, experience with rehabilitation, length of time playing a sport, the particular time in the season, or the meaning of the sport to the athlete.

DEALING WITH A CAREER-ENDING INJURY

One of the hardest adjustments an athlete has to make is when to end participation in a sport. It does appear to matter if this is an abrupt ending (injury, illness, cut from team) or one with some advance warning (retirement, age, ability).[17] For the athlete whose career ends unexpectedly, there is a feeling of not being able to complete goals due to unexpected termination.[62] The athletes who ended careers voluntarily, who chose the time to leave, and who had played the sport longer had a smoother transition.

Injuries that fall into this category include spinal cord injuries, extensive hardware implants (screws, plates, etc.), multiple surgeries with declining benefits, and persistent debilitating or incapacitating illness.

Reaction to a Career-Ending Injury

Isolation is the primary reaction to termination of sport and is dependent upon the athlete's perception of the importance of participation. Many athletes have spent years as part of a team that has offered a well-defined and meaningful activity. The very nature of sport is one of exact boundaries (rules of play, precise beginnings and endings, codes of conduct, etc.), and the athletes in turn have defined roles within these boundaries (position played, rankings, roles within the team structure, etc.). At the time of termination, the disruption of a significant attachment affiliation, coupled with a large time commitment and expansion of injury, all set these athletes up for the debilitating effects of depression.[17]

The secondary reaction is that these athletes must go through a process of **grief**—grieving for a loss of not only a career, but an identity, an extended family, a place in society where they know the rules and can play the game. Sport for the athlete is a community, where they are productive members, where they excel, where they feel accepted, and where they feel they belong. These athletes grieve for what they no longer have: their place in the group, their place in society, their identity as an athlete, their job or career, their place of comfort, their sense of belonging.

The grief process is an adjustment period, and the form it takes and how long it lasts depend on the indi-

vidual's personality and the importance the sport had in forming that personality. There are many theories of the process of grief. A good review can be found in Baillie and Danish[3] or Evans and Hardy.[18] The grief process is a sequential progression: The grief process must take place before acceptance, the acceptance process must take place before career change, the career change attempts to fill the void created after the end of the dream of competition.

Reaction to Rehabilitation for a Career-Ending Injury

Loss of athletic identity is the primary reaction to rehabilitation of an injury that terminates participation in a sport. It is a feeling of "Who am I? Where do I belong? What is my purpose, my reason for being?" The rehabilitation involves the psychological adjustment to the loss of self. Baillie and Danish[3] suggest that athletes have taken anywhere from 2 to 10 years to adjust to termination from sport.

The athlete enters physical rehabilitation halfheartedly, if at all. The athlete often says, "Who cares?" "What does it matter?" "Who will know?" in response to setting a rehabilitation plan. These athletes might go through the motions of rehabilitation, but the inner spark to get back to competition is missing. At this point the sports therapist must decide whether the athlete needs to be referred to a counselor or sports psychologist. The criterion for referral is usually an established protocol and consists of a determination of whether the athlete is able to maintain a sense of control and an engagement in activities while emotionally working through the grief process.

Intervention in a Career-Ending Injury

Interventions for career-ending injuries are decided on an individual basis. Intervention can have the nature of psychological counseling (stress management, alcohol or drug counseling, etc.), career counseling (school enrollment, job placement etc.), financial planning (investments, tax shelters, etc.), or whatever the athlete needs. Adjustment to termination is better for athletes who had participated longer, were aware of chronic injuries, knew of the possibility of being cut, or had planned on retiring from the team. Poor adjustment is associated with sudden unexpected injury that occurs in the prime of the career and results in a forced retirement.[3]

Reaction to Recovery
from a Career-Ending Injury

The primary reaction to recovery from a terminating injury is to see it as both an ending and beginning. **Closure** and **renewal** are intertwined, with closure being necessary to give full energy to renewal. Once they reach the acceptance stage, these athletes can put closure on a career that has ended and focus their other talents, long overshadowed by athletic prowess, toward a new career. This might be either in the field of athletics (coaching, announcer, sponsor, etc.) or in a totally unrelated field. Baillie and Danish[3] found that Olympic athletes and college athletes were better prepared and made a better adjustment to new careers than did older professional athletes. The reason for this might be better education, more choices of careers, more assistance in career planning—in other words, more options. Many athletes make a satisfactory adjustment to termination from sport when it is in their time frame and of their choosing, but termination forced by an unexpected event such as injury is received with less than enthusiasm.

COMPLIANCE AND ADHERENCE
TO REHABILITATION

Compliance to athletic injury rehabilitation programs is abysmal, considering the purpose of rehabilitation.[19,25,51] The goal of athletic rehabilitation is to return the athlete to the level of performance present prior to injury. The primary treatment is exercise to retrain the muscles that have been damaged due to injury. The psychological ramification of unsuccessful rehabilitation is that the athlete tends to focus on the injury, resulting in guarding or muscle tension and/or lack of attentional focus, setting up the scenario for reinjury. In what follows, we discuss, first, definitions of compliance and adherence; second, incidents of compliance in other fields; third, measures of compliance; fourth, deterrents to compliance; and fifth, incentives to increase compliance.

Compliance and Adherence Defined

According to Miechenbaum and Turk,[40] *compliance* is a term from the medical profession and means obedience of the patient to the physician's or health caregiver's instruction. The concept of compliance is more passive than active, and carries the connotation that if patients are noncompliant, they are at fault. This assigns an authoritative position to the caregiver. The implication is: "I tell you what to do, and you do it." The concept of compliance mainly applies to immediate short-term treatment that has been prescribed for a patient. *Adherence* is a term from the exercise discipline and carries the meaning of active voluntary choice, a mutuality in treatment planning. Adherence involves long-term change on a more voluntary basis and suggests a behavioral change sought by the participant. Usually when *adherence* is the term used, it carries the implication that the service was sought out as opposed to being prescribed—for instance, when people seek an exercise program or a weight-loss program, instead of being ordered by the physician to enroll in one. These are usually long-term commitments.

For the purpose of this discussion about rehabilitation, the term *compliance* will be used, but either is acceptable. The term *compliance* has been chosen because there are certain guidelines for treatments that produce the desired result of rehabilitation of an injury. The athlete needs to comply with a certain regimen for the short-term to facilitate healing, then adhere to a program of exercise to decrease the risk of reinjury. In rehabilitation, a *comply now—adhere later* approach is the best descriptor for successful return to the previous level of fitness.

Incidences of Compliance
in Other Disciplines

In the field of athletic injury, compliance is the biggest deterrent to successful rehabilitation.[51] The fields of medicine and exercise fare no better. In medicine, compliance is roughly 50 percent, with the rule of thumb being that one-third always comply, one-third sometimes comply, and one-third never comply.[40] In a study of glaucoma (high intraocular fluid pressure), patients were told that if they didn't use drops 3 times a day, they would go blind. Only 42 percent complied with treatment recommended by the physician. Several weeks later at revisit, they were told they were in danger of losing sight in one eye if they did not comply with treatment. Compliance only increased by 16 percent, according to Vincent.[59] In other words, only 58 percent were compliant when the likely result of being noncompliant was to go blind in one eye!

The exercise literature[15] shows similar findings: There is a 30 to 70 percent dropout rate in the first 3 months of exercise programs. Sixty-six percent of Americans do not exercise on a regular basis; 44 percent do not exercise at all.[15] Self-improvement programs do not fare any better. The dropout rate for obesity, smoking, and stress management programs is 20 to 80 percent. Only 16 to 59 percent of people wear seat belts. There is limited literature on the compliance rate for athletes. Before all hope is lost, it should be understood that maybe

100 percent compliance is not necessary to achieve total rehabilitation. In medicine it was found that less than 100 percent compliance was adequate to bring about desired results.[40] It is important to keep in mind that we are looking at a range, not an absolute. Is the athlete who gets back to preinjury standards without doing 100 percent of treatments noncompliant? They are only if 100 percent compliance is considered to be the gold standard.

Measurements of Compliance

How compliance is measured might be an indicator of the problem. In medicine and exercise, compliance is usually measured in one of three ways: self-report, attendance, and therapeutic outcome.[40] Self-report consists of just asking whether the person has been compliant, through either a structured questionnaire, self-monitoring with record keeping, or corroboration (someone else keeps track). These methods can be inaccurate due to poor memory, trying to please the investigator, or channeling the behavior to please the investigator. Keeping track of attendance is the most common and most direct method. The problem with attendance is that it doesn't say what was done, it just indicates that the athletes showed up. The athletes could be doing exercises somewhere else, or forget to sign in, or sign in and then leave without exercising, or do only a portion of the prescribed rehabilitation exercises. Therapeutic outcome is not completely reliable, as it can be confounded by other factors. In a weight-loss program the athlete could be gaining muscle weight but losing fat weight, could lose weight due to exercising but not due to recommended changes in eating habits, or could lose weight because of illness without exercising or change in eating habits.

In order to start at the beginning of measuring compliance, the Hedgpeth/Gansneder Athletic Rehabilitation Indicators[26] was designed to determine what treatments were used, and what percentage of the time were they used, in a Division I University. The basic areas assessed are aerobic conditioning, strength conditioning, balance, modalities, and long-term strategies (bracing, taping, protective equipment). Athletes are asked what percentage of the time the treatment was done. A range of compliance is measured, with 0–10 percent being the lowest compliance, and 91–100 percent being the highest compliance. A category of N/A was included to indicate that the sports therapist had not suggested the treatment. At the same time, sports therapists were asked to complete the indicator. Preliminary reports suggest a 87 percent reliability rate for the indicator. Until such a time as what is being done in the athletic training room setting is determined, it is premature to discuss why it is or is not being done.

Factors Influencing Compliance

Shank[52] found that athletes who are committed to the rehabilitation program work harder and thus return to competition more quickly with better results than those who are nonadherents. Their pain tolerance is greater and of less concern, and they are more self-motivated, as opposed to the apathy of the nonadherents.

Also, support from peers, coaches, and rehabilitation staff is important in influencing compliance. Athletes with support show a greater effort to fit the rehabilitation effort into their schedules. They are more likely to keep commitments to those who support them. Athletes who are nonadherents respond better to support and motivation from their support group than do the adherents. Thus extra encouragement from this support group for the nonadherent athletes can really pay dividends in getting them motivated to successfully complete their rehabilitation.

Attitude is another important consideration when dealing with injured athletes. If the sports therapist expects the athlete to be nonadherent, this can create the self-fulfilling prophecy.[61] If the sports therapist feels the athlete is going to be nonadherent, then it is less likely that the sports therapist will work to motivate the athlete to comply with the treatment program. Webborn et al.[61] suggest that if instructions are written down—even in the face of the athlete's denial of the need for written instruction—the more likely it is that the athlete will follow through with the treatment plan. Sports therapists have an impact on compliance through enhancing the athlete's belief in the efficacy of the treatment as well as providing a supportive environment[16] (Figure 3-7).

Athletes are expected to report for rehabilitation, but the coach is the disciplinarian, not the sports therapist, and the coach institutes punishment for lack of participation in the rehabilitation process. The coach must support the rehabilitation concept. Athletes soon know that rehabilitation is not a priority with the coach and begin to lose interest if they are not highly motivated to return to competition.

The real challenge of rehabilitation is how to motivate athletes to do their best in the rehabilitation process. Athletes who are not reporting for rehabilitation have a reason. Everything is done for some need. The rehabilitation program must be established within these needs. If athletes are not reporting for rehabilitation, either something is more important to them than a hastened recovery, or they have not had the importance of the process adequately explained to them. Reexamine the program and the athlete's goals. If the program has not been well explained and the athlete is not committed to the program, the program either is doomed to failure

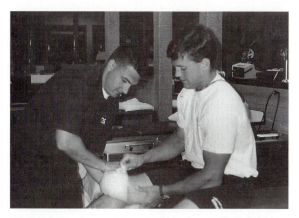

Figure 3-7   A supportive environment and a belief in the effectiveness of the treatment improves compliance.

or will be less than successful. Motivation must come from within, but the sports therapist can provide the encouragement and positive reinforcement necessary for the athlete to make a commitment.

Lack of commitment might indicate frustration, boredom, or feelings of a lack of progress. In this case, further explanations or changes in routine are necessary. The athlete might need the opportunity to comment on the program and make a commitment to the rehabilitation before being structured into a strict regimen of rehabilitative procedures.

The sports therapist should keep in mind that athletes may have many activities in their daily schedules, and fitting the rehabilitation to their schedules rather than the reverse can also encourage compliance. The more the athlete is allowed input and flexibility, the more successful the compliance will be.

Another aspect of compliance has to do with athletes' perception of their ability. Athletes who perceive themselves as continuing on to a more advanced level of competition tend to shirk rehabilitation. They usually are the better athletes. They do not have to work as hard as, but perform better than, their peers, so they assume the same attitude about rehabilitation. With this attitude, these good athletes never become truly great athletes because of their lack of commitment to their sport. Once they have risen to the top level where most athletes have the same skills, the work habit is not there to put them in the top of the elite athletic group.

Other factors of compliance for student athletes are the length of time at a particular school, semester grade-point average, perception of class load, career goals, amount of participation time in contests, perception of time available for treatments, and previous experience

with rehabilitation programs. The more formal education a person has, the higher the level of compliance to treatments; the higher the semester grade-point average, the higher the treatment compliance. Interestingly enough, an inverse relationship exists between athletes' perception of difficulty of their class load and compliance. Often athletes do better academically during the season than at other times, possibly because they budget their time with better discipline during the season, and this approach carries over into the rehabilitation setting. Athletes who have better-defined career goals and those who have the greatest amount of participation time have higher levels of compliance, as do those who perceive they have a greater amount of time available for treatments and those who have previous experience with rehabilitation programs.

PAIN AS A DETERRENT TO COMPLIANCE

Almost all rehabilitation should be pain-free, and what is not is usually detrimental to the return to competition. Painful exercise, therefore, is not only harmful but also reduces compliance, especially in the nonadherent athlete.[19] Rehabilitation programs should be examined to determine the aspects that may be painful.

Pain is subjective, and the caregivers must assume that the pain is as severe or persistent as the athlete says it is. Although the symptoms of pain must be treated to ensure compliance, the cause needs to be addressed. In general, it is more productive in the long run for the sports therapist to determine the cause of pain than to treat the symptoms and disregard the cause. For instance, if swelling is the cause of the pain, then treatment to reduce the swelling is of a more lasting benefit than treating the pain and disregarding or masking the underlying cause of the pain. Pain that persists and does not respond to adjustments in the rehabilitation process (e.g., decreases in the amount of weights, number of sets, or number of repetitions) should be reevaluated by a sports therapist or team physician.

Athletes often say "You can play hurt, you can't play injured." But the difference is in what pain means to the athlete. There is the pain of performance, the pain of training, the pain of rehabilitation, the pain of acute injury, and the chronic pain of overuse. Pain can be assessed across intensity (0 = none to 10 = worst) and quality (burning, aching, stabbing, stinging, etc.), but pain is subjective. Factors affecting pain can be culture,[65] type (contact verses noncontact) of sport,[33] and individual verses team sport.[37]

One technique for pain management that is frequently used and easy to apply is disassociation.[10,57] Disassociation involves thinking about something other than the pain, such as a favorite location, a mountain cabin with the smell of fresh crisp air and the magnificent view of mountains, or a beach cottage with the feel and smell of the salty breeze and the calming rhythmic sound of the surf. Another tactic is one Norman Cousins[10] used to distract his thoughts from intractable pain from cancer as well as to prolong the action of pain medication. He watched funny, vintage, slapstick movies such as Laurel and Hardy, the Three Stooges, and Abbott and Costello. Any activity that engages the mind can be used. The athlete could visualize playing a round of golf from tee to green, playing a football game from kickoff to the final whistle, or playing a final NCAA basketball game from tip-off until the buzzer.

Goal Setting as a Motivator to Compliance

Goal setting in and of itself has been shown to be an effective motivator for compliance to rehabilitation of an athletic injury[13,22] as well as reaching goals in a general sport setting.[9,36] Athletes have been setting goals since they started competing, usually from an early age. They set goals to run faster, jump higher, shoot straighter, throw longer, hit harder, and so on. These goals have all had one thing in common, and that is that they were not achieved with one burst of effort but came as the result of many short-term goals having been met prior to the achievement of the long-term goal. For a comprehensive explanation on goal setting in general, see Locke,[35] or for goal setting specifically in sport, see Locke and Lathman.[36] Heil[27] suggests nine guides for goal setting: It should be specific and measurable; use positive rather than negative language; be challenging but realistic; have a timetable; integrate short-, medium-, and long-term goals; link outcome to process; involve internalized goals; involve monitoring and evaluating goals and sport goals linked to life goals.

In athletic rehabilitation, athletes need to know exactly what the goal is and have a sense that it can be met. This could be accomplished by, for instance, telling an athlete that by a certain day the athlete should be partial weight bearing with crutches. However, this is neither specific or measurable. It is more effective to say that by achieving a certain range of motion and strength level, the foot can be placed on the ground with weight bearing. The measurement of success is that the partial weight bearing is to be without pain. The goal must be a challenge, but one that the athlete can reach with rea-sonable rehabilitation effort. Goals that are easily reached have no reward in success. Goals must be personal and internally satisfying, not imposed on the athlete by the coach or sports therapist. The setting of goals needs to be a joint venture between the athlete and the sports therapist to be successful.[14] The athlete has to take responsibility for the progress of the injury and be responsible for doing the necessary rehabilitation.

Goal setting incorporates a multitude of other motivating factors that intuitively appear to up the odds of compliance by reducing the stress associated with injury rehabilitation. These buffers incorporated within the goal-setting paradigm include: positive reinforcement when goals are met, time management for incorporating goals into a lifestyle, a feeling of social support when goals are set with the sports therapist, the feelings of increased self-efficacy when goals are achieved, etc. Goals should be easily understood by athletes, be concrete, be active events, and be a natural part of their sport that requires no additional time commitment.[8] Goals can be daily for a sense of accomplishment, weekly for a sense of progress, and monthly or yearly for long-term achievement.

RETURN TO COMPETITION

The saying "You have to play with pain" has been interpreted more literally to mean that the athlete has to play through an injury. The difference is that some injuries may be mild and only somewhat painful, resulting in no reinjury in competition, whereas a more severe injury is made worse by continuing to compete. The competitive athlete might be more "body aware" than the general public and therefore more apt to respond to injury with the use of rest, ice, compression, and elevation (RICE) in order to promote healing. The general public, on the other hand, is more likely to respond to the pain of injury rather than the healing process.[44] Therefore the athlete might want to return to competition in spite of pain, whereas the nonathlete wants the pain to be treated before engaging in any activity. The importance of a certified sports therapist for making the decision of when it is safe to compete and when reinjury is a possibility is obvious.

Unfortunately, untrained personnel, such as fellow teammates, parents, and coaches, assume this responsibility when no sports therapist is present or when the sports therapist is easily intimidated by the coach and not backed up by the athletic director. Either situation results in poor medical care and leaves the management vulnerable to legal action as a result of negligence. Courts expect competent medical care to be provided to the athletes (Figure 3-8). That care can be provided only by a qualified sports therapist or a physician.

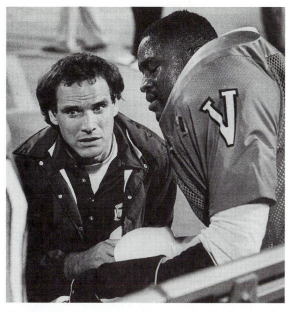

Figure 3-8 Courts expect competent medical care to be provided to athletes by a certified athletic trainer or physician.

Flint and Weiss[21] found that coaches returned players on the basis of status and game situation, whereas sports therapists' decisions were determined by the player's injury. Players who feel that a missed practice or a game will relegate them to the bench for the year, or those who have been encouraged to play no matter what, are candidates for injury and reinjury. Usually what happens, however, is that they are performing poorly because they are not at full strength, thus they only reinforce the coach's decision to play someone else. The role of the sports therapist is to determine when the player is functioning at optimal physical fitness without risk of injury or reinjury and to keep the coach abreast of the player's status. It is important that the athlete have a clear perception of the injury and its limitations.[11] An important role of the sports therapist is to inform the athlete of the difference between pain and injury.

The athlete who continues to play with an unhealed or poorly rehabilitated injury is constantly reducing her or his chances for a healthy life of physical activity. The athlete has to live past the few years of competition. Most athletes, however, have difficulty seeing past the present season, or at best have the goal of participating in their sport until they can no longer compete, regardless of the consequences. The rewards of competition and the admiration of others take sports out of perspective and retard a healthy attitude toward sports. The athlete's attitude is

"Give it up for the sport" and "I'm invincible." Lack of this attitude is viewed by some as weakness or not being a team player. Athletes with this attitude have difficulty adjusting to injury, especially a career-ending one.

Neglecting injured athletes or giving them the perception that they are "outcasts" also can contribute to injury and reinjury. Coaches who foster this attitude are saying to the players that they have no worth if they are injured. Some coaches go so far as to prevent team contact with injured players until they are ready to return, or to belittle them in front of their peers, believing that this will make the athlete want to get back to competition quicker. This tactic might work with some players with minor injuries, but it only causes major adjustment difficulties for athletes who suffer severe injury.

Some coaches refuse to talk to the injured athlete, or tell others that the athlete really doesn't want to play or isn't tough enough. The coach and athlete are experiencing frustration with the injury. Counseling the coach in this situation to point out the effects of such attitudes may be helpful. Unfortunately, these coaches are not in the minority. During this period, either the athletic staff shows its concern for the athlete and in return wins the athlete's loyalty and dedication down the road, or they undermine the athlete's trust and set up a future situation to be let down when the athlete gets in the position of controlling the outcome of a contest—the athlete might underperform out of spite. Commitment is a two-way street. The sports therapy staff has to show their commitment to the athlete to receive commitment from the athlete. By the same token the sports therapist must not become the power broker and in essence say "He can't play because I say so." Showing the coach that the athlete who usually has 4.5 speed can presently run only a 5.0 illustrates to the coach that the athlete is not ready for competition. It will also illustrate to the athlete that more time and effort are necessary to get ready to return.

INTERPERSONAL RELATIONSHIP BETWEEN ATHLETE AND SPORTS THERAPIST

The sports therapist is often the first person athletes interact with after injury and the one who will direct the recovery. As a result, the sports therapist has to deal with the athlete as a person and not as just an injury. When athletes enter the treatment setting, they should get the perception that the sports therapist cares for the athlete as a person and not just as part of the job. Their perception of the sports therapist makes a difference in terms of recovery time and effort. First they have to respect the

Type of therapist	Knowledgeable	Convincing	Sincerely concerned
Great sports therapist	X	X	X
Good sports therapist	X	X	O
Fair sports therapist	X	O	O
Quack	O	X	O
Bad sports therapist	O	O	O

Figure 3-9   The effectiveness of sports therapists is based on three factors.

sports therapist as a person before they can trust the sports therapist in the rehabilitative setting. Successful communication between the sports therapist and the athlete is essential for effective rehabilitation. Taking an interest in athletes before injuries have occurred enables the sports therapist to know the athletes' personalities and be able to work with them in helping to build their confidence.

Active listening is one of the sports therapist's most important skills. One must learn to listen to the athlete beyond the complaining. The sports therapist should listen for fear, anger, depression, or anxiety in the athlete and his or her voice. With fear, the athlete might be wondering what the pain means in terms of function and whether she or he will be accepted by peers. Anger is often a feeling of being victimized by the injury and the unfairness of it. A depressed athlete will have an overwhelming feeling of hopelessness or loneliness. Athletes who feel anxiety wonder how they can survive the injury and what will happen if they cannot return to full competition.[46]

Body language is important as well. The sports therapist who continues to work on paperwork while talking to the athlete is sending a message of noncaring. The therapist needs to be concerned, and look athletes in the eye with a genuine interest in their problems. This will go a long way toward gaining confidence and respect.

It is important for the sports therapist to consider the athlete as an individual instead of the "sprained ankle." If the injury is the only consideration, the athlete becomes just an injury and not a person. As a result the attitude projected to the athlete is just that, thus the sports therapist is perceived as caring for the athlete only superficially (Figure 3-9).

The relationship between the sports therapist and the athlete should be one of person to person and not of a coach to a player or one of a judgmental nature. When the athlete is treated as an equal, the relationship is improved, and it helps the athlete accept responsibility for his or her own rehabilitation. With injury athletes lose control over their physical efforts. They have gone from 4 or 5 hours a day of practice or competition to no activity. They are in a temporary lifestyle change. Their feelings are going to affect the success or failure of the rehabilitation process. The sports therapist must establish rapport and a sense of genuine concern and caring for the athlete, who is not fooled by superficiality.

During an injury evaluation, the sports therapist should allow the athlete to provide as much input about her or his injury as possible. Paraphrasing or restating the information to the athlete will be invaluable to the sports therapist who is unsure of the mechanism of injury or its results. Statements such as "I see" or "Go ahead" or simple silence to allow athletes to fully express themselves are of value. One of the most important bits of information can be the question posed at the end of gathering subjective information: "What else have I not asked you or do I need to know about this injury?" Then give the athlete input into the decision of where to go from here.

The sports therapist is often the person who effectively explains the injury to the athlete. Care should be taken to explain the situation to the athlete in understandable terms. In most cases the simplest explanation acceptable to the athlete is the best. With mild and moderate injuries, the use of the term *sprain, strain,* or *bruise* suffices. The example of a sprained knee and torn ligaments of the knee can be descriptions of the same grade II injury, but the athlete might interpret the two terms altogether differently and react in a totally different way to the explanation.

Athletes must have injuries explained to them to their satisfaction. Disseminating injury information appropriate to athlete's emotional and intellectual level can be a real challenge. The rate and degree of acceptance is not the same with all athletes. Severity of injury is certainly important, but the athlete's perception of that severity is what matters in the rehabilitation process.[11] Thus the physiological must be interrelated with the psychological. In working with athletes, the sports therapist should be not only empathetic but also nonjudgmental.

The addition of a sport psychologist to the rehabilitation team can facilitate the athlete's transition from the sport culture into the rehabilitation culture. Each culture has specific rules as well as defined roles that the members of that culture must follow. An understanding of the different rules and roles can assist the athlete's transition after the injury from the sport culture to the rehabilitation culture. The role of the sports psychologist is to understand the impact this transition has on the athlete who is injured and has to assimilate into a totally new environment, follow new rules, and assume a new role. For example, the concept of pain in the football culture is entirely different from the concept of pain in the rehabilitation culture. In the football culture, "Suck it up" and "Play through the pain" are the norm. In the rehabilitation culture, pain can be an indication that needs to be evaluated. The athlete and sports therapist need to reevaluate the rehabilitation exercises or activity level, decrease the amount of repetitions, change the type of exercise, or to consult with the team physician. If the pain is something the athlete must assimilate into his or her lifestyle, then the sports psychologist can teach the athlete how to deal with it. This can be done through pain management (dissociation) or pain perceptions (pain versus soreness).

The amount of stress associated with playing a sport, and the meaning the sport has to the athlete, can impact the athlete's compliance with rehabilitation.[2] The athlete has a more successful rehabilitation when engaged fully in the activity of rehabilitation, much as the athlete will have a more successful sport career when more interested and involved in the sport. Stress can be a deterrent to engaging in rehabilitation. Several techniques the sport psychologist can use (relaxation, imagery, cognitive restructuring, thought stopping) can lessen the stressful reaction to injury. Often a change in the athlete's perception of the injury and rehabilitation can affect outcome. Systematic rationalization[56] can facilitate changing the athlete's reaction to injury and rehabilitation through changing how the athlete perceives events.

Returning to competition is another area where the sports psychologist can help the athlete. Often athletes perceive themselves as ready to return but not being allowed to, or as being forced to return before ready. The sports psychologist can assist the athlete to make a decision based on the facts and not clouded by emotions.

The addition of a sports psychologist to the sports medicine team can be an effective link when athletes are unable or unwilling to continue to participate in their sport. Frequently an athlete's identify is intertwined with the sport played. The transition into a completely different culture can be a traumatic experience. It is stressful to enter a culture and not know one's place or identity in that culture. To not know what the game is and what the rules are is frustrating for the injured athlete.

The treatment of athletic injury and rehabilitation involves more than the physical, emotional, and psychological aspects of the individual. The impact of the environment, the support of the athletic community, and the culture in which the athlete resides at the time of injury combine to influence the course the athlete takes from injury, through rehabilitation, to return to competition. Treating the athlete's physical injury and attending to the extraneous factors influencing the injured athlete are the challenges facing the sports medicine team.

Summary

1. There are no absolutes when it comes to how an athlete will react to an injury. However, there are some guidelines for progressive reactions to injury based on length of rehabilitation. These guidelines allow the sports therapist to conceptualize individual stress reactions to injury and to implement psychological interventions to facilitate successful rehabilitation.

2. The athlete must take responsibility for rehabilitating his or her injury, but the interpersonal relationship between the athlete and the sports medicine team can promote a positive adjustment to the rehabilitation process.

3. The use of psychological techniques such as disassociation for pain management, the use of buffers for stress reduction, and goal setting for motivation can assist the athlete in taking control of and managing her or his successful rehabilitation.

4. The key to successful rehabilitation is compliance. Advances in the field of medicine have allowed injuries that 10 years ago would have ended an athlete's career to now be successfully repaired. Without compliance to the rehabilitation process, these medical advances are moot.

References

1. American Academy of Orthopaedic Surgeons. 1991. *Athletic training and sports medicine.* 2d ed. Park Ridge, IL: American Academy of Orthopaedic Surgeons.

2. Andersen, M. B., and J. M. Williams. 1988. A model of stress and athletic injury: Predictions and prevention. *J Sport Exerc Physiology* 10:294–306.

3. Baillie, P. H. F., and S. J. Danish. 1992. Understanding the career transition of athletes. *Sport Psychologist* 6:77–98.

4. Benson, H. 1976. *The relaxation response.* New York: Morrow.

5. Block, N. 1981. *Imagery.* Boston: MIT Press.

6. Bramwell, S. T., M. Masuda, N. N. Wagnor, and T. H. Holmes. 1975. Psychosocial factors in athletic injuries: Development and application of the social and athletic readjustment rating scale. *Journal of Human Stress* 1:6–20.

7. Brewer, B. W. 1994. Review and critique of models of psychological adjustment to athletic injury. *Journal of Applied Sport Psychology* 6:87–100.

8. Brewer, B. W., K. E. Jeffers, A. J. Petitpas, and J. L. VanRault. 1994. Perceptions of psychological interventions in the context of sport injury rehabilitation. *Sport Psychologist* 8:176–88.

9. Carron, A. V. 1984. *Motivation: Implications for coaching and teaching.* London, Ontario: Pear Creative.

10. Cousins, N. 1981. *Anatomy of an illness as perceived by the patient: Reflections on healing and regeneration.* New York: Bantam.

11. Crossman, J., and J. Jamieson. 1985. Differences in perceptions of seriousness and disrupting effects of athletic injury as viewed by athletes and their trainer. *Perceptual and Motor Skills* 61:1131–34.

12. Cryan, P. D., and W. F. Alles. 1983. The relationship between stress and college football injuries. *Journal of Sports Medicine* 23:52–58.

13. Danish, S. 1986. Psychological aspects in the care and treatment of athletic injuries. In *Sports injuries: The unthwarted epidemic,* 2d ed., edited by P. E. Vineger, and E. F. Hoerner. Boston, 1986, PSG.

14. DePalma, M. T., and B. DePalma. 1989. The use of instruction and the behavioral approach to facilitate injury rehabilitation. *Athletic Training* 24:217–19.

15. Dishman, R. K. 1982. Compliance/adherence in health related exercise. *Health Psychology* 3:237–67.

16. Duda, J. L., A. E. Smart, and M. K. Tappe. 1989. Predicators of adherence in the rehabilitation of athletic injuries: An application of personal investment theory. *J Sport Exerc Psychology* 11:367–81.

17. Ermler, K. L., and C. E. Thomas. 1990. Interventions for the alienating effects of injury. *Athletic Training* 25:269–71.

18. Evans, L., and L. Hardy. 1995. Sport injury and grief response: A review. *J Sport Exerc Psychology* 17:227–45.

19. Fisher, A. C. 1990. Adherence to sport injury rehabilitation programs. *Sports Medicine* 9:151–58.

20. Flint, F. A. 1993. Seeing helps believing: Modeling in injury rehabilitation. In *Psychological bases of sport injuries,* edited by D. Pargman. Morgantown, WV: Fitness Information Technology.

21. Flint, F. A., and M. R. Weiss. 1992. Returning injured athletes to competition: A role and ethical dilemma. *Canadian J Sport Sci* 17:34–40.

22. Fordyce, W. E. 1988. Pain and suffering: A reappraisal. *American Psychologist* 43:276–83.

23. Green, L. B. 1992. Imagery in the rehabilitation of injured athletes. *Sport Psychologist* 6:416–28.

24. Grove, D. 1987. Why do some athletes choose high risk sports? *Physician and Sports Medicine* 15:190–93.

25. Grove, J. R., R. M. L. Stewart, and S. Gordon. 1990. *Emotional reactions of athletes to knee rehabilitation.* Paper presented at the annual meeting of Australian Sports Medicine Federation (abstract).

26. Hedgpeth, E. G. *Hedgpeth/Gansneder Athletic Rehabilitation Indicator* (unpublished).

27. Heil, J. 1993. *Psychology of sport injury.* Champaign, IL: Human Kinetics.

28. Holmes, T. H., and R. H. Rahe. 1976. The social readjustment rating scale. *J Psychosom Res* 11:213.

29. Ievleva, L., and T. Orlick. 1991. Mental links to enhanced healing: An exploratory study. *Sport Psychologist* 5:25–40.

30. Jackson, D. W., H. Jarrett, D. Bailey, J. Kausek, J. Swanson, and J. Powell. 1978. Injury prediction in the young athlete: A primary report. *American Journal of Sports Medicine* 6:6–14.

31. Jacobsen, E. 1929. *Progressive relaxation.* Chicago: University of Chicago Press.

32. Jacobsen, E. 1931. Variation of specific muscles contracting during muscle imagination. *American Journal of Physiology* 96:101–2.

33. Jaremko, M. E., L. Silbert, and T. Mann. 1981. The differential ability of athletes and non-athletes to cope with two types of pain: A radical behavioral model. *Psychological Record* 31:265–75.

34. Kerr, G., and H. Minden. 1988. Psychological factors related to the occurrence of athletic injuries. *J Sport Exerc Psychology* 10:167–73.

35. Locke, E. A. 1968. Toward a theory of task motivation and incentives. *Organizational Behavior and Human Performance* 3:157–58.

36. Locke, E. A., and G. P. Latham. 1985. The application of goal setting to sport. *Journal of Sport Psychology* 7:205–22.

37. Martens, R., and D. M. Landers. 1969. Coaction effects on a muscular endurance task. *Res Q* 40:733–36.

38. McGinnis, J. 1992. The public health burden of a sedentary lifestyle. *Medicine and Science in Sports and Exercise* 24(suppl.):S196–S200.

39. McNair, D. M., M. Lorr, and L. F. Droppleman. 1971. *Profiles of mood states.* San Diego: Educational and Industrial Testing Service.

40. Meichenbaum, D., and D. C. Turk. 1987. *Facilitating treatment adherence: A practitioners guidebook.* New York: Plenum Press.

41. Michener, J. 1976. *Sports in America.* New York: Random House.

42. Morgan, W. P. 1980. Test of champions: The iceberg profile. *Psychology Today,* pp. 92, 93, 99,102,108.

43. Morgan, W. P., and M. L. Pollock. 1977. Psychological characterizations of the elite distance runner. *Annals of the New York Academy of Science* 301:382–403.

44. Norris, C. 1993. *Psychological aspects of sports injury: Diagnosis and management for physiotherapists.* London: Butterworth Heinemann.

45. Petrie, T. A. 1992. Psychosocial antecedents of athletic injury: The effects of life stress and social support on women collegiate gymnasts. *Behav Med* 18:127–38.

46. Pitt, R. 1992. *Phy Ther Forum,* 16, September.

47. Requa, R. K., L. N. DeAvilla, and J. G. Garrick. 1993. Injuries in recreational adult fitness activities. *American Journal of Sports Medicine* 21:461–67.

48. Reilly, T. 1975. *An ergonomic evaluation of occupational stress in professional football.* Unpublished doctoral thesis. Polytechnic University, Liverpool, England.

49. Rotella, R. J. 1985. Psychological care of the injured athlete. In *The injured athlete,* 2d ed., edited by D. Kuland. Philadelphia: Lippincott.

50. Sanderson, F. H. 1992. Psychology and injury prone athletes. *British Journal of Sports Medicine* 11:56–57.

51. Saterfield, M. J., D. Dowden, and K. Yasumura. 1990. Patient compliance for successful stress fracture rehabilitation. *Journal of Orthopaedic and Sports Physical Therapy* 11:321–24.

52. Shank, R. H. 1989. Academic and athletic factors related to predicting compliance by athletes for treatment. *Athletic Training* 24:123.

53. Smith, A. M., and E. K. Milliner. 1994. Injured athletes and the risk of suicide. *Journal of Athletic Training* 29:337.

54. Smith, A. M., S. G. Scott, W. M. O'Fallon, and M. L. Young. 1990. Emotional responses of athletes to injury. *Mayo Clinic Proceedings* 65:38–40.

55. Smith, A. M., M. J. Stuart, D. M. Wiese-Bjornstal, E. K. Milliner, W. M. O'Fallon, and C. S. Crowson. 1993. Competitive athletes: Preinjury and postinjury mood states and self-esteem. *Mayo Clinic Proceedings* 68:939–47.

56. Sowa, C. J. 1992. Understanding clients' perceptions of stress. *Journal of Counseling Development* 71:179–83.

57. Turk, D. C., D. Meichenbaum, and M. Genest. 1983. *Pain and behavioral medicine: A cognitive behavioral perspective.* New York: Guilford Press.

58. Valiant, P. M. 1981. Personality and injury in competitive runners. *Perceptual and Motor Skills* 53:251–53.

59. Vincent, P. 1971. Factors influencing patient compliance: A theoretical approach. *Nursing Research* 20:509–16.

60. Vinokur, A., and M. L. Selzer. 1975. Desirable versus undesirable life events: Their relationship to stress and distress. *Journal of Personality and Social Psychology* 32:329–37.

61. Webborn, A. D. J., R. J. Carbon, and B. P. Miller. 1997. Injury rehabilitation programs: "What are we talking about?" *Journal of Sport Rehabilitation* 6:54–61.

62. Werthner, P., and T. Orlick. 1986. Retirement experiences of successful athletes. *International Journal of Sport Psychology* 17:337–63.

63. Wiese, D. M., and M. R. Weiss. 1987. Psychological rehabilitation and physical injury: Implications for the sports medicine team. *Sport Psychologist* 1:318–30.

64. Williams, J. M., T. D. Hogan, and M. B. Andersen. 1993. Positive states of mind and injury risk. *Psychosomatic Medicine* 55:468–72.

65. Wolff, B. B. 1985. Ethnocultural factors influencing pain and illness behavior. *Clin J Pain* 1:23–30.

66. Wortman, C. B., and R. C. Silver. 1989. The myth of coping with loss. *Journal of Consulting and Clinical Psychology* 57:349–57.

CHAPTER 4

Restoring Range of Motion and Improving Flexibility

William E. Prentice

After completion of this chapter, the student should be able to do the following:

- Define flexibility, and describe its importance in injury rehabilitation.

- Identify factors that limit flexibility.

- Differentiate between active and passive range of motion.

- Explain the difference between ballistic, static, and PNF stretching.

- Discuss the neurophysiological principles of stretching.

- Describe stretching exercises that may be used to improve flexibility at specific joints throughout the body.

WHY IS RESTORING RANGE OF MOTION CRITICAL IN THE REHABILITATION PROCESS?

When injury occurs, there is almost always some associated loss of the ability to move normally. Loss of motion may by due to pain, swelling, muscle guarding or spasm, inactivity resulting in shortening of connective tissue and muscle; or some combination of these factors. Restoring normal range of motion following injury is one of the primary goals in any rehabilitation program.[66] Thus the sports therapist must routinely include stretching exercises designed to restore normal range of motion to regain normal function.

Flexibility has been defined as the ability to move a joint or series of joints through a full, nonrestricted, pain-free range of motion.[1,2,18,27,31,48,59] Flexibility is dependent on a combination of (1) joint range of motion, which can be limited by the shape of the articulating surfaces and by capsular and ligamentous structures surrounding that joint, and (2) by muscle flexibility, or the ability of the musculotendinous unit to lengthen.[67] In this chapter we will concentrate primarily on rehabilitative stretching techniques used to increase the length of the musculotendinous unit. Joint mobilization and traction techniques used to address tightness in the joint capsule and surrounding ligaments will be discussed in Chapter 12.

THE IMPORTANCE OF FLEXIBILITY TO THE ATHLETE

For the sports therapist, the restoration of, or improvement in, normal preinjury range of motion is an important goal

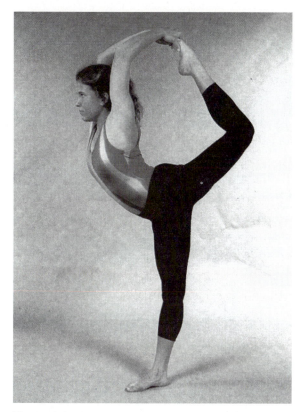

Figure 4-1   Sport activities require superior levels of flexibility.

Flexibility can be discussed in relation to movement involving only one joint, such as the knees, or movement involving a whole series of joints, such as the spinal vertebral joints, which must all move together to allow smooth bending or rotation of the trunk. Flexibility is specific to a given joint or movement. A person might have good range of motion in the ankles, knees, hips, back, and one shoulder joint but lack normal movement in the other shoulder joint; this is a problem that needs to be corrected before the person can function normally.[9]

ANATOMICAL FACTORS THAT LIMIT FLEXIBILITY

A number of anatomic factors can limit the ability of a joint to move through a full, unrestricted range of motion. **Muscles** and their tendons, along with their surrounding fascial sheaths, are most often responsible for limiting range of motion. When performing stretching exercises to improve flexibility about a particular joint, you are attempting to take advantage of the highly elastic properties of a muscle. Over time it is possible to increase the elasticity, or the length that a given muscle can be stretched. Persons who have a good deal of movement at a particular joint tend to have highly elastic and flexible muscles.

Connective tissue surrounding the joint, such as ligaments on the joint capsule, can be subject to contractures. Ligaments and joint capsules have some elasticity; however, if a joint is immobilized for a period of time, these structures tend to lose some elasticity and actually shorten. This condition is most commonly seen after surgical repair of an unstable joint, but it can also result from long periods of inactivity.

It is also possible for a person to have relatively slack ligaments and joint capsules. These people are generally referred to as being loose-jointed. Examples of this trait would be an elbow or knee that hyperextends beyond 180 degrees (Figure 4-2). Frequently there is instability associated with loose-jointedness that can present as great a problem in movement as ligamentous or capsular contractures.

Bony structure can restrict the end point in the range. An elbow that has been fractured through the joint might lay down excess calcium in the joint space, causing the joint to lose its ability to fully extend. However, in many instances we rely on bony prominences to stop movements at normal end points in the range.

Fat can also limit the ability to move through a full range of motion. A person who has a large amount of fat on the abdomen might have severely restricted trunk flexion when asked to bend forward and touch the toes. The fat can act as a wedge between two lever arms, restricting movement wherever it is found.

of any rehabilitation program.[57,65] Most sport activities require relatively "normal" amounts of flexibility. However, some activities, such as gymnastics, ballet, diving, and karate, require increased flexibility for superior performance (Figure 4-1). For an athlete who has a restricted range of motion, performance capabilities will probably decrease.[10] For example, a sprinter with tight, inelastic hamstring muscles probably loses some speed because the hamstring muscles restrict the ability to flex the hip joint and thus shorten stride length. Lack of flexibility can also result in uncoordinated or awkward movement patterns.

Most sports therapists would agree that good flexibility is essential to successful physical performance, although their ideas are based primarily on observation rather than scientific research. Likewise, they also believe that maintaining good flexibility is important in prevention of injury to the musculotendinous unit, and they will generally insist that stretching exercises be included as part of the warm-up before engaging in strenuous activity,[15,42,52] although little or no research evidence is available to support this practice.

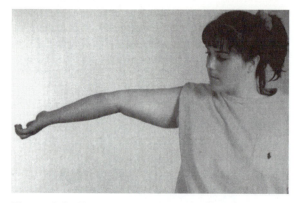

Figure 4-2 Excessive joint motion, such as the hyperextended elbow, can predispose a joint to injury.

Skin might also be responsible for limiting movement. For example, a person who has had some type of injury or surgery involving a tearing incision or laceration of the skin, particularly over a joint, will have inelastic scar tissue formed at that site. This scar tissue is incapable of stretching with joint movement.

Over time, skin contractures caused by scarring of ligaments, joint capsules, and musculotendinous units are capable of improving elasticity to varying degrees through stretching. With the exception of bone structure, age, and gender, all the other factors that limit flexibility can be altered to increase range of joint motion.

ACTIVE AND PASSIVE RANGE OF MOTION

Active range of motion, also called *dynamic flexibility*, refers to the degree to which a joint can be moved by a muscle contraction, usually through the midrange of movement. Dynamic flexibility is not necessarily a good indicator of the stiffness or looseness of a joint, because it applies to the ability to move a joint efficiently, with little resistance to motion.[25]

Passive range of motion, sometimes called *static flexibility*, refers to the degree to which a joint can be passively moved to the end points in the range of motion. No muscle contraction is involved to move a joint through a passive range.

When a muscle actively contracts, it produces a joint movement through a specific range of motion.[48,56] However, if passive pressure is applied to an extremity, it is capable of moving farther in the range of motion. It is essential in sport activities that an extremity be capable of moving through a nonrestricted range of motion.[50] For example, a hurdler who cannot fully extend the knee joint in a normal stride is at considerable disadvantage,

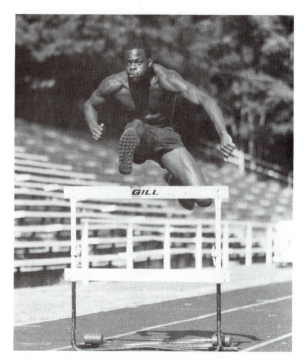

Figure 4-3 Flexibility is an essential component of many sport-related activities.

because stride length and thus speed will be reduced significantly (Figure 4-3).

Passive range of motion is important for injury prevention. There are many situations in sports in which a muscle is forced to stretch beyond its normal active limits. If the muscle does not have enough elasticity to compensate for this additional stretch, it is likely that the musculotendinous unit will be injured.

Assessment of Active and Passive Range of Motion

Accurate measurement of active and passive range of joint motion is difficult.[28] Various devices have been designed to accommodate variations in the size of the joints, as well as the complexity of movements in articulations that involve more than one joint.[30] Of these devices, the simplest and most widely used is the **goniometer** (Figure 4-4).

A goniometer is a large protractor with measurements in degrees. By aligning the individual arms of the goniometer parallel to the longitudinal axis of the two segments involved in motion about a specific joint, it is possible to obtain reasonably accurate measurement of range of movement. To enhance reliability, standardization of measurement techniques and methods of recording active and passive ranges of motion are critical in in-

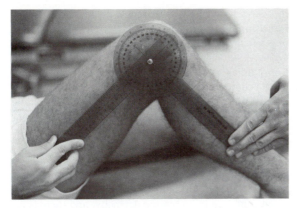

Figure 4-4 Measurement of active knee joint flexion using a goniometer.

■ **TABLE 4-1** Active Ranges of Joint Motions

Joint	Action	Degrees of Motion
Shoulder	Flexion	0–180 degrees
	Extension	0–50 degrees
	Abduction	0–180 degrees
	Medical rotation	0–90 degrees
	Lateral rotation	0–90 degrees
Elbow	Flexion	0–160 degrees
Forearm	Pronation	0–90 degrees
	Supination	0–90 degrees
Wrist	Flexion	0–90 degrees
	Extension	0–70 degrees
	Abduction	0–25 degrees
	Adduction	0–65 degrees
Hip	Flexion	0–125 degrees
	Extension	0–15 degrees
	Abduction	0–45 degrees
	Adduction	0–15 degrees
	Medical rotation	0–45 degrees
	Lateral rotation	0–45 degrees
Knee	Flexion	0–140 degrees
Ankle	Plantarflexion	0–45 degrees
	Dorsiflexion	0–20 degrees
Foot	Inversion	0–30 degrees
	Eversion	0–10 degrees

dividual clinics where successive measurements might be taken by different sports therapists to assess progress. Table 4-1 provides a list of what would be considered normal active ranges for movements at various joints.

The goniometer has an important place in a rehabilitation setting, where it is essential to assess improvement in joint flexibility to modify injury rehabilitation programs.

STRETCHING TECHNIQUES

Flexibility has been defined as the range of motion possible about a single joint or through a series of articulations. The maintenance of a full, nonrestricted range of motion has long been recognized as an essential component of athletic fitness.[11,12,13] Flexibility is important not only for successful physical performance but also for the prevention of injury.[2,7,8,43,60] The goal of any effective flexibility program should be to improve the range of motion at a given articulation by altering the extensibility of the musculotendinous units that produce movement at that joint. It is well documented that exercises that stretch these musculotendinous units over time will increase the range of movement possible about a given joint.[23,45]

Stretching techniques for improving flexibility have evolved over the years.[33] The oldest technique for stretching is called **ballistic stretching,** which makes use of repetitive bouncing motions. A second technique, known as **static stretching,** involves stretching a muscle to the point of discomfort and then holding it at that point for an extended time. This technique has been used for many years. More recently, another group of stretching techniques known collectively as **proprioceptive neuromuscular facilitation (PNF)** techniques, involving alternating contractions and stretches, has also been recommended.[34,62] Researchers have had considerable

discussion about which of these techniques is most effective for improving range of motion, and no clear-cut consensus currently exists.[23,37,45,49,63]

Agonist Versus Antagonist Muscles

Before discussing the three different stretching techniques, it is essential to define the terms **agonist muscle** and **antagonist muscle.** Most joints in the body are capable of more than one movement. The knee joint, for example, is capable of flexion and extension. Contraction of the quadriceps group of muscles on the front of the thigh causes knee extension, whereas contraction of the hamstring muscles on the back of the thigh produces knee flexion.

To achieve knee extension, the quadriceps group contracts while the hamstring muscles relax and stretch. Muscles that work in concert with one another in this manner are called synergistic muscle groups.[5] The muscle that contracts to produce a movement, in this case the quadriceps, is referred to as the agonist muscle. The muscle being stretched in response to contraction of the agonist muscle is called the antagonist muscle.[22] In this example of knee extension, the antagonist muscle would be the hamstring group. Some degree of balance in strength must exist between agonist and antagonist muscle groups. This balance is necessary for normal, smooth, coordinated movement, as well as for reducing the likelihood of muscle strain caused by muscular imbalance. Comprehension of this synergistic muscle action is essential to understanding the three techniques of stretching.

Ballistic Stretching

If you were to walk out to the track on any spring or fall afternoon and watch people who are warming up with stretching exercises before they run, you would probably see them use bouncing movements to stretch a particular muscle. This bouncing technique is more appropriately known as ballistic stretching, in which repetitive contractions of the agonist muscle are used to produce quick stretches of the antagonist muscle.

Over the years, many fitness experts have questioned the safety of the ballistic stretching technique.[3,32] Their concerns have been primarily based on the idea that ballistic stretching creates somewhat uncontrolled forces within the muscle that can exceed the extensibility limits of the muscle fiber, thus producing small microtears within the musculotendinous unit.[19,20,21,41,67] Certainly this might be true in sedentary individuals or perhaps in athletes who have sustained muscle injuries.

Most sport activities are dynamic and require ballistic-type movements. For example, forcefully kicking a soccer ball 50 times involves a repeated dynamic contraction of the agonist quadriceps muscle. The antagonist hamstrings are contracting eccentrically to decelerate the lower leg. Ballistic stretching of the hamstring muscle before engaging in this type of activity should allow the muscle to gradually adapt to the imposed demands and reduce the likelihood of injury. Because ballistic stretching is more functional, it should be integrated into a reconditioning program during the later stages of healing when appropriate.

Static Stretching

The static stretching technique is another extremely effective and widely used technique of stretching.[26] This technique involves passively stretching a given antagonist muscle by placing it in a maximal position of stretch and holding it there for an extended time. Recommendations for the optimal time for holding this stretched position vary, ranging from as little as 3 seconds to as much as 60 seconds.[25] Several studies have indicated that hold-

ing a stretch for 15 to 30 seconds is the most effective for increasing muscle flexibility.[4,35,38] Stretches lasting for longer than 30 seconds seem to be uncomfortable for the athlete. A static stretch of each muscle should be repeated 3 or 4 times. A static stretch can be accomplished by using a contraction of the agonist muscle to place the antagonist muscle in a position of stretch. A passive static stretch requires the use of body weight, assistance from the sports therapist or partner, or use of a T-bar, primarily for stretching the upper extremity.

Much research has been done comparing ballistic and static stretching techniques for the improvement of flexibility. Static and ballistic stretching appear to be equally effective in increasing flexibility, and there is no significant difference between the two.[20,51] However, much of the literature states that with static stretching there is less danger of exceeding the extensibility limits of the involved joints because the stretch is more controlled. Most of the literature indicates that ballistic stretching is apt to cause muscular soreness, especially in sedentary individuals, whereas static stretching generally does not cause soreness and is commonly used in injury rehabilitation of sore or strained muscles.[19,64] Static stretching is likely a much safer stretching technique, especially for sedentary or untrained individuals. However, because many physical activities involve dynamic movement, stretching in a warm-up should begin with static stretching followed by ballistic stretching, which more closely resembles the dynamic activity.

A progressive velocity flexibility program (PVFP) has been proposed that takes the athlete through a series of stretching exercises where the velocity of the stretch and the range of lengthening are progressively controlled.[67] The stretching exercises progress from slow static stretching; to slow, short, end-range stretching; to slow, full-range stretching; to fast, short, end-range stretching; to fast, full-range stretching. This program allows the athlete to control both the range and the speed with no assistance from a sports therapist.

PNF Stretching Techniques

PNF techniques were first used by physical therapists for treating patients who had various neuromuscular disorders.[34] More recently, PNF stretching exercises have increasingly been used as a stretching technique for improving flexibility.[14,39,44,46]

There are three different PNF techniques currently being used for stretching: slow-reversal-hold-relax, contract-relax, and hold-relax techniques.[58] All three techniques involve some combination of alternating isometric or isotonic contractions and relaxation of both agonist and antagonist muscles (a 10-second pushing phase followed by a 10-second relaxing phase).

Contract-relax (CR) is a stretching technique that moves the body part passively into the agonist pattern. The patient is instructed to push by contracting the antagonist (the muscle that will be stretched) isotonically against the resistance of the sports therapist. The patient then relaxes the antagonist while the therapist moves the part passively through as much range as possible to the point where limitation is again felt. This contract-relax technique is beneficial when range of motion is limited by muscle tightness.

Hold-relax (HR) is very similar to the contract-relax technique. It begins with an isometric contraction of the antagonist (the muscle that will be stretched) against resistance, followed by a concentric contraction of the agonist muscle combined with light pressure from the sports therapist to produce maximal stretch of the antagonist. This technique is appropriate when there is muscle tension on one side of a joint and may be used with either the agonist or the antagonist.

Slow reversal-hold-relax (SRHR) also occasionally referred to as the *contract-relax-agonist-contraction (CRAC)*, technique begins with an isotonic contraction of the agonist, which often limits range of motion in the agonist pattern, followed by an isometric contraction of the antagonist (the muscle that will be stretched) during the push phase. During the relax phase, the antagonists are relaxed while the agonists are contracting, causing movement in the direction of the agonist pattern and thus stretching the antagonist. This technique, like the contract-relax and hold-relax, is useful for increasing range of motion when the primary limiting factor is the antagonistic muscle group.

PNF stretching techniques can be used to stretch any muscle in the body.[16,17,44,47,39,41,49,58,63] PNF stretching techniques are perhaps best performed with a partner, although they may also be done using a wall as resistance.

NEUROPHYSIOLOGICAL BASIS OF STRETCHING

All three stretching techniques are based on a neurophysiological phenomenon involving the **stretch reflex** (see Fig. 13-1, p. 199).[46] Every muscle in the body contains various types of mechanoreceptors that, when stimulated, inform the central nervous system of what is happening with that muscle. Two of these mechanoreceptors are important in the stretch reflex: the **muscle spindle** and the **Golgi tendon organ.** Both types of receptors are sensitive to changes in muscle length. The Golgi tendon organs are also affected by changes in muscle tension.

When a muscle is stretched, both the muscle spindles and Golgi tendon organs immediately begin sending a volley of sensory impulses to the spinal cord. Initially impulses coming from the muscle spindles inform the central nervous system that the muscle is being stretched. Impulses return to the muscle from the spinal cord, causing the muscle to reflexively contract, thus resisting the stretch.[46] The Golgi tendon organs respond to the change in length and the increase in tension by firing off sensory impulses of their own to the spinal cord. If the stretch of the muscle continues for an extended period of time (at least 6 seconds), impulses from the Golgi tendon organs begin to override muscle spindle impulses. The impulses from the Golgi tendon organs, unlike the signals from the muscle spindle, cause a reflex relaxation of the antagonist muscle. This reflex relaxation serves as a protective mechanism that will allow the muscle to stretch through relaxation without exceeding the extensibility limits, which could damage the muscle fibers.[61]

With the jerking, bouncing motion of ballistic stretching, the muscle spindles are being repetitively stretched; thus there is continuous resistance by the muscle to further stretch. The ballistic stretch is not continued long enough to allow the Golgi tendon organs to have a relaxing effect.

The static stretch involves a continuous sustained stretch lasting anywhere from 6 to 60 seconds, which is sufficient time for the Golgi tendon organs to begin responding to the increase in tension. The impulses from the Golgi tendon organs can override the impulses coming from the muscle spindles, allowing the muscle to reflexively relax after the initial reflex resistance to the change in length. Thus lengthening the muscle and allowing it to remain in a stretched position for an extended period of time is unlikely to produce any injury to the muscle.

The effectiveness of the PNF techniques can be attributed in part to these same neurophysiological principles. The slow-reversal-hold-relax technique discussed previously takes advantage of two additional neurophysiological phenomena.[44]

The maximal isometric contraction of the muscle that will be stretched during the 10-second "push" phase again causes an increase in tension that stimulates the Golgi tendon organs to effect a reflex relaxation of the antagonist even before the muscle is placed in a position of stretch. This relaxation of the antagonist muscle during contractions is referred to as **autogenic inhibition.**

During the relaxing phase the antagonist is relaxed and passively stretched while there is a maximal isotonic contraction of the agonist muscle pulling the extremity further into the agonist pattern. In any synergistic muscle group, a contraction of the agonist causes a reflex relaxation in the antagonist muscle, allowing it to stretch and protecting it from injury. This phenomenon is referred to as reciprocal inhibition[53] (see Fig. 13-2, p. 200).

Thus, with the PNF techniques the additive effects of autogenic and reciprocal inhibition should theoretically allow the muscle to be stretched to a greater degree than is possible with static or ballistic stretching.[46]

THE EFFECT OF STRETCHING ON THE PHYSICAL AND MECHANICAL PROPERTIES OF MUSCLE

The neurophysiological mechanisms of both autogenic and reciprocal inhibition result in reflex relaxation with subsequent lengthening of a muscle. Thus the mechanical properties of that muscle that physically allow lengthening to occur are dictated via neural input.

Both muscle and tendon are composed largely of noncontractile collagen and elastin fibers. (The physical and mechanical properties of collagen and elastin were discussed in Chapter 2.) Collagen enables a tissue to resist mechanical forces and deformation, whereas elastin composes highly elastic tissues that assist in recovery from deformation.

Unlike tendon, muscle also has active contractile components which are the actin and myosin myofilaments. Collectively the contractile and noncontractile elements determine the muscle's capability of deforming and recovering from deformation.[67]

Both the contractile and the noncontractile components appear to resist deformation when a muscle is stretched or lengthened. The percentage of their individual contribution to resisting deformation depends on the degree to which the muscle is stretched or deformed and on the velocity of deformation. The noncontractile elements are primarily resistant to the degree of lengthening, while the contractile elements limit high-velocity deformation. The greater the stretch, the more the noncontractile components contribute.

Lengthening of a muscle via stretching, which is maintained for a period long enough to allow for autogenic inhibition to reflexively relax the muscle, allows for viscoelastic and plastic changes to occur in the collagen and elastin fibers. The viscoelastic changes that allow slow deformation with imperfect recovery are not permanent. However, plastic changes, although difficult to achieve, result in residual or permanent change in length due to deformation created by long periods of stretching.

The greater the velocity of deformation, the greater the chance for exceeding that tissue's capability to undergo viscoelastic and plastic change.[67]

PRACTICAL APPLICATION

Although all three stretching techniques have been demonstrated to effectively improve flexibility, there is still considerable debate as to which technique produces the greatest increases in range of movement. The ballistic technique is recommended for any athlete who is involved in dynamic activity, despite its potential for causing muscle soreness in the sedentary or untrained individual. In highly trained individuals, it is unlikely that ballistic stretching will result in muscle soreness.

Static stretching is perhaps the most widely used technique. It is a simple technique and does not require a partner. A fully nonrestricted range of motion can be attained through static stretching over time. PNF stretching techniques are capable of producing dramatic increases in range of motion during one stretching session. Studies comparing static and PNF stretching suggest that PNF stretching is capable of producing greater improvement in flexibility over an extended training period.[24,47] The major disadvantage of PNF stretching is that a partner is usually required to assist with the stretch, although stretching with a partner can have some motivational advantages. More and more athletic teams seem to be adopting the PNF technique as the method of choice for improving flexibility.

How long increases in muscle flexibility can be sustained once stretching stops is debatable.[63,68] One study indicated that a significant loss of flexibility was evident after only 2 weeks.[68] It was recommended that flexibility can be maintained by engaging in stretching activities at least once a week. However, to see improvement in flexibility, stretching must be done 3 to 5 times per week.[63]

The Importance of Warm-Up Prior to Stretching

To most effectively stretch a muscle during a program of rehabilitation, intramuscular temperature should be increased prior to stretching.[42] Increasing the temperature has a positive effect on the ability of the collagen and elastin components within the musculotendinous unit to deform. Also, the capability of the Golgi tendon organs to reflexively relax the muscle through autogenic inhibition is enhanced when the muscle is heated. It appears that the optimal temperature of muscle to achieve these beneficial effects is 39° C, or 103° F. This increase in intramuscular temperature can be achieved either through low-intensity warm-up type exercise or through the use of various therapeutic modalities.[52] It is recommended that exercise be used as the primary means for increasing intramuscular temperature.

The use of cold prior to stretching has also been recommended. Cold appears to be most useful when there is some muscle guarding associated with delayed-onset muscle soreness.[47]

THE RELATIONSHIP BETWEEN STRENGTH AND FLEXIBILITY

We often hear about the negative effects that strength training has on flexibility. For example, someone who develops large bulk through strength training is often referred to as "muscle bound." The expression *muscle bound* has negative connotations in terms of the person's ability to move. We tend to think of people who have highly developed muscles as having lost much of their ability to move freely through a full range of motion.[36]

Occasionally a person develops so much bulk that the physical size of the muscle prevents a normal range of motion. Strength training that is not properly done can impair movement. However, there is no reason to believe that weight training, if done properly through a full range of motion, will impair flexibility. Therefore, during a rehabilitation program the athlete must be encouraged to strength-train through a full, pain-free range of motion progressing as rapidly as pain decreases will allow. Proper strength training probably improves dynamic flexibility and, if combined with a rigorous stretching program, can greatly enhance powerful and coordinated movements that are essential for success in many athletic activities. In all cases a heavy weight-training program should be accompanied by a strong flexibility program (Figure 4-5).

GUIDELINES AND PRECAUTIONS FOR STRETCHING

The following guidelines and precautions should be incorporated into a sound stretching program:[6,43,54,55]

- Warm up using a slow jog or fast walk before stretching vigorously.
- To increase flexibility, the muscle must be overloaded or stretched beyond its normal range but not to the point of pain.
- Stretch only to the point where tightness or resistance to stretch, or perhaps some discomfort, is felt. Stretching should not be painful.[6]

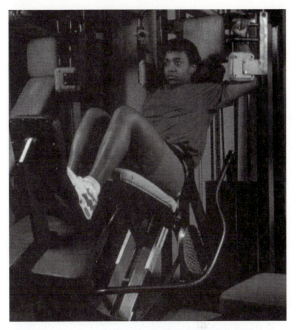

Figure 4-5 Strength training through a full range of motion will not impair, and might improve, flexibility.

- Increases in range of motion will be specific to whatever muscle or joint is being stretched.
- Exercise caution when stretching muscles that surround painful joints. Pain is an indication that something is wrong and should not be ignored.
- Avoid overstretching the ligaments and capsules that surround joints.
- Exercise caution when stretching the low back and neck. Exercises that compress the vertebrae and their discs can cause damage.
- Stretching from a seated rather than a standing position takes stress off the low back and decreases the chances of back injury.
- Be sure to continue normal breathing during a stretch. Do not hold your breath.
- Static and PNF techniques are most often recommended for individuals who want to improve their range of motion.
- Ballistic stretching should be done only by those who are already flexible or accustomed to stretching, and should be done only after static stretching.
- Stretching should be done at least 3 times per week to see minimal improvement. It is recommended to stretch between 5 and 6 times per week to see maximum results.

SPECIFIC STRETCHING EXERCISES

Chapters 19 through 26 will include examples of various stretching exercises that may be used to improve flexibility at specific joints or in specific muscle groups through-out the body. The exercises described may be done statically or with slight modification; they may also be done with a partner using a PNF technique. There are many possible variations to each of these exercises.[29] The exercises selected are those that seem to be the most effective for stretching of various muscle groups.

Summary

1. Flexibility is the ability to move a joint or a series of joints smoothly through a full range of motion.
2. Flexibility is specific to a given joint, and the term *good flexibility* implies that there are no joint abnormalities restricting movement.
3. Flexibility can be limited by muscles and tendons, joint capsules or ligaments, fat, bone structure, or skin.
4. *Passive range of motion* refers to the degree to which a joint can be passively moved to the end points in the range of motion. *Active range of motion* refers to movement through the midrange of motion resulting from active contraction.
5. Measurement of joint flexibility is accomplished through the use of a goniometer.
6. An agonist muscle is one that contracts to produce joint motion; the antagonist muscle is stretched with contraction of the agonist.
7. Ballistic, static, and proprioceptive neuromuscular facilitation (PNF) techniques have all been used as stretching techniques for improving flexibility.
8. Each of these stretching techniques is based on the neurophysiological phenomena involving the muscle spindles and Golgi tendon organs. PNF techniques appear to be the most effective in producing increases in flexibility.
9. Stretching should be included as part of the warm-up period to prepare the muscles for what they are going to be asked to do and to prevent injury, as well as in the cool-down period to help reduce injury. Stretching after an activity can prevent muscle soreness and will help increase flexibility by stretching a loose, warmed-up muscle.
10. Strength training, if done correctly through full range of motion, will likely improve flexibility.

References

1. Alter, M. J. 1988. *The science of stretching.* Champaign, IL: Human Kinetics.
2. Arnheim, D. D., and W. E. Prentice. 1997. *Principles of athletic training.* Madison, WI: Brown & Benchmark.
3. Astrand, P. O., and K. Rodahl. 1986. *Textbook of work physiology.* New York: McGraw-Hill.
4. Bandy, W. D., and J. M. Irion. 1994. The effect of time of static stretch on the flexibility of the hamstring muscles. *Physical Therapy* 74:845–52.
5. Basmajian, J. 1984. *Therapeutic exercise.* 4th ed. Baltimore: Williams & Wilkins.
6. Bealieu, J. E. 1981. Developing a stretching program. *Physician and Sports Medicine* 9(11): 59.
7. Bealieu, J. E. 1980. *Stretching for all sports.* Pasadena, CA: Athletic Press.
8. Blanke, D. 1994. Flexibility. In *Sports medicine secrets,* edited by M. Mellion. Philadelphia: Hanley & Belfus.
9. Chapman, E. A., H. A. deVries, and R. Swezey. 1972. Joint stiffness: Effect of exercise on young and old men. Journal of Gerontology 27:218.
10. Condon, S. A., and R. S. Hutton. 1987. Soleus muscle EMG activity and ankle dorsiflexion range of motion from stretching procedures. *Physical Therapy* 67:24–30.
11. Corbin, C., and K. Fox. 1985. Flexibility: The forgotten part of fitness. *Journal of Physical Education* 16(6): 191.
12. Corbin, C., and L. Noble. 1980. Flexibility. *Journal of Physical Education, Recreation and Dance* 51:23.
13. Corbin, C., and L. Noble. 1985. Flexibility: A major component of physical fitness. In *Implementation of health fitness exercise programs,* edited by D. E. Cundiff. Reston, VA: American Alliance for Health, Physical Education, Recreation and Dance.
14. Cornelius, W., and A. Jackson. 1984. The effects of cryotherapy and PNF on hip extensor flexibility. *Journal of Athletic Training* 19:183–84.
15. Cornelius, W. L., R. W. Hagemann, Jr., and A. W. Jackson. 1988. A study on placement of stretching within a workout. *Journal of Sports Medicine and Physical Fitness* 28(3): 234.
16. Cornelius, W. L. 1986. *PNF and other flexibility techniques.* Arlington, Va: Computer Microfilm International. (microfiche; 20 fr.)
17. Cornelius, W. L. 1981. Two effective flexibility methods. *Athletic Training* 16(1): 23.
18. Couch, J. 1982. *Runners world yoga book.* Mountain View, CA: World.

19. deVries, H. 1986. *Physiology of exercise for physical education and athletics.* Dubuque, IA: Wm. C. Brown.

20. deVries, H. A. 1962. Evaluation of static stretching procedures for improvement of flexibility. *Res Q* 3:222–29.

21. Entyre, B. R., and L. D. Abraham. 1986. Ache-reflex changes during static stretching and two variations of proprioceptive neuromuscular facilitation techniques. *Electroencephalogr Clin Neurophysiol* 63:174–79.

22. Entyre, B. R., and L. D. Abraham. 1988. Antagonist muscle activity during stretching: A paradox reassessed. *Medicine and Science in Sports and Exercise* 20:285–89.

23. Entyre, B. R., and E. J. Lee. 1988. Chronic and acute flexibility of men and women using three different stretching techniques. *Research Quarterly for Exercise and Sport.* 59:222–28.

24. Godges, J. J., H. MacRae, C. Longdon, et al. 1989. The effects of two stretching procedures on hip range of motion and joint economy. *Journal of Orthopaedic and Sports Physical Therapy* 11:350–57.

25. Herling, J. 1981. It's time to add strength training to our fitness programs. *J Phys Educ Program* 79:17.

26. Hubley, C. L., J. W. Kozey, and W. D. Stanish. 1984. The effects of static stretching exercises and stationary cycling on range of motion at the hip joint. *J Orthop Sports Phys Ther* 6:104–09.

27. Humphrey, L. D. 1981. Flexibility. *Journal of Physical Education, Recreation and Dance* 52:41.

28. Hutinger, P. 1974. How flexible are you? *Aquatic World Magazine,* January.

29. Ishii, D. K. 1976. Flexibility strexercises for co-ed groups. *Scholastic Coach* 45:31.

30. Jackson, A. W., and A. A. Baker. 1986. The relationship of the sit-and-reach test to criterion measures of hamstring and back flexibility in young females. *Research Quarterly for Exercise and Sport* 57(3): 183.

31. Jensen, C., and G. Fisher. 1979. *Scientific basis of athletic conditioning.* Philadelphia: Lea & Febiger.

32. Johnson, P. 1975. *Sport, exercise and you.* New York: Holt, Rinehart & Winston.

33. Knortz, K., and C. Ringel. 1985. Flexibility techniques. *National Strength and Conditioning Association Journal* 7(2): 50.

34. Knott, M., and P. Voss. 1985. Proprioceptive neuromuscular facilitation. 3d ed. New York: Harper & Row.

35. Lentell, G., T. Hetherington, J. Eagan, et al. 1992. The use of thermal agents to influence the effectiveness of a low-load prolonged stretch. *J Ortho Sports Phys Ther* 5:200–07.

36. Liemohn, W. 1988. Flexibility and muscular strength. *Journal of Physical Education, Recreation and Dance* 59(7): 37.

37. Louden, K. L., C. E. Bolier, K. A. Allison, et al. 1985. Effects of two stretching methods on the flexibility and retention of flexibility at the ankle joint in runners. *Physical Therapy* 65:698.

38. Madding, S. W., J. G. Wong, and A. Hallum. 1987. Effects of duration of passive stretching on hip abduction range of motion. *J Orthop Sports Phys Ther* 8:409–16.

39. Markos, P. D. 1979. Ipsilateral and contralateral effects of proprioceptive neuromuscular facilitation techniques on hip motion and electromyographic activity. *Physical Therapy* 59:1366–73.

40. McAtee, R. 1993. *Facilitated stretching.* Champaign, IL: Human Kinetics.

41. Moore, M., and R. Hutton. 1980. Electromyographic investigation of muscle stretching techniques. *Medicine and Science in Sports and Exercise* 12:322–29.

42. Murphy, P. 1986. Warming up before stretching advised. *Physician and Sports Medicine* 14(3): 45.

43. Norris, C. 1994. *Flexibility principles and practices.* London: A&C Black.

44. Prentice, W. E., and E. Kooima. 1986. The use of PNF techniques in rehabilitation of sport-related injury. *Athletic Training* 21(1):26-31.

45. Prentice, W. E. 1983. A comparison of static stretching and PNF stretching for improving hip joint flexibility. *Journal of Athletic Training* 18:56–59.

46. Prentice, W. E. 1989. A review of PNF techniques—Implications for athletic rehabilitation and performance. *Forum Medicum* (51): 1–13.

47. Prentice, W. E. 1982. An electromyographic analysis of heat or cold and stretching for inducing muscular relaxation. *J Orthop Sports Phys Ther* 3:133–40.

48. Rasch, P. 1989. *Kinesiology and applied anatomy.* Philadelphia: Lea & Febiger.

49. Sady, S. P., M. Wortman, and D. Blanke. 1982. Flexibility training: Ballistic, static, or proprioceptive neuromuscular facilitation? *Archives of Physical Medicine and Rehabilitation* 63:261–63.

50. Sapega, A. A., T. Quedenfeld, R. Moyer, et al. 1981. Biophysical factors in range-of-motion exercise. *Physician and Sports Medicine* 9(12): 57.

51. Schultz, P. 1979. Flexibility: Day of the static stretch. *Physician and Sports Medicine* 8:73–77.

52. Shellock, F., and W. E. Prentice. 1985. Warm-up and stretching for improved physical performance and prevention of sport related injury. *Sports Med* 2:267–78.

53. Shindo, M., H. Harayama, K. Kondo, et al. 1984. Changes in reciprocal Ia inhibition during voluntary contraction in man. *Exp Brain Res* 53:400–08.

54. St. George, F. 1994. *The stretching handbook: Ten steps to muscle fitness.* Roseville, IL: Simon & Schuster.

55. Stamford, B. 1994. A stretching primer. *Physician and Sports Medicine* 22(9): 85–86.

56. *Staying flexible: The full range of motion.* 1987. Alexandria, VA: Time Life Books.

57. Surburg, P. 1995. Flexibility training program design. In Miller P:*Fitness programming and physical disability,* edited by P. Miller. Champaign, IL: Human Kinetics.

58. Tanigawa, M. C. 1972. Comparison of the hold relax procedure and passive mobilization on increasing muscle length. *Physical Therapy* 52:725.

59. Tobias, M., and J. P. Sullivan. 1992. *Complete stretching.* New York: Knopf.

60. van Mechelen, P. 1993. Prevention of running injuries by warm-up, cool-down, and stretching. *American Journal of Sports Medicine* 21(5): 711–19.

61. Verrill, D., and R. Pate. 1982. Relationship between duration of static stretch in the sit and reach position and biceps femoris electromyographic activity. *Medicine and Science in Sports and Exercise* 14:124.

62. Voss, D. E., M. K. Lonta, and G. J. Myers. 1985. *Proprioceptive neuromuscular facilitation: Patterns and techniques.* 3d ed. Philadelphia: Lippincott.

63. Wallin, D., B. Ekblom, and R. Grahn. 1985. Improvement of muscle flexibility: A comparison between two techniques. *American Journal of Sports Medicine* 13:263–68.

64. Wessel, J., and A. Wan. 1984. Effect of stretching on intensity of delayed-onset muscle soreness. *Journal of Sports Medicine* 2:83–87.

65. Wiktorsson-Moeller, M., B. Oberg, and J. Ekstrand. 1983. Effects of warming-up, massage, and stretching on range of motion and muscle strength in the lower extremity. *American Journal of Sports Medicine* 11:249–52.

66. Worrell, T., T. Smith, and J. Winegardner. 1994. Effect of hamstring stretching on hamstring muscle performance. *J Ortho Sports Phys Ther* 20(3): 154–59.

67. Zachewski, J. 1990. Flexibility for sports. In *Sports physical therapy,* edited by B. Sanders. Norwalk, CT: Appleton & Lange.

68. Zebas, C. J., and M. L. Rivera. 1985. Retention of flexibility in selected joints after cessation of a stretching exercise program. In *Exercise physiology: Current selected research topics,* edited by C. O. Dotson and J. H. Humphrey. New York: AMS Press.

CHAPTER 5

Regaining Muscular Strength, Endurance, and Power

William E. Prentice

After completion of this chapter, the student should be able to do the following:

- Define muscular strength, endurance, and power and discuss their importance in a program of rehabilitation following injury.

- Discuss the anatomy and physiology of skeletal muscle.

- Discuss the physiology of strength development and factors that determine strength.

- Describe specific methods for improving muscular strength.

- Differentiate between muscle strength and muscle endurance.

- Discuss differences between males and females in terms of strength development.

WHY IS REGAINING STRENGTH, ENDURANCE, AND POWER ESSENTIAL TO THE REHABILITATION PROCESS?

Developing muscular strength, endurance, and power is an essential element in any training and conditioning program for the athlete. From the perspective of the sports therapist supervising a rehabilitation program, regaining—and in many instances improving—levels of strength, endurance, and power is critical not only for achieving a competitive fitness level but also for returning the athlete to a competitive functional level following injury.

By definition, **muscular strength** is the ability of a muscle to generate force against some resistance. Maintenance of at least a normal level of strength in a given muscle or muscle group is important for normal healthy living. Muscle weakness or imbalance can result in abnormal movement or gait and can impair normal functional movement. Developing muscle strength is critical to athletic performance.

Muscular strength is closely associated with muscular endurance. **Muscular endurance** is the ability to perform repetitive muscular contractions against some resistance for an extended period of time. As we will see later, as muscular strength increases, endurance tends to increase. For the average person in the population, developing muscular endurance is likely more important than developing muscular strength or power, because muscular endurance is probably more critical in carrying out the everyday activities of living. This becomes increasingly true with age.

Most movements in sport are explosive and must include elements of both strength and speed if they are to be

73

effective. If a large amount of force is generated quickly, the movement can be referred to as a **power** movement. Without the ability to generate power, an athlete will be limited in his or her performance capabilities.[35] Resistance training plays a critical role in achieving competitive fitness levels and also in injury rehabilitation.

TYPES OF SKELETAL MUSCLE CONTRACTION

Skeletal muscle is capable of three different types of contraction: (1) **isometric contraction,** (2) **concentric contraction,** and (3) **eccentric contraction.** An isometric contraction occurs when the muscle contracts to produce tension but there is no change in muscle length. Considerable force can be generated against some immovable resistance even though no movement occurs. In a concentric contraction the muscle shortens in length while tension increases to overcome or move some resistance. In an eccentric contraction, the resistance is greater than the muscular force being produced, and the muscle lengthens while producing tension. Concentric and eccentric contractions are considered dynamic movements.[46]

Recently, an **econcentric contraction** which combines both a controlled concentric and a concurrent eccentric contraction of the same muscle over two separate joints, has been introduced.[15,26] An econcentric contraction is possible only in muscles that cross at least two joints. An example of an econcentric contraction would be a prone, open-kinetic-chain hamstring curl. The hamstrings contract concentrically to flex the knee, while the hip tends to flex eccentrically, lengthening the hamstring. Rehabilitation exercises have traditionally concentrated on strengthening isolated single-joint motions, despite the fact that the same muscle is functioning at a second joint simultaneously. Therefore it has been recommended that the strengthening program included exercises that strengthen the muscle in the manner in which it contracts functionally.

Fast-Twitch versus Slow-Twitch Fibers

All fibers in a particular motor unit are either **slow-twitch fibers** or **fast-twitch fibers.** Each kind has distinctive metabolic and contractile capabilities.

Slow-Twitch Fibers. Slow-twitch fibers are also referred to as *type I* or *slow-oxidative (SO)* fibers. They are more resistant to fatigue than fast-twitch fibers; however, the time required to generate force is much greater in slow-twitch fibers.[25] Because they are relatively fatigue resistant, slow-twitch fibers are associated primarily with long-duration, aerobic-type activities.

Fast-Twitch Fibers. Fast-twitch fibers are capable of producing quick, forceful contractions but have a tendency to fatigue more rapidly than slow-twitch fibers. Fast-twitch fibers are useful in short-term, high-intensity activities, which mainly involve the anaerobic system. Fast-twitch fibers are capable of producing powerful contractions, whereas slow-twitch fibers produce a long-endurance force. There are two subdivisions of fast-twitch fibers. While both types of fast-twitch fibers are capable of rapid contraction, type *IIa fibers* or *fast-oxidative glycolytic (FOG)* fibers are moderately resistant to fatigue, while *type IIb fibers* or *fast-glycolytic (FG) fibers* fatigue rapidly and are considered the "true" fast-twitch fibers. Recently, a third group of fast-twitch fibers, *type IIx,* has been identified in animal models. Type IIx fibers are fatigue resistant and are thought to have a maximum power capacity less than that of type IIb but greater than that of type IIa fibers.[36]

Ratio in Muscle. Within a particular muscle are both types of fibers, and the ratio of the two types in an individual muscle varies with each person.[28] Muscles whose primary function is to maintain posture against gravity require more endurance and have a higher percentage of slow-twitch fibers. Muscles that produce powerful, rapid, explosive strength movements tend to have a much higher percentage of fast-twitch fibers.

Because this ratio is genetically determined, it can play a large role in determining ability for a given sport activity. Sprinters and weight lifters, for example, have a large percentage of fast-twitch fibers in relation to slow-twitch fibers.[12] Conversely, marathon runners generally have a higher percentage of slow-twitch fibers. The question of whether fiber types can change as a result of training has to date not been conclusively resolved.[9] However, both types of fibers can improve their metabolic capabilities through specific strength and endurance training.[6]

FACTORS THAT DETERMINE LEVELS OF MUSCULAR STRENGTH, ENDURANCE, AND POWER

Size of the Muscle

Muscular strength is proportional to the cross-sectional diameter of the muscle fibers. The greater the cross-sectional diameter or the bigger a particular muscle, the stronger it is, and thus the more force it is capable of generating. The size of a muscle tends to increase in cross-sectional diameter with resistance training. This increase in muscle size is referred to as **hypertrophy.**[33] A decrease in the size of a muscle is referred to as **atrophy.**

Number of Muscle Fibers

Strength is a function of the number and diameter of muscle fibers composing a given muscle. The number of fibers is an inherited characteristic; thus a person with a large number of muscle fibers to begin with has the potential to hypertrophy to a much greater degree than does someone with relatively few fibers.[31]

Neuromuscular Efficiency

Strength is also directly related to the efficiency of the neuromuscular system and the function of the motor unit in producing muscular force.[37] As will be indicated later in this chapter, initial increases in strength during the first 8 to 10 weeks of a resistance training program can be attributed primarily to increased neuromuscular efficiency.[49] Resistance training will increase neuromuscular efficiency in three ways: there is an increase in the number of motor units being recruited, in the firing rate of each motor unit, and in the synchronization of motor unit firing.[6]

Biomechanical Considerations

Strength in a given muscle is determined not only by the physical properties of the muscle but also by biomechanical factors that dictate how much force can be generated through a system of levers to an external object.[27,31,51]

Position of Tendon Attachment. If we think of the elbow joint as one of these lever systems, we would have the biceps muscle producing flexion of this joint (Figure 5-1). The position of attachment of the biceps muscle on the forearm will largely determine how much force this muscle is capable of generating. If there are two athletes, A and B, and A has a biceps attachment that is closer to the fulcrum (the elbow joint) than B's, then A must produce a greater effort with the biceps muscle to hold the weight at a right angle because, the length of the effort arm will be greater than for B.

Length-Tension Relationship. The length of a muscle determines the tension that can be generated. By varying the length of a muscle, different tensions can be produced.[27] This length-tension relationship is illustrated in Figure 5-2. At position B in the curve, the interaction of the crossbridges between the actin and myosin myofilaments within the sarcomere is at maximum. Setting a muscle at this particular length will produce the greatest amount of tension. At position A the muscle is shortened, and at position C the muscle is lengthened. In either case the interaction between the actin and myosin myofilaments through the crossbridges is greatly re-

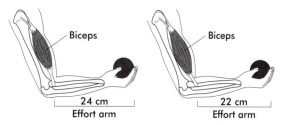

Figure 5-1 The position of attachment of the muscle tendon on the lever arm can affect the ability of that muscle to generate force. **B** should be able to generate greater force than **A** because the tendon attachment on the lever arm is closer to the resistance.

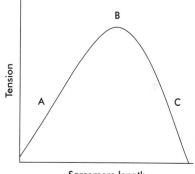

Figure 5-2 The length-tension relation of the muscle. Greatest tension is developed at point B, with less tension developed at points A and C.

duced, thus the muscle is not capable of generating significant tension.

Age

The ability to generate muscular force is also related to age.[2] Both men and women seem to be able to increase strength throughout puberty and adolescence, reaching a peak around 20 to 25 years of age, at which time this ability begins to level off and in some cases decline. After about age 25 a person generally loses an average of 1 percent of his or her maximal remaining strength each year. Thus at age 65 a person would have only about 60 percent of the strength he or she had at age 25.[36] This loss in muscle strength is definitely related to individual levels of physical activity. People who are more active, or perhaps continue to strength-train, considerably decrease this tendency toward declining muscle strength. In addition to retarding this decrease in muscular

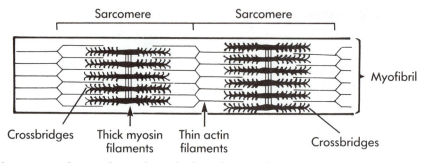

Figure 5-3   Muscles contract when an electrical impulse from the central nervous system causes the myofilaments in a muscle fiber to move closer together.

strength, exercise can also have an effect in slowing the decrease in cardiorespiratory endurance and flexibility, as well as slowing increases in body fat. Thus strength maintenance is important for all athletes regardless of age or the level of competition for achieving total wellness and good health and in rehabilitation after injury.[50]

Overtraining

Overtraining can have a negative effect on the development of muscular strength. Overtraining is an imbalance between exercise and recovery in which the training program exceeds the body's physiological and psychological limits. Overtraining can result in psychological breakdown (staleness) or physiological breakdown, which can involve musculoskeletal injury, fatigue, or sickness. Engaging in proper and efficient resistance training, eating a proper diet, and getting appropriate rest can all minimize the potential negative effects of overtraining.

THE PHYSIOLOGY OF STRENGTH DEVELOPMENT

Muscle Hypertrophy

There is no question that resistance training to improve muscular strength results in an increased size, or hypertrophy, of a muscle. What causes a muscle to hypertrophy? A number of theories have been proposed to explain this increase in muscle size.[18]

Some evidence exists that there is an *increase in the number of muscle fibers (hyperplasia)* due to fibers splitting in response to training.[24] However, this research has been conducted in animals and should not be generalized to humans. It is generally accepted that the number of fibers is genetically determined and does not seem to increase with training.

Second, it has been hypothesized that because the muscle is working harder in resistance training, more blood is required to supply that muscle with oxygen and other nutrients. Thus it is thought that *the number of capillaries is increased.* This hypothesis is only partially correct; *no new* capillaries are formed during resistance training; however, a number of dormant capillaries might well become filled with blood to meet this increased demand for blood supply.[36]

A third theory to explain this increase in muscle size seems the most credible. Muscle fibers are composed primarily of small protein filaments, called myofilaments, which are contractile elements in muscle. **Myofilaments** are small contractile elements of protein within the sarcomere. There are two distinct types of myofilaments: thin **actin** myofilaments and thicker **myosin** myofilaments. Fingerlike projections, or crossbridges, connect the actin and myosin myofilaments. When a muscle is stimulated to contract, the crossbridges pull the myofilaments closer together, thus shortening the muscle and producing movement at the joint that the muscle crosses[4] (Figure 5-3).

These *myofilaments increase in size and number* as a result of resistance training, causing the individual muscle fibers to increase in cross-sectional diameter.[48] This increase is particularly present in men, although women will also see some increase in muscle size. More research is needed to further clarify and determine the specific reasons for muscle hypertrophy.

Reversibility.   If resistance training is discontinued or interrupted, the muscle will atrophy, decreasing in both strength and mass. Adaptations in skeletal muscle that occur in response to resistance training can begin to reverse in as little as 48 hours. It does appear that consistent exercise of a muscle is essential to prevent reversal of the hypertrophy that occurs due to strength training.

Other Physiological Adaptations to Resistance Exercise

In addition to muscle hypertrophy, there are a number of other physiological adaptations to resistance training. The strength of noncontractile structures, including tendons and ligaments, is increased. The mineral content of bone is increased, thus making the bone stronger and more resistant to fracture. Maximal oxygen uptake is improved when resistance training is of sufficient intensity to elicit heart rates at or above training levels. However, it must be emphasized that these increases are minimal and that, if increased maximal oxygen uptake is the goal, aerobic exercise rather than resistance training is recommended. There is also an increase in several enzymes important in aerobic and anaerobic metabolism.[1,21,22] All of these adaptations contribute to strength and endurance.

TECHNIQUES OF RESISTANCE TRAINING

There are a number of different techniques of resistance training for strength improvement, including isometric exercise, progressive resistive exercise, isokinetic training, circuit training, and plyometric exercise.

The Overload Principle

Regardless of which of these techniques is used, one basic principle of reconditioning is extremely important. For a muscle to improve in strength, it must be forced to work at a higher level than it is accustomed to. In other words, the muscle must be overloaded. Without overload the muscle will be able to maintain strength as long as training is continued against a resistance to which the muscle is accustomed, but, no additional strength gains will be realized. This maintenance of existing levels of muscular strength may be more important in resistance programs that emphasize muscular endurance rather than strength gains. Many individuals can benefit more in terms of overall health by concentrating on improving muscular endurance. However, to most effectively build muscular strength, resistance training requires a consistent, increasing effort against progressively increasing resistance.[31,46]

Resistive exercise is based primarily on the principles of overload and progression. If these principles are applied, all of the following resistance training techniques will produce improvement of muscular strength over time.

In a rehabilitation setting, progressive overload is limited to some degree by the healing process. Because

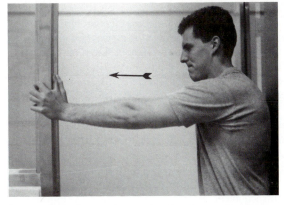

Figure 5-4 Isometric exercises involve contraction against some immovable resistance.

the sports therapist takes an aggressive approach to rehabilitation, the rate of progression is perhaps best determined by the injured athlete's response to a specific exercise. Exacerbation of pain or increased swelling should signal the sports therapist that their rate of progression is too aggressive.

Isometric Exercise

An **isometric exercise** involves a muscle contraction in which the length of the muscle remains constant while tension develops toward a maximal force against an immovable resistance[5] (Figure 5-4). Isometric exercises are capable of increasing muscular strength.[44] However, strength gains are relatively specific, with as much as a 20 percent overflow to the joint angle at which training is performed. At other angles, the strength curve drops off dramatically because of a lack of motor activity at that angle. Thus, strength is increased at the specific angle of exertion, but there is no corresponding increase in strength at other positions in the range of motion.

Another major disadvantage of these isometric exercises is that they tend to produce a spike in systolic blood pressure that can result in potentially life-threatening cardiovascular accidents.[25] This sharp increase in systolic blood pressure results from a Valsalva maneuver, which increases intrathoracic pressure. To avoid or minimize this effect, it is recommended that breathing be done during the maximal contraction to prevent this increase in pressure.

The use of isometric exercises in injury rehabilitation or reconditioning is widely practiced. There are a number of conditions or ailments resulting from trauma or overuse that must be treated with strengthening exercises. Unfortunately, these problems can be exacerbated with full range-of-motion resistance exercises. It might be more desirable to make use of positional or functional isometric exercises that involve the application of isometric force at multiple angles throughout the range of motion. Functional isometrics should be used until the healing process has progressed to the point that full-range activities can be performed.

During rehabilitation, it is often recommended that a muscle be contracted isometrically for 10 seconds at a time at a frequency of 10 or more contractions per hour. Isometric exercises can also offer significant benefit in a strengthening program.[52]

There are certain instances in which an isometric contraction can greatly enhance a particular movement. For example, one of the exercises in power weight lifting is a squat. A squat is an exercise in which the weight is supported on the shoulders in a standing position. The knees are then flexed, and the weight is lowered to a three-quarter squat position, from which the lifter must stand completely straight once again.

It is not uncommon for there to be one particular angle in the range of motion at which smooth movement is difficult because of insufficient strength. This joint angle is referred to as a sticking point. A power lifter will typically use an isometric contraction against some immovable resistance to increase strength at this sticking point. If strength can be improved at this joint angle, then a smooth, coordinated power lift can be performed through a full range of movement.

Progressive Resistive Exercise

A second technique of resistance training is perhaps the most commonly used and most popular technique among sports therapists for improving muscular strength in a rehabilitation program. **Progressive resistive exercise** training uses exercises that strengthen muscles through a contraction that overcomes some fixed resistance such as with dumbbells, barbells, various exercise machines, or resistive elastic tubing. Progressive resistive exercise uses isotonic, or *isodynamic,* contractions in which force is generated while the muscle is changing in length.

Concentric versus Eccentric Contractions. Isotonic contractions can be concentric or eccentric. In performing a bicep curl, to lift the weight from the starting position the biceps muscle must contract and shorten in length. This shortening contraction is referred to as a concentric or positive contraction. If the biceps muscle does not remain contracted when the weight is being lowered, gravity would cause this weight to simply fall back to the starting position. Thus, to control the weight as it is being lowered, the biceps muscle must continue to contract while at the same time gradually lengthening. A contraction in which the muscle is lengthening while still applying force is called an eccentric or negative contraction.

It is possible to generate greater amounts of force against resistance with an eccentric contraction than with a concentric contraction, because eccentric contractions require a much lower level of motor unit activity to achieve a certain force than do concentric contractions. Because fewer motor units are firing to produce a specific force, additional motor units can be recruited to generate increased force. In addition, oxygen use is much lower during eccentric exercise than in comparable concentric exercise. Thus eccentric contractions are less resistant to fatigue than are concentric contractions. The mechanical efficiency of eccentric exercise can be several times higher than that of concentric exercise.[46]

Traditionally, progressive resistive exercise has concentrated primarily on the concentric component without paying much attention to the importance of the eccentric component.[46] The use of eccentric contractions, particularly in rehabilitation of various sport-related injuries, has received considerable emphasis in recent years. Eccentric contractions are critical for deceleration of limb motion, especially during high-velocity dynamic activities. For example, a baseball pitcher relies on an eccentric contraction of the external rotators of the glenohumeral joint to decelerate the humerus, which might be internally rotating at speeds as high as 8,000 degrees per second. Certainly, strength deficits or an inability of a muscle to tolerate these eccentric forces can predispose an injury. Thus, in a rehabilitation program the sports therapist should incorporate eccentric strengthening exercises. Eccentric contractions are possible with all free weights, with the majority of isotonic exercise machines, and with most isokinetic devices. Eccentric contractions are used with plyometric exercise discussed in Chapter 10 and can also be incorporated with functional PNF strengthening patterns discussed in Chapter 12.

In progressive resistive exercise it is essential to incorporate both concentric and eccentric contractions.[29] Research has clearly demonstrated that the muscle should be overloaded and fatigued both concentrically and eccentrically for the greatest strength improvement to occur.[2,18,36] When training specifically for the development of muscular strength, the concentric portion of the exercise should require 1 to 2 seconds, while the eccentric portion of the lift should require 2 to 4 seconds. The ratio of the concentric component to the eccentric component should be approximately 1 to 2. Physiologically the muscle will fatigue much more rapidly concentrically than eccentrically.

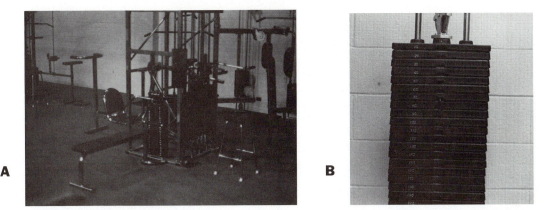

Figure 5-5   Isotonic equipment. **A,** Most exercise machines are isotonic. **B,** Resistance can be easily changed by changing the key in the stack of weights.

Free Weights versus Exercise Machines.   Various types of exercise equipment can be used with progressive resistive exercise, including free weights (barbells and dumbbells) or exercise machines such as Cybex, Universal, Nautilus, Eagle, Body Master, Keiser, Paramount, Continental, Pyramid, Sprint, Hydrafitness, Dynatrac, Future, and Bull. Dumbbells and barbells require the use of iron plates of varying weights that can be easily changed by adding or subtracting equal amounts of weight to both sides of the bar. The exercise machines for the most part have stacks of weights that are lifted through a series of levers or pulleys. The stack of weights slides up and down on a pair of bars that restrict the movement to only one plane. Weight can be increased or decreased simply by changing the position of a weight key (Figure 5-5).

There are advantages and disadvantages to free weights and machines. The exercise machines are relatively safe to use in comparison with free weights. For example, a bench press with free weights requires a partner to help lift the weight back onto the support racks if the lifter does not have enough strength to complete the lift; otherwise the weight might be dropped on the chest. With the machines the weight can be easily and safely dropped without fear of injury.

It is also a simple process to increase or decrease the weight by moving a single weight key with the exercise machines, although changes can generally be made only in increments of 10 or 15 pounds. With free weights, iron plates must be added or removed from each side of the barbell.

Athletes who have strength-trained using free weights and exercise machines realize the difference in the amount of weight that can be lifted. Unlike the ma-

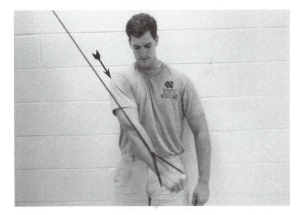

Figure 5-6   Strengthening exercises using surgical tubing are widely used in sport injury rehabilitation.

chines, free weights have no restricted motion and can thus move in many different directions, depending on the forces applied. With free weights, an element of muscular control on the part of the lifter to prevent the weight from moving in any other direction than vertical will usually decrease the amount of weight that can be lifted.[54]

Surgical Tubing or Theraband.   Surgical tubing or Theraband, as a means of providing resistance, has been widely used in sports medicine (Figure 5-6). The advantage of exercising with surgical tubing or Theraband is that the direction of movement is less restricted than with free weights or exercise machines. Thus exercise can be done against resistance in more functional movement planes. The use of surgical tubing exercise in plyometrics and PNF strengthening techniques will be discussed in

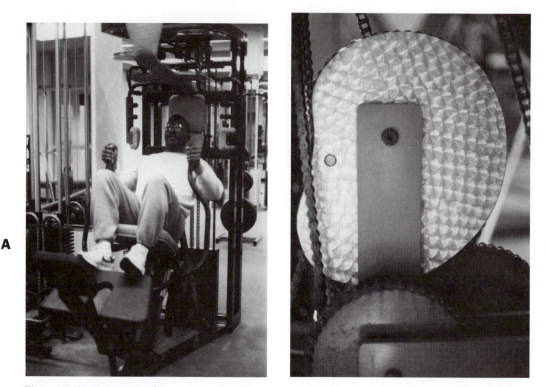

Figure 5-7   Exercise machines. **A,** Bench-press machine. **B,** The cam is designed to equalize resistance throughout the full range of motion.

Chapters 10 and 12. Surgical tubing can be used to provide resistance with the majority of the strengthening exercises shown in Chapters 19 through 26.

Regardless of which type of equipment is used, the same principles of progressive resistive exercise may be applied.

Variable Resistance.   One problem often mentioned in relation to progressive resistive exercise reconditioning is that the amount of force necessary to move a weight through a range of motion changes according to the angle of pull of the contracting muscle. It is greatest when the angle of pull is approximately 90 degrees. In addition, once the inertia of the weight has been overcome and momentum has been established, the force required to move the resistance varies according to the force the muscle can produce through the range of motion. Thus it has been argued that a disadvantage of any type of isotonic exercise is that the force required to move the resistance is constantly changing throughout the range of movement. This change in resistance at different points in the range of motion has been labeled **accommodating resistance** or **variable resistance.**

A number of exercise machine manufacturers have attempted to alleviate this problem of changing force capa-

bilities by using a cam in its pulley system (Figure 5-7). The cam is individually designed for each piece of equipment so that the resistance is variable throughout the movement. The cam is intended to alter resistance so that the muscle can handle a greater load, but at the points where the joint angle or muscle length is mechanically disadvantageous, it reduces the resistance to muscle movement. Whether this design does what it claims is debatable.

Progressive Resistive Exercise Techniques. Perhaps the single most confusing aspect of progressive resistive exercise is the terminology used to describe specific programs.[28] The following list of terms with their operational definitions may help clarify the confusion:

Repetitions: The number of times you repeat a specific movement

Repetition maximum (RM): The maximum number of repetitions at a given weight

Set: A particular number of repetitions

Intensity: The amount of weight or resistance lifted

Recovery period: The rest interval between sets

Frequency: The number of times an exercise is done in a week's period

Recommended Techniques of Resistance Training.   Specific recommendations for techniques of improving muscular strength are controversial among sports therapists. A considerable amount of research has been done in the area of resistance training relative to (1) the amount of weight to be used, (2) the number of repetitions, (3) the number of sets, and (4) the frequency of training.

A variety of specific programs have been proposed that recommend the optimal amount of weight, number of sets, number of repetitions, and frequency for producing maximal gains in levels of muscular strength. However, regardless of the techniques used, the healing process must dictate the specifics of any strength-training program. Certainly, to improve strength, the muscle must be progressively overloaded. The amount of weight used and the number of repetitions must be sufficient to make the muscle work at higher intensity than it is accustomed to. This factor is the most critical in any resistance training program. The resistance training program must also be designed to ultimately meet the specific competitive needs of the athlete.

One of the first widely accepted strength-development programs to be used in a rehabilitation program was developed by DeLorme and was based on a repetition maximum of 10 (10 RM).[14] The amount of weight used is what can be lifted exactly 10 times (Table 5-1).

Zinovieff proposed the Oxford technique, which, like DeLorme's program, was designed to be used in beginning, intermediate, and advanced levels of rehabilitation.[56] The only difference is that the percentage of maximum was reversed in the three sets (Table 5-2). MacQueen's technique[39] differentiates between beginning to intermediate and advanced levels, as is shown in Table 5-3.

Sanders' program (Table 5-4) was designed to be used in the advanced stages of rehabilitation and was based on a formula that used a percentage of body weight to determine starting weights.[46] The percentages below represent median starting points for different exercises:

Barbell squat—45% of body weight
Barbell bench press—30% of body weight
Leg extension—20% of body weight
Universal bench press—30% of body weight
Universal leg extension—20% of body weight
Universal leg curl—10 to 15% of body weight
Universal leg press—50% of body weight
Upright rowing—20% of body weight

Knight applied the concept of progressive resistive exercise in rehabilitation. His DAPRE (daily adjusted progressive resistive exercise) program (Tables 5-5 and 5-6) allows for individual differences in the rates at which patients progress in their rehabilitation programs.[30]

■ **TABLE 5-1**   DeLorme's Program

Set	Amount of Weight	Repetitions
1	50% of 10 RM	10
2	75% of 10 RM	10
3	100% of 10 RM	10

■ **TABLE 5-2**   The Oxford Technique

Set	Amount of Weight	Repetitions
1	50% of 10 RM	10
2	75% of 10 RM	10
3	100% of 10 RM	10

■ **TABLE 5-3**   McQueen's Technique

Sets	Amount of Weight	Repetitions
3 (Beginning/ intermediate)	100% of 10 RM	10
4–5 (Advanced)	100% of 2–3 RM	2–3

■ **TABLE 5-4**   Sanders' Program

Sets	Amount of Weight	Repetitions
Total of 4 sets (3 times per week)	100% of 5 RM	5
Day 1—4 sets	100% of 5 RM	5
Day 2—4 sets	100% of 3 RM	5
Day 3—1 sets	100% of 5 RM	5
2 sets	100% of 3 RM	5
2 sets	100% of 2 RM	5

Berger has proposed a technique that is adjustable within individual limitations (Table 5-7). For any given exercise, the amount of weight selected should be sufficient to allow 6 to 8 RM in each of the three sets, with a recovery period of 60 to 90 seconds between sets. Initial selection of a starting weight might require some trial and error to achieve this 6 to 8 RM range. If at least three sets of 6 RM cannot be completed, the weight is too heavy and should be reduced. If it is possible to do more than three sets of 8 RM, the weight is too light and should be increased.[7] Progression to heavier

■ **TABLE 5-5**   Knight's DAPRE Program

Set	Amount of Weight	Repetitions
1	50% of RM	10
2	75% of RM	6
3	100% of RM	Maximum
4	Adjusted working weight*	Maximum

*See Table 5-6.

■ **TABLE 5-6**   DAPRE Adjusted Working Weight

Number of Repetitions Performed During Third Set	Adjusted Working Weight During Fourth Set	Next Exercise Session
0–2	–5–10 lb	–5–10 lb
3–4	–0–5 lb	Same weight
5–6	Same weight	+5–10 lb
7–10	+5–10 lb	+5–15 lb
11	+10–15 lb	+10–20 lb

■ **TABLE 5-7**   Berger's Adjustment Technique

Sets	Amount of Weight	Repetitions
3	100% of 10 RM	6–8

weights is then determined by the ability to perform at least 8 RM in each of three sets. When progressing weight, an increase of about 10 percent of the current weight being lifted should still allow at least 6 RM in each of three sets.[8]

For rehabilitation purposes, strengthening exercises should be performed on a daily basis initially, with the amount of weight, number of sets, and number of repetitions governed by the injured athlete's response to the exercise. As the healing process progresses and pain or swelling is no longer an issue, a particular muscle or muscle group should be exercised consistently every other day. At that point the frequency of weight training should be at least 3 times per week but no more than 4 times per week. It is common for serious weight lifters to lift every day; however, they exercise different muscle groups on successive days. For example, Monday, Wednesday, and Friday might be used for upper-body muscles, with Tuesday, Thursday, and Saturday spent on lower-body muscles.

It has been suggested that if training is done properly, using both concentric and eccentric contractions, resistance training is necessary only twice each week. However, this schedule has not been sufficiently documented.

Isokinetic Exercise

An **isokinetic exercise** involves a muscle contraction in which the length of the muscle is changing while the contraction is performed at a constant velocity. In theory, maximal resistance is provided throughout the range of motion by the machine. The resistance provided by the machine will move only at some preset speed, regardless of the torque applied to it by the individual. Thus the key to isokinetic exercise is not the resistance but the speed at which resistance can be moved.

Several isokinetic devices are available commercially; Cybex, Orthotron, Biodex, and Kin-Com, are among the more common isokinetic devices (Figure 5-8). In general, they rely on hydraulic, pneumatic, and mechanical pressure systems to produce this constant velocity of motion. Most isokinetic devices are capable of resisting concentric and eccentric contractions at a fixed speed to exercise a muscle.

Isokinetics as a Conditioning Tool.   Isokinetic devices are designed so that regardless of the amount of force applied against a resistance, it can only be moved at a certain speed. That speed will be the same whether maximal force or only half the maximal force is applied. Consequently, in isokinetic training, it is absolutely necessary to exert as much force against the resistance as possible (maximal effort) for maximal strength gains to occur. Maximal effort is one of the major problems with an isokinetic strength-training program.

Anyone who has been involved in a resistance training program knows that on some days it is difficult to find the motivation to work out. Because isokinetic training requires a maximal effort, it is very easy to "cheat" and not go through the workout at a high level of intensity. In a progressive resistive exercise program, the athlete knows how much weight has to be lifted for how many repetitions. Thus isokinetic training is often more effective if a partner system is used, primarily as a means of motivation toward a maximal effort. When isokinetic training is done properly with a maximal effort, it is theoretically possible that maximal strength gains are best achieved through the isokinetic training method in which the velocity and force of the resistance are equal throughout the range of motion. However, there is no conclusive research to support this theory.

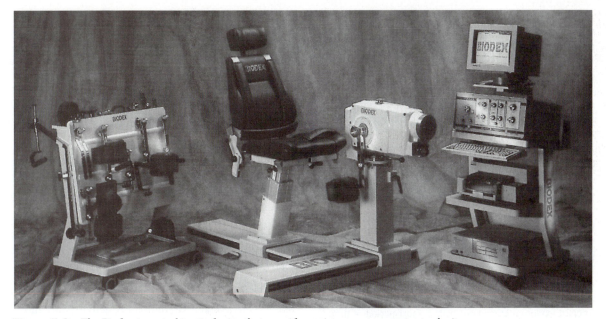

Figure 5-8   The Biodex is an isokinetic device that provides resistance at a constant velocity.

Whether this changing force capability is a deterrent to improving the ability to generate force against some resistance is debatable. In real life it does not matter whether the resistance is changing; what is important is that an individual develops enough strength to move objects from one place to another. The amount of strength necessary for athletes is largely dependent on their level of competition.

Another major disadvantage of using isokinetic devices as a conditioning tool is their cost. With initial purchase costs ranging between \$40,000 and \$60,000 and the necessity of regular maintenance and software upgrades, the use of an isokinetic device for general conditioning or resistance training is for the most part unrealistic. Thus isokinetic exercises are primarily used as a diagnostic and rehabilitative tool.

Isokinetics in Rehabilitation. Isokinetic strength testing gained a great deal of popularity throughout the 1980s in rehabilitation settings. This trend stems from its providing an objective means of quantifying existing levels of muscular strength and thus becoming useful as a diagnostic tool.[40]

Because the capability exists for training at specific speeds, comparisons have been made regarding the relative advantages of training at fast or slow speeds in a rehabilitation program. The research literature seems to indicate that strength increases from slow-speed training are relatively specific to the velocity used in training. Conversely, training at faster speeds seems to produce a more generalized increase in torque values at all velocities. Minimal hypertrophy was observed only while training at fast speeds, affecting only type II or fast-twitch fibers.[13,43] An increase in neuromuscular efficiency caused by more effective motor unit firing patterns has been demonstrated with slow-speed training.[36]

During the early 1990s, the value of isokinetic devices for quantifying torque values at functional speeds has been questioned. This issue, in addition to the theory and use of isokinetic exercise in a rehabilitation setting, will be discussed in detail in Chapter 9.

Circuit Training as a Rehabilitation Technique

Circuit training is a technique that might help the sports therapist maintain or perhaps improve levels of muscular strength or endurance in other parts of the body while the athlete allows for healing and reconditioning of an injured body part. Circuit training uses a series of exercise stations that consist of various combinations of weight training, flexibility, calisthenics, and brief aerobic exercises. Circuits can be designed to accomplish many different training goals. With circuit training the athlete moves rapidly from one station to the next, performing whatever exercise is to be done at that station within a specified time period. A typical circuit would consist of 8 to 12 stations, and the entire circuit would be repeated three times.

Circuit training is most definitely an effective technique for improving strength and flexibility. Certainly if the pace or time interval between stations is rapid and if work load is maintained at a high level of intensity with heart rates at or above target training levels, the cardiorespiratory system can benefit from this circuit. However, there is little research evidence that shows that circuit training is very effective in improving cardiorespiratory endurance. It should be, and is most often, used as a technique for developing and improving muscular strength and endurance.[23]

Plyometric Exercise

Plyometric exercise is a technique that is being increasingly incorporated into later stages of the rehabilitation program by the sports therapist. Plyometric training includes specific exercises that encompass a rapid stretch of a muscle eccentrically, followed immediately by a rapid concentric contraction of that muscle to facilitate and develop a forceful explosive movement over a short period of time.[16] The greater the stretch put on the muscle from its resting length immediately before the concentric contraction, the greater the resistance the muscle can overcome. Plyometrics emphasize the speed of the eccentric phase. The rate of stretch is more critical than the magnitude of the stretch. An advantage to using plyometric exercises is that they can help to develop eccentric control in dynamic movements.[34]

Plyometric exercises involve hops, bounds, and depth jumping for the lower extremity and the use of medicine balls and other types of weighted equipment for the upper extremity.[10,11] Depth jumping is an example of a plyometric exercise in which an individual jumps to the ground from a specified height and then quickly jumps again as soon as ground contact is made.[3]

Plyometrics tend to place a great deal of stress on the musculoskeletal system. The learning and perfection of specific jumping skills and other plyometric exercises must be technically correct and specific to one's age, activity, physical, and skill development. Plyometric exercise will be discussed in detail in Chapter 10.

OPEN- VERSUS CLOSED-KINETIC-CHAIN EXERCISES

The concept of the kinetic chain deals with the anatomical functional relationships that exist in the upper and lower extremities. In a weight-bearing position, the lower-extremity kinetic chain involves the transmission of forces among the foot, ankle, lower leg, knee, thigh, and hip. In the upper extremity, when the hand is in contact with a weight-bearing surface, forces are transmitted to the wrist, forearm, elbow, upper arm, and shoulder girdle.

An **open kinetic chain** exists when the foot or hand is not in contact with the ground or some other surface. In a **closed kinetic chain,** the foot or hand is weight bearing. Movements of the more proximal anatomical segments are affected by these open- versus closed-kinetic-chain positions. For example, the rotational components of the ankle, knee, and hip reverse direction when changing from open- to closed-kinetic-chain activity. In a closed kinetic chain the forces begin at the ground and work their way up through each joint. Also, in a closed kinetic chain, forces must be absorbed by various tissues and anatomical structures rather than simply dissipating as would occur in an open chain.

In rehabilitation, the use of closed-chain strengthening techniques has become a treatment of choice for many sports therapists. Most sport activities involve some aspect of weight bearing with the foot in contact with the ground or the hand in a weight-bearing position, so closed-kinetic-chain strengthening activities are more functional than open-chain activities. Therefore rehabilitative exercises should be incorporated that emphasize strengthening of the entire kinetic chain rather than an isolated body segment. Chapter 11 will discuss closed-kinetic-chain activities in detail.

TRAINING FOR MUSCULAR STRENGTH VERSUS MUSCULAR ENDURANCE

Muscular endurance was defined as the ability to perform repeated muscle contractions against resistance for an extended period of time. Most resistance training experts believe that muscular strength and muscular endurance are closely related.[17,41,47] As one improves, there is a tendency for the other to improve also.

It is generally accepted that when resistance training for strength, heavier weights with a lower number of repetitions should be used.[53] Conversely, endurance training uses relatively lighter weights with a greater number of repetitions.

It has been suggested that endurance training should consist of three sets of 10 to 15 repetitions,[8] using the same criteria for weight selection progression and frequency as recommended for progressive resistive exercise. Thus, suggested training regimens for muscular strength and endurance are similar in terms of sets and numbers of repetitions.[55] Persons who possess great levels of strength tend to also exhibit greater muscular endurance when asked to perform repeated contractions against resistance.[39]

RESISTANCE TRAINING DIFFERENCES BETWEEN MALES AND FEMALES

Resistance training is absolutely essential for an athlete. The approach to strength training is no different for female than for male athletes. However, some obvious physiological differences exist between the sexes.

The average woman will not build significant muscle bulk through resistance training. Significant muscle hypertrophy is dependent on the presence of the steroidal hormone **testosterone.** Testosterone is considered a male hormone, although all females possess some level of testosterone in their systems. Women with higher testosterone levels tend to have more masculine characteristics, such as increased facial and body hair, a deeper voice, and the potential to develop a little more muscle bulk.[19,41] For the average female athlete, developing large, bulky muscles through strength training is unlikely, although muscle tone can be improved. Muscle tone basically refers to the firmness of tension of the muscle during a resting state.

The initial stages of a resistance training program are likely to rapidly produce dramatic increases in levels of strength. For a muscle to contract, an impulse must be transmitted from the nervous system to the muscle. Each muscle fiber is innervated by a specific motor unit. By overloading a particular muscle, as in weight training, the muscle is forced to work more efficiently. Efficiency is achieved by getting more motor units to fire, thus causing more muscle fibers to contract, which results in a stronger contraction of the muscle. Consequently, both women and men often see extremely rapid gains in strength when a weight-training program is first begun. In the female, these initial strength gains, which can be attributed to improved neuromuscular efficiency, tend to plateau, and minimal improvement in muscular strength is realized during a continuing resistance training program. These initial neuromuscular strength gains are also seen in men, although their strength continues to increase with appropriate training. Again, women who possess higher testosterone levels have the potential to increase their strength further because they are able to develop greater muscle bulk.

Differences in strength levels between males and females are best illustrated when strength is expressed in relation to body weight minus fat. The reduced *strength/body weight ratio* in women is the result of their percentage of body fat. The strength/body weight ratio can be significantly improved through resistance training by decreasing the body fat percentage while increasing lean weight.[36]

The absolute strength differences are considerably reduced when body size and composition are considered. Leg strength can actually be stronger in the female than in the male, although upper-extremity strength is much greater in the male.[36]

RESISTANCE TRAINING IN THE YOUNG ATHLETE

The principles of resistance training discussed previously may be applied to the young athlete. There are certainly a number of sociological questions regarding the advantages and disadvantages of younger, in particular prepubescent, athletes engaging in rigorous strength-training programs. From a physiological perspective, experts have for years debated the value of strength training in young athletes. Recently, a number of studies have indicated that if properly supervised, young athletes can improve strength, power, endurance, balance, and proprioception; develop a positive body image; improve sport performance; and prevent injuries.[32] A prepubescent child can experience gains in levels of muscle strength without muscle hypertrophy.[42]

A sports therapist supervising a rehabilitation program for an injured young athlete should certainly incorporate resistive exercise into the program. However, close supervision, proper instruction, and appropriate modification of progression and intensity based on the extent of physical maturation of the individual is critical to the effectiveness of the resistive exercises.[32]

SPECIFIC RESISTIVE EXERCISES USED IN REHABILITATION

Because muscle contractions result in joint movement, the goal of resistance training in a rehabilitation program should be to either regain and perhaps increase the strength of a specific muscle that has been injured or to increase the efficiency of movement about a given joint.[36]

The exercises included throughout Chapter 19-26 show exercises for all motions about a particular joint rather than for each specific muscle. These exercises are demonstrated using free weights (dumbbells or bar weights) and some exercise machines. Other strengthening techniques widely used for injury rehabilitation involving isokinetic exercise, plyometrics, closed kinetic chain exercises, and PNF strengthening techniques will be discussed in greater detail in subsequent chapters.

Summary

1. Muscular strength may be defined as the maximal force that can be generated against resistance by a muscle during a single maximal contraction.
2. Muscular endurance is the ability to perform repeated isotonic or isokinetic muscle contractions or to sustain an isometric contraction without undue fatigue.
3. Muscular endurance tends to improve with muscular strength, thus training techniques for these two components are similar.
4. Muscular strength and endurance are essential components of any rehabilitation program.
5. Muscular power involves the speed with which a forceful muscle contraction is performed.
6. The ability to generate force is dependent on the physical properties of the muscle, neuromuscular efficiency, as well as the mechanical factors that dictate how much force can be generated through the lever system to an external object.
7. Hypertrophy of a muscle is caused by increases in the size and perhaps the number of actin and myosin protein myofilaments, which result in an increased cross-sectional diameter of the muscle.
8. The key to improving strength through resistance training is using the principle of overload within the constraints of the healing process.
9. Five resistance training techniques that can improve muscular strength are isometric exercise, progressive resistive exercise, isokinetic training, circuit training, and plyometric training.
10. Improvements in strength with isometric exercise occur at specific joint angles.
11. Progressive resistive exercise is the most common strengthening technique used by the sports therapist for rehabilitation after injury.
12. Circuit training involves a series of exercise stations consisting of resistance training, flexibility, and calisthenic exercises that can be designed to maintain fitness while reconditioning an injured body part.
13. Isokinetic training provides resistance to a muscle at a fixed speed.
14. Plyometric exercise uses a quick eccentric stretch to facilitate a concentric contraction.
15. Closed-kinetic-chain exercises might provide a more functional technique for strengthening of injured muscles and joints in the athletic population.
16. Women can significantly increase their strength levels but generally will not build muscle bulk as a result of strength training because of their relative lack of the hormone testosterone.

References

1. Alway, S. E., D. MacDougall, G. Sale, et al. 1988. Functional and structural adaptations in skeletal muscle of trained athletes. *Journal of Applied Physiology* 64:1114.
2. Astrand, P. O., and K. Rodahl. 1986. *Textbook of work physiology.* New York: McGraw-Hill.
3. Arnheim, D., and W. E. Prentice. 1997. *Principles of athletic training.* Madison, WI: Brown & Benchmark.
4. Baechle, T., and B. Groves. 1992. *Weight training: Steps to Success.* Champaign, IL: Leisure Press.
5. Baker, D., G. Wilson, and B. Carlyon. 1994. Generality vs. specificity: A comparison of dynamic and isometric measures of strength and speed-strength. *European Journal of Applied Physiology* 68:350–55.
6. Bandy, W., V. Lovelace-Chandler, B. Bandy, et al. 1990. Adaptation of skeletal muscle to resistance training. *Journal of Orthopaedic and Sports Physical Therapy* 12(6): 248–55.
7. Berger, R. 1973. *Conditioning for men.* Boston: Allyn & Bacon.
8. Berger, R. 1962. Effect of varied weight training programs on strength. *Research Quarterly for Exercise and Sport* 33:168.
9. Booth, F., and D. Thomason. 1991. Molecular and cellular adaptation of muscle in response to exercise: Perspectives of various models. *Physiol Rev* 71:541–85.
10. Chu, D. 1992. *Jumping into plyometrics.* Champaign, IL: Human Kinetics.
11. Chu, D. 1989. *Plyometric exercise with the medicine ball.* Livermore, CA: Bittersweet.
12. Costill, D., J. Daniels, W. Evan, et al. 1976. Skeletal muscle enzymes and fiber compositions in male and female track athletes. *Journal of Applied Physiology* 40:149.
13. Coyle, E., D. Feiring, T. Rotkis, et al. 1981. Specificity of power improvements through slow and fast speed isokinetic training. *Journal of Applied Physiology* 51:1437.
14. DeLorme, T., and A. Wilkins. 1951. *Progressive resistance exercise.* New York: Appleton-Century-Crofts.
15. Deudsinger, R. H. 1984. Biomechanics in clinical practice. *Phys Ther* 64:1860–68.
16. Duda, M. 1988. Plyometrics: A legitimate form of power training. *Physician and Sports Medicine* 16:213.
17. Dudley, G. A., and S. J. Fleck. 1987. Strength and endurance training: Are they mutually exclusive? [Review] *Sports Medicine* 4(2): 79.
18. Etheridge, G., and T. Thomas. 1982. Physiological and biomedical changes of human skeletal muscle induced by different strength training programs. *Medicine and Science in Sports and Exercise.* 14:141.

19. Fahey, T. 1994. *Basic weight training for men and women.* Mountain View, CA: Mayfield.

20. Faulkner, J., H. Green, and T. White. 1994. Response and adaptation of skeletal muscle to changes in physical activity. In *Physical activity, fitness, and health,* edited by C. Bouchard, R. Shepard, J. Stephens. Champaign, IL: Human Kinetics.

21. Fleck, S. J., and W. J. Kramer. 1988. Resistance training: Physiological responses and adaptations. *Physician and Sports Medicine* 16:108.

22. Gettman, L., P. Ward, and R. Hagan. 1982. A comparison of combined running and weight training with circuit weight training. *Medicine and Science in Sports and Exercise* 14:229.

23. Gettman, L. 1981. Circuit weight training: A critical review of its physiological benefits. *Physician and Sports Medicine* 9(1): 44.

24. Gonyea, W. 1980. Role of exercise in inducing increases in skeletal muscle fiber number. Journal of Applied Physiology 48:421.

25. Graves, J. E., M. Pollack, A. Jones, et al. 1989. Specificity of limited range of motion variable resistance training. *Medicine and Science in Sports and Exercise* 21:84.

26. Gray, G. W. 1996. Ecocentrics—A theoretical model for muscle function. (Manuscript submitted for publication.)

27. Harmen, E. 1994. The biomechanics of resistance training. In *Essentials of strength training and conditioning,* edited by T. Baechle. Champaign, IL: Human Kinetics.

28. Hickson, R., C. Hidaka, and C. Foster. 1994. Skeletal muscle fiber type, resistance training and strength-related performance. *Medicine and Science in Sports and Exercise* 26:593–98.

29. Hortobagyi, T., and F. I. Katch. 1990. Role of concentric force in limiting improvement in muscular strength. *Journal of Applied Physiology* 68:650.

30. Knight, K. 1979. Knee rehabilitation by the DAPRE technique. *American Journal of Sports Medicine and Physical Fitness* 7:336.

31. Komi, P. 1992. *Strength and power in sport.* London: Blackwell Scientific.

32. Kraemer, W. J., and S. J. Fleck. 1993. *Strength training for young athletes.* Champaign, IL: Human Kinetics.

33. Kraemer, W. J. 1994. General adaptations to resistance and endurance training programs. In *Essentials of strength training and conditioning,* edited by T. Baechle. Champaign, IL: Human Kinetics.

34. Kramer, J., A. Morrow, and A. Leger. 1993. Changes in rowing ergometer, weight lifting, vertical jump and isokinetic performance in response to standard and standard plus plyometric training programs. *International Journal of Sports Medicine* 14(8): 440–54.

35. Mastropolo, J. 1992. A test of maximum power theory for strength. *European Journal of Applied Physiology* 65:415-20.

36. McArdle, W., F. Katch, and V. Katch. 1994. *Exercise physiology, energy, nutrition, and human performance.* Philadelphia: Lea & Febiger.

37. McComas, A. 1994. Human neuromuscular adaptations that accompany changes in activity. *Medicine and Science in Sports and Exercise* 26(12): 1498–1509.

38. McGlynn, G. H. 1972. A reevaluation of isometric training. *Journal of Sports Medicine and Physical Fitness* 12:258.

39. MacQueen, I. 1954. Recent advance in the techniques of progressive resistance. *British Medical Journal* 11:11993.

40. Nicholas, J. J. 1989. Isokinetic testing in young nonathletic able-bodied subjects [Review]. *Archives of Physical Medicine and Rehabilitation* 70(3): 210.

41. Nygard, C. H., T. Luophaarui, T. Suurnakki, et al. 1988. Muscle strength and muscle endurance of middle-aged women and men associated to type, duration and intensity of muscular load at work. *Int Arch Occup Environ Health* 60(4): 291.

42. Ozmun, J., A. Mikesky, and P. Surburg. 1994. Neuromuscular adaptations following prepubescent strength training. *Medicine and Science in Sports and Exercise* 26:514.

43. Pipes, T., and J. Wilmore. 1975. Isokinetic vs. isotonic strength training in adult men. *Medicine and Science in Sports and Exercise* 7:262.

44. Rehfeldt, H., G. Caffiber, H. Kramer, et al. 1989. Force, endurance time, and cardiovascular responses in voluntary isometric contractions of different muscle groups. *Biomed Biochim Acta* 48(5–6): S509.

45. Sale, D., and D. MacDougall. 1981. Specificity in strength training: A review for the coach and athlete. *Canadian Journal of Applied Sports Science* 6:87.

46. Sanders, M. 1990. Weight training and conditioning. In *Sports physical therapy,* edited by B. Sanders. Norwalk, CT: Appleton & Lange.

47. Smith, T. K. 1981. Developing local and general muscular endurance. *Athletic Journal* 62:42.

48. Soest, A., and M. Bobbert. 1993. The role of muscle properties in control of explosive movements. *Biol Cybern* 69:195–204.

49. Staron, R. S., D. L. Karapondo, and W. J. Kreamer. 1994. Skeletal muscle adaptations during early phase of heavy resistance training in men and women. *Journal of Applied Physiology* 76:1247–55.

50. Stone, M., S. Fleck, and N. Triplett. 1991. Health and performance related potential of resistance training. *Sports Medicine* 11:210–31.

51. Strauss, R. H., ed. 1991. *Sportsmedicine.* Philadelphia: W. B. Saunders.

52. Ulmer, H., W. Knierman, T. Warlow, et al. 1989. Interindividual variability of isometric endurance with regard to the endurance performance limit for static work. *Biomed Biochim Acta* 48(5–6): S504.

53. Van Etten, L., E. Verstappen, and K. Westerterp. 1994. Effect of body building on weight training induced adaptations in body composition and muscular strength. *Medicine and Science in Sports and Exercise* 26:515–21.

54. Weltman, A., and B. Stamford. 1982. Strength training: Free weights vs. machines. *Physician and Sports Medicine* 10:197.

55. Yates, J. W. 1987. Recovery of dynamic muscular endurance. *European Journal of Applied Physiology* 56(6): 662.

56. Zinovieff, A. 1951. Heavy resistance exercise: The Oxford technique. *Br. J. Physiol Med* 14:129.

CHAPTER 6

Reestablishing Neuromuscular Control

Scott Lephart
C. Buz Swanik
Freddie Fu

After completion of this chapter, the student should be able to do the following:

- Explain why neuromuscular control is essential in the rehabilitation process.

- Define proprioception, kinesthesia, and neuromuscular control.

- Discuss the physiology of articular and tenomuscular mechanoreceptors.

- Discuss the neural pathways of the peripheral efferent pathways.

- Discuss the importance of feed-forward and feedback neuromuscular control.

- Discuss the various techniques for reestablishing neuromuscular control in both the upper and the lower extremities.

WHY IS NEUROMUSCULAR CONTROL CRITICAL TO THE REHABILITATION PROCESS?

Reestablishing neuromuscular control is a critical component in the rehabilitation of pathological joints. The objective of the neuromuscular control activities is to integrate peripheral sensations relative to joint loads and process these signals into coordinated motor responses. This muscle activity serves to protect joint structures from excessive strain and provides a prophylactic mechanism to recurrent injury. Neuromuscular control activities are intended to complement traditional rehabilitation protocols, which encompass the modulation of pain and inflammation as well as regaining flexibility, strength, and endurance.

In the domain of joint motion and position awareness, basic science research has provided insight into the sensory and/or motor characteristics of structures regulating neuromuscular control. Peripheral mechanoreceptors within articular and tenomuscular structures mediate neuromuscular control by conveying joint motion and position sense to the individual. The primary roles of articular structures such as the capsule, ligaments, menisci, and labrum are to stabilize and guide skeletal segments while providing mechanical restraint to abnormal joint movements.[101] However, capsuloligamentous tissue also has a sensory role essential for detecting joint motion and position.[27,51,87] Tenomuscular receptors contribute to joint motion and position sensation via changes in muscle length, and have been implicated in the regulation of muscle stiffness.[3,45,46,80] Increased muscle stiffness, prior to joint loading, is another mechanism utilized for dynamic restraint of joints.[24] Muscles preactivated

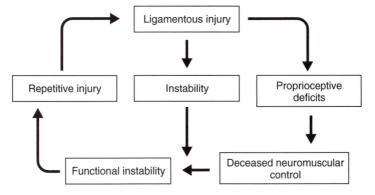

Figure 6-1 Functional stability paradigm depicting the influence of mechanical instability and proprioceptive deficits on neuromuscular control and functional stability, which predisposes the knee to repetitive injury.

might have a greater impact on knee stability than previously anticipated. Recently, the interaction between joint and muscle receptors has received even greater appreciation for contributing to the dynamic restraint system prior to and succeeding joint pathology.[19,27,46]

Injury to articular structures results not only in a mechanical disturbance, but also in a loss of joint sensation, due to deafferentation of peripheral mechanoreceptors.[47,85,90] This partial deafferentation disrupts sensory feedback necessary for reflexive joint stabilization and neuromuscular coordination. There is substantial evidence suggesting that the aberrations in muscle activity subsequent to joint injury are a result of disrupted reflex pathways.[11,17,47,63,83,94,98] Therefore, joint pathology not only reduces mechanical stability, it often diminishes the capability of the dynamic restraint system, rendering the joint functionally unstable (Figure 6-1).

Reconstructive surgery combined with rehabilitation restores the mechanical stability and partially reestablishes the neuromuscular characteristic associated with the dynamic restraint system.[9,66,68] Clinical research has revealed a number of activities that promote these characteristics and are beneficial to developing neuromuscular control. To accomplish this, clinicians must identify the peripheral and central neuromuscular characteristics that compensate for mechanical insufficiencies and encourage these adaptations, restoring functional stability.

Rehabilitation of the pathological joint should address the anticipatory (feed-forward) and reflexive (feedback) neuromuscular control mechanisms required for joint stability. Four elements crucial for reestablishing neuromuscular control and functional stability are joint proprioception and kinesthesia, dynamic stability, preparatory and reactive muscle characteristics, and conscious and unconscious functional motor patterns.[67]

The following sections will define the sensory receptors and neural pathways that contribute to normal joint stabilization. The theoretical framework for reestablishing neuromuscular control will be presented, followed by specific activities designed to encourage the peripheral, spinal, and cortical adaptations crucial for improving functional stability.

WHAT IS NEUROMUSCULAR CONTROL?

Proprioception refers to conscious and unconscious appreciation of joint position, while **kinesthesia** is the sensation of joint motion or acceleration.[79] Proprioceptive and kinesthetic signals are transmitted to the spinal cord via afferent (sensory) pathways. Conscious awareness of joint motion and position is essential for proper joint function in sport and activities of daily living, while unconscious proprioception modulates muscle function and initiates reflex stabilization. The efferent (motor) response to sensory information is termed **neuromuscular control**.[49] Two motor control mechanisms are involved with interpreting afferent information and coordinating efferent responses.[23,50] *Feed-forward neuromuscular control* involves planning movements based on sensory information from past experiences.[23,59] The *feedback* process continuously regulates motor control through reflex pathways. Feed-forward mechanisms are responsible for preparatory muscle activity; feedback processes are associated with reactive muscle activity. Because of skeletal muscle's orientation and activation characteristics, a diverse array of movement capabilities can be coordinated involving concentric, eccentric, and isometric contractions, while excessive joint motion is restricted. Therefore dynamic restraint is achieved through preparatory and reflexive neuromuscular control.[22,23,33,36,42]

The level of muscle activation, whether it is preparatory or reactive, greatly modifies its stiffness properties.[80,85] From a mechanical perspective, **muscle stiffness** is the ratio in the change of force to the change in length.[3,22,24] In essence, muscles that are more stiff resist stretching episodes more effectively, have greater tone, and provide more effective dynamic restraint to joint displacement.[3,74]

Clinical studies addressing the role of muscle stiffness in the dynamic restraint system have been limited. In the knee, McNair[74] demonstrated that increased hamstring muscle activation also significantly increased hamstring stiffness, and that there is a moderate correlation between the degree of muscle stiffness in ACL-deficient athletes and their functional ability.[74] Therefore athletes with greater hamstring stiffness were more functional. Efficient regulation of muscle stiffness might embody all of the components in the dynamic restraint system, and thus be vital for restoring functional stability.

THE PHYSIOLOGY OF MECHANORECEPTORS

Articular Mechanoreceptors

The dynamic restraint system is mediated by specialized nerve endings called mechanoreceptors.[35] A mechanoreceptor functions by transducing mechanical deformation of tissue into frequency-modulated neural signals.[35] An increased stimulus of deformation is coded by an increased afferent discharge rate or a rise in the quantity of mechanoreceptors activated.[35,38] These signals provide sensory information concerning internal and external forces acting on the joint. Three morphological types of mechanoreceptors have been identified in the knee: Pacinian corpuscles, Meissner corpuscles, and free nerve endings.[27,35,53] These mechanoreceptors are classified as either quick adapting (QA), because they cease discharging shortly after the onset of a stimulus, or slow adapting (SA), because they continue to discharge while the stimulus is present.[18,27,35,51,86] In healthy joints, QA mechanoreceptors are believed to provide conscious and unconscious kinesthetic sensations in response to joint movement or acceleration while SA mechanoreceptors provide continuous feedback and thus proprioceptive in-

formation relative to joint position.[18,29,35,89] Debate exists over the relative contribution of articular afferents in the dynamic restraint system, because mechanoreceptors in articular structures appear to be stimulated only when under considerable loads.[92] Sensory organs in the musculotendinous unit largely provide continuous feedback during submaximal loading.

Tenomuscular Mechanoreceptors

Changes in joint position are accompanied by simultaneous alterations in muscle length and tension. Muscle spindles, embedded within skeletal muscle, detect length and rate of length changes, transmitting these signals by way of afferent nerves.[4,19,38] Muscle spindles are also innervated by small motor fibers called gamma efferents.[4,38,62] This independent arrangement of sensory and motor fibers permits the muscle spindle to accommodate for muscle length and rate of length changes while continuously transmitting afferent signals.[4,38] Muscle spindle afferents project directly on skeletal motoneurons through very fast monosynaptic reflexes.[100] When muscle spindles are stimulated, they elicit a reflex contraction in the agonist muscle. Increased signals from the gamma motor nerves heighten the stretch sensitivity of muscle spindles.[45,46] This is the mechanism (stretch reflex) whereby muscle spindles have the capacity to mediate muscle activity.[45,76,100]

Golgi tendon organs (GTO) are also capable of regulating muscle activity and are responsible for monitoring muscle tension.[43] Located within the tendon and tenomuscular junction, GTOs serve to protect the tenomuscular unit by reflexively inhibiting muscle activation when excessive tension might cause damage. Therefore GTOs have the opposite effect of muscle spindles by producing a reflex inhibition (relaxation) in the muscle being loaded.[35,43]

NEURAL PATHWAYS OF PERIPHERAL AFFERENTS

Understanding the extent to which articular and tenomuscular sensory information is utilized requires analysis of the reflexive and cortical pathways employed by peripheral afferents. Encoded signals concerning joint motion and position are transmitted from peripheral receptors, via afferent pathways, to the central nervous system (CNS).[25,27] Ascending pathways to the cerebral cortex provide conscious appreciation of proprioception and kinesthesia. Two reflexive pathways couple articular receptors with motor nerves and tenomuscular receptors by way of interneurons in the spinal column. A third monosynaptic reflex pathway links the muscle spindles directly with motor nerves. Sensory information from the periphery is utilized by cerebral cortex for somatosensory awareness and feed-forward neuromuscular control, whereas balance and postural control are processed at the brain stem.[19,29,38,50] Balance is influenced by the same peripheral afferent mechanism that mediates joint proprioception and is partially dependent upon the inherent ability to integrate joint position sense with neuromuscular control. Balance, therefore, is frequently used to measure functional joint stability, and deficits can result from aberrations in the afferent feedback loop of the lower extremity.

Synapses at the spinal level link afferent fibers from articular and tenomuscular receptors with efferent motor nerves, constituting the reflex loops between sensory information and motor responses. This reflexive neuromotor link contributes to dynamic stability by utilizing the feedback process for reactive muscular activation.[13,83,92] Interneurons within the spinal column connect articular receptors and GTOs with large motor nerves innervating muscles and small gamma motor nerves innervating muscle spindles. Johansson[46] contends that articular afferent pathways do not exert as much influence directly on skeletal motoneurons as previously reported, but rather they have more frequent and potent effects on muscle spindles. Muscle spindles, in turn, regulate muscle activation through the monosynaptic stretch reflex. Articular afferents therefore have some influence on the large skeletal motor nerves as well as the tenomuscular receptors, via gamma motor nerves.[45,46,47]

This sophisticated articular-tenomuscular link has been described as the "final common input."[2,47] The final common input suggests that muscle spindles integrate peripheral afferent information and transmit a final modified signal to the (CNS).[2,47] This feedback loop is responsible for continuously modifying muscle activity during locomotion via the muscle spindle's stretch reflex arc.[40,80] By coordinating reflexive and descending motor commands, muscle stiffness is modified and dynamic stability is maintained.[47,56]

FEED-FORWARD AND FEEDBACK NEUROMUSCULAR CONTROL

The efferent response of muscles transforming neural information into physical energy is termed neuromuscular control.[49] Traditional beliefs about the processing of afferent signals into efferent responses for dynamic stabilization were based on reactive or feedback neuromuscular control pathways.[62] More-contemporary theories emphasize the significance of preactivated muscle tension in anticipation of movements and joint loads. The preac-

tivation theory suggests that prior sensory feedback (experience) concerning the task is utilized to preprogram muscle activation patterns. This process is described as feed-forward neuromuscular control.[22,24,34,59] Feed-forward motor control utilizes advance information about a task, usually from experience, to preprogram muscle activity.[23,59] These centrally generated motor commands are responsible for preparatory muscle activity and high-velocity movements.[50]

Preparatory muscle activity serves several functions that contribute to the dynamic restraint system. By increasing muscle activation levels, the stiffness properties of the entire tenomuscular unit are increased.[77] This increased muscle activation and stiffness can drastically improve the stretch sensitivity of the muscle spindle system while reducing the electromechanical delay required to develop muscle tension.[20,22,36,42,47,74,77,85] Clinical research has also shown that the stretch reflex can increase muscle stiffness one to three times.[39,69] Heightened stretch sensitivity and stiffness could improve the reactive capabilities of muscle by providing additional sensory feedback and superimposing stretch reflexes onto descending motor commands.[22,48,75]

Whether muscle stiffness increases stretch sensitivity or decreases electromechanical delay, it appears to be crucial for dynamic restraint and functional stability (Figure 6-2). Preactivated muscles therefore can provide quick compensation for external loads and are critical for dynamic joint stability.[22,36] Sensory information about the task is then used to evaluate the results and help arrange future muscle activation strategies.

The feedback mechanism of motor control is characterized by numerous reflex pathways continuously adjusting ongoing muscle activity.[14,23,62,76] Information from joint and muscle receptors reflexively coordinates muscle activity toward the completion of a task. This feedback process, however, results in long conduction delays and is best equipped for maintaining posture and regulating slow movements.[50] The efficacy of reflex-mediated dynamic stabilization is therefore related to the speed and magnitude of joint perturbations. It is unclear what relative contribution feedback mediated muscle reflexes provide when in vivo loads are placed on joints.

Both feed-forward and feedback neuromuscular control can enhance dynamic stability if the sensory and motor pathways are frequently stimulated. Each time a signal passes through a sequence of synapses, the synapses become more capable of transmitting the same signal.[38,41] When these pathways are "facilitated" regularly, memory of that signal is created and can be recalled to program future movements.[38] Frequent facilitation therefore enhances both the memory about tasks for

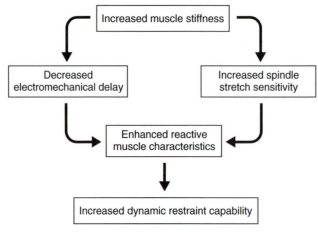

Figure 6-2 Diagram depicting the influence of muscle stiffness on electromechanical delay and muscle spindle sensitivity, which enhances the reactive characteristics of muscle for dynamic joint restraint.

preprogrammed motor control and reflex pathways for reactive neuromuscular control.

REESTABLISHING NEUROMUSCULAR CONTROL

Athletes who have sustained damage to the articular structures in the upper or lower extremities exhibit distinctive proprioceptive, kinesthetic, and neuromuscular deficits.[5,11,13,61,63,68,70,88,89,91,98] Although identifying these abnormalities might be difficult in a clinical setting, a thorough appreciation of the pathoetiology of these conditions is necessary to guide clinicians who are attempting to reestablish neuromuscular control and functional stability.

Most researchers believe that disruption of the articular structures results in some level of deafferentation to ligamentous and probably capsular mechanoreceptors.[21,26,61,63,68,70, 89,91] In the acute phase of healing, joint inflammation and pain can compound sensory deficits; however, this can not account for the chronic deficits in proprioception and kinesthesia associated with pathological joints.[8,53] Research has demonstrated that athletes with congenital or pathological joint laxity have diminished capability for detecting joint motion and position.[28,31,91] These proprioceptive and kinesthetic characteristics, coupled with mechanical instability, lead to functional instability.[62,66]

Developing or reestablishing proprioception, kinesthesia, and neuromuscular control in the injured athletes

will minimize the risk of reinjury. Capsuloligamentous retensioning and reconstruction, coupled with traditional rehabilitation, is one option that appears to restore some kinesthetic awareness, although not equal to that of noninvolved limbs.[10,21,66]

The objective of neuromuscular rehabilitation is to develop or reestablish afferent and efferent characteristics that enhance dynamic restraint capabilities with respect to in vivo loads. Four basic elements are crucial to reestablishing neuromuscular control and functional stability: (1) proprioceptive and kinesthetic sensation, (2) dynamic joint stabilization, (3) reactive neuromuscular control, and (4) functional motor patterns.[62] In the pathological joint these dynamic mechanisms are compensatory for the lack of static restraints, and can result in a functionally stable joint.

Several afferent and efferent characteristics contribute to the efficient regulation of these elements and the maintenance of neuromuscular control. These characteristics include the sensitivity of peripheral receptors and facilitation of afferent pathways, muscle stiffness, the onset rate and magnitude of muscle activity, agonist/antagonist coactivation, reflex muscle activation, and discriminatory muscle activation. Specific rehabilitation techniques allow these characteristics to be modified, significantly impacting dynamic stability and function.[12,44,61,99]

Although clinical research continues, several exercise techniques show promise for inducing beneficial adaptations to these characteristics while the plasticity of the neuromuscular system permits rapid modifications during rehabilitation that enhance preparatory and reactive muscle activity.[12,41,43,44,67,99] The techniques include closed-kinetic-chain activities, balance training, eccentric and high-repetition/low-load exercises, reflex facilitation through reactive training, stretch-shortening activities, and biofeedback training. Traditional rehabilitation, accompanied by these specific techniques, results in beneficial adaptations to the neuromuscular characteristics responsible for dynamic restraint, ultimately enhancing their efficiency for providing a functionally stable joint.

In order to restore dynamic muscle activation necessary for functional stability, one must employ simulated positions of vulnerability that necessitate reactive muscle stabilization. Although there are inherent risks in placing the joint in positions of vulnerability, if this is done in a controlled and progressive fashion, neuromuscular adaptations will occur and subsequently permit the athlete to return to competitive situations with confidence that the dynamic mechanisms will protect the joint from subluxation and reinjury.

Neuromuscular Characteristics

Peripheral Afferent Receptors. The foundation for feedback and feed-forward neuromuscular control is reliable kinesthetic and proprioceptive information. Altered peripheral afferent information can disrupt preparatory and reactive muscle activity, affecting motor control and functional stability. Closed-kinetic-chain exercises create axial loads that maximally stimulate articular receptors while tenomuscular receptors are excited by changes in length and tension.[18,35,47,96,97,102] Chronic athletic participation can also enhance proprioceptive and kinesthetic acuity by repeatedly facilitating afferent pathways from peripheral receptors. Highly conditioned athletes demonstrate greater appreciation of joint kinesthesia and more accurately reproduce limb position than sedentary controls.[6,64,69] Whether this is a congenital anomaly or a training adaptation, greater awareness of joint motion and position can improve feed-forward and feedback neuromuscular control.[64]

Muscle Stiffness. It is evident that muscle stiffness has a significant role in preparatory and reactive dynamic restraint by resisting and absorbing joint loads.[71,73,74] Therefore exercise modes that increase muscle stiffness should be encouraged during rehabilitation. Research by Bulbulian and Pousson[15,84] has established that eccentric loading increases muscle tone and stiffness. Chronic overloading of the musculotendinous unit can result in connective tissue proliferation, desensitizing GTOs and increasing muscle spindle activity.[43] Such evo-lutions impact both the neuromuscular and the tendinous components of stiffness.[15,33,77,84]

Training techniques that emphasize low loads and high repetitions cause connective tissue adaptations similar to those found with eccentric training. However, increased muscle stiffness resulting from this rehabilitation technique can be attributed to fiber type transition.[33,43,57,58] Slow-twitch fibers have longer crossbridge cycle times and can maintain the prolonged, low-intensity contractions necessary for postural control.[58] Goubel[33] found, in the animal model, that low-load/high-repetition training resulted in higher muscle stiffness, compared to strength training. However, Kyrolaninen's[58] analysis of power- and endurance-trained athletes inferred that muscle stiffness was greater in the power-trained individuals, because the onset of muscle preactivation (EMG) was faster and higher prior to joint loading. It appears that endurance training might enhance stiffness by increasing the baseline motor tone and crossbridge formation time, while power training alters the rate and magnitude of muscle tension during preactivation. Both of these adaptations readily adhere to existing principles of progressive rehabilitation, where early strengthening exercises focus on low loads with high repetitions, progressing to shorter, more explosive, sport-specific activities. Research assessing the efficacy of low-load/high-repetition training versus high-load/low-repetition training would be beneficial for optimizing muscle stiffness and functional progression in the injured athlete.

Reflex Muscle Activation. Various training modes also cause neuromuscular adaptations that might account for discrepancies in the reflex latency times between power- and endurance-trained athletes. Sprint- and/or power-trained individuals have more vigorous reflex responses (tendon-tap) relative to sedentary and endurance-trained samples.[54,55,93] McComas[72] suggests that strength training increases descending (cortical) drive to the large motor nerves of skeletal muscle and the small efferent fibers to muscle spindles, referred to as alpha-gamma coactivation. Increasing both muscle tension and efferent drive to muscle spindles results in a heightened sensitivity to stretch, consequently reducing reflex latencies.[43] Melvill-Jones[75] suggests that the stretch reflexes are superimposed on preprogrammed muscle activity from higher centers, illustrating the concomitant use of feed-forward and feedback neuromuscular control for regulating preparatory and reactive muscle stiffness. Therefore, preparatory and reactive muscle activation might improve dynamic stability and function if muscle stiffness is enhanced in a mechanically insufficient or reconstructed joint.

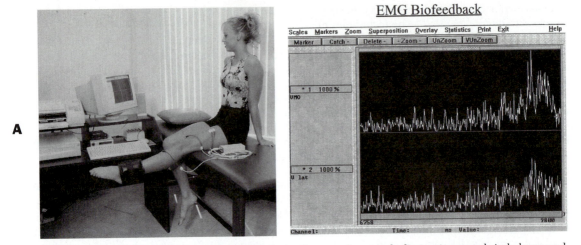

Figure 6-3   Biofeedback training reestablishes discriminative muscle control, eliminating muscle imbalance and promoting functionally specific muscle activation patterns.

A limited number of clinical training studies have been directed at improving reaction times.[12,44,99] Ihara[44] significantly reduced the latency of muscle reactions over a 3-week period by inducing perturbations to athletes on unstable platforms. Several other researchers later confirmed this finding with rehabilitation programs designed to improve reflex muscle activation.[12,99] Beard[12] and Wojtyes[99] suggest that agility-type training, in the lower extremity, produces more-desirable muscle reaction times when compared to strength training. This research has significant implications for reestablishing the reactive capability of the dynamic restraint system. Reducing the electromechanical delay between joint loading and protective muscle activation can increase dynamic stability and function.

Discriminative Muscle Activation.   In addition to reactive muscle firing, unconscious control of muscle activation patterns is critical for balancing internal and external joint forces. This very evident relative to the force couples described for the shoulder complex. Restoring the force couples of agonist and antagonists might initially require conscious, discriminative muscle activation before unconscious control is acquired. Biofeedback training provides instantaneous sensory feedback concerning muscle activation patterns and can help athletes correct errors by consciously altering or redistributing muscle activity.[10,30] The objective of biofeedback training is to reacquire voluntary muscle control and promote functionally specific motor patterns, eventually converting these patterns from conscious to unconscious control[10] (Figure 6-3). Using biofeedback for discriminative muscle control can help eliminate muscle imbalances

while reestablishing preparatory and reactive muscle activity for dynamic joint stability.[23,30]

Elements for Neuromuscular Control

Proprioception and Kinesthesia.   The objective of kinesthetic and proprioceptive training is to restore the neurosensory properties of injured capsuloligamentous structures and enhance the sensitivity of uninvolved peripheral afferents.[67] To what degree this occurs in conservatively managed athletes is unknown; however, ligament retensioning and reconstruction coupled with extensive rehabilitation does appear to normalize joint motion and position sense.[9,66]

Joint compression is believed to maximally stimulate articular receptors and can be accomplished with closed-chain exercises throughout the available ROM.[18,35,47,96,97] Early joint repositioning tasks enhance conscious proprioceptive and kinesthetic awareness, eventually leading to unconscious appreciation of joint motion and position. Applying a neoprene sleeve or elastic bandage can provide additional proprioceptive and kinesthetic information by stimulating cutaneous receptors[9,66,82] (Figure 6-4).

Dynamic Stabilization.   The objective of dynamic joint stabilization exercises is to encourage preparatory agonist/antagonist coactivation. Efficient coactivation restores the force couples necessary to balance joint forces and increase joint congruency, thereby reducing the loads imparted to the static structures. Dynamic stabilization from muscles requires anticipating and reacting to joint loads. This includes placing the joint in positions of

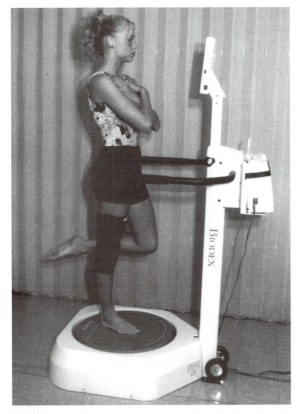

Figure 6-4   Neoprene sleeves stimulate cutaneous receptors, providing additional sensory feedback for joint motion and position awareness.

cises should induce unanticipated joint perturbations if they are expected to facilitate reflex muscle activation. Reflex-mediated muscle activity is a crucial element in the dynamic restraint mechanism and should complement preprogrammed muscle activity to achieve a functionally stable joint.

Functional Activities.   The objective of functional rehabilitation is to return the athlete to preinjury activity level while minimizing the risk of reinjury.[65] This includes restoring functional stability and sport-specific movement patterns or skills, then utilizing functional tests to assess the athlete's readiness to return to full participation. Functional activities incorporate all of the available resources for stimulating peripheral afferents, muscle coactivation, and reflex and preprogrammed motor control. Emphasis should be placed on sport-specific techniques, including positions and maneuvers where the joint is vulnerable. With repetition and controlled intensity, muscle activity (preparatory and reactive) gradually progresses from conscious to unconscious motor control.[50] Implementing these activities will help athletes develop functionally specific movement repertoires, within a controlled setting, decreasing the risk of injury upon completion of rehabilitation.

Understanding the afferent and efferent characteristics that contribute to joint sensation, dynamic stabilization, reflex activity, and functional motor pattern is necessary for reestablishing neuromuscular control and functional stability (Table 6-1).

Lower-Extremity Techniques

Many activities that promote neuromuscular control in the lower extremity exist in traditional rehabilitation schemes. Early kinesthetic training and joint repositioning tasks can begin to reestablish reflex pathways from articular afferents to skeletal motor nerves, the muscle spindle system, and cortical motor control centers, while enhancing muscle stiffness increases the stretch sensitivity of tenomuscular receptors. To induce adaptations in muscle stiffness, exercises should be performed with high repetitions and low rest intervals, focusing on the eccentric phase. Increased muscle stiffness will heighten the stretch sensitivity of tenomuscular receptors, providing additional sensory information concerning joint motion and position.

These techniques should focus on individual muscle groups that require attention and progress from no weight to weight assisted. The use of closed-chain activities is encouraged because they replicate the environment specific to the lower-extremity function. Partial weight bearing, in pools or with unloading devices,

vulnerability where dynamic support is established under controlled conditions. Balance and stretch-shortening exercises both require preparatory and reactive muscle activity through feed-forward and feedback motor control systems, while closed-kinetic-chain exercises are excellent for inducing coactivation and compression.

Reactive Neuromuscular Control.   Reactive neuromuscular training focuses on stimulating the reflex pathways from articular and tenomuscular receptors to skeletal muscle. Although preprogrammed muscle stiffness can enhance the reactive capability of muscles by reducing reflex latency time, the objective is to generate joint perturbations that are not anticipated, stimulating reflex stabilization. The efficacy of reactive neuromuscular exercises was demonstrated nearly a decade ago.[44] Persistent use of these reflex pathways can decrease the response time and develop reactive strategies to unexpected joint loads.[38] Furthermore, Caraffa[16] significantly reduced the incidence of knee injuries in soccer players who performed reactive type training. All reactive exer-

■ **TABLE 6-1** The Elements, Rehabilitation Techniques, and Afferent/Efferent Characteristics Necessary for Restoring Proprioception and Neuromuscular Control

Elements	Rehabilitation Techniques	Afferent/Efferent Characteristics
Proprioception and Kinesthesia	Joint repositioning Functional range of motion Axial loading Closed-kinetic-chain exercises	Peripheral receptor sensitivity Facilitate afferent pathways
Dynamic Stability	Closed-kinetic-chain exercises and translatory forces High-repetition/low-resistance Eccentric loading Stretch-shortening exercises Balance training	Agonist/antagonist coactivation Muscle activation rate and amplitude Peripheral receptor sensitivity Muscle stiffness
Reactive Neuromuscular Control	Reaction to joint perturbation Stretch shortening, plyometrics Balance reacquisition	Reflex facilitation Muscle activation rate and amplitude
Functional Motor Patterns	Biofeedback Sport-specific drills Control-progressive participation	Discriminatory muscle activation Arthrokinematics Coordinated locomotion

simulates the closed-chain environment without subjecting the ankle, knee, or hip to excessive joint loads.[52] The closed-chain nature of these exercises creates joint compression, thus enhancing joint congruency and neurosensory feedback, while minimizing shearing forces on the joints.[81]

Early dynamic joint stabilization exercises begin with balance training and partial weight bearing on stable surfaces, progressing to partial weight bearing on unstable surfaces. Balancing on unstable surfaces is initiated once full weight bearing is achieved. Exercises such as "kickers" also require balance and can begin on stable surfaces, progressing to unstable platforms (Figure 6-5).

Slide board training and basic strength exercises can be instituted to stimulate coactivation while increasing muscular force and endurance. Strength exercises focus on eccentric and endurance-type activities in a closed kinetic orientation, further enhancing dynamic stability through increases in preparatory muscle stiffness and reactive characteristics. Eccentric loading is accomplished by activities such as forward and backward stairclimbing or backward downhill walking. Strength and balance exercises can be combined and executed with light external forces to increase the level of difficulty (Figure 6-6).

Biofeedback can also help athletes trying to develop agonist/antagonist coactivation during strength exercises. Biofeedback provides additional information concerning muscle activation and encourages voluntary muscle activation by facilitating efferent pathways. Reeducating injured athletes through selective muscle activation is necessary for dynamic stabilization and neuromuscular control.

Stretch-shortening exercises are a necessary component for conditioning the neuromuscular apparatus to respond more quickly and forcefully, permitting eccentric deceleration then developing explosive concentric contractions.[1] Stretch-shortening exercises need not be withheld until the late stages of rehabilitation. There is a variety of plyometric activities, and intensity can be controlled by manipulating the load or number of repetitions. Stretch-shortening movements require both preparatory and reactive muscle activities along with the related changes in muscle stiffness. This preparatory muscle activation prior to eccentric loading is considered to be preprogrammed, while activation after ground contact is considered reactive. Plyometric activities such as low-impact hopping may commence once weight bearing is achieved (Figure 6-7). Double-leg bounding is an effective intermediate exercise, because the uninvolved limb can be used for assistance. Stretch-shortening activities are made more difficult with alternate-leg bounding, then single-leg hopping. Subsequent activities such as hopping with rotation, lateral hopping, and hopping onto various surfaces are instituted as tolerated. Plyometric training

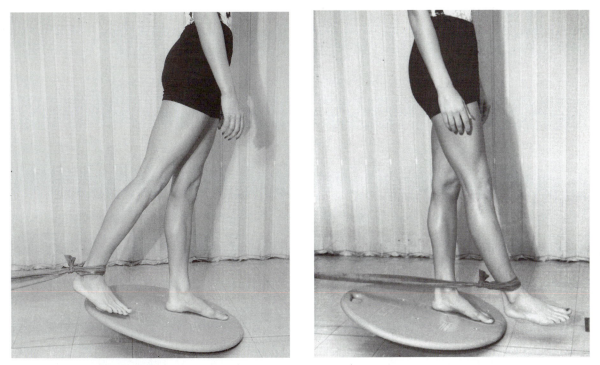

Figure 6-5 "Kickers" use an elastic band fixed to the distal aspect of the involved or uninvolved limb. The athlete attempts to balance while executing short kicks with either knee extension or hip flexion. This exercise is most difficult when performed on unstable surfaces.

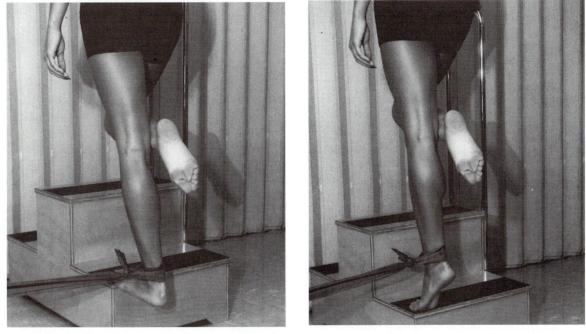

Figure 6-6 Balance and strength exercises are combined by incorporating light external forces and increasing the level of difficulty for balancing while strengthening the muscles required for dynamic stabilization.

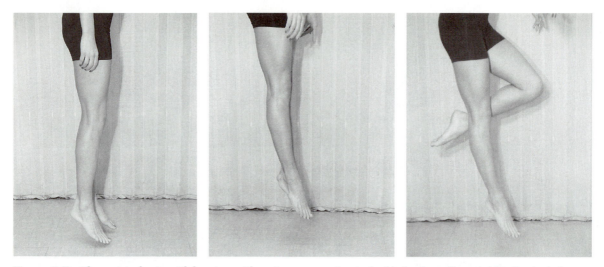

Figure 6-7 Plyometrics begin with low-impact hopping, progressing to double-leg bounding, and finally single-leg hopping.

requires preparatory muscle activation and facilitates reflexive pathways for reactive neuromuscular control.

Rhythmic stabilization exercises should be included during early rehabilitation to enhance lower-extremity neuromuscular coordination and reaction to unexpected joint perturbations. The intensity of rhythmic stabilization is increased by applying greater joint loads and displacements. Foot pass drills are also effective for developing coordinated preparatory and reactive muscle activity; begin with large balls and progress to smaller balls.

Unstable platforms are utilized to manually induce linear and angular perturbations to the joint, altering the athlete's center of gravity while the athlete attempts to balance (Figure 6-8). These exercises can facilitate adaptations to reflex pathways mediated by peripheral afferents, resulting in reactive muscle activation. Ball tossing can be incorporated in conjunction with balance exercises for the purpose of disrupting concentration and inducing unconscious, reactive adaptations. Walking and running in sand also require similar reactive muscle activity and can enhance reflexive joint stabilization.

During the later stages of rehabilitation, reactive neuromuscular activity incorporates trampoline hopping. The athlete begins by hopping and landing on both feet, progressing to hopping on one foot, and hopping with rotation. The most difficult reactive tasks include hopping while catching a ball, or hopping off of a trampoline onto various landing surfaces such as artificial turf, grass, or dirt.

Functional activities begin with restoring normal gait. Clinicians can give verbal instruction or use a mirror

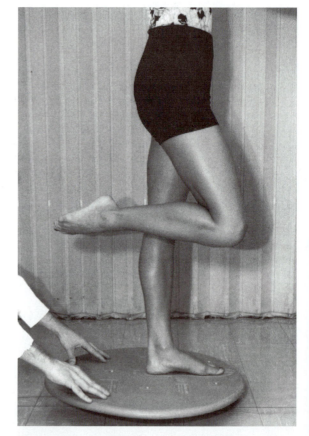

Figure 6- 8 An unstable platform promotes reactive muscle activity when an athlete attempts to balance and a clinician manually perturbs the platform.

to help athletes internalize normal kinematics during the stance and swing phases. This includes backward (retro) walking, which has been shown to further facilitate hamstring activation and balance.[78] If a pool or unloading device is available, crossover walking and figure eights can begin, progressing to jogging and hopping as tolerated. Functional activities during partial weight bearing help restore motor patterns without compromising static restraints. Weight-bearing activities are continued on land with the incorporation of acceleration and deceleration and pivot maneuvers. Drills such as jogging, cutting, and carriocas are initiated, gradually increasing the speed of maneuvers.

The most difficult functional activities are designed to simulate the demands of individual sports and positions. Activities such as shuttle runs, carrioca crossovers, retro sprinting and forward sprinting are implemented with sport-specific drills such as fielding a ball, receiving a pass, and dribbling a soccer ball.

Upper Extremity

Contrary to the lower extremity, the glenohumeral joint lacks inherent stability from capsuloligamentous structures; therefore dynamic mechanisms are even more crucial for maintaining functional stability.[37,95] The difficulty of working with a diverse array of shoulder positions and velocities is compounded by shearing forces associated with manipulating the upper extremity in an open-kinetic-chain environment.[95] Maintaining joint congruency and functional stability requires coordinated muscle activation for dynamic restraint while complex movement repertoires are executed.[67]

Two distinct types of muscle have been identified in the shoulder girdle and are primarily responsible for either stabilization or initiating movement. The orientation and size of the stabilizing muscles, referred to as the rotator cuff, are not suited for creating joint motion but are more capable of steering the humeral head in the glenoid fossa.[65] Larger muscles (primary movers) with insertion sites further from the glenohumeral joint have greater mechanical advantage for initiating joint motion.[65,68,69] Maintaining proper joint kinematics requires balancing the external forces and internal moments while limiting excessive translation of the humeral head on the glenoid fossa.

Injury to the static structures results in altered kinematics and diminished sensory feedback, which can be detrimental to feed-forward and feedback neuromuscular control mechanisms. Moreover, failure of the dynamic restraint system exposes the static structures to excessive or repetitive loads, jeopardizing joint integrity and predisposing the athlete to reinjury. Developing or restoring neuromuscular control in the upper extremity is an important

component to rehabilitation and the eventual return to functional activities. Exercise techniques originally designed to promote neuromuscular control in the lower extremity can be adapted for the upper extremity as well.

Activities to enhance proprioceptive and kinesthetic awareness in the upper extremity emulate techniques discussed for the lower extremity; however, multiplanar joint repositioning tasks are performed actively and passively to maximize the increased range of motion available in the shoulder. Functional positions, such as overhead throwing, should be incorporated and are more sport-specific (Figure 6-9). Closed-kinetic-chain activities can be performed in the upper extremity, although the objective is slightly different. The glenohumeral articulation is not configured to function in closed-chain environments such as weight bearing. However, with significant axial loads and muscle coactivation, the resultant joint approximation stimulates capsuloligamentous mechanoreceptors, similar to lower-extremity activities.[68,96] Therefore, closed-chain activities should be used to promote afferent feedback and coactivation in the upper extremity.

Muscle stiffness can be enhanced by using elastic resistance tubing, concentrating on the eccentric phase, and performing high repetitions with low resistance. These exercises are well established for strengthening and reconditioning the rotator cuff muscles in functional patterns. To complement elastic tubing exercises, clinicians can utilize commercially available upper-extremity ergometers for endurance training.

Like similar exercises for the lower extremity, dynamic stabilization exercises for the shoulder, use unstable platforms to create linear and angular joint displacement, maximally stimulating coactivation. The intensity is controlled by manipulating the degree of joint displacement and loading. Four closed-chain exercises have been described to stimulate coactivation in the shoulder: pushups, horizontal abduction on a slide board, and tracing circular motions on a slide board with the dominant and nondominant arms[65] (Figure 6-10). These exercises accommodate for the individual's tolerance to joint loads by progressing from a quadruped to a push-up position. Multidirectional slide board exercises also require dynamic stabilization while concomitantly using feedforward and feedback neuromuscular control. Plyometric exercises with a heavy ball are also excellent for conditioning preparatory and reactive muscle coactivation (Figure 6-11).

Reactive neuromuscular characteristics are facilitated by manually perturbing the upper extremity while the athlete attempts to maintain a permanent position. During the early phases of rehabilitation, light loads are used with rhythmic stabilization exercises. As the athlete

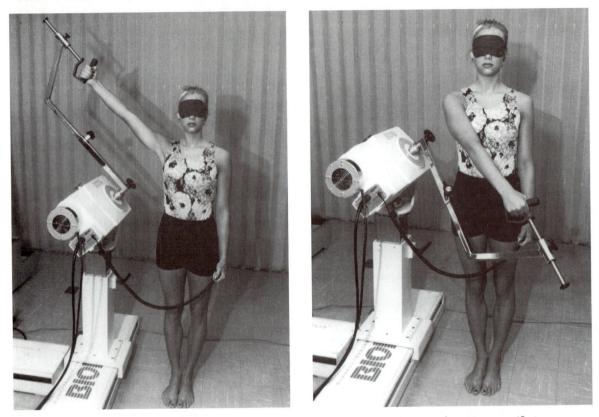

Figure 6-9 Active and passive repositioning activities should be performed in functional positions specific to individual sports.

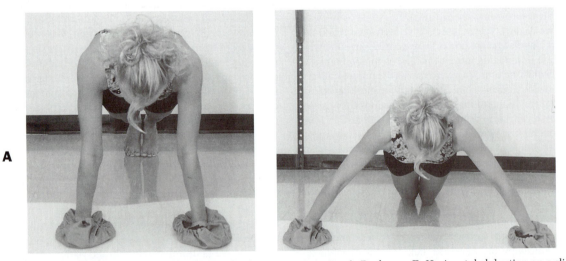

Figure 6-10 Dynamic stabilization exercises for the upper extremity. **A,** Push-ups. **B,** Horizontal abduction on a slide board.

C

D

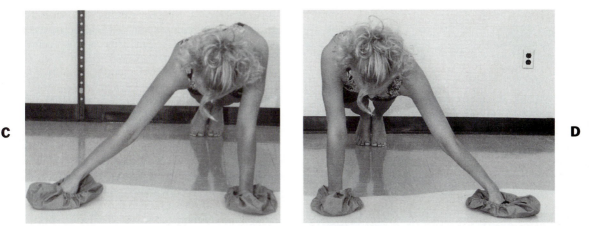

Figure 6-10 (Continued) C, Tracing a circle with the dominant arm on a slide board. **D,** Tracing a circle with the non-dominant arm on a slide board.

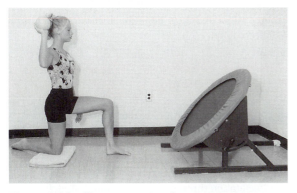

Figure 6-11 Upper-extremity plyometric exercises with a heavy ball require preparatory and reactive muscle activation.

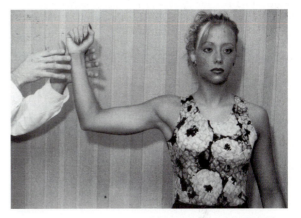

Figure 6-13 Rhythmic stabilization exercises should include simulated positions of vulnerability, promoting neuromuscular adaptations to dynamic stabilization.

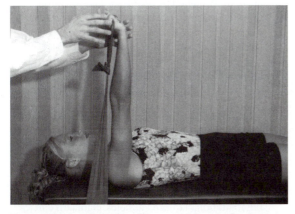

Figure 6-12 Elastic bands are used during rhythmic stabilization exercises to create joint loads and facilitate muscle activation.

progresses, resistance is added to maximize muscle activation (Figure 6-12). Positions where the joint is inherently unstable must be incorporated, but under controlled intensity (Figure 6-13). Increased joint loads during rhythmic stabilization exercises mimic closed-chain environments and conditions the athlete for more difficult reactive drills under weighted conditions on stable surfaces and unstable platforms (Figure 6-14).

Functional training for the upper extremity most often involves developing motor patterns in the *overhead position,* whether it be shooting a basketball, throwing, or hitting as in volleyball and tennis. However, special considerations are necessary for other sports, like rowing, wrestling, and swimming, that rely heavily on the upper extremity. Functional activities need to reproduce the

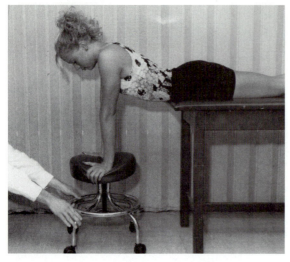

Figure 6-14   Linear displacements produced by a clinician facilitate reflex pathways for dynamic stabilization in the upper extremity.

demands of specific events, beginning with slower velocities and conscious control and eventually progressing to functional speeds and unconscious control. Technique, rather than speed, should be emphasized to promote the appropriate muscle activation patterns and avoid faulty kinematics. Reeducating functional motor patterns involves all of the elements for dynamic restraint and neuromuscular control and will minimize the risk of reinjury upon returning to full participation.

The speed and complexity of movements in athletic competition requires rapid integration of sensory information by feed-forward and feedback neuromuscular control systems. While many peripheral, spinal, and cortical elements contribute to the neuromuscular control system, dynamic joint stabilization is contingent upon both cortically programmed preactivation and reflex-mediated muscle activation. Disrupted joint kinematics, muscle activation patterns, and conditioning can contribute to disruption of the dynamic restraint system and must be reestablished for functional stability.

Summary

1. The efferent response to peripheral afferent information is termed neuromuscular control.
2. Injury to capsuloligamentous structures compromises both the static and the dynamic restraining mechanisms of joints.
3. The primary role of articular structures is to guide skeletal segments providing static restraint, but they also contain mechanoreceptors that mediate the dynamic restraint mechanism.
4. Articular sensations are coupled with information from tenomuscular mechanoreceptors, via cortical and reflex pathways, providing conscious and unconscious appreciation of joint motion and position.
5. Muscle spindles have received special consideration for their capacity to integrate peripheral afferent information and reflexively modify muscle activity.
6. Feed-forward and feedback neuromuscular controls utilize sensory information for preparatory and reactive muscle activity.
7. The degree of muscle activation largely determines a muscle's resistance to stretching or stiffness. Muscle with increased stiffness can assist the dynamic restraint mechanism by resisting excessive joint translation.

8. To reestablish neuromuscular control and functional stability, clinicians may utilize specific rehabilitation techniques—including, closed-kinetic-chain activities, balance training, eccentric and high-repetition/low-load exercises, reflex facilitation through reactive training, stretch-shortening activities, and biofeedback training.
9. Rehabilitative techniques produce adaptations in the sensitivity of peripheral receptors and facilitation of afferent pathways, agonist/antagonist coactivation, muscle stiffness, the onset rate and magnitude of muscle activity, reflex muscle activation, and discriminatory muscle activation.
10. Afferent and efferent characteristics regulate the four elements critical to neuromuscular control and functional stability: proprioception and kinesthesia, dynamic stabilization, reflex muscle activation, and functional motor patterns.
11. Each phase of traditional rehabilitation can incorporate the appropriate activities, emphasizing each of the four elements, according to the individual's tolerance and functional progression. By integrating these elements into the rehabilitation of injured athletes, clinicians can maximize the contributions of the dynamic restraint mechanisms to functional stability.

References

1. Abott, J. C., J. B. Saunders, and M. Dec. 1944. Injuries to the ligaments of the knee joint. *Journal of Bone Joint Surgery* 26:503–21.

2. Appleberg, B., H. Johansson, M. Hulliger, and P. Sojka. 1986. Actions on φ motoneurons elicited by electrical stimulation of group III muscle afferent fibers in the hind limb of the cat. *Journal of Physiology* (London) 375:137–52.

3. Bach, T. M., A. E. Chapman, and T. W. Calvert. 1983. Mechanical resonance of the human body during voluntary oscillations about the ankle. *Journal of Biomechanics* 16:85–90.

4. Barker, D. 1974. The morphology of muscle receptors. In *Handbook of sensory physiology,* edited by C. C. Hunt, pp. 191–234. Berlin: Springer-Verlag.

5. Barrack, R. L., H. B. Skinner, M. E. Brunet, and S. D. Cook. 1983. Joint laxity and proprioception in the knee. *Physician and Sports Medicine* 11:130–35.

6. Barrack, R. L., H. B. Skinner, M. E. Brunet, and S. D. Cook. 1984. Joint kinesthesia in the highly trained knee. *Journal of Sports Medicine* 24:18–20.

7. Barrack, R. L., H. B. Skinner, S. D. Cook, and J. R. Haddad. 1983. Effect of articular disease and total arthroplasty on knee joint-position sense. *Journal of Neurophysiology* 50:684–87.

8. Barrett, D. S., A. G. Cobb, and G. Bentley, G. 1991. Joint proprioception in normal, osteoarthritic, and replaced knees. *Journal of Bone Joint Surgery* 73-B:53–56.

9. Barrett, D. S. 1991. Proprioception and function after anterior cruciate reconstruction. *Journal of Bone Joint Surgery* 73-B:83–87.

10. Basmajian, J. V., ed. 1979. *Biofeedback: Principles and practice for clinicians.* Baltimore: Williams & Wilkins.

11. Beard, D. J., P. J. Kyberd, C. M. Fergusson, and C. A. F. Dodd. 1993. Proprioception after rupture of the anterior cruciate ligament. *Journal of Bone Joint Surgery* 75-B:311–15.

12. Beard, D. J., C. A. F. Dodd, H. R. Trundle, A. Hamish, and R. W. Simpson. 1994. Proprioception enhancement for anterior cruciate ligament deficiency. *Journal of Bone Joint Surgery* 76-B(4): 654–59.

13. Branch, T., R. Hunter, and M. Donath. 1989. Dynamic EMG analysis of the anterior cruciate ligament deficient legs with and without bracing during cutting. *American Journal of Sports Medicine* 17(1): 35–41.

14. Brener, J. 1977. Sensory and perceptual determinants of voluntary visceral control In *Biofeedback: Theory and Research,* edited by G. E. Schwartz & J. Beatty. New York: Academic Press.

15. Bulbulian, R., and D. K. Bowles. 1992. Effect of downhill running on motoneuron pool excitability. *Journal of Applied Physiology* 73(3): 968–73.

16. Caraffa, A., G. Cerulli, M. Proietti, G. Aisa, and A. Rizzo. 1995. Prevention of anterior cruciate ligament in soccer: A prospective controlled study of proprioceptive training. *Knee Surgery Sports Traumatol., Arthroscopy* 4(1): 19–21.

17. Ciccotti, M., R. Kerlain, J. Perry, and M. Pink. 1994. An electromyographic analysis of the knee during functional activities: II. The anterior cruciate ligament-deficient knee and reconstructed profiles. *American Journal of Sports Medicine* 22(5): 651–58.

18. Clark, F. J., and P. R. Burgess. 1975. Slowly adapting receptors in cat knee joint: Can they signal joint angle? *Journal of Neurophysiology* 38:1448–63.

19. Clark, F. J., R. C. Burgess, J. W. Chapin, and W. T. Lipscomb. 1985. Role of intramuscular receptors in the awareness of limb position. *Journal of Neurophysiology* 54(6): 1529–40.

20. Colebatch, J. G., and D. I. McClosky. 1987. Maintenance of constant arm position or force: Reflex and volitional components in man. *Journal of Physiology* 386:247–61.

21. Corrigan, J. P., W. F. Cashmen, and M. P. Brady. 1992. Proprioception in the cruciate deficient knee. *Journal of Bone Joint Surgery* 74-B:247–50.

22. Dietz, V., J. Noth, and D. Schmidtbleicher. 1981. Interaction between pre-activity and stretch reflex in human tricepts brachii during landing from forward falls. *Journal of Physiology* 311:113–25.

23. Dunn, T. G., S. E. Gillig, S. E. Ponser, and N. Weil. 1986. The learning process in biofeedback: Is it feed-forward or feedback? *Biofeedback Self. Reg.* 11(2): 143–55.

24. Dyhre-Poulsen, P., B. Simonsen, and M. Voigt. 1991. Dynamic control of muscle stiffness and H reflex modulation during hopping and jumping in man. *Journal of Physiology* 437:287–304.

25. Eccles, R.M., and A. Lindberg. 1959. Synaptic actions in motoneurons by afferents which may evoke the flexion reflex. *Extrait. Arch. Ital. Biol.* 97:199–221.

26. Finsterbush, A., and B. Friedman. 1975. The effects of sensory denervation on rabbits' knee joints. *Journal of Bone Joint Surgery* 57-A:949–56.

27. Freeman, M. A. R., and B. Wyke. 1966. Articular contributions to limb reflexes. *British Journal of Surgery* 53:61–9.

28. Forwell, L. A., and H. Carnahan. 1996. Proprioception during manual aiming in individuals with shoulder instability and controls. *Journal of Orthopaedic and Sports Physical Therapy* 23(2): 111–19.

29. Gardner, E., F. Latimer, and D. Stiwell. 1949. Central connections for afferent fibers from the knee joint of a cat. *American Journal of Physiology* 159:195–98.

30. Glaros, A. G., and K. Hanson. 1990. EMG biofeedback and discriminative muscle control. *Biofeedback Self. Reg.* 15(2): 135–43.

31. Glencross, D., and E. Thornton. 1981. Position sense following joint injury. *Journal of Sports Medicine and Physical Fitness* 21:23–7.

32. Gollhofer, A., and H. Kyrolaninen. 1991. Neuromuscular control of the human leg extensor muscles in jump exercises under various stretch-load conditions. *International Journal of Sports Medicine* 12:34–40.

33. Goubel, F., and J. F. Marini. 1987. Fiber type transition and stiffness modification of soleus muscle of trained rats. *European Journal of Physiology* 410:321–25.

34. Greenwood, R., and A. Hopkins. 1976. Landing from an unexpected fall and a voluntary step. *Brain* 99:375–86.

35. Grigg, P. 1994. Peripheral neural mechanisms in proprioception. *Journal of Sport Rehabilitation* 3:1–17.

36. Griller, S. 1972. A role for muscle stiffness in meeting the changing postural and locomotor requirements for force development by ankle extensors. *Acta. Physiol. Scand.* 86:92–108.

37. Guanche, C., T. Knatt, M. Solomonow, Y. Lu, and R. Baratta. 1995. The synergistic action of the capsule and the shoulder muscles. *American Journal of Sports Medicine* 23(3): 301–6.

38. Guyton, A. C. 1981. *Textbook of medical physiology.* 6th ed. Philadelphia, W.B. Saunders Co.

39. Hagood. S., M. Solomonow, R. Baratta, B. H. Zhou, and R. D'Ambrosia. 1990. The effect of joint velocity on the contribution of the antagonist musculature to knee stiffness and laxity. *American Journal of Sports Medicine* 18(2): 182–87.

40. Hoffer, J. A., and S. Andreassen. 1981. Regulation of soleus muscle stiffness in premammillary cats: Intrinsic and reflex components. *Journal of Neurophysiology* 45:267-85.

41. Hodgson, J. A., R. R. Roy, R. DeLeon, B. Dobkin, and R. V. Edgerton. 1994. Can the mammalian lumbar spinal cord learn a motor task? *Medicine and Science in Sports and Exercise* 26(12): 1491–97.

42. Houk, J. C., P. E. Crago, and W. Z. Rymer. 1981. Function of the dynamic response in stiffness regulation: A predictive mechanism provided by non-linear feedback. In *Muscle receptors and movement,* edited by A. Taylor, and A. Prochazka. London: Macmillan.

43. Hutton, R. S., and S. W. Atwater. 1992. Acute and chronic adaptations of muscle proprioceptors in response to increased use. *Sports Med.* 14(6): 406–21.

44. Ihara, H., and A. Nakayama. 1986. Dynamic joint control training for knee ligament injuries. *Am. J. Sports Med.* 14(4): 309–15.

45. Johansson, H. 1981. Reflex control of γ-motorneurons. *Umea Univ Med Diss:* New Series No., pp. 70.

46. Johansson, H., P. Sjolander, and P. Sojka. 1986. Actions on γ-motorneurons elicited by electrical stimulation of joint afferent fibers in the hind limb of the cat. *Journal of Physiology* (London) 375:137–52.

47. Johansson, H., P. Sjolander, and P. Sojka. 1991. A sensory role for the cruciate ligaments. *Clin. Orthop.* 268:161–78.

48. Johansson, H., P. Sjolander, and P. Sojka. 1991. The receptors in the knee joint ligaments and their role in the biomechanics of the joint. *Biomed. Eng.* 18:341–68.

49. Jonsson, H., J. Karrholm, and L. G. Elmquist. 1989. Kinematics of active knee extension after tear of the anterior cruciate ligament. *American Journal of Sports Medicine* 17:796–802.

50. Kandell, E. R., J. H. Schwartz, and T. M. Jessell. 1996. *Principles of neural science.* 3rd ed. Norwalk, CT: Appleton & Lange

51. Katonis, P. G., A. P. Assimakopoulos, M. V. Agapitos, and E. I. Exarchou. 1991. Mechanoreceptors in the posterior cruciate ligament. *Acta. Orthop. Scand.* 62(3): 276–78.

52. Kelsey, D. D., and E. Tyson. 1994. A new method of training for the lower extremity using unloading. *J. Orthop. Sports Phys. Ther.* 19(4): 218–23.

53. Kennedy, J. C., I. J. Alexander, and K. C. Hayes. 1982. Nerve supply of the human knee and its functional importance. *American Journal of Sports Medicine* 103:329–35.

54. Koceja, D. M., and G. Kamen. 1988. Conditioned patellar tendon reflexes in sprint and endurance-trained athletes. *Medicine and Science in Sports and Exercise* 20:172–77.

55. Koceja, D. M., J. R. Burke, and G. Kamen. 1991. Organization of segmental reflexes in trained dancers. *International Journal of Sports Medicine* 12:285–89.

56. Kochner, M. S., F. H. Fu, and C. D. Harner. 1994. Neuropathophysiology. In *Knee surgery,* vol. 1, edited by F. H. Fu, and C. D. Harner. Baltimore: Williams & Wilkins.

57. Kovanen, V., H. Suominen, and E. Heikkinen. 1984. Mechanical properties of fast and slow skeletal muscle with special reference to collagen and endurance training. *Journal of Biomechanics* 17(10): 725–35.

58. Kyrolaninen, H., and P. V. Komi. 1995. The function of neuromuscular system in maximal stretch-shortening cycle exercises: Comparison between power- and endurance-trained athletes. *J. Electromyogr. Kinesiol.* 5:15–25.

59. La Croix, J. M. 1981. The acquisition of autonomic control through biofeedback: The case against an afferent process and a two-process alternative. *Psychophysiology* 18:573–87.

60. Konradsen, L., M. Voigt, and C. Hojsgaard. 1997. Ankle inversion injuries: The role of the dynamic defense mechanism. *American Journal of Sports Medicine* 25(1): 54–8.

61. Leanderson, J., E. Eriksson, C. Nilsson, and A. Wykman. 1996. Proprioception in classical ballet dancers: A prospective study of the influence of an ankle sprain on proprioception in the ankle joint. *American Journal of Sports Medicine* 24(3): 370–74.

62. Leksell, L. 1945. The action potential and excitatory effects of the small ventral root fibers to skeletal muscle. *Acta. Physiol. Scand.* 10;Suppl (31): 1–84.

63. Lephart, S. M. 1997. *EMG profile of the functional ACL deficient patient during dynamic activities.* Paper presented at the American Orthopaedic Society for Sports Medicine, San Francisco, CA: February.

64. Lephart, S. M., J. L. Giraldo, P. A. Borsa, and F. A. Fu. 1996. Knee joint proprioception: A comparison between female intercollegiate gymnasts and controls. *Knee Surg. Sports Traumatol., Arthroscopy* 4:121–24.

65. Lephart, S. M., and T. J. Henry. 1996. The physiological basis for open and closed kinetic chain rehabilitation for the upper extremity. *Journal of Sport Rehabilitation* 5:71–87.

66. Lephart, S. M., M. S. Kocher, F. H. Fu, P. A. Borsa, and C. D. Harner. 1992. Proprioception following ACL reconstruction. *Journal of Sport Rehabilitation* 1:188–96.

67. Lephart, S. M., D. M. Pincivero, J. L. Giraldo, and F. H. Fu. 1997. The role of proprioception in the management and rehabilitation of athletic injuries. *American Journal of Sports Medicine* 25(1): 130–37.

68. Lephart, S. M., J. J. P. Warner, P. A. Borsa, and F. H. Fu. 1994. Proprioception of the shoulder joint in healthy, unstable, and surgically repaired shoulders. *Journal of Shoulder Elbow Surgery* 3:371–80.

69. Lieber, R. L., and J. Friden. 1992. Neuromuscular stabilization of the shoulder girdle. In *The shoulder: A balance of mobility and stability,* edited by F. A. Matsen, pp. 91–106. Rosemont, IL: American Academy of Orthopaedic Surgeons.

70. Lynch, S. A., U. Eklund, D. Gottlieb, P. A. F. H. Renstrom and B. Beynnon. 1996. Electromyographic latency changes in the ankle musculature during inversion moments. *American Journal of Sports Medicine* 24(3): 362–69.

71. Mair, S. D., A. V. Seaber, R. R. Glisson, and W. E. Garrett. 1996. The role of fatigue in susceptibility to acute muscle strain injury. *American Journal of Sports Medicine* 24(2): 137–43.

72. McComas, A. J. 1994. Human neuromuscular adaptations that accompany changes in activity. *Medicine and Science in Sports and Exercise* 26(12): 1498–1509.

73. McNair, P. J., and R. N. Marshall. 1994. Landing characteristics in subjects with normal and anterior cruciate ligament deficient knee joints. *Archives of Physical Medicine and Rehabilitation* 75:584–89.

74. McNair, P. J., G. A. Wood, and R. N. Marshall. 1992. Stiffness of the hamstring muscles and its relationship to function in anterior cruciate deficient individuals. *Clin. Biomech.* 7:131–73.

75. Melvill-Jones, G. M., and G. D. Watt. 1971. Observations of the control of stepping and hopping in man. *Journal of Physiology* 219:709–27.

76. Merton, P. A. 1953. Speculations on the servo-control of movement. In *The spinal cord,* edited by G. E. W. Wolstenholme. London: Churchill.

77. Morgan, D. L. 1977. Separation of active and passive components of short-range stiffness of muscle. *American Journal of Physiology* 32(1): 45–9.

78. Morton, C. 1986. Running backwards may help athletes move forward. *Physician and Sports Medicine* 14(12): 149–52.

79. Mountcastle, V. S. 1980. *Medical Physiology.* 14th ed. St. Louis: Mosby.

80. Nichols, T. R., and J. C. Houk. 1976. Improvements in linearity and regulation of stiffness that results from actions of stretch reflex. *Journal of Neurophysiology* 39:119–42.

81. Palmitier, R. A., A. N. Ka, S. G. Scott, and E. Y. S. Choa. 1991. Kinetic chain exercises in knee rehabilitation. *Sports Medicine* 11:402–13.

82. Perlau, R., C. Frank, and G. Fick. 1995. The effects of elastic bandages on human knee proprioception in the uninjured population. *American Journal of Sports Medicine* 23(2): 251–55.

83. Pope, M. H., R. J. Johnson, D. W. Brown, and C. Tighe. 1972. The role of the musculature in injuries to the medials collateral ligament. *Journal of Bone Joint Surgery* 61-A(3): 398–402.

84. Pousson, M., J. V. Hoecke, and F. Goubel. 1990. Changes in elastic characteristics of human muscle induced by eccentric exercise. *Journal of Biomechanics* 23(4): 343–48.

85. Rack, P. M. H., and D. R. Westbury. 1974. The short range stiffness of active mammalian muscle and its effect on mechanical properties. *Journal of Physiology* 240:331–50.

86. Schultz, R. A., D. C. Miller, C. S. Kerr, and L. Misceli. 1984. Mechanoreceptors in human cruciate ligaments. *Journal of Bone Joint Surgery* 66-A:1072–76.

87. Sherrington, C. S. 1911. *The integrative action of the nervous system.* New Haven: Yale University Press.

88. Sinkjἒr, T., and L. Arendt-Nielsen. 1991. Knee stability and muscle coordination in patients with anterior cruciate ligament injuries: An electromyographic approach. *J. Electromyogr. Kinesiol.* 1(3): 209–17.

89. Skinner, H. B., and R. L. Barrack. 1991. Joint position sense in the normal and pathologic knee joint. *J. Electromyogr. Kinesiol.* 1(3): 180–90.

90. Skinner, H. B., R. L. Barrack, S. D. Cook, and R. J. Haddad. 1984. Joint position sense in total knee arthroplasty. *J. Orthop. Res.* 1:276–83.

91. Smith, R. L., and J. Brunolli. 1989. Shoulder kinesthesia after anterior glenohumeral joint dislocation. *Physical Therapy* 69(2): 106–12.

92. Solomonow, M., R. Baratta, B. H. Zhou, H. Sholi, W. Bose, C. Beck, and R. D'Ambrosia. 1987. The synergistic action of the anterior cruciate ligament and thigh muscles in maintaining joint stability. *American Journal of Sports Medicine* 15(3): 207–13.

93. Upton, A. R. M., and P. F. Radford. 1975. Motorneuron excitability in elite sprinters. In *Biomechanics,* V-A, edited by P. V. Komi, pp. 82–7. Baltimore: University Park.

94. Walla, D. J., J. P. Albright, E. McAuley, et al. 1985. Hamstring control and the unstable anterior cruciate ligament-deficient knee. *American Journal of Sports Medicine* 13:34–9.

95. Warner, J. J. P., S. M. Lephart, and F. H. Fu. 1996. Role of proprioception in pathoetiology of shoulder instability. *Clin. Orthop.* 330:35–39.

96. Wilk, K. E., C. A. Arrigo, and J. R. Andrews. 1996. Closed and open chain exercises for the upper extremity. *Journal of Sport Rehabilitation* 5:88–102.

97. Wilk, K. E., R. F. Escamilla, G. S. Fleisig, S. W. Barrentine, J. R. Andrews, and M. L. Boyd. 1996. A comparison of tibiofemoral joint forces and electromyographic activity during open and closed kinetic chain exercises. *American Journal of Sports Medicine* 24(4): 518–27.

98. Wojtys, E., and L. Huston. 1994. Neuromuscular performance in normal and anterior cruciate ligament-deficient lower extremities. *American Journal of Sports Medicine* 22:89–104.

99. Wojtys, E., L. Huston, P. D. Taylor, and S. D. Bastian. 1996. Neuromuscular adaptations in isokinetic, isotonic, and agility training programs. *American Journal of Sports Medicine* 24(2): 187–92.

100. Wolf, S. L., and R. L. Segal. 1990. Conditioning of the spinal stretch reflex: Implications for rehabilitation. *Physical Therapy* 70:652–56.

101. Woo, S. L., R. A. Z. Sofranko, and J. P. Jamison. 1994. Biomechanics of knee ligaments relating to sports medicine. In *Sports injuries, mechanism, prevention, treatment,* edited by F. F. Fu, and D. A. Stone. Baltimore: Williams & Wilkins.

102. Yack, H. J., C. E. Collins, and T. J. Wieldon. 1993. Comparison of closed and open kinetic chain exercises in the anterior cruciate ligament-deficient knee. *American Journal of Sports Medicine* 21(1): 49–54.

CHAPTER 7

Regaining Balance and Postural Equilibrium

Kevin M. Guskiewicz

After completion of this chapter, the student should be able to do the following:

- Define and explain the role of the three sensory modalities responsible for maintaining balance.

- Explain how movement strategies along the closed kinetic chain help maintain the center of gravity in a safe and stable area.

- Differentiate between subjective and objective balance assessment.

- Differentiate between static and dynamic balance assessment.

- Explain the effect that injury to the ankle, knee, and head has on balance and postural equilibrium.

- Discuss the goals of each phase of balance training, and how to progress the athlete through each phase.

- Discuss the difference between static, semidynamic and dynamic balance-training exercises.

WHY IS BALANCE IMPORTANT IN THE REHABILITATION PROCESS?

Although maintaining balance while standing might appear to be a rather simple motor skill for able-bodied athletes, this feat cannot be taken for granted in an athlete with musculoskeletal dysfunction. Muscular weakness, proprioceptive deficits, and range of motion (ROM) deficits can challenge an athlete's ability to maintain their center of gravity within the body's base of support, or in other words, cause them to lose their balance. Balance is the single most important element dictating movement strategies within the closed kinetic chain. Acquisition of effective strategies for maintaining balance is therefore essential for athletic performance. Although balance is often thought of as a static process, it's actually a highly integrative dynamic process involving multiple neurological pathways. *Balance* is the more commonly used term; the broader term **postural equilibrium** refers to the alignment of joint segments in an effort to maintain the COG within an optimal range of the maximum limits of stability (LOS), which will be discussed later.

Despite being classified at the end of the continuum of goals associated with therapeutic exercise,[45] maintenance of balance is a vital component in the rehabilitation of joint injuries and should not be overlooked. Traditionally, orthopedic rehabilitation has emphasized isolated joint mechanics, such as improving ROM and flexibility, and increasing muscle strength and endurance, rather than afferent information obtained by the joint(s) to be processed by the postural control system. More recently, however, research in the area of proprioception and kinesthesia has emphasized the need to

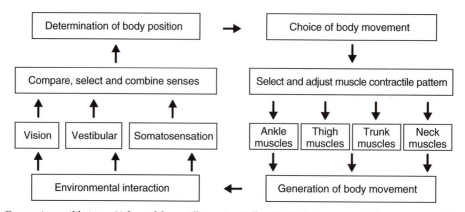

Figure 7-1 Dynamic equilibrium. (Adapted from Allison, L., Fuller, R. Hedenberg, et al. *Contemporary Management of Balance Deficits.* Clackamas, OR: NeuroCom International, 1994; with permission)

train the joint's neural system[46–50] (see Chapter 6). Joint position sense, proprioception, and kinesthesia are vital to all athletic performance, but particularly those athletic activities requiring balance. Current rehabilitation protocols are therefore focusing more on closed-kinetic-chain exercises, and **balance training** is receiving more attention in the sports medicine community. This chapter focuses on the postural control system, various balance-training techniques, and technological advancements that are enabling sports medicine clinicians to assess and treat balance deficits in physically active people.

POSTURAL CONTROL SYSTEM

The sports therapist must first have an understanding of the postural control system and its various components. The postural control system utilizes complex processes involving both sensory and motor components. Maintenance of postural equilibrium includes sensory detection of body motions, integration of sensorimotor information within the central nervous system (CNS), and execution of appropriate musculoskeletal responses. Most daily activities, such as walking, climbing stairs, reaching, or throwing a ball, require static foot placement with controlled balance shifts, especially if a favorable outcome is to be attained. So, balance should be considered both a dynamic and a static process. The successful accomplishment of static and dynamic balance is based on the interaction between body and environment.[44] The complexity of this dynamic process can be seen in Figure 7-1. From a clinical perspective, separating the sensory and motor processes of balance means that a person can have impaired balance for one or two reasons: (1) The position of

the center of gravity (COG) relative to the base of support is not accurately sensed; (2) the automatic movements required to bring the COG to a balanced position are not timely or effectively coordinated.[60]

The position of the body in relation to gravity and its surroundings is sensed by combining visual, vestibular, and somatosensory inputs. Balance movements also involve motions of the ankle, knee, and hip joints, which are controlled by coordinated actions along the kinetic chain (Figure 7-2). These processes are all vital for producing fluid sport-related movements.

CONTROL OF BALANCE

The human body is a very tall structure balanced on a relatively small base, and its COG is quite high, being just above the pelvis.[76] Many factors enter into the task of controlling balance within the base of support. Balance control involves a complex network of neural connections and centers that are related by peripheral and central feedback mechanisms.[34]

The postural control system operates as a feedback control circuit between the brain and the musculoskeletal system. The sources of afferent information supplied to the postural control system collectively come from visual, vestibular, and somatosensory inputs. Involvement of the central nervous system (CNS) in maintaining upright posture can be divided into two components. The first component, **sensory organization,** involves those processes that determine the timing, direction, and amplitude of corrective postural actions based upon information obtained from the vestibular, visual, and somatosensory (proprioceptive) inputs.[56] Despite the

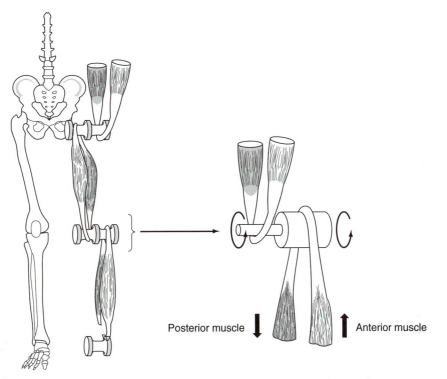

Figure 7-2 Paired relationships between major postural musculatures that execute coordinated actions along the kinetic chain to control the center of gravity.

Posterior muscle ↓   Anterior muscle ↑

availability of multiple sensory inputs, the central nervous system generally relies on only one sense at a time for orientation information. For healthy adults, the preferred source of information for balance control is somatosensory (i.e., feet in contact with the support surface, and detection of joint movement).[37,56] In considering orthopedic injuries, the somatosensory system is of most importance and will be the focus of this chapter.

The second component, **muscle coordination,** is the collection of processes that determine the temporal sequencing and distribution of contractile activity among the muscles of the legs and trunk that generate supportive reactions for maintaining balance. Research suggests that balance deficiencies in people with neurological problems can result from inappropriate interaction among the three sensory inputs that provide orientation information to the postural control system. A patient might be inappropriately dependent on one sense for situations presenting intersensory conflict.[56,69]

From a clinical perspective, stabilization of upright posture requires the integration of afferent information from the three senses, which work in combination and

are all critical to the execution of coordinated postural corrections. Impairment of one component is usually compensated for by the remaining two. Often, one of the systems provides faulty or inadequate information such as different surfaces and/or changes in visual acuity and/or peripheral vision. In this case it is crucial that one of the other senses provide accurate and adequate information so that balance can be maintained. For example, when somatosensory conflict is present such as a moving platform or a compliant foam surface, balance is significantly decreased with the eyes closed as compared to with the eyes open.

Somatosensory inputs provide information concerning the orientation of body parts to one another and to the support surface.[21,60] **Vision** measures the orientation of the eyes and head in relation to surrounding objects, and plays an important role in the maintenance of balance. On a stable surface, closing the eyes should cause only minimal increases in postural sway in healthy subjects. However, if somatosensory input is disrupted due to ligamentous injury, closing the eyes will increase sway significantly.[12,16,37,38,60] The **vestibular** apparatus supplies information that measures gravitational, linear, and angular accelerations of the head in relation to inertial space. It does not, however, provide orientation information in relation to external objects, and therefore plays only a minor role in the maintenance of balance when the visual and somatosensory systems are providing accurate information.[60]

SOMATOSENSATION AS IT RELATES TO BALANCE

The terms *somatosensation, proprioception, kinesthesia,* and *balance* are often used to denote similar phenomena. *Somatosensation* is the more global term; proprioceptive mechanisms related to postural control. Somatosensation is best defined as a specialized variation of the sensory modality of touch that encompasses the sensation of joint movement (kinesthesia) and joint position (joint position sense).[46,50] As previously discussed, *balance* refers to the ability to maintain the body's COG within the base of support provided by the feet. Somatosensation and balance work closely together, as the postural control system utilizes sensory information related to movement and posture from peripheral sensory receptors (e.g., muscle spindles, Golgi tendon organs, joint afferents, cutaneous receptors). So the question remains, how does proprioception influence postural equilibrium and balance?

Somatosensory input is received from mechanoreceptors, but it is unclear whether the tactile senses, the muscle spindles, or the Golgi tendon organs (GTOs) are more responsible for controlling balance. Nashner[55] concluded, after using electromyography (EMG) responses following platform perturbations, that other pathways had to be involved in the responses they recorded because the latencies were longer than those normally associated with a classic myotatic reflex. The stretch-related reflex is the earliest mechanism for increasing the activation level of muscles about a joint following an externally imposed rotation of the joint. Rotation of the ankles is the most probable stimulus of the myotatic reflex that occurs in many persons. It appears to be the first useful phase of activity in the leg muscles after a change in erect posture.[55] The myotatic reflex can be seen when perturbations of gait or posture automatically evoke functionally directed responses in the leg muscles to compensate for imbalance or increased postural sway.[14,55] Muscle spindles sense a stretching of the agonist, thus sending information along its afferent fibers to the spinal cord. There the information is transferred to alpha and gamma motor neurons that carry information back to the muscle fibers and muscle spindle, respectively, and contract the muscle to prevent or control additional postural sway.[14]

Postural sway was assessed on a platform moving into a toes-up and toes-down position, and a stretch reflex was found in the triceps surae after a sudden ramp displacement into the toes-up position.[13] A medium latency response was observed in the stretched muscle, followed by a delayed response of the antagonistic anterior tibialis muscle. The investigators also blocked afferent proprioceptive information in an attempt to study the role of proprioceptive information from the legs for the maintenance of upright posture. These results suggested that proprioceptive information from pressure and/or joint receptors of the foot (ischemia applied at ankle) plays an important role in postural stabilization during low frequencies of movement, but is of minor importance for the compensation of rapid displacements. The experiment also included a "visual" component, as subjects were tested with eyes closed, followed by eyes open. Results suggested that when subjects were tested with eyes open, visual information compensated for the loss of proprioceptive input.

Another study[14] used compensatory EMG responses during impulsive disturbance of the limbs during stance on a treadmill to describe the myotatic reflex. Results revealed that during backward movement of the treadmill, ankle dorsiflexion caused the COG to be shifted anteriorly, thus evoking a stretch reflex in the gastrocnemius muscle, followed by weak anterior tibialis activation. In another trial, the movement was reversed (plantar flexion), thus shifting the COG posteriorly and evoking a stretch reflex of the anterior tibialis muscle. Both of these studies suggest that stretch reflex responses help to control the body's COG, and that the vestibular system is unlikely to be directly involved in the generation of the necessary responses.

Elimination of all sensory information from the feet and ankles revealed that proprioceptors in the leg muscles (gastrocnemius and tibialis anterior) were capable of providing sufficient sensory information for stable standing.[20] Researchers speculated that group I or group II muscle spindle afferents, and group Ib afferents from GTOs were the probable sources of this proprioceptive information. The study demonstrated that normal subjects can stand in a stable manner when receptors in the leg muscles are the only source of information about postural sway.

Other studies[38,5] have examined the role of somatosensory information by altering or limiting somatosensory input through the use of platform sway referencing or foam platforms. These studies reported that subjects still responded with well-coordinated movements but the movements were often either ineffective or inefficient for the environmental context in which they were used.

BALANCE AS IT RELATES TO THE CLOSED KINETIC CHAIN

Balance is the process of maintaining the center of gravity (COG) within the body's base of support. The human body's center of gravity is quite high, just above the pelvis.[76] Many factors enter into the task of controlling balance within this designated area. One component often overlooked is the role balance plays within the **kinetic chain.** Ongoing debates as to how the kinetic chain should be defined and whether open- or closed-kinetic-chain exercises are best has caused many sports therapists to lose sight of what is most important. An understanding of the postural control system as well as the theory of the kinetic (segmental) chain about the lower extremity helps conceptualize the role of the chain in maintaining balance. Within the kinetic chain, each moving segment transmits forces to every other segment along the chain, and its motions are influenced by forces transmitted from other segments[10] (see Chapter 11). The act of maintaining equilibrium or balance is associated with the closed kinetic chain, as the distal segment (foot) is fixed beneath the base of support.

The coordination of automatic postural movements during the act of balancing is not determined solely by the muscles acting directly about the joint. Leg and trunk muscles exert indirect forces on neighboring joints through the inertial interaction forces among body segments.[57,58] A combination of one or more strategies (ankle, knee, hip) are used to coordinate movement of the COG back to a stable or balanced position when a person's balance is disrupted by an external perturbation. Injury to any one of the joints or corresponding muscles along the kinetic chain can result in a loss of appropriate feedback for maintaining balance.

BALANCE DISRUPTION

Let's say, for example, that a basketball player goes up for a rebound and collides with another player, causing her to land in an unexpected position, therefore compromising her normal balance. In order to prevent a fall from occurring, the body must correct itself by returning the COG to a position within safer limits of stability (LOS). Afferent mechanoreceptor inputs from the hip, knee, and ankle joints are responsible for initiating automatic postural responses through the use of one of three possible movement strategies.

Selection of Movement Strategies

Three principle joint systems (ankles, knees, and hips) are located between the base of support and the COG. This allows for a wide variety of postures that can be assumed, while the COG is still positioned above the base of support. As described by Nashner,[60] motions about a given joint are controlled by the combined actions of at least one pair of muscles working in opposition. When forces exerted by pairs of opposing muscle about a joint (e.g., anterior tibialis and gastrocnemius/soleus) are combined, the effect is to resist rotation of the joint relative to a resting position. The degree to which the joint resists rotation is called joint stiffness. The resting position and the stiffness of the joint are each altered independently by changing the activation levels of one or both muscle groups.[39,60] Joint resting position and joint stiffness are by themselves an inadequate basis for controlling postural movements, and it is theorized that the myotatic stretch reflex is the earliest mechanism for increasing the activation level of the muscles of a joint following an externally imposed rotation of the joint.[60]

When a person's balance is disrupted by an external perturbation, movement strategies involving joints of the lower extremity coordinate movement of the COG back to a balanced position. Three strategies (ankle, hip, stepping) have been identified along a continuum.[37] In general, the relative effectiveness of ankle, hip, and stepping strategies in repositioning the COG over the base of support depends on the configuration of the base of support, the COG alignment in relation to the LOS, and the speed of the postural movement.[37,38]

The **ankle strategy** shifts the COG while maintaining the placement of the feet by rotating the body as a rigid mass about the ankle joints. This is achieved by contracting either the gastrocnemius or the anterior tibialis muscles to generate torque about the ankle joints. Anterior sway of the body is counteracted by gastrocnemius activity, which pulls the body posteriorly. Conversely, posterior sway of the body is counteracted by contraction of the tibialis anterior. Thus, the importance of these muscles should not be underestimated when designing the rehabilitation program. The ankle strategy is most effective in executing relatively slow COG movements when the base of support is firm and the COG is well within the LOS perimeter. The ankle strategy is also believed to be effective in maintaining a static posture with the COG offset from the center. The thigh and lower trunk muscles contract and thereby resist the destabilization of these proximal joints due to the indirect effects of the ankle muscles on the proximal joints (Table 7-1). Under normal sensory conditions, activation of ankle musculature is almost exclusively selected to maintain equilibrium. However, there are subtle differences associated with loss of somatosensation and with vestibular dysfunction in terms of postural control strategies. Persons with somatosensory loss appear to rely on their hip

■ **TABLE 7-1** Function Anatomy of Muscles Involved in Balance Movements

Joint	Extension		Flexion	
	Anatomic	**Function**	**Anatomic**	**Function**
Hip	Paraspinals Hamstrings	Paraspinals Hamstrings Tibialis	Abdominal Quadriceps	Abdominals Quadriceps Gastrocnemius
Knee	Quadriceps	Paraspinals Quadriceps Gastrocnemius	Hamstrings Gastrocnemius	Abdominals Hamstrings Tibialis
Ankle	Gastrocnemius	Abdominals Quadriceps Gastrocnemius	Tibialis	Paraspinals Hamstrings Tibialis

Adapted from Nashner, L. M. 1993. Physiology of Balance. In *Handbook of Balance Function and Testing,* edited by G. Jacobson, C. Newman, and J. Kartush, pp. 261–79. St. Louis: Mosby Yearbook.

musculature to retain their COG while experiencing forward or backward perturbation or with different support surface lengths.[21]

If the ankle strategy is not capable of controlling excessive sway, the **hip strategy** is available to help control motion of the COG through the initiation of large and rapid motions at the hip joints with antiphase rotation of the ankles. It is most effective when the COG is located near the LOS perimeter, and when the LOS boundaries are contracted by a narrowed base of support. Finally, when the COG is displaced beyond the LOS, a step or stumble **(stepping strategy)** is the only strategy that can be used to prevent a fall.[58,60]

It is proposed that LOS and COG alignment are altered in individuals exhibiting a musculoskeletal abnormality such as an ankle or knee sprain. For example, weakness of ligaments following acute or chronic sprain about these joints is likely to reduce range of motion, therefore shrinking LOS and placing the person at greater risk for a fall with a relatively smaller sway envelope.[58] Pintsaar et al[67] revealed that impaired function was related to a change from ankle synergy toward hip synergy for postural adjustments among athletes with functional ankle instability. This finding, which was consistent with previous results reported by Tropp et al.,[74] suggests that sensory proprioceptive function for the injured athletes was affected.

ASSESSMENT OF BALANCE

Several methods of balance assessment have been proposed for clinical use. Many of the techniques have been criticized for offering only a subjective ("qualitative")

measurement of balance rather than an objective ("quantitative") measure.

Subjective Assessment

Prior to the mid 1980s, there were very few methods for systematic and controlled assessment of balance. The assessment of static balance in athletes has traditionally been performed through the use of the standing Romberg test. This test is performed standing with feet together, arms at the side, and eyes closed. Normally a person can stand motionless in this position; the tendency to sway or fall to one side is considered a positive Romberg's sign indicating a loss of proprioception.[8] The Romberg test has, however, been criticized for its lack of sensitivity and objectivity. It is considered to be a rather qualitative assessment of static balance because a considerable amount of stress is required to make the subject sway enough for an observer to characterize the sway.[42] Other tests of static balance include a single-leg stance test, which includes balancing on one leg for a specified amount of time with eyes open or closed. The Tandem Romberg test[19] requires placement of one foot in front of the other (heel to toe).

Semidynamic and dynamic balance assessment can be performed through functional reach tests, timed agility tests such as the figure eight test,[15,19,78] carioca or hop test,[40,78] Bass Test for Dynamic Balance,[75] timed "T-Band kicks," and timed balance beam walking with the eyes open or closed. The objective in most of these tests is to decrease the size of the base of support, in an attempt to determine an athlete's ability to control upright posture while moving. Many of these tests have been criticized for failing to quantify balance adequately, as they

Static Systems	Dynamic Systems
Chattecx Balance System	Biodex Stability System
EquiTest	Chattecx Balance System
Forceplate	EquiTest
Pro Balance Master	EquiTest with EMG
Smart Balance Master	Forceplate
	Kinesthetic Ability Trainer (KAT)
	Pro Balance Master
	Smart Balance Master

■ TABLE 7-2   High-Technology Balance Assessment Systems

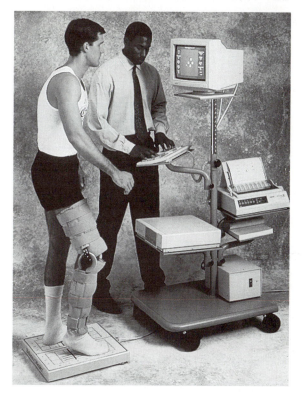

Figure 7-3   Athlete training on the Balance Master.

merely report the length of time a particular posture is maintained, angular displacement, or the distance covered after walking.[6,21,46,60] At any rate, they can often provide the clinician with valuable information about an athlete's function and/or readiness to return to play.

Objective Assessment

More recently, advancements in technology have provided the medical community with commercially available balance systems (Table 7-2) for quantitatively assessing and training static and dynamic balance. These systems provide easy, practical, and cost-effective methods of quantitatively assessing and training functional balance through analysis of postural stability. Thus, the potential exists to assess injured athletes and (1) identify possible abnormalities that might be associated with injury, (2) isolate various systems that are affected, (3) develop recovery curves based on quantitative measures for determining readiness to return to activity, and (4) train the injured athlete.

Most manufacturers use computer-interfaced forceplate technology consisting of a flat, rigid surface supported on three or more points by independent force-measuring devices. As the athlete stands on the forceplate surface, the position of the center of vertical forces exerted on the forceplate over time is calculated (Figure 7-3). The center of vertical force movements provides an indirect measure of postural sway activity.[59] The Kistler forceplate was used for much of the early work in the area of postural stability and balance.[6,17,27,52,54] Manufacturers such as Chattecx Corporation (Hixson, TN) and NeuroCom International, Inc. (Clackamas, OR) have developed more sophisticated systems with expanded diagnostic and training capabilities. Clinicians must be aware that the manufacturers often use conflicting terminology to describe various balance parameters.

These inconsistencies have created confusion in the literature, because what some manufacturers classify as *dynamic balance*, others claim is really *static balance*. Our classification system (see the section "Balance Training") will hopefully clear up some of the confusion and allow for a more consistent labeling of the numerous balance-related exercises.

Force platforms generally evaluate three aspects of postural control: steadiness, symmetry, and dynamic stability. **Steadiness** is the ability to keep the body as motionless as possible. This is a measure of postural sway. **Symmetry** is the ability to distribute weight evenly between the two feet in an upright stance. This is a measure of center of pressure (COP), center of balance (COB), or center of force (COF) depending which testing system you are using. Although inconsistent with our classification system, **dynamic stability** is the ability to transfer the vertical projection of the COG around a stationary supporting base.[27] This is often referred to as a measure of one's perception of one's "safe" limits of stability, as the goal is to lean or reach as far possible without losing one's balance. Some manufacturers measure dynamic stability by assessing a person's postural response to external perturbations from a moving platform in one of

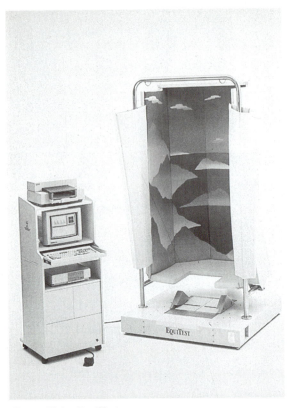

Figure 7-4 EquiTest.

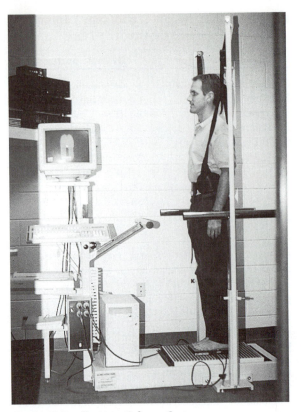

Figure 7-5 Chattecx Balance System.

four directions: tilting toes up, tilting toes down, shifting medial-lateral (M-L), and shifting anterior posterior (A-P). Platform perturbation on some systems is unpredictable and determined by the positioning and sway movement of the subject. In such cases, a person's reaction response can be determined (Figure 7-4). Other systems have a more predictable sinusoidal waveform, which remains constant regardless of subject positioning (Figure 7-5).

Many of these force platform systems measure the vertical ground reaction force and provide a means of computing the center of pressure (COP). The COP represents the center of the distribution of the total force applied to the supporting surface. The COP is calculated from horizontal movement and vertical force data generated by triaxial force platforms. Center of balance (COB), in the case of the Chattecx Balance System, is the point between the feet where the ball and heel of each foot each has 25 percent of the body weight. This point is referred to as the relative weight positioning over the four load cells as measured only by vertical forces. The center of vertical force (COF), on NeuroCom's EquiTest, is the cen-

ter of the vertical force exerted by the feet against the support surface. In any case (COP, COB, COF), the total force applied to the force platform fluctuates because it includes both body weight and the inertial effects of the slightest movements of the body, which occur even when one attempts to stand motionless. The movements of these force-based reference points are theorized to vary according to the movement of the body's COG and the distribution of muscle forces required to control posture. Ideally, healthy athletes should maintain their COP very near the A-P and M-L midlines.

Once the COP, COB, or COF is calculated, several other balance parameters can be attained. Deviation from this point in any direction represents a person's postural sway. Postural sway can be measured in various ways, depending on which system is being used. Mean displacement, length of sway path, length of sway area, amplitude, frequency, and direction with respect to the COP can be calculated on most systems. An equilibrium score, comparing the angular difference between the calculated maximum anterior to posterior COG displacements to a theoretical maximum displacement, is unique to Neuro-

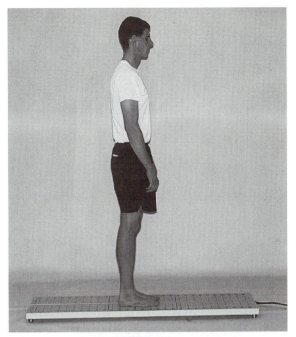

Figure 7-6 Balance Master with accessory 5-foot forceplate.

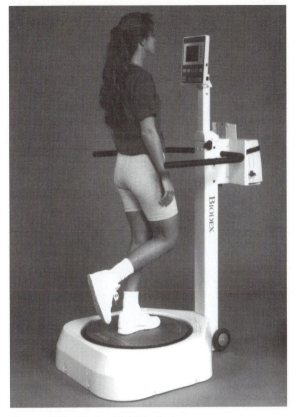

Figure 7-7 Biodex Stability System.

Com International's EquiTest. Sway index (SI), representing the degree of scatter of data about the COB, is unique to the Chattecx Balance System.

Forceplate technology allows for quantitative analysis and understanding of a subject's postural instability. These systems are fully integrated with hardware/software systems for quickly and quantitatively assessing and rehabilitating balance disorders. Most manufacturers allow for both static and dynamic balance assessment in either double- or single-leg stances, with eyes open or eyes closed. NeuroCom's EquiTest System is equipped with a moving visual surround (wall) that allows for the most sophisticated technology available for isolating and assessing sensory modality interaction.

Long forceplates have been developed by some manufacturers in an attempt to combat criticism that balance assessment is not functional. This newer variation on some systems (Figure 7-6) adds a vast array of dynamic balance exercises for training, such as walking, step up and over, side and crossover steps, hopping, leaping and lunging. These important return-to-sport activities can be practiced and perfected through the use of the computer's visual feedback.

Biodex Medical Systems (Shirley, NY) and Breg, Inc. (Vista, CA) both manufacture dynamic multiaxial tilting platforms that offer computer-generated data similar to those from a forceplate system. The Biodex Stability System (Figure 7-7) utilizes a dynamic multiaxial platform that allows up to 20 degrees of deflection in any direction. It is theorized that this degree of deflection is sufficient to stress joint mechanoreceptors that provide proprioceptive feedback (at end ranges of motion) necessary for balance control. Clinicians can therefore assess deficits in dynamic muscular control of posture relative to joint pathology. The patient's ability to control the platform's angle of tilt is quantified as a variance from center, as well as degrees of deflection over time, at various stability levels. A large variance is indicative of poor muscle response. The Kinesthetic Ability Trainer or KAT (Figure 7-8) is similar to the Biodex Stability System, in that it utilizes a multiaxial unstable platform. Exercises performed on these multiaxial unstable systems are similar to those of the BAP system and are especially effective for regaining proprioception and balance following injury to the ankle joint.

The FASTEX system (Cybex Division of Lumex, Inc., Ronkonkoma, NY) is another device available for assessing and training functional balance. The FASTEX consists of

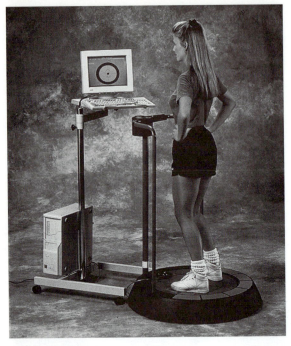

Figure 7-8 KAT.

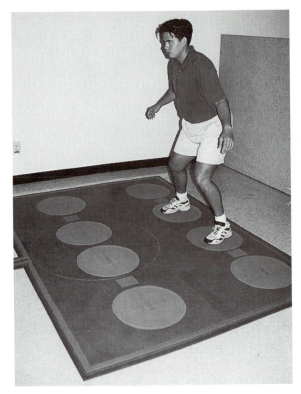

Figure 7-9 FASTEX.

eight deformable force platforms that include piezoelectric sensors. The sensor encircles each platform, which allows it to capture the entire shock wave from each impact (Figure 7-9). On impact, a measurable electric impulse is produced and translated into one of several quantitative variables. This system is not a forceplate capable of measuring COG alignment or postural sway, but it can assess reaction time, mobility, and time to stability.[75]

INJURY AND BALANCE

It has long been theorized that failure of stretched or damaged ligaments to provide adequate neural feedback in an injured extremity can contribute to decreased proprioceptive mechanisms necessary for maintenance of proper balance. Research has revealed these impairments in individuals with ankle injury[23,31,73] and anterior cruciate ligament (ACL) injury.[4,65] A lack of proprioceptive feedback resulting from such injuries might allow excessive or inappropriate loading of a joint. Furthermore, although the presence of a capsular lesion might interfere with the transmission of afferent impulses from the joint, a more important effect might be alteration of the afferent neural code that is conveyed to the CNS.[80] Decreased reflex excitation of motor neurons can result from either or both of the following events: (a) a decrease in propriocep-

tive input to the CNS, and (b) an increase in the activation of inhibitory interneurons within the spinal cord. All of these factors can lead to progressive degeneration of the joint and continued deficits in joint dynamics, balance, and coordination.

Ankle Injuries

Joint proprioceptors are believed to be damaged during injury to the lateral ligaments of the ankle because joint receptor fibers possess less tensile strength than the ligament fibers. Damage to the joint receptors is believed to cause joint deafferentation, therefore diminishing the supply of messages from the injured joint up the afferent pathway, disrupting proprioceptive function.[24] Freeman et al[24] were the first to report a decrease in the frequency of functional instability following ankle sprains when coordination exercises were performed as part of rehabilitation. Thus the term *articular deafferentation* was introduced to designate the mechanism that they believed to be the cause of functional instability of the ankle. This finding led to the inclusion of balance training in ankle rehabilitation programs.

Since 1965, Freeman[23] has theorized that if ankle injuries cause partial deafferentation and functional instability, a person's postural sway would be altered due to a proprioception deficit. Although some studies[72,73] have not supported Freeman's theory, other more recent studies using high-tech equipment (forceplate, kinesthesiometer, etc.) have revealed balance deficits in ankles following acute sprains[25,31,66] and/or in ankles with chronic instabilities.[9,22,26,67]

Differences were identified between injured and uninjured ankles in 14 ankle-injured subjects using a computerized strain gauge forceplate.[25] Four of five possible postural sway parameters (standard deviation of the mean center of pressure dispersion, mean sway amplitude, average speed, and number of sway amplitudes exceeding 5 and 10 mm) taken in the frontal plane from a single-leg stance position were reported to discriminate between injured and noninjured ankles. The authors reported that the application of an ankle brace eliminated the differences between injury status when tested on each parameter, therefore improving balance performance. More importantly this study suggests that the stabilometry technique of selectively analyzing postural sway movements in the frontal plane, where the diameter of the supporting area is smallest, leads to higher sensitivity. Because difficulties of maintaining balance after a ligament lesion involves the subtalar axis, it is proposed that increased sway movements of the different body segments would be found primarily in the frontal plane. The authors speculated that this could explain nonsignificant findings of earlier stabilometry studies[72,73] involving injured ankles.

Orthotic intervention and postural sway was studied in 13 subjects with acute inversion ankle sprains and 12 uninjured subjects under two treatment conditions (orthotic, nonorthotic) and four platform movements (stable, inversion/eversion, plantar flexion/dorsiflexion, medial/lateral perturbations).[31] Results revealed that ankle-injured subjects swayed more than uninjured subjects when assessed in a single-leg test on the Chattecx Balance System. The analysis also revealed that custom-fit orthotics can restrict undesirable motion at the foot and ankle, and enhance joint mechanoreceptors to detect perturbations and provide structural support for detecting and controlling postural sway in ankle injured subjects. A similar study[66] reported improvements in static balance for injured subjects while wearing custom-made orthotics.

Studies involving subjects with chronic ankle instabilities[9,22,26,67] indicate that individuals with a history of inversion ankle sprain are less stable in single-limb stance on the involved leg as compared to the uninvolved leg

and/or noninjured subjects. Significant differences between injured and uninjured subjects for sway amplitude but not sway frequency using a standard forceplate were revealed.[9] The effect of stance perturbation on frontal plane postural control was studied[67] in three groups of subjects: (1) control (no previous ankle injury); (2) functional ankle instability and 8-week training program; and (3) mechanical instability without functional instability (without shoe, with shoe, with brace and shoe). Results revealed a relative change from ankle to hip synergy at medially directed translations of the support surface on the NeuroCom EquiTest. The impairment was restored after 8 weeks of ankle disk training. The effect of a shoe and brace did not exceed the effect of the shoe alone. Impaired ankle function was shown to be related to coordination, as subjects changed from ankle toward hip strategies for postural adjustments.

Similarly, researchers[36] reported that lateral ankle joint anesthesia does not alter postural sway or passive joint position sense, but affects the center of balance position (similar to center of pressure) during both static and dynamic testing. This suggests the presence of an adaptive mechanism to compensate for the loss of afferent stimuli from the region of the lateral ankle ligaments.[36] Subjects tended to shift their center of balance medially during dynamic balance testing and slightly laterally during static balance testing. The authors speculated that center-of-balance shifting might provide additional proprioceptive input from cutaneous receptors in the sole of the foot/or stretch receptors in the peroneal muscle tendon unit that therefore prevents increased postural sway.

Increased postural sway frequency and latencies are parameters thought to be indicative of impaired ankle joint proprioception.[13,68] Cornwall et al[9] and Pintsaar et al,[67] however, found no differences between chronically injured subjects and control subjects on these measures. This raises the question as to whether postural sway was in fact caused by a proprioceptive deficit. Increased postural sway amplitudes in the absence of sway frequencies might suggest that chronically injured subjects recover their ankle joint proprioception over time. Thus, more research is warranted for investigating loss of joint proprioception and postural sway frequency.[9]

In summary, results of studies involving both chronic and acute ankle sprains suggest that increased postural sway and/or balance instability might be due not to a single factor but to disruption of both neurological and biomechanical factors at the ankle joint. Loss of balance might result from abnormal or altered biomechanical alignment of the body, thus affecting the transmission of somatosensory information from the ankle joint. It is possible that observed postural sway amplitudes following injury are a result of joint instability along the kinetic chain rather than deafferentation. Thus, the orthotic intervention[31,61,62] may have provided more optimal joint alignment.

Knee Injuries

Ligamentous injury to the knee has proven to affect the ability of subjects to accurately detect position.[2,3,4,46,49,50] The general consensus among numerous investigators performing proprioceptive testing is that a clinical proprioception deficit occurs in most patients after an ACL rupture who have functional instability and that this deficit seems to persist to some degree after an ACL reconstruction.[2] Because of the relationships between proprioception (somatosensation) and balance, it has been suggested that the patient's ability to balance on the ACL-injured leg might also be decreased.[4,65]

Studies have evaluated the effects of ACL ruptures on standing balance using forceplate technology, and although some studies have revealed balance deficits,[25,53] others have not.[18,35] Thus, there appear to be conflicting results from these studies, depending on which parameters are measured. Mizuta et al.[53] found significant differences in postural sway when measuring center of pressure and sway distance area between 11 functionally stable and 15 functionally unstable subjects who had unilateral ACL-deficient knees. Faculjak et al.,[18] however, found no differences in postural stability between 8 ACL-deficient subjects and 10 normal subjects when measuring average latency and response strength on an EquiTest System.

Several potential reasons for this discrepancy exist. First, it has been suggested that there might be a link between static balance and isometric strength of the musculature at the ankle and knee. Isometric muscle strength could therefore compensate for any somatosensory deficit present in the involved knee during a closed chain static balance test. Second, many studies fail to discriminate between functionally unstable ACL-deficient knees and knees that were not functionally unstable. This presents a design flaw, especially considering that functionally stable knees would most likely provide adequate balance despite ligamentous pathology. Another suggested reason for not seeing differences between injured knees and uninjured knees on static balance measures could be explained by the role that joint mechanoreceptors play. Neurophysiological studies[28,29,43,46] have revealed that joint mechanoreceptors provide enhanced kinesthetic awareness in the near-terminal range of motion or extremes of motion. Therefore, it could be speculated that if the maximum LOS are never reached during a static bal-

ance test, damaged mechanoreceptors (muscle or joint) might not even become a factor. Dynamic balance tests or functional hop tests that involve dynamic balance could challenge the postural control system (ankle strategies are taken over by hip and/or stepping strategies), requiring more mechanoreceptor input. These tests would most likely discriminate between functionally unstable ACL-deficient knees and normal knees.

Head Injury

Neurological status following mild head injury has been assessed using balance as a criterion variable. Athletic trainers and team physicians have long evaluated head injuries using the Romberg tests of sensory modality function to test balance. This is an easy and effective sideline test, however, the literature suggests there is more to posture control than just balance and sensory modality,[55,56,61,64,69] especially when assessing people with head injury.[30,33] The postural control system, which is responsible for linking brain to body communication, is often affected as a result of mild head injury. Recent studies have identified postural stability deficits in athletes up to 3 days post-injury using commercially available balance systems.[30,33] It appears that this deficit is related to a sensory interaction problem, whereby the injured athlete fails to use the visual system effectively. This research suggests that objective balance assessment can be used for establishing recovery curves for making return-to-play decisions in concussed athletes. Rehabilitation of concussed athletes using balance techniques has yet to be studied.

BALANCE TRAINING

Developing a rehabilitation program that includes exercises for improving balance and postural equilibrium is vital for a successful return to competition from a lower-extremity injury. Regardless of whether the athlete has sustained a quadriceps strain or an ankle sprain, the injury has caused a disruption at some point between the body's COG and base of support. This is likely to have caused compensatory weight shifts and gait changes along the kinetic chain that have resulted in balance deficits. These deficits can be detected through the use of functional assessment tests and/or computerized instrumentation previously discussed for assessing balance. Having the advanced technology available to quantify balance deficits is an amenity, but not a necessity. Imagination and creativity are often the best tools available to clinicians with limited resources who are trying to design balance-training protocols.

Because virtually all sport activities involve closed-chain lower-extremity function, functional rehabilitation should be performed in the closed kinetic chain. However, ROM, movement speed, and additional resistance might be more easily controlled in the open chain initially. Therefore, adequate, safe function in an open chain might be the first step in the rehabilitation process, but it should not be the focus of the rehabilitation plan. The sports medicine clinician should attempt to progress the athlete to functional closed-chain exercises quickly and safely. Depending on severity of injury, this could be as early as 1 day post-injury.

As previously mentioned, there is a close relationship between somatosensation, kinesthesia, and balance. Therefore, many of the exercises proposed for kinesthetic training indirectly enhance balance. Several methods of regaining balance have been proposed in the literature and are included in the most current rehabilitation protocols for ankle injury[41,71,80] and knee injury.[11,40,51,70,79]

A variety of activities can be used to improve balance, but the sports medicine clinicians should first consider five general rules before beginning:

- The exercises must be safe yet challenging.
- Stress multiple planes of motion.
- Incorporate a multisensory approach.
- Begin with static, bilateral, and stable surfaces and progress to dynamic, unilateral, and unstable surfaces.
- Progress to sport specific exercises.

There are several ways in which the clinician can meet these goals. Balance exercises should be performed in an open area, where the athlete will not be injured in the event of a fall. It is best to perform exercises with an assistive device within arm's reach (e.g., chair, railing, table, wall), especially during the initial phase of rehabilitation. When considering exercise duration for balance exercises, the clinician can use either sets and repetitions or a time-based protocol. The athlete can perform 2 or 3 sets of 15 repetitions and progress to 30 repetitions as tolerated, or perform 10 of the exercises for a 15-second period and progress to 30-second periods later in the program.

Classification of Balance Exercises

Static balance is when the COG is maintained over a fixed base of support (unilateral or bilateral) while standing on a stable surface. Examples of static exercises are a single-leg, double-leg, or Tandem stance Romberg task. *Semidynamic* balance involves one of two possible activities: (1) The person maintains their COG over a fixed base of support while standing on a moving surface (Chattecx Bal-

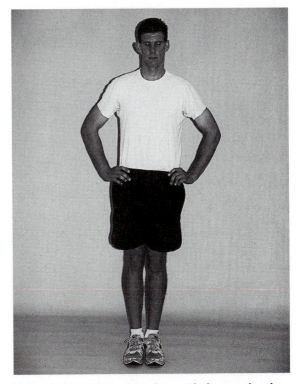

Figure 7-10   Bilateral Romberg with the eyes closed.

ance System or EquiTest) or unstable surface (Biodex Stability System, KAT, BAPS, medium-density foam or minitramp); or (2) the person transfers their COG over a fixed base of support to selected ranges and/or directions within the LOS while standing on a stable surface (Balance Master's LOS, functional reach tests, minisquats, or T-Band kicks). *Dynamic* balance involves the maintenance of the COG within the LOS over a moving base of support (feet), usually while on a stable surface. These tasks require the use of a stepping strategy. The base of support is always changing its position, therefore forcing the COG to be adjusted with each movement. Examples of dynamic exercises are walking on a balance beam, step up and over, or bounding). *Functional* balance tasks are the same as dynamic tasks with the inclusion of sport-specific tasks such as throwing and catching.

Phase I

The progression of activities during this phase should include nonballistic types of drills. Training for static balance can be initiated once the athlete is able to bear weight on the extremity. The athlete should first be asked to perform a bilateral 20-second Romberg test (Figure 7-10), followed

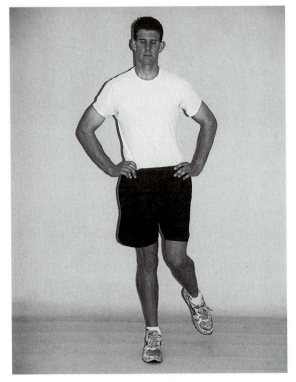

Figure 7-11 Unilateral Romberg with the eyes closed.

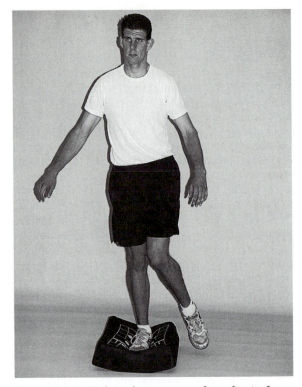

Figure 7-12 Unilateral stance on medium-density foam.

by a unilateral test (Figure 7-11) on both the involved and the uninvolved extremity. The clinician should make comparisons from these tests to determine the athlete's ability to balance bilaterally and unilaterally. It should be noted that even though this is termed "static" balance, the athlete does not remain perfectly motionless. In order to maintain static balance, the athlete must make many small corrections at the ankle, hip, trunk, arms, or head as previously discussed (see "Selection of Muscle Strategies"). An athlete who is having difficulties performing these activities should not be progressed. Repetitions of modified Romberg tests can be performed by first using the arms as a counterbalance, then attempting the activity without using the arms. Static balance activities should be used as a precurser to more dynamic activities. The general progression of these exercises should be from bilateral to unilateral, with eyes open to eyes closed. The exercises should attempt to eliminate or alter the various sensory information (visual, vestibular, and somatosensory) in order to challenge the other systems. In most orthopedic rehabilitation situations, this is going to involve eye closure and changes in the support surface so the somatosensory system can be overloaded or stressed. This theory is synonymous with the overload principle in therapeutic exercise. Research suggests that balance activities, both with and

without visual input, will enhance motor function at the brain stem level.[7,71] However, as the athlete becomes more efficient at performing activities involving static balance, eye closure is recommended so that only the somatosensory system is left to control balance.

As improvement occurs on a firm surface, static balance drills should progress to more semidynamic exercises on an unstable surface such as foam (Figure 7-12), minitramp (Figure 7-13), BAPS board (Figure 7-14), or rocker board (Figure 7-15). Additionally, the clinician can introduce light shoulder, back, or chest taps in an attempt to challenge the athlete's ability to maintain balance (Figure 7-16). Finally, the use of multiaxial devices such as the Biodex Stability System or Kinesthetic Ability Trainer on a relatively easy level can be initiated during the later part of Phase I. These exercises increase awareness of the location of the COG under a challenged condition, thereby helping to increase ankle strength in the closed kinetic chain. Such training can also increase sensitivity of the muscle spindle and thereby increase proprioceptive input to the spinal cord, which might provide compensation for altered joint afference.[46]

Static exercises and semidynamic exercises are likely not very functional for most sport activities, but they are the first step toward regaining proprioceptive awareness,

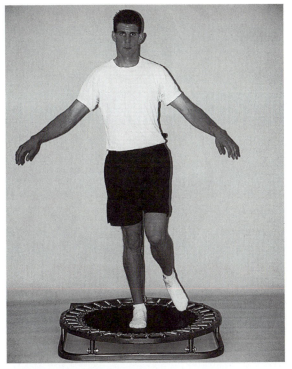

Figure 7-13   Unilateral stance on minitramp.

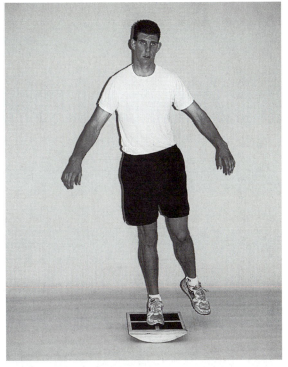

Figure 7-15   Unilateral stance on rocker board.

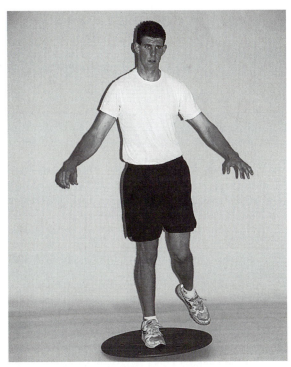

Figure 7-14   Unilateral stance on BAPS board.

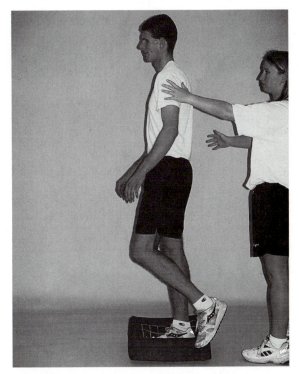

Figure 7-16   Clinician causing perturbations using shoulder taps.

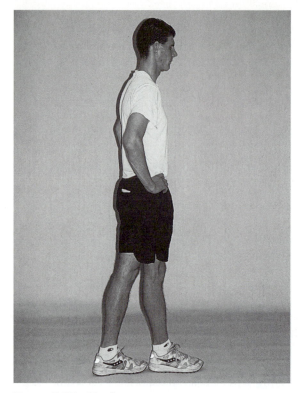

Figure 7-17   Tandem stance.

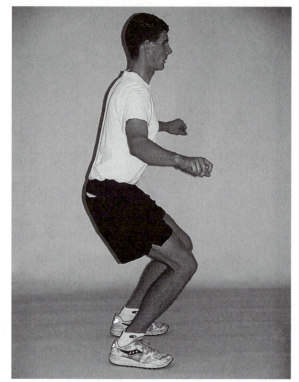

Figure 7-18   Minisquat.

reflex stabilization, and postural orientation. The athlete should attempt to assume a functional stance while performing static balance drills. Training in different positions places a variety of demands on the musculotendinous structures about the ankle, knee, and hip joints. For example, a gymnast should practice static balance with the hip in neutral and external rotation, as well as during a tandem stance (Figure 7-17), in order to mimic performance on a balance beam. A basketball player should perform these drills in the "ready position" on the balls of the feet with the hips and knees slightly flexed. Athletes requiring a significant amount of static balance for performing their sport include gymnasts, cheerleaders, and football linemen.[41]

Phase II

Phase II should be considered the transition phase from static to more dynamic balance activities. Dynamic balance will be especially important for athletes who perform activities such as running, jumping, and cutting—which encompasses about 95 percent of all athletes. Such activities require the athlete to repetitively lose and gain balance to perform their sport without falling or becoming injured.[41] Dynamic balance activities should be in-

corporated into the rehabilitation program only when sufficient healing has occurred and the athlete has adequate ROM, muscle strength, and endurance. This could be as early as a few days post-injury in the case of a grade 1 ankle sprain, or as late as 6 weeks postsurgery in the case of an anterior cruciate reconstruction. Before clinicians progress the athlete to challenging dynamic and sport specific balance drills, several semidynamic (intermediate) exercises should be introduced.

These semidynamic balance drills involve displacement or perturbation of the COG away from the base of support. The athlete is challenged to return and/or steady the COG above the base of support throughout several repetitions of the exercise. Some of these exercises involve a bilateral stance, some involve a unilateral stance, and others involve transferring of weight from one extremity to the other.

The bilateral-stance balance drills include the minisquat, which is performed with the feet shoulder-width apart and the COG centered over a stable base of support. The trunk should be positioned upright over the legs as the athlete slowly flexes the hips and knees into a partial squat approximately 45 to 60 degrees of knee flexion (Figure 7-18). The athlete then returns to the starting posi-

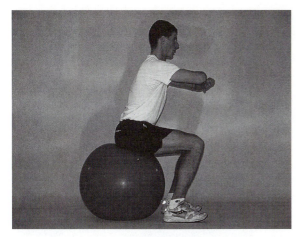

Figure 7-19 Sit-to-stand using Physioball.

tion and repeats the task several times. Once ROM, strength, and stability have improved, the athlete can progress to a full squat, which approaches 90 degrees of knee flexion. These should be performed in front of a mirror so the athlete can observe the amount of stability on return to the extended position. A large PhysioBall can also be used to perform sit-to-stand activities (Figure 7-19). These exercises are important in the rehabilitation of knee and hip injuries, as they help improve weight transfer, COG sway velocity, and left/right weight symmetry.

The lunge is a more specific bilateral drill that begins to simulate sport-specific moves. The exercise decreases the base of support and increases the stress to one extremity at a given moment. ROM can be stressed to a higher degree than with the squatting exercises. When lunges are used to improve balance, it is important that the athlete perform the drill slowly so that the COG can be steadied over each support leg. When performing the forward lunge, the athlete may use exaggerated extension movements of the lumbar region to assist weak or uncoordinated hip extension (Figure 7-20). This substitution is not produced during the squatting exercises.[77] Normal lunge distances should approach, but not reach, the athlete's total height.

Forward Lunge. The athlete's hands should be placed on the hips, while the involved leg is placed forward and the uninvolved backward. The progression for lunges should be from standard short lunges without tubing, to assisted lunges and resisted lunges using tubing. During the **assisted forward lunge,** the athlete faces away from the tubing, which descends at a sharp angle (approximately 60 degrees) and wraps around the waist. The tubing's angle parallels the athlete's COG, which moves forward and down (Figure 7-21), thereby assisting the athlete up from the lowest point. The assistance also

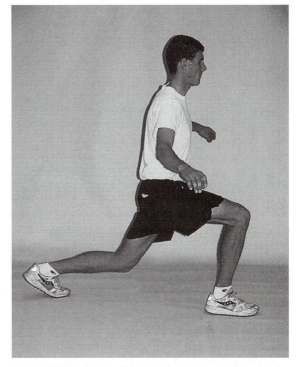

Figure 7-20 Forward lunge.

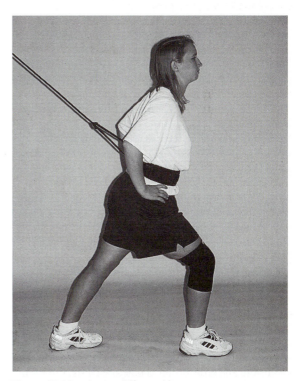

Figure 7-21 Assisted forward lunge.

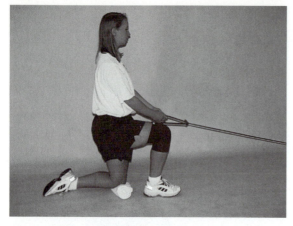

Figure 7-22   Resisted forward lunge with block.

minimizes eccentric demands for deceleration when lowering and improves balance by helping the athlete focus on the COG.[77]

During the **resisted forward lunge** the uninvolved leg remains forward. The athlete faces the tubing, which is now ascending from the floor to the level of the waist. The athlete should position her- or himself far enough from the tubing so that tension is created when kneeling on the uninvolved (back) leg (Figure 7-22). During the upward movement the focus should be on hip extension and not knee extension. The athlete should initiate movement from the hip and not from lumbar hyperextension or excessive knee extension.[71,77] During the downward movement, the tubing will increase the eccentric loading on the quadriceps.

Lateral Lunge.   The **assisted lateral lunge** positions the involved leg opposite the side of the tubing (Figure 7-23). The tubing reduces relative body weight while allowing closed-kinetic-chain function in a lateral direction. The uninvolved extremity initiates movement of the COG over the involved extremity, followed by an assisted push-off from the involved extremity toward the uninvolved side. The **resisted lateral lunge** positions the involved leg on the same side as the tubing (Figure 7-24). During this drill, the involved leg initiates the movement and acts as the primary weight-bearing extremity. Like the forward resisted lunge, it provides overloading on the involved extremity.[71,77]

The clinician has a variety of options for unilateral semidynamic balance exercises. A unilateral minisquat is a good starting point. These can be performed while holding on to a chair or support rail with the uninvolved knee flexed to 45 degrees. The athlete should emphasize controlled hip and knee flexion, followed by a smooth return

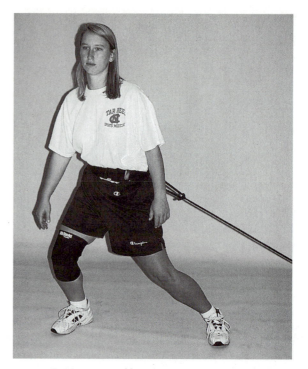

Figure 7-23   Assisted lateral lunge.

to the starting position on the involved extremity. Once this skill is mastered, the athlete can progress to more dynamic exercises, such as a step-up. Step-ups can be performed either in the saggital plane (forward step-up) or in the transverse plane (lateral step-up). These drills should begin with the heel of the uninvolved extremity on the floor. Using a 2 count, the athlete should shift body weight toward the involved side and use the involved extremity to slowly raise the body onto the step.[71] The involved knee should not be "locked" into full extension. Instead, the knee should be positioned in approximately 5 degrees of flexion, while balancing on the step for 3 seconds. Following the 3 count, the body weight should be shifted toward the uninvolved side and lowered to the heel of the uninvolved side (Figures 7-25 and 7-26). **Step-up-and-over** activities are similar to step-ups, but involve more dynamic transfer of the COG. These can be performed by having the athlete either both ascend and descend using the involved extremity (Figure 7-27) or ascend with the involved extremity and descend with the uninvolved extremity forcing the involved leg to support the body on the descend (Figure 7-28).

The sports therapist can also introduce the athlete to more challenging static tests during this phase. For example, foam padding can be used in conjunction with the

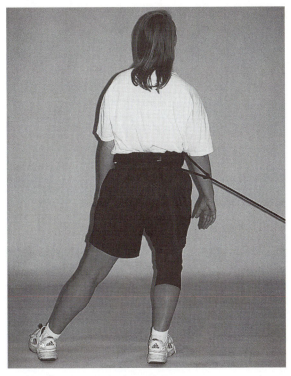

Figure 7-24 Resisted lateral lunge.

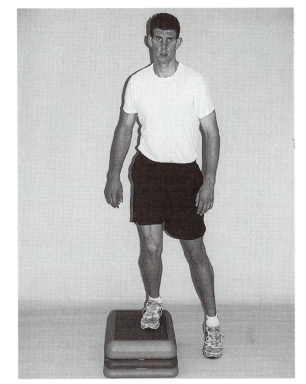

Figure 7-26 Lateral step-up.

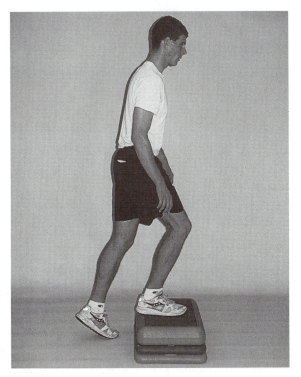

Figure 7-25 Forward step-up.

rocker board (Figure 7-29). A slant board can be used to stretch the heel cord while attempting to balance (Figure 7-30). Finally, the very popular TheraBand kicks (T-Band kicks, or steamboats) are excellent for improving balance. TheraBand kicks are performed with an elastic material (attached to the ankle of the uninvolved leg) serving as a resistance against a relatively fast kicking motion. The athlete's balance on the involved extremity is challenged by perturbations caused by the kicking motion of the uninvolved leg (Figure 7-31). Four sets of these exercises should be performed, one for each of four possible kicking motions: hip flexion, hip extension, hip abduction, and hip adduction. T-Band kicks can also be performed on foam or a minitramp if additional somatosensory challenges are desired.[70]

Phase III

Once the athlete can successfully complete the semidynamic and simple dynamic exercises presented in phase II, they should be ready to perform more dynamic and functional types of exercises. The general progression for activities to develop dynamic balance and control is from

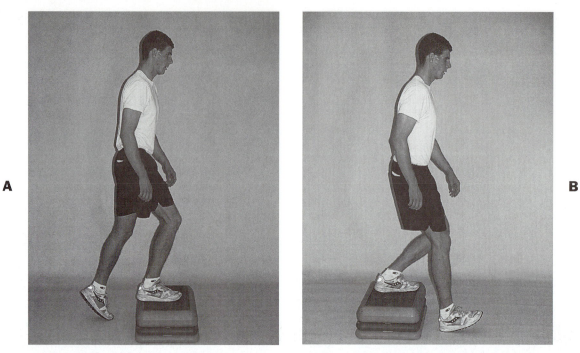

Figure 7-27   Step up and over. **A,** Ascending on the uninvolved extremity. **B,** Descending on the involved extremity.

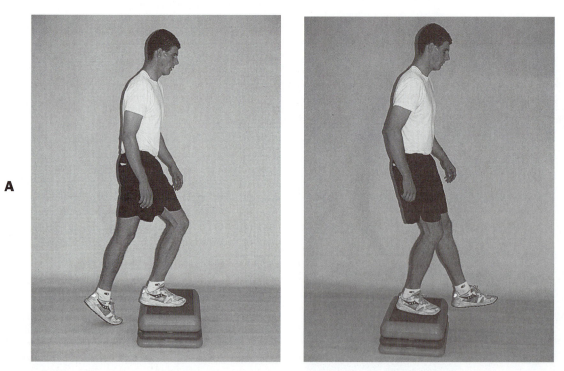

Figure 7-28   Step up and over. **A,** Ascending on the involved extremity. **B,** Descending on the uninvolved extremity.

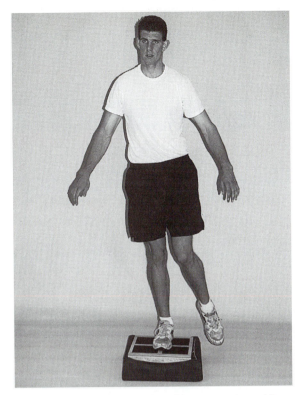

Figure 7-29   Rocker board used in conjunction with foam padding.

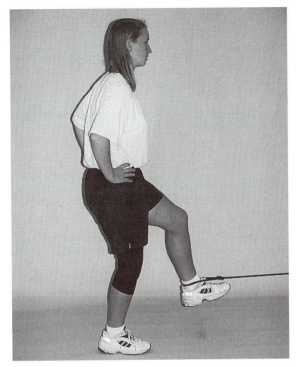

Figure 7-31   T-Band kicks.

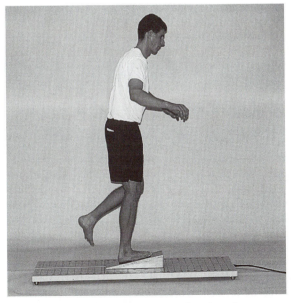

Figure 7-30   Unilateral stance on slant board.

slow-speed to fast-speed activities, from low-force to high-force activities, and from controlled to uncontrolled activities.[41] In other words, the athlete should be working toward sport-specific drills that will allow for a safe return to sport activity. These exercises will likely be different depending on which sport the person plays. For example, drills to improve lateral weight shifting and sidestepping should be incorporated into a program for a tennis player, whereas drills to improve jumping and landing are going to be more important for a track athlete who performs the long jump. As previously mentioned, clinicians often need to use their imagination to develop the best protocols for their athletes.

Bilateral jumping drills are a good place to begin once the athlete has reached Phase III. These can be performed either front to back or side to side. The athlete should concentrate on landing on each side of the line as quickly as possible [70,71] (Figure 7-32). As the athlete progresses through these exercises, eye closure can be used to further challenge the athlete's somatosensation. After mastering these straight-plane jumping patterns, the athlete can begin diagonal jumping patterns through the use of a cross on the floor formed by two pieces of tape (Figure 7-33). The intersecting lines create four quadrants that can be numbered and used to perform

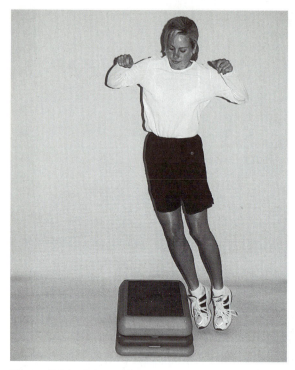

Figure 7-32   Bilateral hops.

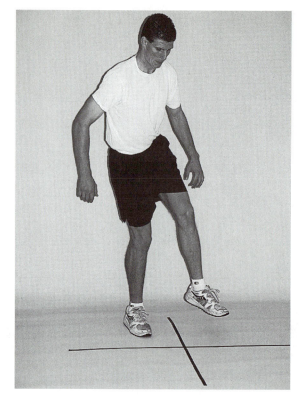

Figure 7-33   Diagonal hops.

different jumping sequences, such as 1,3,2,4 for the first set and 1,4,2,3 for the second set.[70,71] A larger grid can be designed to allow for longer sequences and longer jumps, both of which require additional strength, endurance, and balance control.

Bilateral dynamic balance exercises should progress to unilateral dynamic balance exercises as quickly as possible during Phase III. At this stage of the rehabilitation, pain and fatigue should not be as much of a factor. All jumping drills performed bilaterally should now be performed unilaterally, by practicing first on the uninvolved extremity (Figure 7-33). If additional challenges are needed, a vertical component can be added by having the athlete jump over a box or another suitable object (Figure 7-34).

Tubing can be used to add resistance to dynamic unilateral training exercises. The athlete can perform stationary running against the tube's resistance, followed by lateral and diagonal bounding exercises. Diagonal bounding, which involves jumping from one foot to another, places greater emphasis on lateral movements. It is recommended that the athlete first learn the bounding exercise without tubing, and then attempt the exercise with tubing. A foam roll, towel, or other obstacle can be used to increase jump height and/or distance[77] (Figure 7-35). The

final step in trying to improve dynamic balance should involve the incorporation of sport-related activities such as throwing and catching a ball. At this stage of the rehabilitation program, the athlete should be able to safely concentrate on the functional activity (catching and throwing), while subconsciously controlling dynamic balance (Figure 7-36).

CLINICAL VALUE OF HIGH-TECH TRAINING AND ASSESSMENT

The benefit of using the commercially available balance systems is that not only can deficits be detected, but progress can be charted with quantitatively through the computer generated results. For example, NeuroCom's New Balance Master 6.0 is capable of assessing an athlete's ability to perform coordinated movements essential for sport performance. The system, equipped with a 5-foot-long force platform, is capable of identifying specific components underlying performance of several functional tasks. Exercises are also available on the system that help to improve the deficits.[62]

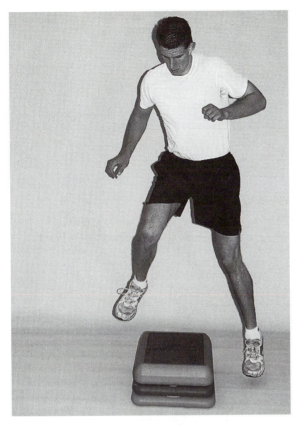

Figure 7-34 Lateral jumps over box.

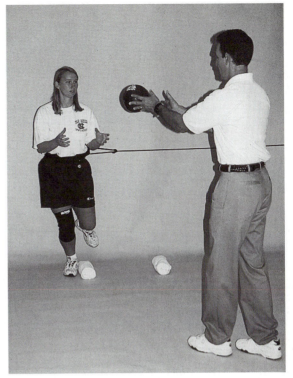

Figure 7-36 Control dynamic balance while throwing and catching a ball.

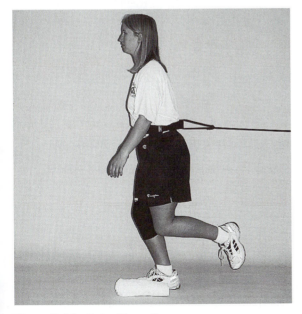

Figure 7-35 Lateral bounding.

Results of a step-up-and-over test are presented in Figure 7-37. The components analyzed in this particular task are (1) **lift-up index,** which quantifies the maximum lifting (concentric) force exerted by the leading leg and is expressed as a percentage of the person's weight; (2) **movement time,** which quantifies the number of seconds required to complete the task, beginning with initial weight shift to the nonstepping leg and ending with impact of the lagging leg onto the surface; and (3) **impact index,** which quantifies the maximum vertical impact force (percentage of body weight) as the lagging leg lands on the surface.[62]

Early research on the clinical applicability of these measures has revealed interesting results. Preliminary observations from two studies in progress suggest that deficits in impact control are a common feature of patients with ACL injuries, even when strength and range of motion of the involved knee are within normal limits. Several other performance assessments are available on this system, including *sit to stand, walk test, step and quick turn, forward lunge, weight bearing/squat, rhythmic weight shift.*

Name:	Doe, John J	Diagnosis:	ACL Tear L Knee	File:	HBM1.QBM
ID:	ATID00001	Operator ID:	Jodi Bower	Date:	03/06/97
DOB:	11/22/55	Referred by:	Dr. Tom Merkle	Time:	6:35:06 PM
Height:	5'11"	Comments:	DOI: 7/4/96; DOS: 7/6/96		

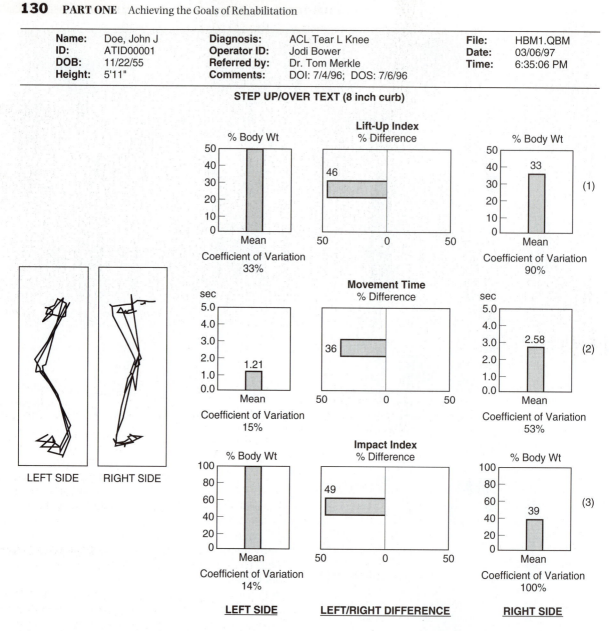

STEP UP/OVER TEXT (8 inch curb)

Figure 7-37   Results from a step-up-and-over protocol on the New Balance Master 6.0.

Summary

1. There are very close relationships among proprioception, kinesthesia, and balance.
2. The most common form of proprioception training involves unilateral balance drills on challenging surfaces.
3. Exercises performed on foam or multiaxial devices are good precursors for more dynamic balance exercises such as lunges, lateral bounding, and unilateral hopping drills.
4. The goal of any rehabilitation program should be to move safely through a progression of balance exercises (phase I through phase III).
5. The use of commercially manufactured balance systems adds a nice feature to balance training and assessment, allowing the sports therapist to quantify progress.
6. With a little creativity, the sports therapist can design low-cost, yet very effective exercises for regaining balance.

References

1. Balogun, J. A., C. O. Adesinasi, and D. K. Marzouk. 1992. The effects of a wobble board exercise training program on static balance performance and strength of lower extremity muscle. *Physiotherapy Canada* 44:23–30.
2. Barrack, R. L., P. Lund, and H. Skinner. 1994. Knee joint proprioception revisited. *Journal of Sport Rehabilitation* 3:18–42.
3. Barrack, R. L., H. B. Skinner, and S. L. Buckley. 1989. Proprioception in the anterior cruciate deficient knee. *American Journal of Sports Medicine* 17:1–6.
4. Barrett, D. 1991. Proprioception and function after anterior cruciate reconstruction. *Journal of Bone and Joint Surgery* [Br] 73:833–37.
5. Black, F., C. Wall, and L. Nashner. 1983. Effect of visual and support surface orientations upon postural control in vestibular deficient subjects. *Acta Otolaryngol* 95:199–210.
6. Black, O., C. Wall, H. Rockette, and R. Kitch. 1982. Normal subject postural sway during the Romberg test. *American Journal of Otolaryngology* 3(5): 309–18.
7. Blackburn, T., and M. Voight. 1995. Single leg stance: Development of a reliable testing procedure. *Proceedings of the 12th International Congress of the World Confederation for Physical Therapy.*
8. Booher, J., and G. Thibodeau. 1995. *Athletic injury assessment.* St. Louis: Times Mirror/Mosby College.
9. Cornwall, M., and P. Murrell. 1991. Postural sway following inversion sprain of the ankle. *J. American Podiatric. Med. Assoc.* 81:243–47.
10. Davies, G. 1995. The need for critical thinking in rehabilitation. *Journal of Sport Rehabilitation* 4(1): 1–22.
11. DeCarlo, M., T. Klootwyk, and K. Shelbourne. 1997. ACL surgery and accelerated rehabilitation: Revisited. *Journal of Sport Rehabilitation* 6(2): 144–56.
12. Diener, H., J. Dichgans, B. Guschlbauer, et al. 1986. Role of visual and static vestibular influences on dynamic posture control. *Hum. Neurobiol.* 5:105–13.
13. Diener, H., J. Dichgans, B. Guschlbauer, and H. Mau. 1984. The significance of proprioception on postural stabilization as assessed by ischemia. *Brain Research* 296:103–9.
14. Dietz, V., G. Horstmann, and W. Berger. 1989. Significance of proprioceptive mechanisms in the regulation of stance. *Progress in Brain Research* 80:419–23.
15. Donahoe, B., D. Turner, and T. Worrell. 1993. The use of functional reach as a measurement of balance in healthy boys and girls ages 5–15. *Physical Therapy* 73(6): S71.
16. Dornan, J., G. Fernie, and P. Holliday. 1978. Visual input: Its importance in the control of postural sway. *Archives of Physical Medicine and Rehabilitation* 59:586–91.
17. Ekdahl, C., G. Jarnlo, and S. Anderson. 1989. Standing balance in healthy subjects: Evaluation of a quantitative test battery on a force platform. *Scandanavian Journal of Rehabilitation Medicine* 21:187–95.
18. Faculjak, P., K. Firoozbakshsh, D. Wausher, and M. McGuire. 1993. Balance characteristics of normal and anterior cruciate ligament deficient knees. *Physical Therapy* 73:S22.
19. Fisher, A., S. Wietlisbach, and J. Wilberger. 1988. Adult performance on three tests of equilibrium. *American Journal of Occupational Therapy* 42(1): 30–35.
20. Fitzpatrick, R., D. K. Rogers, and D. I. McCloskey. 1994. Stable human standing with lower-limb muscle afferents providing the only sensory input. *Journal of Physiology* 480(2): 395–403.
21. Flores, A. 1992. Objective measures of standing balance. *Neurology Report - Am. Phys. Ther. Assoc.* 16(1): 17–21.
22. Forkin, D. M., C. Koczur, R. Battle, and R. A. Newton. 1996. Evaluation of kinesthetic deficits indicative of balance control in gymnasts with unilateral chronic ankle sprains. *Journal of Orthopaedic and Sports Physical Therapy* 23(4): 245–50.
23. Freeman, M. 1965. Instability of the foot after injuries to the lateral ligament of the ankle. *Journal of Bone and Joint Surgery* 47B:678–85.
24. Freeman, M., M. Dean, and I. Hanham. 1965. The etiology and prevention of functional instability of the foot. *J. Bone Joint Surg.* 47B: 669–77.
25. Friden, T., R. Zatterstrom, A. Lindstrand, and U. Moritz. 1989. A stabilometric technique for evaluation of lower limb instabilities. *American Journal of Sports Medicine* 17(1): 118–22.

26. Garn, S. N., and R. A. Newton. 1988. Kinesthetic awareness in subjects with multiple ankle sprains. *Physical Therapy* 68:1667–71.

27. Goldie, P., T. Bach, and O. Evans. 1989. Force platform measures for evaluating postural control: Reliability and validity. *Archives of Physical Medicine and Rehabilitation* 70:510–17.

28. Grigg, P. 1975. Mechanical factors influencing response of joint afferent neurons from cat knee. *Journal of Neurophysiology* 38:1473–84.

29. Grigg, P. 1976. Response of joint afferent neurons in cat medial articular nerve to active and passive movements of the knee. *Brain Research* 118:482–85.

30. Guskiewicz, K. M., D. H. Perrin, and B. Gansneder. 1996. Effect of mild head injury on postural stability. *Journal of Athletic Training* 31(4): 300–306.

31. Guskiewicz, K. M., and D. H. Perrin. 1996. Perrin. Effect of orthotics on postural sway following inversion ankle sprain. *Journal of Orthopaedic and Sports Physical Therapy* 23(5): 326–31.

32. Guskiewicz, K. M., and D. M. Perrin. 1996. Research and clinical applications of assessing balance. *Journal of Sport Rehabilitation* 5:45–63.

33. Guskiewicz, K. M., B. L. Riemann, D. H. Riemann, and L. M. Nashner. 1997. Alternative approaches to the assessment of mild head injury in athletes. *Medicine and Science in Sports and Exercise* 29(7): S213–S221.

34. Guyton, A. 1991. *Textbook of medical physiology*. 8th ed. Philadelphia: W. B. Saunders.

35. Harrison, E., N. Duenkel, R. Dunlop, and G. Russell. 1994. Evaluation of single-leg standing following anterior cruciate ligament surgery and rehabilitation. *Physical Therapy* 74(3): 245–52.

36. Hertel, J. N., K. M. Guskiewicz, D. M. Kahler, and D. H. Perrin. 1996. Effect of lateral ankle joint anesthesia on center of balance, postural sway and joint position sense. *Journal of Sport Rehabilitation* 5:111–19.

37. Horak, F. B., L. M. Nashner, and H. C. Diener. 1990. Postural strategies associated with somatosensory and vestibular loss. *Exp. Brain. Res.* 82:167–77.

38. Horak, F., and L. Nashner. 1986. Central programming of postural movements: Adaptation to altered support surface configurations. *Journal of Neurophysiology* 55:1369–81.

39. Houk, J. 1979. Regulation of stiffness by skeleto-motor reflexes. *Annual Review of Physiology* 41:99–114.

40. Irrgang, J., and C. Harner. 1997. Recent advances in ACL rehabilitation: Clinical factors. *Journal of Sport Rehabilitation* 6(2): 111–24.

41. Irrgang, J., S. Whitney, and E. Cox. 1994. Balance and proprioceptive training for rehabilitation of the lower extremity. *Journal of Sport Rehabilitation* 3:68–83.

42. Jansen, E., R. Larsen, and B. Mogens. 1982. Quantitative Romberg's test: Measurement and computer calculations of postural stability. *Acta Neurol. Scand.* 66:93–99.

43. Johansson, H., I. J. Alexander, and K. C. Hayes. 1982. Nerve supply of the human knee and its functional importance. *American Journal of Sports Medicine* 10:329–35.

44. Kauffman, T. L., L. M. Nashner, and L. K. Allison. 1997. Balance is a critical parameter in orthopedic rehabilitation. *Orthopaedic Phys. Ther. Clin. North America* 6(1): 43–78.

45. Kisner, C., and L. A. Colby. 1996. *Therapeutic exercise: foundations and techniques.* 3d ed. Philadelphia: F. A. Davis.

46. Lephart, S. M. 1993. Re-establishing proprioception, kinesthesia, joint position sense, and neuromuscular control in rehabilitation. In *Rehabilitation techniques in sports*, 2d ed., edited by W. E. Prentice, pp. 118–37. St. Louis: Times Mirror/Mosby College.

47. Lephart, S. M., and T. J. Henry. 1995. Functional rehabilitation for the upper and lower extremity. *Orthopedic Clin. North America* 26(3): 579–92.

48. Lephart, S. M., and M. S. Kocher. 1993. The role of exercise in the prevention of shoulder disorders. In *The shoulder: A balance of mobility and stability*, edited by F. A. Matsen, F. H. Fu, and R. J. Hawkins, pp. 597–620. Rosemont, IL: American Academy of Orthopaedic Surgeons.

49. Lephart, S. M., M. S. Kocher, F. H. Fu, et al. 1992. Proprioception following ACL reconstruction. *Journal of Sport Rehabilitation* 1:186–96.

50. Lephart, S. M., D. Pincivero, J. Giraldo, and F. Fu. 1997. The role of proprioception in the management and rehabilitation of athletic injuries. *American Journal of Sports Medicine* 25:130–37.

51. Mangine, R., and T. Kremchek. 1997. Evaluation-based protocol of the anterior cruciate ligament. *Journal of Sport Rehabilitation* 6(2): 157–81.

52. Mauritz, K., J. Dichgans, and A. Hufschmidt. 1979. Quantitative analysis of stance in late cortical cerebellar atrophy of the anterior lobe and other forms of cerebellar ataxia. *Brain* 102, 461–82.

53. Mizuta, H., M. Shiraishi, K. Kubota, K. Kai, and K. Takagi. 1992. A stabilometric technique for evaluation of functional instability in the anterior cruciate ligament deficient knee. *Clin. J. Sports Med.* 2:235–39.

54. Murray, M., A. Seireg, and S. Sepic. 1975. Normal postural stability: Qualitative assessment. *J. Bone Joint Surg.* 57A(4): 510–16.

55. Nashner, L. 1976. Adapting reflexes controlling the human posture. *Exploring Brain Research* 26:59–72.

56. Nashner, L. 1982. Adaptation of human movement to altered environments. *Trends in Neuroscience* 5:358–61.

57. Nashner, L. 1985. A functional approach to understanding spasticity. In *Electromyography and evoked potentials*, edited by A. Struppler and A. Weindl, pp. 22–29. Berlin: Springer-Verlag.

58. Nashner, L. 1989. Sensory, neuromuscular and biomechanical contributions to human balance. In *Balance: Proceedings of the APTA Forum, June 13–15, 1989*, edited by P. Duncan, pp. 5–12. Alexandria, VA: American Physical Therapy Association.

59. Nashner, L. 1993. Computerized dynamic posturography. In *Handbook of balance function and testing*, edited by G. Jacobson, C. Newman, and J. Kartush, pp. 280–307. St. Louis: Mosby Yearbook.

60. Nashner, L. 1993. Practical biomechanics and physiology of balance. In *Handbook of balance function and testing,* edited by G. Jacobson, C. Newman, and J. Kartush, pp. 261–79. St. Louis: Mosby Yearbook.

61. Nashner, L., F. Black, and C. Wall, III. 1982. Adaptation to altered support and visual conditions during stance: Patients with vestibular deficits. *Journal of Neuroscience* 2(5): 536–44.

62. NeuroCom International, Inc. 1997. *The objective quantification of daily life tasks: The NEW Balance Master 6.0* [manual]. Clackamas, OR.

63. Newton, R. 1992. Review of tests of standing balance abilities. *Brain Injury* 3:335–43.

64. Norre, M. 1993. Sensory interaction testing in platform posturography. *J. Laryngol. and Otol.* 107:496–501.

65. Noyes, F., S. Barber, and R. Mangine. 1991. Abnormal lower limb symmetry determined by function hop test after anterior cruciate ligament rupture. *American Journal of Sports Medicine* 19(5): 516–18.

66. Orteza, L., W. Vogelbach, and C. Denegar. 1992. The effect of molded and unmolded orthotics on balance and pain while jogging following inversion ankle sprain. *Journal of Athletic Training* 27(1): 80–84.

67. Pintsaar, A., J. Brynhildsen, and H. Tropp. 1996. Postural corrections after standardised perturbations of single limp stance: Effect of training and orthotic devices in patients with ankle instability. *British Journal of Sports Medicine* 30:151–155.

68. Shambers, G. M. 1969. Influence of the fusimotor system on stance and volitional movement in normal man. *American Journal of Physical Medicine* 48:225–27.

69. Shumway-Cook, A., and F. Horak. 1986. Assessing the influence of sensory interaction on balance. *Physical Therapy* 66(10): 1548–50.

70. Swanik, C. B., S. M. Lephart, F. P. Giannantonio, and F. H. Fu. 1997. Reestablishing proprioception and neuromuscular control in the ACL-injured athlete. *Journal of Sport Rehabilitation* 6(2): 182–206.

71. Tippett, S., and M. Voight. 1995. *Functional progression for sports rehabilitation.* Champaign, IL: Human Kinetics.

72. Tropp, H., J. Ekstrand, and J. Gillquist. 1984. Factors affecting stabilometry recordings of single limb stance. *American Journal of Sports Medicine* 12:185–88.

73. Tropp, H., J. Ekstrand, and J. Gillquist. 1984. Stabilometry in functional instability of the ankle and its value in predicting injury. *Medicine and Science in Sports and Exercise* 16:64–66.

74. Tropp, H., and P. Odenrick. 1988. Postural control in single limb stance. *J. Orthop. Res.* 6:833–39.

75. Trulock, S. C. 1996. *A comparison of static, dynamic and functional methods of objective balance assessment.* Master's thesis, University of North Carolina, Chapel Hill.

76. Vander, A., J. Sherman, and D. Luciano. 1990. *Human physiology: The mechanisms of Body Function.* 5th ed. New York: McGraw-Hill.

77. Voight, M., and G. Cook. 1996. Clinical application of closed kinetic chain exercise. *Journal of Sport Rehabilitation* 5(1): 25–44.

78. Whitney, S. 1994. Clinical and high tech alternatives to assessing postural sway in athletes. Paper presented at the annual meeting of the National Athletic Trainers' Association, Dallas, 11, June.

79. Wilk, K., N. Zheng, G. Fleisig, J. Andrews, and W. Clancy. 1997. Kinetic chain exercise: Implications for the anterior cruciate ligament patient. *Journal of Sport Rehabilitation* 6(2): 125–43.

80. Wilkerson, G., and J. Nitz. 1994. Dynamic ankle stability: Mechanical and neuromuscular interrelationships. *Journal of Sport Rehabilitation* 3:43–57.

CHAPTER 8

Maintaining Cardiorespiratory Fitness during Rehabilitation

William E. Prentice

After completion of this chapter, the student should be able to do the following:

- Explain the relationships between heart rate, stroke volume, cardiac output, and rate of oxygen use.

- Describe the function of the heart, blood vessels, and lungs in oxygen transport.

- Describe the oxygen transport system and the concept of maximal rate of oxygen use.

- Describe the principles of continuous, interval, fartlek, and par cours training and the potential of each technique for improving cardiorespiratory endurance.

- Describe the differences between aerobic and anaerobic activity.

- Identify methods for assessing cardiorespiratory endurance.

- Demonstrate a method for assessing cardiorespiratory endurance.

WHY IS IT IMPORTANT TO MAINTAIN CARDIORESPIRATORY FITNESS DURING REHABILITATION PROCESS?

Although strength and flexibility are commonly regarded as essential components in any injury rehabilitation program, often relatively little consideration is given to maintaining levels of cardiorespiratory endurance. An athlete spends a considerable amount of time preparing the cardiorespiratory system to be able to handle the increased demands made upon it during a competitive season. When injury occurs and the athlete is forced to miss training time, levels of cardiorespiratory endurance can decrease rapidly. Thus the sports therapist must design or substitute alternative activities that allow the individual to maintain existing levels of fitness during the rehabilitation period.

By definition, **cardiorespiratory endurance** is the ability to perform whole-body activities for extended periods of time without undue fatigue.[10,15] The cardiorespiratory system supplies oxygen to the various tissues of the body. Without oxygen, the cells in the human body cannot possibly function, and ultimately death will occur. Thus the cardiorespiratory system is the basic life-support system of the body.[10]

TRAINING EFFECTS ON THE CARDIORESPIRATORY SYSTEM

Basically, transport of oxygen throughout the body involves the coordinated function of four components: (1) the heart, (2) the blood vessels, (3) the blood, and (4) the lungs. The improvement of cardiorespiratory endurance through training occurs because of increased capability of each of these four elements in providing necessary oxygen to the working tissues.[42] A basic discussion of the training effects and response to exercise that occur in the heart, blood vessels, blood, and lungs should make it easier to understand why the training techniques to be discussed later are so effective in improving cardiorespiratory endurance.

Adaptation of the Heart to Exercise

The heart is the main pumping mechanism and circulates oxygenated blood throughout the body to the working tissues. The heart receives deoxygenated blood from the venous system and then pumps the blood through the pulmonary vessels to the lungs, where carbon dioxide is exchanged for oxygen. The oxygenated blood then returns to the heart, from which it exits through the aorta to the arterial system and is circulated throughout the body, supplying oxygen to the tissues.

Heart Rate.   As the body begins to exercise, the muscles use the oxygen at a much higher rate, and the heart must pump more oxygenated blood to meet this increased demand. The heart is capable of adapting to this increased demand through several mechanisms. **Heart rate** shows a gradual adaptation to an increased workload by increasing proportionally to the intensity of the exercise, and it will plateau at a given level after about 2 to 3 minutes (Figure 8-1).

Monitoring heart rate is an indirect method of estimating oxygen consumption.[15] In general, heart rate and oxygen consumption have a linear relationship, although at very low intensities as well as at high intensities this linear relationship breaks down[2] (Figure 8-2). During higher-intensity activities, maximal heart rate might be achieved before maximum oxygen consumption, which will continue to rise.[31] The greater the intensity of the exercise, the higher the heart rate. Because of these existing relationships, it should become apparent that the rate of oxygen consumption can be estimated by taking the heart rate.[12]

Stroke Volume.   A second mechanism by which the heart is able to adapt to increased demands during exercise is to increase the **stroke volume,** the volume of blood being pumped out with each beat. The heart pumps out approximately 70 ml of blood per beat. Stroke volume can continue to increase only to the point at which there is simply not enough time between beats for the heart to fill up. This occurs at about 40 to 50 percent of maximal oxygen consumption or at a heart rate of 110 to 120 beats per minute; above this level, increases in the volume of blood being pumped

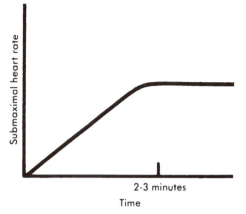

Figure 8-1   For the heart rate to plateau at a given level, 2 to 3 minutes are required.

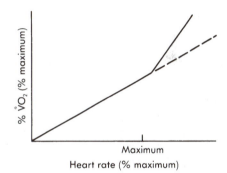

Figure 8-2   Maximum heart rate is achieved at about the same time as $\dot{V}O_2$max.

out per unit of time must be caused entirely by increases in heart rate[11] (Figure 8-3).

Cardiac Output.   Stroke volume and heart rate collectively determine the volume of blood being pumped through the heart in a given unit of time. Approximately 5 L of blood are pumped through the heart during each minute at rest. This is referred to as the **cardiac output,** which indicates how much blood the heart is capable of pumping in exactly 1 minute. Thus, cardiac output is the primary determinant of the maximal rate of oxygen consumption possible (Figure 8-4). During exercise, cardiac output increases to approximately four times that experienced during rest (i.e., to about 20 L) in the normal individual and can increase as much as six times (i.e., to about 30 L) in the elite endurance athlete.

$$\text{Cardiac output} = \text{stroke volume} \cdot \text{heart rate}$$

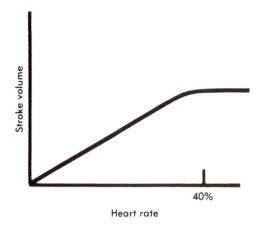

Figure 8-3 Stroke volume plateaus at about 40 percent of maximal heart rate.

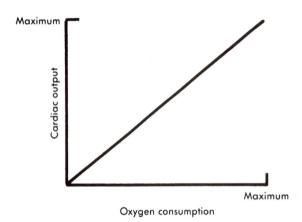

Figure 8-4 Cardiac output limits $\dot{V}O_2$max.

A training effect that occurs with regard to cardiac output of the heart is that the stroke volume increases while exercise heart rate is reduced at a given standard exercise load. The heart becomes more efficient because it is capable of pumping more blood with each stroke. Because the heart is a muscle, it will hypertrophy, or increase in size and strength, to some extent, but this is in no way a negative effect of training.

Training Effect
Increased stroke volume × decreased heart rate
= cardiac output

During exercise, females tend to have a 5 to 10 percent higher cardiac output than males do, at all intensities. This is likely due to a lower concentration of hemoglobin in the female, which is compensated for during exercise by an increased cardiac output.[45]

Adaptation in Blood Flow. The amount of blood flowing to the various organs increases during exercise. However, there is a change in overall distribution of cardiac output; the percentage of total cardiac output to the nonessential organs is decreased, whereas it is increased to active skeletal muscle. Volume of blood flow to the heart muscle or myocardium increases substantially during exercise, even though the percentage of total cardiac output supplying the heart muscle remains unchanged. In skeletal muscle there is increased formation of blood vessels or capillaries, although it is not clear whether new ones form or dormant ones simply open up and fill with blood.[38]

The total peripheral resistance is the sum of all forces that resist blood flow within the vascular system. Total peripheral resistance decreases during exercise primarily because of vessel vasodilation in the active skeletal muscles.

Blood Pressure. Blood pressure in the arterial system is determined by the cardiac output in relation to total peripheral resistance to blood flow. Blood pressure is created by contraction of the heart muscle. Contraction of the ventricles of the heart creates systolic pressure, and relaxation of the heart creates diastolic pressure. During exercise, there is a decrease in total peripheral resistance and an increase in cardiac output.[9] Systolic pressure increases in proportion to oxygen consumption and cardiac output, whereas diastolic pressure shows little or no increase.[5] Blood pressure falls below preexercise levels after exercise and might stay low for several hours. There is general agreement that engaging in consistent aerobic exercise will produce modest reductions in both systolic and diastolic blood pressure at rest as well as during submaximal exercise.[14]

Adaptations in the Blood. Oxygen is transported throughout the system bound to **hemoglobin.** Found in red blood cells, hemoglobin is an iron-containing protein that has the capability of easily accepting or giving up molecules of oxygen as needed. Training for improvement of cardiorespiratory endurance produces an increase in total blood volume, with a corresponding increase in the amount of hemoglobin. The concentration of hemoglobin in circulating blood does not change with training; it might actually decrease slightly.

Adaptation of the Lungs. As a result of training, pulmonary function is improved in the trained individual relative to the untrained individual. The volume of air that can be inspired in a single maximal ventilation is increased. The diffusing capacity of the lungs is also increased, facilitating the exchange of oxygen and carbon dioxide. Pulmonary resistance to air flow is also decreased.[29] The following list summarizes the effects of training on the cardiorespiratory system:

- Decreased resting heart rate
- Decreased heart rate at specific workloads
- Increased stroke volume
- Unchanged cardiac output
- Decrease in recovery time
- Increased capillarization
- Increased functional capacity in the lungs
- Decreased muscle glycogen use

MAXIMAL OXYGEN CONSUMPTION

The maximal amount of oxygen that can be used during exercise is referred to as **maximal oxygen consumption ($\dot{V}O_2$max).** It is considered to be the best indicator of the level of cardiorespiratory endurance. $\dot{V}O_2$max is most often presented in terms of the volume of oxygen used relative to body weight per unit of time (ml•kg^{-1}• min^{-1}).[2] A normal $\dot{V}O_2$max for most collegiate men and women athletes would fall in the range of 50 to 60 ml•kg^{-1}• min^{-1}. A world-class male marathon runner might have a $\dot{V}O_2$max in the 70 to 80 ml•kg^{-1}• min^{-1} range, whereas a world-class female marathoner will have a 60 to 70 ml•kg^{-1}• min^{-1} range.[31]

Rate of Oxygen Consumption

The performance of any activity requires a certain rate of oxygen consumption that is about the same for all persons, depending on their present level of fitness. Generally the greater the rate or intensity of the performance of an activity, the greater will be the oxygen consumption. Each person has his or her own maximal rate of oxygen consumption. That person's ability to perform an activity is closely related to the amount of oxygen required by that activity. This ability is limited by the maximal rate of oxygen consumption the person is capable of delivering into the lungs. Fatigue occurs when insufficient oxygen is supplied to muscles. It should be apparent that the greater percentage of maximal oxygen consumption required during an activity, the less time the activity can be performed (Figure 8-5).

Three factors determine the maximal rate at which oxygen can be used: (1) external respiration, involving the ventilatory process, or pulmonary function; (2) gas transport, which is accomplished by the cardiovascular system (that is, the heart, blood vessels, and blood); and (3) internal respiration, which involves the use of oxygen by the cells to produce energy. Of these three factors the most limiting is generally the ability to transport oxygen through the system; thus the cardiovascular system limits the overall rate of oxygen consumption. A high

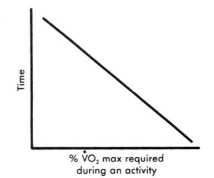

Figure 8-5 The greater the percentage of $\dot{V}O_2$max required during an activity, the less time an activity can be performed.

$\dot{V}O_2$max within a person's range indicates that all three systems are working well.

$\dot{V}O_2$max: An Inherited Characteristic

The maximal rate at which oxygen can be used is a genetically determined characteristic; we inherit a certain range of $\dot{V}O_2$max, and the more active we are, the higher the existing $\dot{V}O_2$max will be within that range.[37,44] A training program is capable of increasing $\dot{V}O_2$max only to its highest limit within our range.[44]

Fast-Twitch versus Slow-Twitch Muscle Fibers. The range of maximal oxygen consumption that is inherited is largely determined by the metabolic and functional properties of skeletal muscle fibers. As discussed in detail in Chapter 5, there are two distinct types of muscle fibers: **slow-twitch** and **fast-twitch** fibers, each of which has distinctive metabolic as well as contractile capabilities. Because they are relatively fatigue resistant, slow-twitch fibers are associated primarily with long-duration, aerobic-type activities. Fast-twitch fibers are useful in short-term, high-intensity activities, which mainly involve the anaerobic system. In general, if an athlete has a high ratio of slow-twitch to fast-twitch muscle fibers, he or she will be able to utilize oxygen more efficiently and thus will have a higher $\dot{V}O_2$max.

Cardiorespiratory Endurance and Work Ability

Cardiorespiratory endurance plays a critical role in our ability to carry out normal daily activities.[35] Fatigue is closely related to the percentage of $\dot{V}O_2$max that a particular workload demands.[43] For example, Figure 8-6 presents two persons, A and B. A has a $\dot{V}O_2$max of 50 ml/kg/min, whereas B has a $\dot{V}O_2$max of only

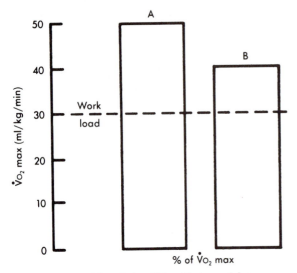

Figure 8-6 Athlete A should be able to work longer than athlete B as a result of a lower percentage use of $\dot{V}O_2$max.

40 ml/kg/min. If both A and B are exercising at the same intensity, then A will be working at a much lower percentage of $\dot{V}O_2$max than B is. Consequently, A should be able to sustain his or her activity over a much longer period of time. Everyday activities can be adversely affected if the ability to use oxygen efficiently is impaired. Thus, improvement of cardiorespiratory endurance should be an essential component of any conditioning program and must be included as part of the rehabilitation program for the injured athlete.[8]

Regardless of the training technique used for the improvement of cardiorespiratory endurance, one principal goal remains the same: **to increase the ability of the cardiorespiratory system to supply a sufficient amount of oxygen to working muscles.** Without oxygen, the body is incapable of producing energy for an extended period of time.

PRODUCING ENERGY FOR EXERCISE

All living systems need to perform a variety of activities such as growing, generating energy, repairing damaged tissues, and eliminating wastes. All of these activities are referred to as metabolic or cellular **metabolism.**

Muscles are metabolically active and must generate energy to move. Energy is produced from the breakdown of certain nutrients from foodstuffs. This energy is stored in a compound called adenosine triphosphate (ATP), which is the ultimate usable form of energy for muscular

activity. ATP is produced in the muscle tissue from blood glucose or glycogen. Fats and proteins can also be metabolized to generate ATP. Glucose not needed immediately is stored as glycogen in the resting muscle and liver. Stored glycogen in the liver can later be converted back to glucose and transferred to the blood to meet the body's energy needs.[6]

If the duration or intensity of the exercise increases, the body relies more heavily on fats stored in adipose tissue to meet its energy needs. The longer the duration of an activity, the greater the amount of fat used, especially during the later stages of endurance events. During rest and submaximal exertion, both fat and carbohydrates are used to provide energy in approximately a 60 to 40 percent ratio. Carbohydrate must be available, to use fat. If glycogen is totally depleted, fat cannot be completely metabolized. Regardless of the nutrient source that produces ATP, it is always available in the cell as an immediate energy source. When all available sources of ATP are used, more must be regenerated for muscular contraction to continue.[7,24]

Various sport activities involve specific demands for energy. For example, sprinting and jumping are high-energy-output activities, requiring a relatively large production of energy for a short time. Long-distance running and swimming, on the other hand, are mostly low-energy-output activities per unit of time, requiring energy production for a prolonged time. Other physical activities demand a blend of both high and low energy output. These various energy demands can be met by the different processes in which energy can be supplied to the skeletal muscles.[16]

Anaerobic versus Aerobic Metabolism

Two major energy-generating systems function in muscle tissue: anaerobic metabolism and aerobic metabolism. Each of these systems produces ATP.[19] During sudden outbursts of activity in intensive, short-term exercise, ATP can be rapidly metabolized to meet energy needs. After a few seconds of intensive exercise, however, the small stores of ATP are used up. The body then turns to stored glycogen as an energy source. Glycogen can be broken down to supply glucose, which is then metabolized within the muscle cells to generate ATP for muscle contractions.[31]

Glucose can be metabolized to generate small amounts of ATP energy without the need for oxygen. This energy system is referred to as **anaerobic metabolism** (*anaerobic* = occurring in the absence of oxygen). As exercise continues, the body must rely on a more complex form of carbohydrate and fat metabolism to generate

ATP. This second energy system requires oxygen and is therefore referred to as **aerobic metabolism** (*aerobic = occurring in the presence of oxygen*). The aerobic system of producing energy generates considerably more ATP than the anaerobic one.

In most activities, both aerobic and anaerobic systems function simultaneously. The degree to which the two major energy systems are involved is determined by the intensity and duration of the activity.[41] If the intensity of the activity is such that sufficient oxygen can be supplied to meet the demands of working tissues, the activity is considered to be **aerobic.** If the activity is of high enough intensity or the duration is such that there is insufficient oxygen available to meet energy demands, the activity becomes **anaerobic.**[45]

Excess Postexercise Oxygen Consumption (Oxygen Deficit). As the intensity of the exercise increases and insufficient amounts of oxygen are available to the tissues, an oxygen deficit is incurred. Oxygen deficit occurs in the beginning of exercise (within the first 2 or 3 minutes) when the oxygen demand is greater than the oxygen supplied. It has been hypothesized that this oxygen debt is caused by lactic acid produced during anaerobic activity and that this "debt" must be "paid back" during the postexercise period. However, currently there is a different rationale for this oxygen deficit, referred to as "excess postexercise oxygen consumption." According to this theory, the deficit is caused by disturbances in mitochondral function due to an increase in temperature.[31]

TECHNIQUES FOR MAINTAINING CARDIORESPIRATORY ENDURANCE

There are several different training techniques that may be incorporated into a rehabilitation program through which cardiorespiratory endurance can be maintained. Certainly, a primary consideration for the sports therapist would be whether the injury involves the upper or lower extremity. With injuries that involve the upper extremity, weight-bearing activities, such as walking, running, stair climbing, and modified aerobics, may be used. However, if the injury is to the lower extremity, alternative non-weight-bearing activities, such as swimming or stationary cycling, might be necessary. In a sport, such as soccer, that requires a considerable amount of running, training using appropriate non-weight-bearing activities will not keep the athlete "match fit." The only way to achieve match fitness is to engage in functional activities specific to that sport. The goal of the sports therapist in substituting alternative activities during rehabilitation is

to try to maintain a cardiorespiratory endurance base so that the athlete can quickly regain match fitness once the injury has healed.

The principles of the training techniques discussed below can be applied to running, cycling, swimming, stair climbing, or any other activity designed to maintain levels of cardiorespiratory fitness.

Continuous Training

Continuous training involves the FITT principles:

The **F**requency of the activity
The **I**ntensity of the activity
The **T**ype of activity
The **T**ime (duration) of the activity

Frequency of Training. To see at least minimal improvement in cardiorespiratory endurance, it is necessary for the average person to engage in no less than three sessions per week. A competitive athlete should be prepared to train as often as six times per week. Everyone should take off at least 1 day per week to give damaged tissues a chance to repair themselves.

Intensity of Training. The intensity of exercise is also a critical factor, though recommendations regarding training intensities vary.[22] This is particularly true in the early stages of training, when the body is forced to make a lot of adjustments to increased workload demands. Because heart rate is linearly related to the intensity of the exercise and to the rate of oxygen consumption, it becomes a relatively simple process to identify a specific workload (pace) that will make the heart rate plateau at the desired level.[40] By monitoring heart rate, we know whether the pace is too fast or too slow to get the heart rate into a target range.[27]

Monitoring heart rate. There are several points at which heart rate is easily measured. The most reliable is the radial artery. The carotid artery is simple to find, especially during exercise. However, there are pressure receptors located in the carotid artery that, if subjected to hard pressure from the two fingers, will slow down the heart rate, giving a false indication of exactly what the heart rate is. Thus the pulse at the radial artery proves the most accurate measure of heart rate. Regardless of where the heart rate is taken, it should be monitored within 15 seconds after stopping exercise.

Another factor must be considered when measuring heart rate during exercise. The athlete is trying to elevate heart rate to a specific target rate and maintain it at that level during the entire workout.[20] Heart rate can be increased or decreased by speeding up or slowing down the pace. It has already been indicated that heart rate increases proportionately with the intensity of the workload and will plateau after 2 to 3 minutes of activity. Thus the athlete should be actively engaged in the workout for 2 to 3 minutes before measuring pulse.[47]

There are several formulas that will easily allow the sports therapist to identify a target training heart rate.[39] Exact determination of maximal heart rate involves exercising an athlete at a maximal level and monitoring the heart rate using an electrocardiogram. This process is difficult outside of a laboratory. However, an approximate estimate of maximal heart rate (MHR) for both males and females in the population is thought to be about 220 beats per minute.[36] MHR is related to age. As you get older, your MHR decreases.[28] Thus a relatively simple estimate of MHR would be MHR = 220 – age. For a 20-year-old athlete, MHR would be about 200 beats per minute (220 – 20 = 200). If you are interested in working at 70 percent of your maximal heart rate, the target heart rate can be calculated by multiplying $0.7 \cdot (220 - \text{age})$. Again using a 20-year-old as an example, a target heart rate would be 140 beats per minute $(0.7 \cdot [220 - 20] = 140)$.

Another commonly used formula that takes into account your current level of fitness is the Karvonen equation:[23,25]

Target training HR =
Resting HR + (0.6 [Maximum HR – Resting HR])

Resting heart rate generally falls between 60 to 80 beats per minute. A 20-year-old athlete with a resting pulse of 70 beats per minute, according to the Karvonen equation, would have a target training heart rate of 148 beats per minute (70 + 0.6 [200 – 70] = 148).

Regardless of the formula used, to see minimal improvement in cardiorespiratory endurance, the athlete must train with the heart rate elevated to at least 60 percent of its maximal rate.[1,21,26] The American College of Sports Medicine (ACSM)[3] recommends that the collegiate athlete train in the 60 to 90 percent range when training continuously. Exercising at a 70 percent level is considered moderate, because activity can be continued for a long period of time with little discomfort and still produce a training effect.[32] In a trained individual it is not difficult to sustain a heart rate at the 85 percent level.[13]

Rating of perceived exertion. Rating of perceived exertion (RPE) can be used in addition to monitoring heart rate to indicate exercise intensity.[4] During exercise, individuals are asked to rate subjectively, on a numerical scale from 6 to 20, exactly how they feel relative to their level of exertion (Table 8-1). More intense exercise that requires a higher level of oxygen consumption and energy expenditure is directly related to higher subjective ratings of perceived exertion. Over a period of

■ **TABLE 8-1** Rating of Perceived Exertion

Scale	Verbal Rating
6	
7	Very, very light
8	
9	Very light
10	
11	Fairly light
12	
13	Somewhat hard
14	
15	Hard
16	
17	Very hard
18	
19	Very, very hard
20	

From G. A. Borg, Psychophysical basis of perceived exertion, *Medicine and Science in Sports and Exercise* 14:377 (1982).

time, athletes can be taught to exercise at a specific RPE that relates directly to more objective measures of exercise intensity.[18,33]

Type of Exercise. The type of activity used in continuous training must be aerobic. Aerobic activities are activities that generally involve repetitive, whole-body, large-muscle movements that are rhythmical in nature and that use large amounts of oxygen, elevate the heart rate, and maintain it at that level for an extended period of time. Examples of aerobic activities are walking, running, jogging, cycling, swimming, rope skipping, stepping, aerobic dance exercise, rollerblading, and cross-country skiing.

The advantage of these aerobic activities as opposed to more intermittent activities, such as racquetball, squash, basketball, or tennis, is that it is easy to regulate their intensity by either speeding up or slowing down the pace.[30] Because we already know that the given intensity of the workload elicits a given heart rate, these aerobic activities allow us to maintain heart rate at a specified or target level.[46] Intermittent activities involve variable speeds and intensities that cause the heart rate to fluctuate considerably. Although these intermittent activities will improve cardiorespiratory endurance, they are much more difficult to monitor in terms of intensity. It is important to point out that any type of activity, from gardening to aerobic exercise, can improve fitness.[34]

Time (Duration). For minimal improvement to occur, a person must participate in at least 20 minutes of continuous activity with the heart rate elevated to its working level. ACSM recommends 20 to 60 minutes of workout/activity with the heart rate elevated to training levels.[3] Generally, the greater the duration of the workout, the greater the improvement in cardiorespiratory endurance. The competitive athlete should train for at least 45 minutes.

Interval Training

Unlike continuous training, **interval training** involves activities that are more intermittent. Interval training consists of alternating periods of relatively intense work and active recovery. It allows for performance of much more work at a more intense workload over a longer period of time than if working continuously. We have stated that it is most desirable in continuous training to work at an intensity of about 60 to 80 percent of maximal heart rate. Obviously, sustaining activity at a relatively high intensity over a 20-minute period would be extremely difficult. The advantage of interval training is that it allows work at this 80 percent or higher level for a short period of time followed by an active period of recovery during which the individual works at only 30 to 45 percent of maximal heart rate. Thus the intensity of the workout and its duration can be greater than with continuous training.

Most sports (for example, football, basketball, soccer, or tennis) are anaerobic, involving short bursts of intense activity followed by a sort of active recovery period. Training with the interval technique allows a more sport-specific workout. Interval training allows application of the overload principle, making the training period much more intense. There are several important considerations in interval training. The training period is the amount of time during which continuous activity is actually being performed, and the recovery period is the time between training periods. A set is a group of combined training and recovery periods, and a repetition is the number of training/recovery periods per set. Training time or distance refers to the rate or distance of the training period. The training/recovery ratio indicates a time ratio for training versus recovery.

An example of interval training would be a soccer player running sprints. An interval workout would involve running two sets of four 400-meter dashes in under 70 seconds, with a 2-minute 20-second walking recovery period between each dash. During this training session the soccer player's heart rate would probably increase to 85 to 95 percent of maximal level during the dash and should probably fall to the 35 to 45 percent level during the recovery period.

Older adults should exercise some caution when using interval training as a method for improving cardiorespiratory endurance. The intensity levels attained during the active periods might be too high for the older adult.

Combining Continuous and Interval Training. As indicated previously, most sport activities involve some combination of aerobic and anaerobic metabolism.[47] Continuous training is generally done at an intensity level that primarily uses the aerobic system. In interval training the intensity is sufficient to necessitate a greater percentage of anaerobic metabolism.[17] Therefore the sports therapist should incorporate both training techniques into a rehabilitation program to maximize cardiorespiratory fitness.

Fartlek Training

The **fartlek** training technique is a type of cross-country running that originated in Sweden. *Fartlek* literally means "speed play." It is similar to interval training in that the athlete must run for a specified period of time; however, specific pace and speed are not identified. It is recommended that the course for a fartlek workout be some type of varied terrain with some level running, some uphill and downhill running, and some running through a course with obstacles such as trees or rocks. The object is to put surges into a running workout, varying the length of the surges according to individual purposes. One advantage of fartlek training is that because the pace and terrain always change, the training session is less regimented and provides a refreshing change of pace in the training routine.

Again, if fartlek training is going to improve cardiorespiratory endurance, it must elevate the heart rate to at least minimal training levels. Fartlek might best be used as an off-season conditioning activity or as a change-of-pace activity to counteract the boredom of training using the same activity day after day.

Par Cours

Par cours is a technique for improving cardiorespiratory endurance that basically combines continuous training and circuit training. This technique involves jogging a short distance from station to station and performing a designated exercise at each station according to guidelines and directions provided on an instruction board located at that station. Par cours circuits provide an excellent means for gaining some aerobic benefits while incorporating some of the benefits of calisthenics. Par cours circuits are found most typically in parks or recreational areas within metropolitan areas.

Summary

1. The sports therapist should routinely incorporate into the rehabilitation program activities that will help maintain levels of cardiorespiratory endurance.

2. Cardiorespiratory endurance involves the coordinated function of the heart, lungs, blood, and blood vessels to supply sufficient amounts of oxygen to the working tissues.

3. The best indicator of how efficiently the cardiorespiratory system functions is the maximal rate at which oxygen can be used by the tissues.

4. Heart rate is directly related to the rate of oxygen consumption. It is therefore possible to predict the intensity of the work in terms of the rate of oxygen use by monitoring heart rate.

5. Aerobic exercise involves activity in which the level of intensity and duration is low enough to provide a sufficient amount of oxygen to supply the demands of the working tissues.

6. In anaerobic exercise the intensity of the activity is so high that oxygen is being used more quickly than it can be supplied, thus an oxygen debt is incurred that must be repaid before working tissue can return to its normal resting state.

7. Continuous or sustained training for maintenance of cardiorespiratory endurance involves selecting an activity that is aerobic in nature and training at least three times per week for a time period of no less than 20 minutes with the heart rate elevated to at least 60 percent of maximal rate.

8. Interval training involves alternating periods of relatively intense work followed by active recovery periods. Interval training allows performance of more work at a relatively higher workload than in continuous training.

9. During rehabilitation, continuous and interval training techniques should be incorporated.

10. Fartlek makes use of jogging or running over varying types of terrain at changing speeds.

11. Par cours is a training technique that combines continuous training with exercises done at stations along the course.

References

1. Åstrand, P. O., and K. Rodahl. 1986. *Textbook of work physiology.* New York: McGraw-Hill.

2. Åstrand, P. O. 1954. Åstrand-Rhyming nomogram for calculation of aerobic capacity from pulse rate during submaximal work. *Journal of Applied Physiology* 7:218.

3. American College of Sports Medicine. 1995. *Guidelines for exercise testing and prescription.* Philadelphia: Lea & Febiger.

4. Borg, G. A. 1982. Psychophysical basis of perceived exertion. *Medicine and Science in Sports and Exercise* 14:377.

5. Brooks, G., T. Fahey, and T. White. 1996. *Exercise physiology: Human bioenergetics and its applications.* Mountain View, CA: Mayfield.

6. Brooks, G., and J. Mercier. 1994. The balance of carbohydrate and lipid utilization during exercise: The crossover concept. *Journal of Applied Physiology* 76:2253–61.

7. Cerretelli, P. 1992. Energy sources for muscle contraction. *Sports Medicine* 13:S106–S110.

8. Chillag, S. A. 1986. Endurance athletes: Physiologic changes and nonorthopedic problems [Review]. *South Med J* 79(10):1264.

9. Convertino, V. A. 1987. Aerobic fitness, endurance training, and orthostatic intolerance [Review]. *Exercise and Sport Sciences Reviews* 15:223.

10. Cooper, K. H. 1982. *The aerobics program for total well-being.* New York: Bantam Books.

11. Cox, M. 1991. Exercise training programs and cardiorespiratory adaptation. *Clinical Sports Medicine* 10(1): 19–32.

12. deVries, H. 1986. *Physiology of exercise for physical education and athletics.* Dubuque, IA: Wm. C. Brown.

13. Dicarlo, L., P. Sparling, and M. Millard-Stafford. 1991. Peak heart rates during maximal running and swimming: Implications for exercise prescription. *International Journal of Sport Education* 12:309–12.

14. Durstein, L., R. Pate, and D. Branch. 1993. Cardiorespiratory responses to acute exercise. In *American College of Sports Medicine: Resource manual for guidelines for exercise testing and prescription.* Philadelphia: Lea & Febiger.

15. Fahey, T. 1995. *Encyclopedia of sports medicine and exercise physiology.* New York: Garland.

16. Fox, E., R. Bowers, and M. Foss. 1981. *The physiological basis of physical education and athletics.* Philadelphia: W. B. Saunders.

17. Gaesser, G. A., and L. A. Wilson. 1988. Effects of continuous and interval training on the parameters of the power-endurance time relationship for high-intensity exercise. *International Journal of Sports Medicine* 9(6): 417.

18. Glass, S., M. Whaley, and M. Wegner. 1991. A comparison between ratings of perceived exertion among standard protocols and steady state running. *International Journal of Sports Education* 12:77–82.

19. Green, J., and A. Patla. 1992. Maximal aerobic power: Neuromuscular and metabolic considerations. *Medicine and Science in Sports and Exercise* 24:38–46.

20. Greer, N., and F. Katch. 1982. Validity of palpation recovery pulse rate to estimate exercise heart rate following four intensities of bench step exercise. *Research Quarterly for Exercise and Sport* 53:340.

21. Hage, P. 1982. Exercise guidelines: Which to believe? *Physician and Sports Medicine* 10:23.

22. Hawley, J., K. Myburgh, and T. Noakes. 1995. Maximal oxygen consumption: A contemporary perspective. In *Encyclopedia of sports medicine and exercise physiology*, edited by T. Fahey. New York: Garland.

23. Hickson, R. C., C. Foster, M. Pollac, et al. 1985. Reduced training intensities and loss of aerobic power, endurance, and cardiac growth. *Journal of Applied Physiology* 58(2): 492.

24. Honig, C., R. Connett, and T. Gayeski. 1992. O_2 transport and its interaction with metabolism. *Medicine and Science in Sports and Exercise* 24:47–53.

25. Karvonen, M. J., E. Kentala, and O. Mustala. 1957. The effects of training on heart rate: A longitudinal study. *Ann Med Exp Biol* 35:305.

26. Koyanagi, A., K. Yamamoto, and K. Nishijima. 1993. Recommendation for an exercise prescription to prevent coronary heart disease. *Ed Syst* 17:213–17.

27. Levine, G. and G. Balady. 1993. The benefits and risks of exercise testing: The exercise prescription. *Adv Intern Ed* 38:57–79.

28. Londeree, B., and M. Moeschberger. 1992. Effect of age and other factors on maximal heart rate. *Research Quarterly in Exercise and Sport* 53:297.

29. MacDougall, D., and D. Sale. 1981. Continuous vs. interval training: A review for the athlete and coach. *Can J Appl Sport Sci* 6:93.

30. Marcinik, E. J., K. Hogden, K. Mittleman, et al. 1985. Aerobic/calisthenic and aerobic/circuit weight training programs for Navy men: A comparative study. *Medicine and Science in Sports and Exercise* 17(4): 482.

31. McArdle, W., F. Katch, and V. Katch. 1994. *Exercise physiology, energy, nutrition, and human performance.* Philadelphia: Lea & Febiger.

32. Mead, W., and R. Hartwig. 1981. Fitness evaluation and exercise prescription. *Fam Pract* 13:1039.

33. Monahan, T. 1988. Perceived exertion: An old exercise tool finds new applications. *Physician and Sports Medicine* 16:174.

34. Pate, R., M. Pratt and S. Blair. 1995. Physical activity and public health: A recommendation from the CDC and ACSM. *Journal of American Medical Association* 273(5): 402–7.

35. Powers, S. 1993. Fundamentals of exercise metabolism. In *American College of Sports Medicine: Resource manual for guidelines for exercise testing and prescription.* Philadelphia: Lea & Febiger.

36. Rowland, T. W., and G. M. Green. 1989. Anaerobic threshold and the determination of training target heart rates in premenarcheal girls. *Pediatr Cardiol* 10(2): 75.

37. Saltin, B., and S. Strange. 1992. Maximal oxygen uptake: Old and new arguments for a cardiovascular limitation. *Medicine and Science in Sports and Exercise* 24:30–37.

38. Smith, M., and J. Mitchell. 1993. Cardiorespiratory adaptations to exercise training. In *American College of Sports Medicine: Resource manual for guidelines for exercise testing and prescription,* Philadelphia: Lea & Febiger.

39. Stachenfeld, N., M. Eskenazi, and G. Gleim. 1992. Predictive accuracy of criteria used to assess maximal oxygen consumption. *Am Heart J* 123:922–25.

40. Swain, D., K. Abernathy, and C. Smith. 1994. Target heart rates for the development of cardiorespiratory fitness. *Medicine and Science in Sports and Exercise* 26:112–16.

41. Vago, P., M. Mercier, M. Ramonatxo, et al. 1987. Is ventilatory anaerobic threshold a good index of endurance capacity? *International Journal of Sports Medicine* 8(3): 190.

42. Wagner, P. 1991. Central and peripheral aspects of oxygen transport and adaptations with exercise. *Sports Med* 11:133–42.

43. Weltman, A., J. Weltman, R. Ruh, et al. 1989. Percentage of maximal heart rate reserve, and $\dot{V}O_2$ peak for determining endurance training intensity in sedentary women [Review]. *International Journal of Sports Medicine* 10(3): 212.

44. Weymans, M., and T. Reybrouck. 1989. Habitual level of physical activity and cardiorespiratory endurance capacity in children. *Eur J Appl Physiol* 58(8): 803.

45. Williford, H., M. Scharff-Olson, and D. Blessing. 1993. Exercise prescription for women: Special considerations. *Sports Ed* 15:299–311.

46. Wilmore, J., and D. Costill. 1994. *Physiology of sport and exercise.* Champaign, IL: Human Kinetics.

47. Zhang, Y., M. Johnson, and N. Chow. 1991. Effect of exercise testing protocol on parameters of aerobic function. *Medicine and Science in Sport and Exercise* 23:625–30.

PART TWO

The Tools of Rehabilitation

CHAPTER 9

Isokinetics in Rehabilitation

Janine Oman

After completion of this chapter, the student should be able to do the following:

- Describe isokinetic exercise.

- Identify the advantages and disadvantages of isokinetic exercise.

- List the various computerized isokinetic systems.

- Describe the use of isokinetic evaluation in the athletic population.

- Discuss the use of isokinetic exercise as a rehabilitation tool in the athletic population.

ISOKINETIC EXERCISE

The concept of isokinetic exercise was described in 1967 by Hislop and Perrine.[18] **Isokinetic exercise** can best be described as movement that occurs at a constant angular velocity with accommodating resistance. Maximum muscle tension can be generated throughout the range of motion because the resistance is variable to match the muscle tension produced at the various points in the range of motion. Isokinetic machines allow the angular velocity to be preset. Once the specified angular velocity is achieved, the machine provides accommodating resistance throughout the specified range of motion.

Isokinetic evaluation and rehabilitation are limited by the technological advances of isokinetic dynamometers. Isokinetic dynamometers now provide concentric and eccentric resistance. Velocities are variable depending on the machine, although the average range is from zero to 300 degrees/second in the eccentric mode. Some machines allow concentric velocities greater than 500 degrees/second.

Historically, the two primary advantages associated with isokinetic exercise are the ability to work maximally throughout the range of motion and the ability to work at various velocities to simulate functional activity.[38] Care should be taken, however, when inferring functional capacity based on results of dynamic isokinetic testing.[28] Velocities achieved during functional activity greatly exceed the velocity capacities of isokinetic dynamometers. Angular velocities produced by professional baseball pitchers have been shown to range between 6,500 and 7,200 degrees/second.[8] Velocities measured at the hip and knee during a soccer kick exceeded 400 degrees/second and 1,200 degrees/second, respectively.[27] The majority of isokinetic testing is done in a non-weight-bearing position that is not representative of functional activities. However, given these limitations, isokinetic exercise can be a very powerful tool for the sports therapist in the evaluation and rehabilitation of sport-related injuries.

ISOKINETIC DYNAMOMETERS

Various isokinetic dynamometers are commercially available to the sports therapist. The different systems all offer variable types of resistance and velocities. This section is not meant to endorse a particular isokinetic system but is provided to give the sports therapist information on the specifications of some of the more common commercially available isokinetic dynamometers. Table 9-1 provides a comparison of the different dynamometers with information related to the manufacturer's address, exercise modes available, velocities, and torque maximums.

Biodex

The Biodex isokinetic dynamometer allows concentric and eccentric motion (Figure 9-1). This system has isometric, isotonic, CPM, and isokinetic exercise modes. Concentric velocities range from 30 to 500 degrees/second. Eccentric velocities range from 10 to 300 degrees/second. Maximum torque values allowed for safety purposes are 500 ft lb concentrically and 300 ft lb eccentrically.[3] The Biodex also has lift and closed chain attachments.

One advantage of the Biodex is that it allows for high-speed concentric activity while being fairly user friendly. The Biodex also can be set up easily for strengthening in diagonal planes. The Biodex generates a very comprehensive report after isokinetic evaluation. The Biodex does have a lower eccentric maximum, which may be a limitation when used in the athletic population.

Cybex 6000

The Cybex 6000 is the newest dynamometer manufactured by Cybex that allows concentric and eccentric motion (Figure 9-2). All other Cybex dynamometers allow only concentric activity. The 6000 has powered and nonpowered modes. The nonpowered mode allows free limb acceleration with concentric/concentric activity that is similar to previous Cybex dynamometers. The powered mode provides both concentric and eccentric activity and continuous passive motion (CPM). The

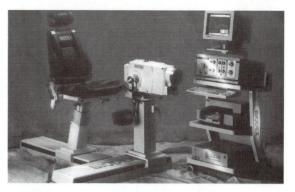

Figure 9-1   Biodex isokinetic dynamometer.

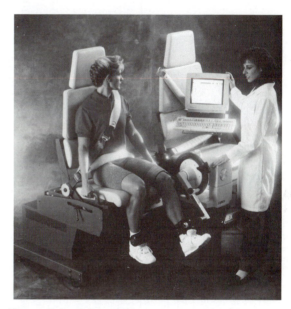

Figure 9-2   Cybex 6000.

Cybex 6000 has 18 exercise/test patterns available. Nonpowered concentric velocities range from 15 to 500 degrees/second. The torque maximum for nonpowered concentric activity is 500 ft lb. Powered concentric velocities range from 15 to 300 degrees/second. The torque maximum for this mode is also 500 ft lb. Powered eccentric velocities range from 15 to 300 degrees/second. The torque maximums vary depending on the velocity in this mode. The torque maximum for velocities between 15 and 55 degrees/second is 250 ft lb. The torque maximum in the eccentric powered mode for velocities between 60 and 300 degrees/second is 300 ft lb. The velocities in the continuous passive motion mode vary between 1 and 300 degrees/second.[6]

■ **TABLE 9-1** Isokinetic Equipment Information

Isokinetic Equipment and Manufacturer	Exercise Modes Available	Speeds	Torque Maximum*
BIODEX Biodex Corporation PO Box S Shirley, NY 11967	Isokinetic (concentric and eccentric) Isometric Continuous Passive Motion (CPM)	Isokinetic: Concentric: 30–450/sec Eccentric: 10–120/sec CPM: 2–120/sec	Concentric: 650 ft lb Eccentric: 300 ft lb
CYBEX Cybex Corporation 2100 Smithtown Ave. PO Box 9003 Ronkonkoma, NY 11779-0903	Isokinetic Concentric: powered and non-powered mode Eccentric: powered mode CPM	Powered Concentric: 15–120/sec Non-powered Concentric: 15–500/sec Powered Eccentric: 30–120/sec CPM: 5–120/sec	Powered Concentric: 500 ft lb Powered Eccentric: 30–55/sec: 250 ft lb 60–120/sec: 300 ft lb
KIN-COM Chattecx Corporation 4717 Adams Road PO Box 489 Hixson, TN 37343	Isometric Isokinetic (concentric and eccentric) Isotonic CPM	Isokinetic: Concentric: 1–250/sec Eccentric: 1–250/sec Isotonic: 1–250/sec CPM: 1–250/sec	Isometric: 450 ft lb Isokinetic: Concentric: 450 ft lb Eccentric: 450 ft lb Isotonic: 2–450 ft lb

*To convert foot-pounds to Newton-meters, multiply by 4.45.

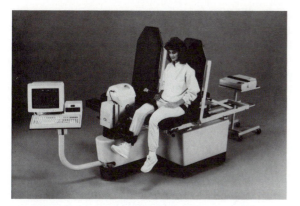

Figure 9-3 Kin-Com 500H isokinetic dynamometer.

One of the primary advantages of this dynamometer is that it is a Cybex product. The nonpowered mode of this dynamometer is the same as previous Cybex dynamometers, so the normative and research data can be used as comparison data with this machine. This machine also is very versatile in that it can be used for many exercise patterns for the upper and lower extremity. Cybex has increased its speeds in the powered concentric and eccentric mode. The nonpowered mode has the highest velocities and torque maximums available. The disadvantage of the Cybex is similar to the Biodex, with lower eccentric torque maximums velocities when used in the athletic population.

Kin-Com

The Kin-Com isokinetic dynamometer was the first active system available that allowed concentric and eccentric activity (Figure 9-3). The Kin-Com has options for a dual-channel EMG system to use in combination with the Kin-Com. It also has a balance station option kit. The Kin-Com dynamometers offer isometric, isotonic, continuous passive motion (CPM), and isokinetic modes. The velocities for isotonic, CPM, and isokinetic (concentric and eccentric) modes range from 1 to 250 degrees/second. The force maximums are 450 ft lb (2000 Newtons) for all of the exercise modes. All of the Kin-Com dynamometers are computer controlled.[19]

The Kin-Com dynamometers offer the highest force maximums combined with high velocities for eccentric testing and rehabilitation, which is a distinct advantage in the athletic setting. The Kin-Com is also extremely user friendly. The Kin-Com does not provide as comprehensive a data report as other dynamometers. The Kin-Com is limited to 250 degrees/second in the concentric mode, which is slower than other available isokinetic dynamometers.

ISOKINETIC EVALUATION

Parameters

Various parameters of force and torque are used to compare extremities during isokinetic evaluation. One of the limitations of the isokinetic literature is that many parameters are used in describing isokinetic strength characteristics of muscle. The sports therapist is faced with evaluating the results of specific isokinetic tests and correctly applying the results with normative data that is available in the literature.

Primarily, force or torque data are used in isokinetic literature. Force can best be described as the push or pull produced by the action of one object on another. Force is measured in pounds or Newtons. Torque is the moment of force applied during rotational motion. Torque is measured in foot-pounds or Newton-meters.[22] Either parameter can be used in isokinetic testing, but *force* and *torque* are not interchangeable terms. Most of the isokinetic dynamometers use torque as the measured parameter.

The force and torque parameters in the literature relate to either peak or average force/torque production. Peak force/torque is the point of highest force/torque production.[15] Average force/torque is the force/torque produced across the whole range of motion.[26] Peak and average force/torque can also be compared to body weight for a weight-adjusted force/torque. Work and power parameters are also identified in isokinetic literature. Work is defined as force multiplied by displacement.[22] Work is best represented as the area under the torque or force curve. Power is defined as the rate of performing work. Data relating to power characteristics are best evaluated by identifying the amount of work performed in a specific time period. Endurance parameters are also evaluated in relationship to reductions in peak torque from the first repetition to the last repetition. Another parameter that may be evaluated is the time it takes to drop to 50 percent of peak torque.[10]

Testing

Isokinetic evaluation is dependent on many different variables to produce a reliable test. Two of the variables are speed of testing and the position of the athlete during testing. These variables need to be controlled and should be consistent from test session to test session. The sports therapist needs to test the athlete at specific speeds if comparison to normative data is desired.

The literature provides a vast array of testing speeds for upper- and lower-extremity isokinetic evaluations.[17,20,28] Previous research suggested that testing at different speeds allowed the sports therapist to test different characteristics of muscular strength and power.[7] The current research supports the view that torque, work, and power characteristics are determined independent of test velocity. The results are not indicative of the ability of the individual muscle to perform different strength or power tasks.[26]

Generally, 60 degrees/second has been used as the primary test speed for concentric isokinetic testing. Eccentric testing speeds tend to be more variable. Hageman and Sorenson[15] recommend 150 degrees/second as the upper limit for eccentric testing in the general population and 180 degrees/second as the upper limit in the athletic population. Coactivation of the antagonistic musculature occurs with faster speed testing.[16] This coactivation happens because the antagonistic musculature produces force to slow down the lever arm in preparation for the end point of the range of motion with open kinetic testing. Reciprocal testing of antagonistic musculature might not be accurate at faster speeds because of the increased force produced by the antagonistic musculature.

This coactivation most probably occurs in the nonpowered mode of isokinetic testing because of free acceleration of the lever arm. No resistance is applied until the subject meets the preset velocity. This is the most probable cause of increased antagonistic activity to slow down the lever arm. The powered mode entails the use of a preload. This necessitates the production of a predetermined amount of force before isokinetic contraction can be initiated, eliminating the free acceleration of the lever arm.

Recommended positioning of the athlete during an isokinetic evaluation varies depending on the specific literature reviewed. Positioning of the joint should account for the gravity effect and the healing phase of the injured structures. The gravity effect torque must be calculated if the sports therapist is analyzing reciprocal group ratios such as the quadriceps and hamstrings. Failure to account for this torque skews the agonist/antagonist ratio if the sports therapist tests the two muscles in the same position. An easy way to control this effect is to test the different muscles in different positions so that each muscle is in an antigravity position during testing. Many of the new dynamometers correct for the gravity effect torque if desired. The sports therapist may need to modify the testing position to protect healing structures. For example, early testing of the shoulder musculature after an episode of subluxation/dislocation should be performed with the arm at the side and not in the abducted position. Wilk and Arrigo[34] proposed performing shoulder strengthening initially at 0 degrees of abduction, progressing to the plane of the scapula and finally to 90 degrees of abduction. This progresses the shoulder from a position of max-

imal joint stability to a position of minimal joint stability. The plane of the scapula is achieved by placing the humerus in a position 30 to 45 degrees anterior to the frontal plane.[15] Research has indicated that there is no difference in torque production between the traditional and the scapular plane.[32]

Positioning the tested joint so that it reproduces functional activity can be beneficial for the sports therapist. The effect of hip position on the torque values of the quadriceps and hamstrings has been studied by Worrell et al.[34] Their results indicated that peak torque was greater in the seated position and less in the supine position. However, the authors state that evaluation of peak torque might be more appropriate from the supine position to mimic hip position during functional activity.

The length of the lever arm of the dynamometer affects the ability to produce torque. Torque production is significantly affected when the lever arm is changed in length. The sports therapist can limit torque production early in the healing phase of injury by decreasing the length of the lever arm. However, the length of the lever arm needs to be consistent between testing sessions if the sports therapist is comparing previous testing sessions to the current test. Wilk and Andrews[33] studied the effect of pad placement and angular velocity on tibial displacement. Their results indicated that proximal pad placement resulted in less anterior tibial translation than distal pad placement. With respect to velocity, the greatest amount of tibial translation occurred at 60 degrees/second as compared to 180 degrees/second and 300 degrees/second. The sports therapist should keep this in mind when performing isokinetic evaluations on ACL injuries.

Reliability

It is important that the sports therapist have reliable and reproducible test results. Test reliability is dependent on many factors but is probably the most overlooked aspect of isokinetic evaluation. Because of the wide variety of test protocols in the literature, the clinician should include several essential components within the isokinetic test to facilitate reliability of measurement. The clinician needs to evaluate the use of a warm-up period and a rest period, the number of test repetitions, and test velocity. These variables need to be consistent between testing sessions for comparison data as well as facilitating maximal torque production. Kues[20] recommends that patients have two practice sessions prior to the actual test. Reliability can also be influenced by the testing mode. Eccentric testing especially involves a significant learning curve because of the athlete's unfamiliarity with this exercise mode, but test-retest reliability in this mode has been established.[12]

Testing of multiaxial joints, such as the shoulder and ankle, provides the sports therapist with difficulty in reproducing test results secondary to the complexity of setups, as well as the limitations in aligning the axis of rotation of the limb with the mechanical axis of rotation of the machine. Results have shown very poor reliability between repetitive trials of peak torque for ankle plantarflexion/dorsiflexion.[31] A suggestion to limit the error is to always test both extremities during a testing session. The sports therapist should limit comparisons between testing sessions. The sports therapist needs to recognize the limitations associated with testing multiaxial joints.

Retesting the athlete allows the sports therapist to evaluate the progress made with the rehabilitation program. Broad statements regarding the strength and functional ability of the tested musculature should be limited, because isokinetic evaluation is not correlated with the ability to perform functional activity.[1,13,21] However, retesting of the involved musculature does enable the sports therapist to evaluate the effectiveness of the rehabilitation program. Improvements in test results that occur within 1 week of testing probably do not reflect changes in strength of the involved musculature but are indicative of either the athlete's familiarity with testing or possibly neuromuscular changes within the muscle.[2] True strength changes involving hypertrophic changes in the muscle usually require 4 to 6 weeks of training.[24] Both neuromuscular and hypertrophic strength changes are important to evaluate, but the sports therapist needs to understand that true strength changes of the involved musculature do not occur within a short period of time.

Interpretation of Graphs

Specific ratios of force, torque, work, or power are identified during isokinetic testing to determine differences between the two tested extremities. The most commonly used ratios are peak/average torque ratios between injured/noninjured extremities, agonist/antagonist ratios, and concentric/eccentric ratios. Historically, normal peak and average force/torque ratios comparing the injured to the uninjured extremity typically use the 85 to 90 percent ratio to allow the athlete to return to competition.[25] However, the sports therapist should not use a percentage criterion as the sole indicator for return to activity, because isokinetic strength has not been correlated with the ability to perform functional tasks.[13,21,37]

Agonist/antagonist ratios are another commonly used ratio in isokinetic evaluation. The hamstring/quadriceps ratio is the most analyzed ratio. Historically,

based on Cybex evaluations, a 66 percent ratio between the hamstrings and the quadriceps at 60 degrees/second is described as the normative value.[7] This testing is only done in the concentric mode. The sports therapist needs to be careful in comparing the hamstring/quadriceps ratio. The 66 percent ratio is reflective of testing done in the concentric mode at 60 degrees/second. Likewise, agonist/antagonist ratios have been identified for other muscle groups such as shoulder internal/external rotation. The sports therapist does not need to know all the specifics of the data but does need to know which of the agonist/antagonist musculature is capable of producing the most force. The sports therapist can then evaluate the function of the opposing muscle groups without knowing the specific ratio numbers of the agonist/antagonist. Perrin[26] provides detailed descriptions of normative data for all joints.

Finally, the eccentric/concentric ratio is another parameter to evaluate with isokinetic testing. Blacker[4] reports that eccentric testing should produce a 5 to 70 percent increase in force/torque as compared with concentric testing. Bennett and Stauber[2] identified eccentric to concentric quadriceps torque deficits in approximately 30 percent of their patients with anterior knee pain. The deficit was defined as less than an 85 percent peak torque ratio between eccentric and concentric activity. The researchers felt that the deficit might have been one cause of the subjects' increased pain. The symptoms and isokinetic deficits were reversed through a training program. Trudelle-Jackson et al.,[30] however, tested asymptomatic subjects concentrically and eccentrically and reported a significant percentage of healthy subjects who demonstrated eccentric to concentric deficits of greater than 15 percent. One reason for the difference is that eccentric testing involves a greater variability than concentric testing.[23] The sports therapist needs to evaluate concentric and eccentric force production. The athlete should be able to produce more force eccentrically, but the sports therapist should be aware that a greater variance exists with eccentric testing.

Shape of the Curve

The information provided by evaluation of the curve varies depending on the researcher. Rothstein, Lamb, and Mayhew[28] state that the shape of the torque curve might be due to machine artifact and might not be related to patient performance. These researchers state that the sports therapist should not draw specific conclusions regarding pathological conditions based on the shape of the torque curve. However, there is some evidence that the shape of the torque curve might be related to patient function.

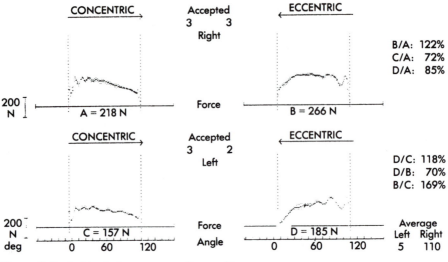

Figure 9-4 Isokinetic torque curve abnormality.

Engle and Faust[11] tested patients with a history of shoulder subluxation. The testing involved performing traditional and diagonal patterns of shoulder motion. The researchers identified consistent torque defects in symptomatic and asymptomatic patients. Torque curve abnormalities were found from 70 to 110 degrees with flexion/abduction/external rotation diagonal in patients with rotator cuff weakness. The abnormalities were seen at 85 degrees in the extension/adduction/internal rotation diagonal in patients with posterior labral tearing. Dvir et al.[9] tested patients with patellofemoral pain. The researchers identified a large percentage of patients who exhibited a break in the torque curve that lasted for 10 degrees at approximately 45 degrees of flexion. The break was associated with a load reduction of approximately 25 percent of the patient's weight. Pain inhibition was hypothesized to be the cause of the break in the curve.

Clinically, deficits in the shape of the curve should be identified. One repetition that produces a torque abnormality should not lead the sports therapist to conclude that the athlete has altered function. Testing should include multiple repetitions to identify consistent torque curve deficits. The sports therapist should then design a specific rehabilitation program to attempt to correct for these deficits.

Figure 9-4 shows a torque curve abnormality. These graphs involve an isokinetic evaluation of a patient who had history of significant patellofemoral pain after an ACL reconstruction. The lower two graphs are of the involved side. Evaluation of the concentric force curve re-

veals consistent deficits between 25 and 60 degrees. The eccentric force curve is very inconsistent with a decrease in force production from 35 to 60 degrees. Pain inhibition was thought to be the contributing factor to these force curve abnormalities. A rehabilitation program was designed to attempt to correct for these deficits and to avoid painful ranges identified on the force curves.

Figure 9-5 shows an isokinetic evaluation of a decathlete with hamstring strain. This athlete had a history of recurrent hamstring strains of both extremities. The lower two graphs are of the involved side. Evaluation of the eccentric force curve reveals a divot bilaterally from 90 to 100 degrees of flexion. The athlete exhibits diminished eccentric control throughout the motion. The eccentric curve also reveals a decay of force from 30 to 50 degrees of flexion. A rehabilitation program was designed that included eccentric control of the hamstrings and eccentric/concentric quick reversals in the standing position for the leg curl motion in addition to traditional strengthening of the hamstrings.

ISOKINETIC TRAINING

Force-Velocity Curve

The use of isokinetic dynamometers should not be limited solely to evaluation purposes. Isokinetic training is a valuable rehabilitation tool and should not be overlooked in designing an exercise program. The force-velocity curve should be the basis for designing an isokinetic training program.

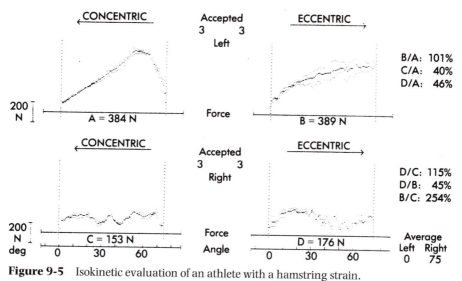

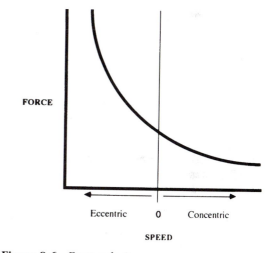

Figure 9-5 Isokinetic evaluation of an athlete with a hamstring strain.

The force-velocity curve identifies two of the major components that sports therapists can control in a rehabilitation program—force and speed. Numerous research studies have been performed that identify the force production with concentric and eccentric activity with changes in velocity of motion. Figure 9-6 is a representation of the force-velocity curve. Force production is located on the *y* axis, and the velocity of motion (speed) is on the *x* axis. Concentric motion is located on the right side of the *x* axis, and eccentric motion is on the left side of the *x* axis. Velocity increases from left to right with concentric motion, and velocity increases from right to left with eccentric motion. Force production decreases with increases in velocity with concentric motion.[5] Conversely, eccentric force production might increase with an increase in the velocity of motion.[35] However, some researchers disagree and feel eccentric torque remains the same with increases in velocity.[5,14] It is important to remember that research relating to specificity of training for speed and mode of exercise is extremely variable.

The sports therapist should use the force-velocity curve as the basis for designing a rehabilitation program. The velocity and the mode of exercise should be chosen with regard to the type of injury and the potential for force production with the different velocities and modes of exercise. In the acute phase of healing after injury, force production should be kept to a minimum to allow appropriate healing of the injured structures. Eccentric isokinetic training is not advised in this phase because of the potential for increased force production.

Figure 9-6 Force-velocity curve.

SAMPLE PROGRESSION

Some of the isokinetic dynamometers offer the ability to provide other types of resistance, such as isotonic, isometric, and passive motion, that allow the sports therapist more flexibility in the use of dynamometers in the rehabilitation program. Progression through the rehabilitation program should be based on the attainment of short-term goals and the phase of healing after injury. In the acute phase of injury, the goals should be related to regaining motion and maintenance of strength. The isokinetic dynamometer can be used in this phase to provide isometric and submaximal isotonic resistance and passive motion if needed. Positioning of the athlete for rehabilitation sessions may need to be altered to lessen the gravity effect torque. As healing progresses and the injury enters the scar proliferation stage (7 to 21 days), graded resistive stresses can be applied to initiate the strengthening phase or rehabilitation. The isokinetic dynamometer can be used for submaximal to maximal isotonics and the initiation of submaximal concentric/eccentric isokinetics. As the injury progresses into the scar remodeling phase (21 days), more aggressive strengthening can be added to the rehabilitation program. The isokinetic dynamometer can be used to alter velocity and force production using traditional and diagonal planes of motion for maximal isotonic and isokinetic resistance.

Hageman and Sorenson[15] describe an eccentric training progression. The authors suggest a good warm-up followed by an orientation to the eccentric isokinetic mode. Training should include one to three sets of ten repetitions beginning at 60 degrees/second in the concentric-eccentric mode. The clinician should advance by 30 degrees/second increments up to 180 degrees/second, continuing with two to three sets of ten repetitions with each advancing speed.

The disadvantage of isokinetics, as was previously mentioned, is that motion is performed in an open isokinetic chain, which is not representative of functional activity. However, some dynamometers can be adjusted to provide closed-kinetic-chain resistance in the form of leg-press motions and standing terminal knee extension or some units have a closed kinetic attachment for use with their dynamometer. The addition of closed kinetic activities makes the dynamometers more versatile in the rehabilitation setting. However, while isokinetic evaluation and training is a valuable tool for the sports therapist, isokinetic testing might not be representative of functional ability in sport-specific activity. The sports therapist needs to evaluate functional ability in the functional setting and use isokinetics as a guide for progression through the rehabilitation program.

Summary

1. Isokinetic exercise is movement that occurs at a constant angular velocity with accommodating resistance.
2. Force can be best described as a push or pull produced by the action of one object on another.
3. Torque is defined as the moment of force applied during rotational motion.
4. Work is defined as force multiplied by displacement. Work is measured as the area under the torque curve.
5. Power is defined as the rate of performing work.
6. The sports therapist needs to be consistent with isokinetic testing from one session to another. Speed and position of the athlete should remain the same.
7. The athlete may need a practice session before isokinetic testing to be familiarized to the testing sequence and the isokinetic dynamometer.
8. Peak/average torque ratios, agonist/antagonist ratios, and eccentric/concentric ratios are commonly used to evaluate the results of isokinetic testing, but the sports therapist should be hesitant to use specific percentage criteria for a return to functional activity.
9. The sports therapist needs to evaluate the shape of the torque curve for consistent abnormalities. A rehabilitation program should be designed to correct specific deficits that are identified.
10. The force-velocity curve should be the basis for designing specific isokinetic training programs.

References

1. Anderson, M., J. Gieck, D. Perrin, et al. 1991. The relationships among isometric, isotonic, and isokinetic concentric and eccentric quadriceps and hamstring force and three components of athletic performance. *Journal of Orthopaedic and Sports Physical Therapy* 14(3): 114–20.
2. Bennett, J., and W. Stauber. 1986. Evaluation and treatment of anterior knee pain using eccentric exercise. *Medicine and Science in Sports and Exercise* 18(5): 526–30.
3. Biodex Informational Packet. Shirley, NY: Biodex Corp.
4. Blacker, H. Measurements predicting outcome in pain treatment. In *Kin-Com Clinical Resource Kit*. Hixson, TN: Chattanooga Corp.
5. Chandler, J., and P. Duncan. 1988. Eccentric versus concentric force-velocity relationships of the quadriceps femoris muscle. *Physical Therapy* 68(5): 800.
6. Cybex Informational Packet. Ronkonkoma, NY: Cybex Corp.
7. Davies, G. 1984. *A compendium of isokinetics in clinical usage*. LaCrosse, WI: S & S.

8. Dillman, C. J., G. S. Fleisig, S. L. Werner, et al. 1990. Biomechanics of the shoulder in sports: Throwing activities, Pennington, NJ, Post Graduate Studies in Physical Therapy, Forum Medicum.

9. Dvir, Z., N. Halperin, A. Snklar, et al. 1991. Quadriceps function and patellofemoral pain syndrome. *Isokinetics Exerc Sci* 1(1): 31–35.

10. Dvir, Z. 1995. *Isokinetic muscle testing, interpretation, and clinical applications.* New York: Churchill Livingstone.

11. Engle, R., and J. Faust. 1991. Isokinetic evaluation in posterior shoulder subluxation. *Isokinetics Exerc Sci* 1(2): 72–74.

12. Frisiello, S., A. Gazaille, J. O'Halloran, W. L. Palmer, and D. Waugh. 1994. Test-retest reliability of eccentric peak torque values for shoulder medial and lateral rotation using the Biodex isokinetic dynamometer. *Journal of Orthopaedic and Sports Physical Therapy* 19(6): 341–44.

13. Greenberger, H. B., and M. V. Paterno. 1995. Relationship of knee extensor strength and hopping test performance in the assessment of lower extremity function. *Journal of Orthopaedic and Sports Physical Therapy* 22(5): 202–6.

14. Hageman, P., D. Gillaspie, and L. Hill. 1988. Effects of speed and limb dominance on eccentric and concentric isokinetic testing of the knee. *Journal of Orthopaedic and Sports Physical Therapy* 10(2): 59-65.

15. Hageman, P., and T. Sorenson. 1995. Eccentric isokinetics. In *Eccentric muscle training in sports and orthopaedics*, 2d ed., edited by M. Albert. New York: Churchill Livingstone.

16. Hagood, S., M. Solomonow, R. Baratta, et al. 1990. The effect of joint velocity on the contribution of the antagonistic musculature to knee stiffness and laxity. *American Journal of Sports Medicine* 18(2): 182–87.

17. Hellwig, E. V., and D. H. Perrin. 1991. A comparison of two positions for assessing shoulder rotator peak torque: The traditional frontal plane versus the plane of the scapula. *Isokinetics Exerc Sci* 1:1–5.

18. Hislop, H., and J. Perrine. 1967. The isokinetic concept of exercise. *Physical Therapy* 47(2): 114–17.

19. Kin-Com Informational Packet. Hixson, TN: Chattanooga Corp.

20. Kues, J. M., J. M. Rothstein, and R. L. Lamb. 1992. Obtaining reliable measurements of knee extensor torque produced during maximal voluntary contractions: An experimental investigation. *Physical Therapy* 72(7): 492–504.

21. Lephart, S. M., D. H. Perrin, F. H. Fu, J. C. Gieck, F. C. McCue, and J. J. Irrgang. 1992. Relationship between selected physical characteristics and functional capacity in the anterior cruciate ligament-insufficient athlete. *Journal of Orthopaedic and Sports Physical Therapy* 16:174–81.

22. Leveau, B. 1992. *Williams and Lister's biomechanics of human motion.* 3d ed. Philadelphia: W. B. Saunders.

23. Malerba, J. L., M. L. Adam, B. A. Harris, and D. E. Krebs. 1992. Reliability of dynamic and isometric testing of shoulder internal and external rotators. *Journal of Orthopaedic and Sports Physical Therapy* 18(4): 543–52.

24. Mathews, P., and D. M. St-Pierre. 1996. Recovery of muscle strength following arthroscopic meniscectomy. *Journal of Orthopaedic and Sports Physical Therapy* 23(1): 18–26.

25. Perrin, D., R. Robertson, and R. Lay. 1987. Bilateral isokinetic peak torque, torque acceleration energy, power, and work relationships in athletes and non-athletes. *Journal of Orthopaedic and Sports Physical Therapy* 9(5): 184–89.

26. Perrin, D. H. 1993. *Isokinetic exercise and assessment.* Champaign, IL: Human Kinetics.

27. Poulmedis, P., G. Rondoyannis, A. Mitsou, et al. 1988. The influence of isokinetic muscle torque exerted in various speeds on soccer ball velocity, *Journal of Orthopaedic and Sports Physical Therapy* 10(3): 93–96.

28. Rothstein, J., L. Lamb, and T. Mayhew. 1987. Clinical uses of isokinetic measurements. *Physical Therapy* 67(12): 1840–44.

29. Sirota, S. C., G. A. Malanga, J. J. Eischen, and E. R. Laskowski. 1997. An eccentric and concentric strength profile of shoulder external and internal rotator muscles in professional baseball pitchers. *American Journal of Sports Medicine* 25(1): 59–64.

30. Trudelle-Jackson, E., N. Meske, C. Highgenboten, et al. Eccentric/concentric torque deficits in the quadriceps muscle. *Journal of Orthopaedic and Sports Physical Therapy* 11(4): 142.

31. Wennerberg, D. 1991. Reliability of an isokinetic dorsiflexion and plantarflexion apparatus. *American Journal of Sports Medicine* 19(5): 519–22.

32. Whitcomb, L. J., M. J. Kelley, and C. I. Leiper. 1995. A comparison of torque production during dynamic strength testing of shoulder abduction in the coronal plane and the plane of the scapula. *Journal of Orthopaedic and Sports Physical Therapy* 21(4): 227–32.

33. Wilk, K. E., and J. R. Andrews. 1993. The effects of pad placement and angular velocity on tibial displacement during isokinetic exercise. *Journal of Orthopaedic and Sports Physical Therapy* 17(1): 24.

34. Wilk, K. E., and C. A. Arrigo. 1993. Current concepts in the rehabilitation of the athletic shoulder. *Journal of Orthopaedic and Sports Physical Therapy* 18: 365.

35. Worrell, T., D. Perrin, and C. Denegar. 1989. The influence of hip position on quadriceps and hamstring peak torque and reciprocal muscle group ratio values. *Journal of Orthopaedic and Sports Physical Therapy* 11(3): 104–7.

36. Worrell, T. W., D. H. Perrin, B. M. Gansneder, and J. H. Gieck. 1991. Comparison of isokinetic strength and flexibility measures between hamstring injured and non-injured athletes. *Journal of Orthopaedic and Sports Physical Therapy* 13: 118–25.

37. Worrell, T. W., B. Borchert, K. Erner, J. Fritz, and P. Leerar. 1993. Effect of a lateral step-up exercise protocol on quadriceps and lower extremity performance. *Journal of Orthopaedic and Sports Physical Therapy* 18(6): 646–53.

38. Wyatt, M., and A. Edwards. 1981. Comparisons of quadriceps and ham-string torque values during isokinetic exercise. *Journal of Orthopaedic and Sports Physical Therapy* 3(2): 48–56.

Suggested Readings

Brown, L. E., M. Whitehurst, R. Gilbert, and D. N. Buchalter. 1995. The effect of velocity and gender on load range during knee extension and flexion exercise on an isokinetic exercise on an isokinetic device. *Journal of Orthopaedic and Sports Physical Therapy* 21(2): 107–12.

Ellenbecker, T. S. 1995. Rehabilitation of shoulder and elbow injuries. *Clinics in Sports Medicine* 14(1): 87–107.

Griffin, J. W., R. E. Tooms, R. vanderZwaag, T. E. Bertorini, and M. L. O'Toole. 1993. Eccentric muscle performance of elbow and knee muscle groups in untrained men and women. *Medicine and Science in Sports and Exercise* 25(8): 936–44

Heiderscheit, B. C., K. P. McLean, and G. J. Davies. 1996. The effects of isokinetic versus plyometric training on the shoulder internal rotators. *Journal of Orthopaedic and Sports Physical Therapy* 23(2): 125–33.

Kang, S. W., J. H. Moon, and S. I. Chun. 1995. Exercise effect of modified contralateral stabilization bar during one-legged isokinetic exercise. *Archives of Physical Medicine and Rehabilitation* 76(2): 177–82.

Kauffman, K. R., K. N. An, and E. Y. Chao. 1995. A comparison of intersegmental joint dynamics to isokinetic dynamometer measurements. *Journal of Biomechanics* 28(10): 1243–56.

Keating, J. L., and T. A. Matyas. 1996. The influence of subject and test design on dynamometric measurements of extremity muscles. *Physical Therapy* 76(8): 866.

Mikesky, A. E., J. E. Edwards, J. K. Wigglesworth, and S. Kunkel. 1995. Eccentric and concentric strength of the shoulder and arm musculature in collegiate baseball pitchers. *American Journal of Sports Medicine* 23(5): 638–42.

Mont, M. A., D. B. Cohen, K. R. Campbell, K. Gravara, and S. K. Mathur. 1994. Isokinetic concentric versus eccentric training of shoulder rotators with functional evaluation of performance enhancement in elite tennis players. *American Journal of Sports Medicine* 22(4): 513–17.

Porter, M. M., A. A. Vandervoort, and J. F. Kramer. 1996. A method of measuring standing isokinetic plantar and dorsiflexion peak torques. *Medicine and Science in Sports and Exercise* 28(4): 516–22.

Schwendner, K. I., A. E. Mikesky, J. K. Wigglesworth, and D. B. Burr. 1995. Recovery of dynamic muscle function following isokinetic fatigue testing. *International Journal of Sports Medicine* 16(3): 185–89.

Weir, J. P., S. A. Evans, and M. L. Housh. 1996. The effect of extraneous movements on peak torque and constant joint angle torque-velocity curves. *Journal of Orthopaedic and Sports Physical Therapy* 23(5): 302–8.

Wilk, K. E., J. R. Andrews, C. A. Arrigo, M. A. Keirns, and D. J. Erber. 1993. The strength characteristics of internal and external rotator muscles in professional baseball pitchers. *American Journal of Sports Medicine* 21(1): 61–66.

Wilk, K. E., W. T. Romaniello, S. M. Soscia, C. A. Arrigo, and J. R. Andrews. 1994. The relationship between subjective knee scores, isokinetic testing, and functional testing in the AL-reconstructed knee. *Journal of Orthopaedic and Sports Physical Therapy* 20(2): 60–73.

CHAPTER 10

Plyometric Exercise in Rehabilitation

Michael Voight
Steve Tippett

After completion of this chapter, the student should be able to do the following:

- Describe the mechanical, neurophysiological, and neuromuscular control mechanisms involved in plyometric training.

- Discuss how biomechanical evaluation, stability, dynamic movement, and flexibility should be assessed before beginning a plyometric program.

- Explain how a plyometric program can be modified by changing intensity, volume, frequency, and recovery.

- Discuss how plyometrics can be integrated into a rehabilitation program.

WHAT IS PLYOMETRIC EXERCISE?

In sports training and rehabilitation of athletic injuries, the concept of specificity has emerged as an important parameter in determining the proper choice and sequence of exercise in a training program. The jumping movement is inherent in numerous sport activities such as basketball, volleyball, gymnastics, and aerobic dancing. Even running is a repeated series of jump-landing cycles. Therefore jump training should be used in the design and implementation in the overall training program.

Peak performance in sport requires technical skill and power. Skill in most activities combines natural athletic ability and learned specialized proficiency in an activity. Success in most activities is dependent upon the speed at which muscular force or power can be generated. Strength and conditioning programs throughout the years have attempted to augment the force production system to maximize the power generated. Because power combines strength and speed, it can be increased by increasing the amount of work or force that is produced by the muscles or by decreasing the amount of time required to produce the force. Although weight training can produce increased gains in strength, the speed of movement is limited. The amount of time required to produce muscular force is an important variable for increasing the power output. A form of training that attempts to combine speed of movement with strength is plyometrics.

The term **plyometric training** is relatively new, but the concept of plyometric training is not new. The roots of plyometric training can be traced to eastern Europe, where it was known simply as jump training. The term *plyometrics* was coined by an American track and field coach, Fred Wilt.[35] The development of the term is confusing. *Plyo-* comes from the Greek word *plythein,* which means "to increase." *Plio* is the Greek word for "more," and *metric* literally means "to measure." Practically, plyometrics is defined as a quick, powerful movement involving prestretching the muscle and activating the stretch-shortening cycle to produce a subsequently stronger concentric contraction. It takes advantage of the length-shortening cycle to increase muscular power.

In the late 1960s and early 1970s when the Eastern Bloc countries began to dominate sports requiring power, their training methods became the focus of attention. After the 1972 Olympics, articles began to appear in coaching magazines outlining a strange new system of jumps and bounds that had been used by the Soviets to increase speed. Valery Borzov, the 100-meter gold medalist, credited plyometric exercise for his success. As it turns out, the Eastern Bloc countries were not the originators of plyometrics, just the organizers. This system of hops and jumps has been used by American coaches for years as a method of conditioning. Both rope jumping and bench hops have been used to improve quickness and reaction times. The organization of this training method has been credited to the legendary Soviet jump coach Yuri Verhoshanski, who during the late 1960s began to tie this method of miscellaneous hops and jumps into an organized training plan.[30]

The main purpose of plyometric training is to heighten the excitability of the nervous system for improved reactive ability of the neuromuscular system.[31] Therefore, any type of exercise that uses the myotatic stretch reflex to produce a more powerful response of the contracting muscle is plyometric in nature. All movement patterns in both athletes and activities of daily living (ADL) involve repeated stretch-shortening cycles. Picture a jumping athlete preparing to transfer forward energy to upward energy. As the final step is taken before jumping, the loaded leg must stop the forward momentum and change it into an upward direction. As this happens, the muscle undergoes a lengthening eccentric contraction to decelerate the movement and prestretch the muscle. This prestretch energy is then immediately released in an equal and opposite reaction, thereby producing kinetic energy. The neuromuscular system must react quickly to produce the concentric shortening contraction to prevent falling and produce the upward change in direction. Most elite athletes will naturally exhibit with great ease this ability to use stored kinetic energy. Less gifted athletes can train this ability and enhance their production of power. Consequently, specific functional exercise to emphasize this rapid change of di-

rection must be used to prepare patients and athletes for return to activity. Because plyometric exercises train specific movements in a biomechanically accurate manner, the muscles, tendons, and ligaments are all strengthened in a functional manner.

Most of the literature to date on plyometric training has been focused on the lower quarter. Because all movements in athletics involve a repeated series of stretch-shortening cycles, adaptation of the plyometric principles can be used to enhance the specificity of training in other sports or activities that require a maximum amount of muscular force in a minimal amount of time. Whether the athlete is jumping or throwing, the musculature around the involved joints must first stretch and then contract to produce the explosive movement. Because of the muscular demands during the overhead throw, plyometrics have been advocated as a form of conditioning for the overhead throwing athlete.[32,34] Although the principles are similar, different forms of plyometric exercises should be applied to the upper extremity to train the stretch-shortening cycle. Additionally, the intensity of the upper extremity plyometric program is usually less than that of the lower extremity, due to the smaller muscle mass and type of muscle function of the upper extremity compared to the lower extremity.

BIOMECHANICAL AND PHYSIOLOGICAL PRINCIPLES OF PLYOMETRIC TRAINING

The goal of plyometric training is to decrease the amount of time required between the yielding eccentric muscle contraction and the initiation of the overcoming concentric contraction. Normal physiological movement rarely begins from a static starting position but rather is preceded by an eccentric prestretch that loads the muscle and prepares it for the ensuing concentric contraction. The coupling of this eccentric-concentric muscle contraction is known as the stretch-shortening cycle. The physiology of this stretch-shortening cycle can be broken down into two components: proprioceptive reflexes and the elastic properties of muscle fibers. These components work together to produce a response, but they will be discussed separately for the purpose of understanding.

Mechanical Characteristics

The mechanical characteristics of a muscle can best be represented by a three-component model (Figure 10-1). A contractile component (CC), series elastic component (SEC), and parallel elastic component (PEC) all interact to

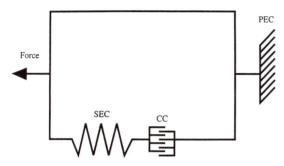

Figure 10-1   Three-component model.

produce a force output. Although the CC is usually the focal point of motor control, the SEC and PEC also play an important role in providing stability and integrity to the individual fibers when a muscle is lengthened. During this lengthening process, energy is stored within the musculature in the form of kinetic energy.

When a muscle contracts in a concentric fashion, most of the force that is produced comes from the muscle fiber filaments sliding past one another. Force is registered externally by being transferred through the SEC. When eccentric contraction occurs, the muscle lengthens like a spring. With this lengthening, the SEC is also stretched and allowed to contribute to the overall force production. Therefore the total force production is the sum of the force produced by the CC and the stretching of the SEC. An analogy would be the stretching of a rubber band. When a stretch is applied, potential energy is stored and applied as it returns to its original length when the stretch is released. Significant increases in concentric muscle force production have been documented when immediately preceded by an eccentric contraction.[2,4,9] This increase might be partly due to the storage of elastic energy, because the muscles are able to use the force produced by the SEC. When the muscle contracts in a concentric manner, the elastic energy that is stored in the SEC can be recovered and used to augment the shortening contraction. The ability to use this stored elastic energy is affected by three variables: time, magnitude of stretch, and velocity of stretch.[17] The concentric contraction can be magnified only if the preceding eccentric contraction is of short range and performed quickly without delay.[2,4,9] Bosco and Komi proved this concept experimentally when they compared damped versus undamped jumps.[4] Undamped jumps produced minimal knee flexion upon landing and were followed by an immediate rebound jump. With damped jumps, the knee flexion angle increased significantly. The power output was much higher with the undamped jumps. The increased knee flexion seen in the damped jumps decreased elastic be-

havior of the muscle, and the potential elastic energy stored in the SEC was lost as heat. Similar investigations produced greater vertical jump height when the movement was preceded by a countermovement as opposed to a static jump.[2,5,6,22]

The type of muscle fiber involved in the contraction can also affect storage of elastic energy. Bosco et al. noted a difference in the recoil of elastic energy in slow-twitch versus fast-twitch muscle fibers.[7] This study indicates that fast-twitch muscle fibers respond to a high-speed, small-amplitude prestretch. The amount of elastic energy used was proportional to the amount stored. When a long, slow stretch is applied to muscle, slow- and fast-twitch fibers exhibit a similar amount of stored elastic energy; however, this stored energy is used to a greater extent with the slow-twitch fibers. This trend would suggest that slow-twitch muscle fibers might be able to use elastic energy more efficiently in ballistic movement characterized by long and slow prestretching in the stretch-shortening cycle.

Neurophysiological Mechanisms

The proprioceptive stretch reflex is the other mechanism by which force can be produced during the stretch-shortening cycle. Mechanoreceptors located within the muscle provide information about the degree of muscular stretch. This information is transmitted to the central nervous system and becomes capable of influencing muscle tone, motor execution programs, and kinesthetic awareness. The mechanoreceptors that are primarily responsible for the stretch reflex are the Golgi tendon organs and muscle spindles.[24] The muscle spindle is a complex stretch receptor that is located in parallel within the muscle fibers. Sensory information regarding the length of the muscle spindle and the rate of the applied stretch is transmitted to the central nervous system. If the length of the surrounding muscle fibers is less than that of the spindle, the frequency of the nerve impulses from the spindle is reduced. When the muscle spindle becomes stretched, an afferent sensory response is produced and transmitted to the central nervous system. Neurological impulses are in turn sent back to the muscle, causing a motor response. As the muscle contracts, the stretch on the muscle spindle is relieved, thereby removing the original stimulus. The strength of the muscle spindle response is determined by the rate of stretch.[24] The more rapidly the load is applied to the muscle, the greater the firing frequency of the spindle and resultant reflexive muscle contraction.

The Golgi tendon organ lies within the muscle tendon near the point of attachment of the muscle fiber to the tendon. Unlike the facilitory action of the muscle spindle, the Golgi tendon organ has an inhibitory effect on the muscle by contributing to a tension limiting reflex. Because the Golgi tendon organs are in series alignment with the contracting muscle fibers, they become activated with tension or stretch within the muscle. Upon activation, sensory impulses are transmitted to the central nervous system. These sensory impulses cause an inhibition of the alpha motor neurons of the contracting muscle and its synergists, thereby limiting the amount of force produced. With a concentric muscle contraction, the activity of the muscle spindle is reduced because the surrounding muscle fibers are shortening. During an eccentric muscle contraction, the muscle stretch reflex generates more tension in the lengthening muscle. When the tension within the muscle reaches a potentially harmful level, the Golgi tendon organ fires, thereby reducing the excitation of the muscle. The muscle spindle and Golgi tendon organ systems oppose each other, and increasing force is produced. The descending neural pathways from the brain help to balance these forces and ultimately control which reflex will dominate.[26]

The degree of muscle fiber elongation is dependent upon three physiological factors. Fiber length is proportional to the amount of stretching force applied to the muscle. The ultimate elongation or deformation is also dependent upon the absolute strength of the individual muscle fibers. The stronger the tensile strength, the less elongation that will occur. The last factor for elongation is the ability of the muscle spindle to produce a neurophysiological response. A muscle spindle with a low sensitivity level will result in a difficulty in overcoming the rapid elongation and therefore produce a less powerful response. Plyometric training will assist in enhancing muscular control within the neurological system.

The increased force production seen during the stretch-shortening cycle is due to the combined effects of the storage of elastic energy and the myotatic reflex activation of the muscle.[2,5,8,9,23,27] The percentage of contribution from each component is unknown.[5] The increased amount of force production is dependent upon the time frame between the eccentric and concentric contractions.[9] This time frame can be defined as the amortization phase.[13] The amortization phase is the electromechanical delay between eccentric and concentric contraction during which time the muscle must switch from overcoming work to acceleration in the opposite direction. Komi found that the greatest amount of tension developed within the muscle during the stretch-shortening cycle occurred during the phase of muscle lengthening just before the concentric contraction.[21] The conclusion from this study was that an increased time in

the amortization phase would lead to a decrease in force production.

Physiological performance can be improved by several mechanisms with plyometric training. Although there has been documented evidence of increased speed of the stretch reflex, the increased intensity of the subsequent muscle contraction might be best attributed to better recruitment of additional motor units.[11] The force-velocity relationship states that the faster a muscle is loaded or lengthened eccentrically, the greater the resultant force output. Eccentric lengthening will also place a load on the elastic components of the muscle fibers. The stretch reflex might also increase the stiffness of the muscular spring by recruiting additional muscle fibers.[11] This additional stiffness might allow the muscular system to use more external stress in the form of elastic recoil.[11]

Another possible mechanism by which plyometric training can increase the force or power output involves the inhibitory effect of the Golgi tendon organs on force production. Because the Golgi tendon organ serves as a tension-limiting reflex, restricting the amount of force that can be produced, the stimulation threshold for the Golgi tendon organ becomes a limiting factor. Bosco and Komi have suggested that plyometric training can desensitize the Golgi tendon organ, thereby raising the level of inhibition.[4] If the level of inhibition is raised, a greater amount of force production and load can be applied to the musculoskeletal system.

Neuromuscular Coordination

The last mechanism in which plyometric training might improve muscular performance centers around neuromuscular coordination (see Chapter 6). The speed of muscular contraction can be limited by neuromuscular coordination. In other words, the body can move only within a set speed range, no matter how strong the muscles are. Training with an explosive prestretch of the muscle can improve the neural efficiency, thereby increasing neuromuscular performance. Plyometric training can promote changes within the neuromuscular system that allow the individual to have better control of the contracting muscle and its synergists, yielding a greater net force even in the absence of morphological adaptation of the muscle. This neural adaptation can increase performance by enhancing the nervous system to become more automatic.

In summary, effective plyometric training relies more on the rate of stretch than on the length of stretch. Emphasis should center on the reduction of the amortization phase. If the amortization phase is slow, the elastic energy is lost as heat and the stretch reflex is not activated. Conversely, the quicker the individual is able to switch from yielding eccentric work to overcoming concentric work, the more powerful the response.

PROGRAM DEVELOPMENT

Specificity is the key concept in any training program. Sport-specific activities should be analyzed and broken down into basic movement patterns. These specific movement patterns should then be stressed in a gradual fashion, based upon individual tolerance to these activities. Development of a plyometric program should begin by establishing an adequate strength base that will allow the body to withstand the large stress that will be placed upon it. A greater strength base will allow for greater force production due to increased muscular cross-sectional area. Additionally, a larger cross-sectional area can contribute to the SEC and subsequently store a greater amount of elastic energy.

Plyometric exercises can be characterized as rapid eccentric loading of the musculoskeletal complex.[11] This type of exercise trains the neuromuscular system by teaching it to more readily accept the increased strength loads.[3] Also, the nervous system is more readily able to react with maximal speed to the lengthening muscle by exploiting the stretch reflex. Plyometric training attempts to fine tune the neuromuscular system, so all training programs should be designed with specificity in mind.[25] This goal will help to ensure that the body is prepared to accept the stress that will be placed upon it during return to function.

Plyometric Prerequisites

Biomechanical Examination. Before beginning a plyometric training program, a cursory biomechanical examination and a battery of functional tests should be performed to identify potential contraindications or precautions. Lower-quarter biomechanics should be sound to help ensure a stable base of support and normal force transmission. Biomechanical abnormalities of the lower quarter are not contraindications for plyometrics but can contribute to stress failure-overuse injury if not addressed. Before initiating plyometric training, an adequate strength base of the stabilizing musculature must be present. Functional tests are very effective to screen for an adequate strength base before initiating plyometrics. Poor strength in the lower extremities will result in a loss of stability when landing and also increase the amount of stress that is absorbed by the weight-bearing tissues with high-impact forces, which will reduce performance and increase the risk of injury. The Eastern Bloc countries arbitrarily placed a one-repetition maximum in the squat at 1.5 to 2 times the individual's body weight before initiating lower-quarter plyometrics.[3] If this were to hold true, a 200-pound individual would have to squat 400 pounds before beginning plyometrics. Unfortunately, not many individuals would meet this minimal criteria. Clinical and practical experience has demonstrated that plyometrics can be started without that kind of leg strength.[11] A simple functional parameter to use in determining whether an individual is strong enough to initiate a plyometric training program has been advocated by Chu.[12] Power squat testing with a weight equal to 60 percent of the individual's body weight is used. The individual is asked to perform five squat repetitions in 5 seconds. If the individual cannot perform this task, emphasis in the training program should again center on the strength-training program to develop an adequate base.

Because eccentric muscle strength is an important component to plyometric training, it is especially important to ensure an adequate eccentric strength base is present. Before an individual is allowed to begin a plyometric regimen, a program of closed-chain stability training that focuses on eccentric lower-quarter strength should be initiated. In addition to strengthening in a functional manner, closed-chain weight-bearing exercises also allow the individual to use functional movement patterns. Once cleared to participate in the plyometric program, precautionary safety tips should be adhered to.

Stability Testing. Stability testing before initiating plyometric training can be divided into two subcategories: static stability and dynamic movement testing. Static stability testing determines the individual's ability to stabilize and control the body. The muscles of postural support must be strong enough to withstand the stress of explosive training. Static stability testing (Figure 10-2) should begin with simple movements of low motor complexity and progress to more difficult high motor skills. The basis for lower-quarter stability centers around single-leg strength. Difficulty can be increased by having the individual close his or her eyes. The basic static tests are one-leg standing and single-leg quarter squats that are held for 30 seconds. An individual should be able to perform one-leg standing for 30 seconds with eyes open and closed before the initiation of plyometric training. The individual should be observed for shaking or wobbling of the extremity joints. If there is more movement of a weight-bearing joint in one direction than the other, the musculature producing the movement in the opposite direction needs to be assessed for specific weakness. If weakness is determined, the individual's program should be limited and emphasis placed on isolated strengthening of the weak muscles. For dynamic jump exercises to be initiated, there should be no wobbling of the support leg during the quarter knee squats.

Plyometric Static Stability Testing

- Single-Leg Stance — 30 sec
  – Eyes open
  – Eyes closed

- Single-Leg 25% Squat — 30 sec
  – Eyes open
  – Eyes closed

- Single-Leg 50% Squat — 30 sec
  – Eyes open
  – Eyes closed

Figure 10-2   Static stability testing.

After an individual has satisfactorily demonstrated both single-leg static stance and a single-leg quarter squat, more dynamic tests of eccentric capabilities can be initiated. Once an individual has stabilization strength, the concern shifts toward developing and evaluating eccentric strength. The limiting factor in high-intensity, high-volume plyometrics is eccentric capabilities. Eccentric strength can be assessed with stabilization jump tests. If an individual has an excessively long amortization phase or a slow switching from eccentric to concentric contractions, the eccentric strength levels are insufficient.

Dynamic Movement Testing.   Dynamic movement testing will assess the individual's ability to produce explosive, coordinated movement. Vertical or single-leg jumping for distance can be used for the lower quarter. Researchers have investigated the use of single-leg hop for distance and a determinant for return to play after knee injury. A passing score on their test is 85 percent in regard to symmetry. The involved leg is tested twice, and the average between the two trials is recorded. The noninvolved leg is tested in the same fashion, and then the scores of the noninvolved leg are divided by the scores of the involved leg and multiplied by 100. This provides the symmetry index score. Another functional test that can be used to determine whether an individual is ready for plyometric training is the ability to long jump a distance equal to the individual's height. In the upper quarter, the medicine ball toss is used as a functional assessment.

Flexibility.   Another important prerequisite for plyometric training is general and specific flexibility, because a high amount of stress is applied to the musculoskeletal system. Therefore all plyometric training sessions should begin with a general warm-up and flexibility exercise program. The warm-up should produce mild sweating.[19] The flexibility exercise program should address muscle groups involved in the plyometric program and should include static and short dynamic stretching techniques.[18]

Chu's Plyometric Categories

- In-place jumping
- Standing jumps
- Multiple-response jumps and hops
- In-depth jumping and box drills
- Bounding
- High-stress sport-specific drills

Figure 10-3   Six categories of plyometric training.

When the individual can demonstrate static and dynamic control of their body weight with single-leg squats, low-intensity in-place plyometrics can be initiated. Plyometric training should consist of low-intensity drills and progress slowly in deliberate fashion. As skill and strength foundation increase, moderate-intensity plyometrics can be introduced. Mature athletes with strong weight-training backgrounds can be introduced to ballistic-reactive plyometric exercises of high intensity.[12] Once the individual has been classified as beginner, intermediate, or advanced, the plyometric program can be planned and initiated. Chu[10,11,13] has divided lower-quarter plyometric training into six categories (Figure 10-3).

PLYOMETRIC PROGRAM DESIGN

As with any conditioning program, the plyometric training program can be manipulated through training variables: i.e., direction of body movement, weight of the athlete, speed of the execution, external load, intensity, volume, frequency, training age, and recovery.

Direction of Body Movement

Horizontal body movement is less stressful than vertical movement. This is dependent upon the weight of the athlete and the technical proficiency demonstrated during the jumps.

Weight of the Athlete

The heavier the athlete, the greater the training demand placed on the athlete. What might be a low-demand in-place jump for a lightweight athlete might be a high-demand activity for a heavyweight athlete.

Speed of Execution of the Exercise

Increased speed of execution on exercises like single-leg hops or alternate-leg bounding raises the training demand on the individual.

External Load

Adding an external load can significantly raise the training demand. Do not raise the external load to a level that will significantly slow the speed of movement.

Intensity

Intensity can be defined as the amount of effort exerted. With traditional weight lifting, intensity can be modified by changing the amount of weight that is lifted. With plyometric training, intensity can be controlled by the type of exercise that is performed. Double-leg jumping is less stressful than single-leg jumping. As with all functional exercise, the plyometric exercise program should progress from simple to complex activities. Intensity can be further increased by altering the specific exercises. The addition of external weight or raising the height of the step or box will also increase the exercise intensity.

Volume

Volume is the total amount of work that is performed in a single workout session. With weight training, volume would be recorded as the total amount of weight that was lifted (weight times repetitions). Volume of plyometric training is measured by counting the total number of foot contacts. The recommended volume of foot contacts in any one session will vary inversely with the intensity of the exercise. A beginner should start with low-intensity exercise with a volume of approximately 75 to 100 foot contacts. As ability is increased, the volume is increased to 200 to 250 foot contacts of low to moderate intensity.

Frequency

Frequency is the number of times an exercise session is performed during a training cycle. With weight training, the frequency of exercise has typically been three times weekly. Unfortunately, research on the frequency of plyometric exercise has not been conducted. Therefore the optimum frequency for increased performance is not known. It has been suggested that 48 to 72 hours of rest are necessary for full recovery before the next training stimulus.[12] Intensity, however, plays a major role in determining the frequency of training. If an adequate recovery period does not occur, muscle fatigue will result with a corresponding increase in neuromuscular reaction times. The beginner should allow at least 48 hours between training sessions.

Training Age

Training age is the number of years an athlete has been in a formal training program. At younger training ages the overall training demand should be kept low.

Recovery

Recovery is the rest time used between exercise sets. Manipulation of this variable will depend on whether the goal is to increase power or muscular endurance. Because plyometric training is anaerobic in nature, a longer recovery period should be used to allow restoration of metabolic stores. With power training, a work rest ratio of 1:3 or 1:4 should be used. This time frame will allow maximal recovery between sets. For endurance training, this work/rest ratio can be shortened to 1:1 or 1:2. Endurance training typically uses circuit training, where the individual moves from one exercise set to another with minimal rest in between.

The beginning plyometric program should emphasize the importance of eccentric versus concentric muscle contractions. The relevance of the stretch-shortening cycle with decreased amortization time should be stressed. Initiation of lower-quarter plyometric training begins with low-intensity in-place and multiple-response jumps. The individual should be instructed in proper exercise technique. The feet should be nearly flat in all landings, and the individual should be encouraged to "touch and go." An analogy would be landing on a hot bed of coals. The goal is to reverse the landing as quickly as possible, spending only a minimal amount of time on the ground.

Success of the plyometric program will depend on how well the training variables are controlled, modified, and manipulated. In general, as the intensity of the exercise is increased, the volume is decreased. The corollary to this is that as volume increases, the intensity is decreased. The overall key to successfully controlling these variables is to be flexible and listen to what the athlete's body is telling you. The body's response to the program will dictate the speed of progression. Whenever in doubt as to the exercise intensity or volume, it is better to underestimate to prevent injury.

Before implementing a plyometric program, the sports therapist should assess the type of athlete that is being rehabilitated and whether plyometrics are suitable for that individual. In most cases, plyometrics should be used in the latter phases of rehabilitation, starting in the advanced strengthening phase once the athlete has obtained an appropriate strength base.[32,34] When utilizing

■ **TABLE 10-1** Upper-Extremity Plyometric Drills

I. Warm-Up Drills

Plyoball trunk rotation
Plyoball side bends
Plyoball wood chops
ER/IR with tubing
PNF D2 pattern with tubing

II. Throwing Movements—Standing Position

Two-hand chest pass
Two-hand overhead soccer throw
Two-hand side throw overhead
Tubing ER/IR (Both at side & 90° abduction)
Tubing PNF D2 pattern
One-hand baseball throw
One-hand IR side throw
One-hand ER side throw
Plyo push-up (against wall)

III. Throwing Movements—Seated Position

Two-hand overhead soccer throw
Two-hand side-to-side throw
Two-hand chest pass
One-hand baseball throw

IV. Trunk Drills

Plyoball sit-ups
Plyoball sit-up and throw
Plyoball back extension
Plyoball long sitting side throws

V. Partner Drills

Overhead soccer throw
Plyoball back-to-back twists
Overhead pullover throw
Kneeling side throw
Backward throw
Chest pass throw

VI. Wall Drills

Two-hand chest throw
Two-hand overhead soccer throw
Two-hand underhand side-to-side throw
One-hand baseball throw
One-hand wall dribble

VII. Endurance Drills

One-hand wall dribble
Around-the-back circles
Figure eight through the legs
Single-arm ball flips

---

plyometric training in the uninjured athlete, the application of plyometric exercise should follow the concept of periodization.[31] The concept of periodization refers to the year-round sequence and progression of strength training, conditioning, and sport-specific skills.[34] There are four specific phases in the year-round periodization model: the competitive season, postseason training, the preparation phase, and the transitional phase.[31] Plyometric exercises should be performed in the latter stages of the preparation phase and during the transitional phase for optimal results and safety. To obtain the benefits of a plyometric program, the athlete should (1) be well conditioned with sufficient strength and endurance, (2) exhibit athletic abilities, (3) exhibit coordination and proprioceptive abilities, and (4) free of pain from any physical injury or condition.

It should be remembered that the plyometric program is not designed to be an exclusive training program for the athlete. Rather, it should be one part of a well-structured training program that includes strength training, flexibility training, cardiovascular fitness, and sport-specific training for skill enhancement and coordination. By combining the plyometric program with other training techniques, the effects of training are greatly enhanced.

Table 10-1 and Table 10-2 suggest upper-extremity and lower-extremity plyometric drills.

GUIDELINES FOR PLYOMETRIC PROGRAMS

The proper execution of the plyometric exercise program must continually be stressed. A sound technical foundation from which higher-intensity work can build should be established. It must be remembered that jumping is a continuous interchange between force reduction and force production. This interchange takes place throughout the entire body: ankle, knee, hip, trunk, and arms. The timing and coordination of these body segments yields a positive ground reaction that will result in a high rate of force production.

■ **TABLE 10-2**   Lower-Extremity Plyometric Drills

I. **Warm-Up Drills**

Double-leg squats
Double-leg leg press
Double-leg squat-jumps
Jumping jacks

II. **Entry Level Drills—Two-Legged**

•Two-Legged Drills
Side to side (floor / line)
Diagonal jumps (floor / 4 corners)
Diagonal jumps (4 spots)
Diagonal zig/zag (6 spots)
Plyo leg press
Plyo leg press (4 corners)

III. **Intermediate Level Drills**

Two-Legged Box Jumps
One-box side jump
Two-box side jumps
Two-box side jumps with foam
Four-box diagonal jumps
Two-box with rotation
One/Two box with catch
One/Two box with catch (foam)
•Single-Leg Movements
Single-leg plyo leg press
Single-leg side jumps (floor)

Single-leg side-to-side jumps (floor/4 corners)
Single-leg diagonal jumps (floor/4 corners)

IV. **Advanced Level Drills**

•Single-Leg Box Jumps
One-box side jumps
Two-box side jumps
Single-leg plyo leg press (4 corners)
Two-box side jumps with foam
Four-box diagonal jumps
One-box side jumps with rotation
Two-box side jumps with rotation
One-box side jump with catch
One-box side jump rotation with catch
Two-box side jump with catch
Two-box side jump rotation with catch

V. **Endurance/Agility Plyometrics**

Side-to-side bounding (20 feet)
Side jump lunges (cone)
Side jump lunges (cone with foam)
Altering rapid step-up (forward)
Lateral step-overs
High stepping (forward)
High stepping (backwards)
Depth jump with rebound jump
Depth jump with catch
Jump and catch (plyoball)

As the plyometric program is initiated, the individual must be made aware of several guidelines.[31] Any deviation from these guidelines will result in minimal improvement and increased risk for injury. These guidelines include the following:

1. Plyometric training should be specific to the individual goals of the athlete. Activity-specific movement patterns should be trained. These sport-specific skills should be broken down and trained in their smaller components and then rebuilt into a coordinated activity-specific movement pattern.
2. The quality of work is more important than the quantity of work. The intensity of the exercise should be kept at a maximal level.
3. The greater the exercise intensity level, the greater the recovery time.
4. Plyometric training can have its greatest benefit at the conclusion of the normal workout. This pattern will best replicate exercise under a partial to total fatigue environment that is specific to activity. Only low- to medium-stress plyometrics should be used at the conclusion of a workout, because of the increased potential of injury with high-stress drills.
5. When proper technique can no longer be demonstrated, maximum volume has been achieved and the exercise must be stopped. Training improperly or with fatigue can lead to injury.
6. The plyometric training program should be progressive in nature. The volume and intensity can be modified in several ways:
   a. Increase the number of exercises.
   b. Increase the number of repetitions and sets.
   c. Decrease the rest period between sets of exercise.

7. Plyometric training sessions should be conducted no more than three times weekly in the preseason phase of training. During this phase, volume should prevail. During the competitive season, the frequency of plyometric training should be reduced to twice weekly, with the intensity of the exercise becoming more important.

8. Dynamic testing of the individual on a regular basis will provide important progression and motivational feedback.

The key element in the execution of proper technique is the eccentric or landing phase. The shock of landing from a jump is not absorbed exclusively by the foot but rather is a combination of the ankle, knee, and hip joints all working together to absorb the shock of landing and then transferring the force.

INTEGRATING PLYOMETRICS INTO THE REHABILITATION PROGRAM: CLINICAL CONCERNS

When used judiciously, plyometrics are a valuable asset in the sports rehabilitation program. As previously stated, the majority of lower-quarter sport function occurs in the closed kinetic chain. Lower-extremity plyometrics are an effective functional closed-chain exercise that can be incorporated into the sports rehabilitation program. According to Davis's law, soft tissue responds to stress imparted upon it to become more resilient along these same lines of stress. As previously mentioned, through the eccentric prestretch, plyometrics place added stress on the tendinous portion of the contractile unit. Eccentric loading is beneficial in the management of tendinitis.[33] Through a gradually progressed eccentric loading program, healing tendinous tissue is stressed, yielding an increase in ultimate tensile strength. This eccentric load can be applied through jump-downs (Figure 10-4).

Clinical plyometrics can be categorized according to the loads applied to the healing tissue. These activities include (1) medial/lateral loading, (2) rotational loading, and (3) shock absorption/deceleration loading. In addition, plyometric drills will be divided into (1) in-place activities (activities that can be performed in essentially the same or small amount of space); (2) dynamic distance drills (activities that occur across a given distance; and (3) depth jumping (jumping down from a predetermined height and performing a variety of activities upon landing). Simple jumping drills (bilateral activities) can be progressed to hopping (unilateral activities).

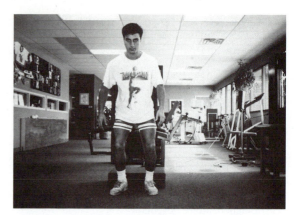

Figure 10-4   Jump-down exercises.

Medial-Lateral Loading

Virtually all sporting activities involve cutting maneuvers. Inherent to cutting activities is adequate function in the medial and lateral directions. A plyometric program designed to stress the athlete's ability to accept weight on the involved lower extremity and then perform cutting activities off that leg is imperative. Individuals who have suffered sprains to the medial or lateral capsular and ligamentous complex of the ankle and knee, as well as the hip abductor/adductor and ankle invertor/evertor muscle strains, are candidates for medial/lateral plyometric loading. Medial/lateral loading drills should be implemented following injury to the medial soft tissue around the knee after a valgus stress. By gradually imparting progressive valgus loads, tissue tensile strength is augmented.[36] In the rehabilitation setting, bilateral support drills can be progressed to unilateral valgus loading efforts. Specifically, lateral jumping drills are progressed to lateral hopping activities. However, the medial structures must also be trained to accept greater valgus loads sustained during cutting activities. As a prerequisite to full-speed cutting, lateral bounding drills should be performed (Figure 10-5). These efforts are progressed to activities that add acceleration, deceleration, and momentum. Lateral sliding activities that require the individual to cover a greater distance can be performed on a slide board. If a slide board is not available, the same movement pattern can be stressed with plyometrics (Figure 10-6).

IN-PLACE ACTIVITIES
Lateral bounding (quick step valgus loading)
Slide bounds

DYNAMIC DISTANCE DRILLS
Crossovers

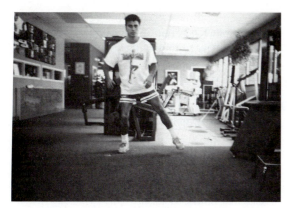

Figure 10-5 Lateral bounding drills.

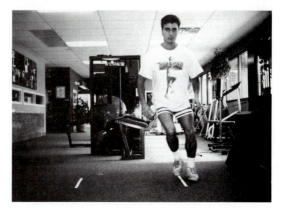

Figure 10-6 Lateral sliding activities.

Rotational Loading

Because rotation in the knee is controlled by the cruciate ligaments, menisci, and capsule, plyometric activities with a rotational component are instrumental in the rehabilitation program after injury to any of these structures. As previously discussed, care must be taken not to exceed healing time constraints when using plyometric training.

IN-PLACE ACTIVITIES
Spin jumps

DYNAMIC DISTANCE DRILLS
Lateral hopping

Shock Absorption (Deceleration Loading)

Perhaps some of the most physically demanding plyometric activities are shock absorption activities, which place a tremendous amount of stress upon muscle, tendon, and articular cartilage. Therefore, in the final preparation for a return to sports involving repetitive jumping and hopping, shock absorption drills should be included in the rehabilitation program.

One way to prepare the athlete for shock absorption drills is to gradually maximize the effects of gravity, such as beginning in a gravity-minimized position and progressing to performance against gravity. Popular activities to minimize gravity include water activities or assisted efforts through unloading.

IN-PLACE ACTIVITIES
Cycle jumps
Five-dot drill

DEPTH JUMPING PREPARATION
Jump downs

The activities listed above are a good starting point from which to develop a clinical plyometric program. Manipulations of volume, frequency, and intensity can advance the program appropriately. Proper progression is of prime importance when using plyometrics in the rehabilitation program. These progressive activities are reinjuries waiting to happen if the progression does not allow for adequate healing or development of an adequate strength base. A close working relationship fostering open communication and acute observation skills is vital in helping ensure that the program is not overly aggressive.

Summary

1. Although the effects of plyometric training are not yet fully understood, it still remains a widely used form of combining strength with speed training to functionally increase power. While the research is somewhat contradictory, the neurophysiological concept of plyometric training is on a sound foundation.

2. A successful plyometric training program should be carefully designed and implemented after establishing an adequate strength base.

3. The effects of this type of high-intensity training can be achieved safely if the individual is supervised by a knowledgeable person who uses common sense and follows the prescribed training regimen.

4. The plyometric training program should use a large variety of different exercises, because year-round training often results in boredom and a lack of motivation.
5. Program variety can be manipulated with different types of equipment or kinds of movement performed.
6. Continued motivation and an organized progression are the keys to successful training.
7. Plyometrics are also a valuable asset in the rehabilitation program after a sport injury.
8. Used after lower-quarter injury, plyometrics are effective in facilitating joint awareness, strengthening tissue during the healing process, and increasing sport-specific strength and power.
9. The most important considerations in the plyometric program are common sense and experience.

References

1. Adams, T. 1984. An investigation of selected plyometric training exercises on muscular leg strength and power. *Track and Field Quarterly Review* 84(1): 36–40.
2. Asmussen, E., and F. Bonde-Peterson. 1974. Storage of elastic energy in skeletal muscles in man. *Acta Physiol Scan* 91:385.
3. Bielik, E., D. Chu, F. Costello, et al. 1986. Roundtable: 1. Practical considerations for utilizing plyometrics. *National Strength and Conditioning Association Journal* 8:14.
4. Bosco, C., and P. V. Komi. 1979. Potentiation of the mechanical behavior of the human skeletal muscle through prestretching. *Acta Physio Scan* 106:467.
5. Bosco, C., and P. V. Komi. 1982. Muscle elasticity in athletes. In *Exercise and sports biology*, edited by P. V. Komi. Champaign, IL: Human Kinetics.
6. Bosco, C., J. Tarkka, and P. V. Komi. 1982. Effect of elastic energy and myoelectric potentiation of triceps surea during stretch-shortening cycle exercise. *International Journal of Sports Medicine* 2:137.
7. Bosco, C., J. Tihanyia, and P. V. Komi, et al. 1987. Store and recoil of elastic energy in slow and fast types of human skeletal muscles. *Acta Physio Scan* 116:343.
8. Cavagna, G. A., B. Dusman, and R. Margaria. 1968. Positive work done by a previously stretched muscle. *Journal of Applied Physiology* 24:21.
9. Cavagna, G., F. Saibene, and R. Margaria. 1965. Effect of negative work on the amount of positive work performed by an isolated muscle. *Journal of Applied Physiology* 20:157.
10. Chu, D. 1984. Plyometric exercise. *National Strength and Conditioning Association Journal* 6:56.
11. Chu, D. 1989. *Conditioning/plyometrics*. Paper presented at 10th Annual Sports Medicine Team Concept Conference, San Francisco, December.
12. Chu, D. 1992. *Jumping into plyometrics*. Champaign, IL: Leisure Press.
13. Chu, D. and L. Plummer. 1984. The language of plyometrics. *National Strength and Conditioning Association Journal* 6:30.
14. Curwin, S., and W. D. Stannish. 1984. *Tendinitis: Its etiology and treatment*. Lexington, MA: Collamore Press.
15. Dunsenev, C. I. 1979. Strength training for jumpers. *Soviet Sports Review* 14:2.
16. Dunsenev, C. I. 1982. Strength training of jumpers. *Track and Field Quarterly* 82:4.
17. Enoka, R. M. 1989. *Neuromechanical basis of kinesiology*. Champaign, IL: Human Kinetics.
18. Javorek, I. 1989. Plyometrics. *National Strength and Conditioning Association Journal* 11:52.
19. Jensen, C. 1975. Pertinent facts about warming. *Athletic Journal* 56:72.
20. Katchajov, S., K. Gomberaze, and A. Revson. 1976. Rebound jumps. *Modern Athlete and Coach* 14(4): 23.
21. Komi, P. V. 1984. Physiological and biomechanical correlates of muscle function: Effects of muscle structure and stretch-shortening cycle on force and speed. In *Exercise and sports sciences review*, edited by Terjung. Lexington, MA: Collamore Press.
22. Komi, P. V., and C. Bosco. 1978. Utilization of stored elastic energy in leg extensor muscles by men and women. *Medicine and Science in Sports and Exercise* 10(4): 261.
23. Komi, P. V., and E. Buskirk. 1972. Effects of eccentric and concentric muscle conditioning on tension and electrical activity of human muscle. *Ergonomics* 15:417.
24. Lundon, P. 1985. A review of plyometric training. *National Strength and Conditioning Association Journal* 7:69.
25. Rach, P. J., M. D. Grabiner, R. J. Gregor, et al. 1989. *Kinesiology and applied anatomy*. 7th ed., Philadelphia: Lea & Febiger.
26. Rowinski, M. 1988. *The role of eccentric exercise*. Biodex Corp, Pro Clinica.
27. Thomas, D. W. 1988. Plyometrics—More than the stretch reflex. *National Strength and Conditioning Association Journal* 10:49.
28. Verhoshanski, Y. 1969. Are depth jumps useful? *Yesis Review of Soviet Physical Education and Sport* 4:74–79.
29. Verkhoshanski, Y. 1969. Perspectives in the improvement of speed-strength preparation of jumpers. *Yesis Review of Soviet Physical Education and Sports* 28–29.
30. Verhoshanski, Y., and G. Chornonson. 1967. Jump exercises in sprint training. *Track and Field Quarterly* 9:1909.
31. Voight, M., and P. Draovitch. 1991. Plyometrics. In *Eccentric muscle training in sports and orthopedics*, edited by M. Albert. New York: Churchill Livingstone.

32. Voight, M., and D. Bradley. 1994. Plyometrics. In *A compendium of isokinetics in clinical usage and rehabilitation techniques* (4th ed), edited by G. J. Davies. Onalaska, WI: S & S.

33. Von Arx, F. 1984. Power development in the high jump. *Track Technique* 88:2818–19.

34. Wilk, K. E., M. L. Voight, M. A. Keirns, V. Gambetta, J. Andrews, and C. J. Dillman. 1993. Stretch-shortening drills for the upper extremities: Theory and clinical application. *Journal of Orthopaedic and Sports Physical Therapy* 17:225–39.

35. Wilt, F. 1975. Plyometrics—What it is and how it works. *Athletic Journal* 55b:76.

36. Woo, S. L., M. Inoue, E. McGurk-Burleson, et al. 1987. Treatment of the medial collateral ligament injury: Structure and function of canine knees in response to differing treatment regimens. *American Journal of Sports Medicine* 15(1): 22–29.

CHAPTER 11

Open- versus Closed-Kinetic-Chain Exercise

William E. Prentice

After completion of this chapter, the student should be able to do the following:

- Differentiate between the concepts of an open kinetic chain and a closed kinetic chain.

- Discuss the advantages and disadvantages of using open- versus closed-kinetic-chain exercise.

- Discuss how closed-kinetic-chain exercises can be used to regain neuromuscular control.

- Describe the biomechanics of closed-kinetic-chain exercise in the lower extremity.

- Discuss how both open- and closed-kinetic-chain exercises should be used in rehabilitation of the lower extremity.

- Identify the various closed-kinetic-chain exercises for the lower extremity.

- Describe the biomechanics of closed-kinetic-chain exercise in the upper extremity.

- Explain how closed-kinetic-chain exercises are used in rehabilitation of the upper extremity.

- Describe the various types of closed-kinetic-chain exercises for the upper extremity.

In recent years the concept of **closed-kinetic-chain exercise** has received considerable attention as a useful and effective technique of rehabilitation, particularly for injuries involving the lower extremity.[45] The ankle, knee, and hip joints constitute the kinetic chain for the lower extremity. When the distal segment of the lower extremity is stabilized or fixed, as is the case when the foot is weight-bearing on the ground, the kinetic chain is said to be closed. Conversely, in an **open kinetic chain**, the distal segment is mobile and is not fixed. Traditionally, rehabilitation strengthening protocols have used open-kinetic-chain exercises such as knee flexion and extension on a knee machine.

Closed-kinetic-chain exercises are used more often in rehabilitation of injuries to the lower extremity, but they are also useful in rehabilitation protocols for certain

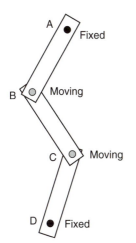

Figure 11-1   If both ends of a link system are fixed, movement at one joint produces predictable movement at all other joints.

upper-extremity activities. For the most part the upper extremity functions in an open kinetic chain with the hand moving freely, as in throwing a baseball. But there are a number of activities in which the upper extremity functions in a closed kinetic chain, as in performing a handstand in gymnastics or assuming a down position in wrestling.

Despite the recent popularity of closed-kinetic-chain exercises, it must be stressed that both open- and closed-kinetic-chain exercises have their place in the rehabilitative process. This chapter will attempt to clarify the role of both open- and closed-kinetic-chain exercises in that process.

THE CONCEPT OF THE KINETIC CHAIN

The concept of the kinetic chain was first proposed in the 1970s and was initially referred to as the *link system* by mechanical engineers.[38] In this link system, pin joints connect a series of overlapping, rigid segments (Figure 11-1). If both ends of this system are connected to an immovable frame, there is no movement of either the proximal or the distal end. In this closed link system, each moving body segment receives forces from and transfers forces to adjacent body segments and thus either affects or is affected by the motion of those components.[17] In a closed link system, movement at one joint produces predictable movement at all other joints.[38] In reality, this type of closed link system does not exist in either the

upper or the lower extremity. However, when the distal segment in an extremity (that is, the foot or hand) meets resistance or is fixed, muscle recruitment patterns and joint movements are different than when the distal segment moves freely.[38] Thus, two systems—a closed system and an open system—have been proposed.

Whenever the foot or the hand meets resistance or is fixed, as is the case in a closed kinetic chain, movement of the more proximal segments occurs in a predictable pattern. If the foot or hand moves freely in space as in an open kinetic chain, movements occurring in other segments within the chain are not necessarily predictable.[6]

To a large extent the term *closed-kinetic-chain exercise* has come to mean "weight-bearing exercise." However, although all weight-bearing exercises involve some elements of closed-kinetic-chain activities, not all closed-kinetic-chain activities are weight-bearing.[37]

Muscle Actions in the Kinetic Chain

Muscle actions that occur during open-kinetic-chain activities are usually reversed during closed-kinetic-chain activities. In open-kinetic-chain exercise, the origin is fixed and muscle contraction produces movement at the insertion. In closed-kinetic-chain exercise, the insertion is fixed and the muscle acts to move the origin. Although this may be important biomechanically, physiologically the muscle can lengthen, shorten, or remain the same length, and thus it makes little difference whether the origin or insertion is moving in terms of the way the muscle contracts.

The Concurrent Shift in a Kinetic Chain

The concept of the **concurrent shift** applies to biarticular muscles that have distinctive muscle actions within the kinetic chain during weight-bearing activities. For example, the rectus femoris shortens as the knee flexes and lengthens as the hip extends. Thus the muscle length changes very little even though significant motion is occurring at both the hip and the knee. Also, the rectus femoris is exhibiting distinct muscle actions involving simultaneous eccentric contraction at the hip and concentric contraction at the knee. This concurrent shift occurs only during closed-kinetic-chain exercises.

The concepts of the reversibility of muscle actions and the concurrent shift are hallmarks of closed-kinetic-chain exercises.[37]

ADVANTAGES AND DISADVANTAGES OF OPEN- VERSUS CLOSED-KINETIC-CHAIN EXERCISES

Open- and closed-kinetic-chain exercises offer distinct advantages and disadvantages in the rehabilitation process. The choice to use one or the other depends on the desired treatment goal. Characteristics of closed-kinetic-chain exercises include increased joint compressive forces; increased joint congruency and thus stability; decreased shear forces; decreased acceleration forces; large resistance forces; stimulation of proprioceptors; and enhanced dynamic stability—all of which are associated with weight bearing. Characteristics of open-kinetic-chain exercises include increased acceleration forces; decreased resistance forces; increased distraction and rotational forces; increased deformation of joint and muscle mechanoreceptors; concentric acceleration and eccentric deceleration forces; and promotion of functional activity. These are typical of non-weight-bearing activities.[25]

From a biomechanical perspective, it has been suggested that closed-kinetic-chain exercises are safer and produce stresses and forces that are potentially less of a threat to healing structures than open-kinetic-chain exercises.[35] Coactivation or **co-contraction** of agonist and antagonist muscles must occur during normal movements to provide joint stabilization. Co-contraction, which occurs during closed-kinetic-chain exercise, decreases the shear forces acting on the joint, thus protecting healing soft tissue structures that might otherwise be damaged by open chain exercises.[17] Additionally, weight-bearing activity increases joint compressive forces, further enhancing joint stability.

It has also been suggested that closed-kinetic-chain exercises, particularly those involving the lower extremity, tend to be more functional than open-kinetic-chain exercises because they involve weight-bearing activities.[44] The majority of activities performed in daily living, such as walking, climbing, and rising to a standing position, as well as in most sport activities, involve a closed-kinetic-chain system. Because the foot is usually in contact with the ground, activities that make use of this closed system are said to be more functional. With the exception of a kicking movement, there is no question that closed-kinetic-chain exercises are more sport- or activity-specific, involving exercise that more closely approximates the desired activity. In a sports medicine setting, specificity of training must be emphasized to maximize carryover to functional activities on the playing field.[37]

With open-kinetic-chain exercises, motion is usually isolated to a single joint. Open-kinetic-chain activities may include exercises to improve strength or range of motion.[19] They may be applied to a single joint manually, as in proprioceptive neuromuscular facilitation or joint mobilization techniques, or through some external resistance using an exercise machine. Isolation-type exercises typically use a contraction of a specific muscle or group of muscles that produces usually single-plane and occasionally multiplanar movement. Isokinetic exercise and testing is usually done in an open kinetic chain and can provide important information relative to the torque production capability of that isolated joint.

When there is some dysfunction associated with injury, the predictable pattern of movement that occurs during closed-kinetic-chain activity might not be possible due to pain, swelling, muscle weakness, or limited range of motion. Thus, movement compensations result that interfere with normal motion and muscle activity. If only closed-kinetic-chain exercise is used, the joints proximal or distal to the injury might not show an existing deficit. Without using open-kinetic-chain exercises that isolate specific joint movements, the deficit might go uncorrected, thus interfering with total rehabilitation.[11] The sports therapist should use the most appropriate open- or closed-kinetic-chain exercise for the given situation.

Closed-kinetic-chain exercises use varying combinations of isometric, concentric, and eccentric contractions that must occur simultaneously in different muscle groups, creating multiplanar motion at each of the joints within the kinetic chain. Closed-kinetic-chain activities require synchronicity of more complex agonist and antagonist muscle actions.[15]

USING CLOSED-KINETIC-CHAIN EXERCISES TO REGAIN NEUROMUSCULAR CONTROL

In Chapter 6 it was stressed that proprioception, joint position sense, and kinesthesia are critical to the neuromuscular control of body segments within the kinetic chain. To perform a motor skill, muscular forces, occurring at the correct moment and magnitude, interact to move body parts in a coordinated manner.[31] Coordinated movement is controlled by the central nervous system that integrates input from joint and muscle mechanoreceptors acting within the kinetic chain. Smooth coordinated movement requires constant integration of receptor, feedback, and control center information.[31]

In the lower extremity, a functional weight-bearing activity requires muscles and joints to work in synchrony and in synergy with one another. For example, taking a single step requires concentric, eccentric, and isometric muscle contractions to produce supination and pronation in the foot; ankle dorsiflexion and plantarflexion; knee flexion, extension, and rotation; and hip flexion, extension, and rotation. Lack of normal motion secondary to injury in one joint will affect the way another joint or segment moves.[31]

To perform this single step in a coordinated manner, all of the joints and muscles must work together. Thus, exercises that act to integrate, rather than isolate, all of these functioning elements would seem to be the most appropriate. Closed-kinetic-chain exercises that recruit foot, ankle, knee, and hip muscles in a manner that reproduces normal loading and movement forces in all of the joints within the kinetic chain, are similar to functional mechanics and would appear to be most useful.[31]

Quite often, open-kinetic-chain exercises are used primarily to develop muscular strength while little attention is given to the importance of including exercises that reestablish proprioception and joint position sense.[1] Closed-kinetic-chain activities facilitate the integration of proprioceptive feedback coming from Pacinian corpuscles, Ruffini endings, Golgi-Mazzoni corpuscles, Golgi-tendon organs, and Golgi-ligament endings through the functional use of multijoint and multiplanar movements.[6]

BIOMECHANICS OF OPEN- VERSUS CLOSED-KINETIC-CHAIN ACTIVITIES IN THE LOWER EXTREMITY

Open- and closed-kinetic-chain exercises have different biomechanical effects on the joints of the lower extremity. Walking and running, along with the ability to change direction, require coordinated joint motion and a complex series of well-timed muscle activations. Biomechanically, shock absorption, foot flexibility, foot stabilization, acceleration and deceleration, multiplanar motion, and joint stabilization must occur in each of the joints in the lower extremity for normal function.[31] Some understanding of how these biomechanical events occur during both open- and closed-kinetic-chain activities is essential for the sports therapist.

The Foot and Ankle

The foot's function in the support phase of weight bearing during gait is twofold. At heel strike, the foot must act as a shock absorber to the impact or ground reaction forces and then adapt to the uneven surfaces. Subsequently, at push-off, the foot functions as a rigid lever to transmit the explosive force from the lower extremity to the ground.[42]

As the foot becomes weight-bearing at heel strike, creating a closed kinetic chain, the subtalar joint moves into a pronated position in which the talus adducts and the plantar flexes while the calcaneous everts. Pronation of the foot unlocks the midtarsal joint and allows the foot to assist in shock absorption. It is important during initial impact to reduce the ground reaction forces and to distribute the load evenly on many different anatomical structures throughout the lower-extremity kinetic chain. As pronation occurs at the subtalar joint, there is obligatory internal rotation of the tibia and slight flexion at the knee. The dorsiflexors contract eccentrically to decelerate plantar flexion. In an open kinetic chain, when the foot pronates, the talus is stationary while the foot everts, abducts, and dorsiflexes. The muscles that evert the foot appear to be most active.[42]

The foot changes its function from being a shock absorber to being a rigid lever system as the foot begins to push off the ground. In weight bearing in a closed kinetic chain, supination consists of the talus abducting and dorsiflexing on the calcaneus while the calcaneus inverts on the talus. The tibia externally rotates and produces knee extension. During supination the plantar flexors stabilize the foot, decelerate the tibia, and flex the knee. In an open kinetic chain, supination consists of the calcaneus inverting as the talus adducts and plantarflexes. The foot moves into adduction, plantarflexion, around the stabilized talus.[42]

The Knee Joint

It is essential for the sports therapist to understand forces that occur around the knee joint. Palmitier et al. have proposed a biomechanical model of the lower extremity that quantifies two critical forces at the knee joint[30] (Figure 11-2). A **shear force** occurs in a posterior direction that would cause the tibia to translate anteriorly if not checked by soft tissue constraints (primarily the anterior cruciate ligament).[7] The second force is a **compressive force** directed along a longitudinal axis of the tibia. Weight-bearing exercises increase joint compression, which enhances joint stability.

In an open-kinetic-chain seated knee joint exercise, as a resistive force is applied to the distal tibia, the shear and compressive forces would be maximized (Figure 11-3A). When a resistive force is applied more proximally, shear force is significantly reduced, as is the compressive force (Figure 11-3B). If the resistive force is applied in a more axial direction, the shear force is also smaller (Figure 11-3C). If a hamstring co-contraction occurs, the shear force is minimized (Figure 11-3D).

Closed-kinetic-chain exercises induce hamstring contraction by creating a flexion moment at both the hip and

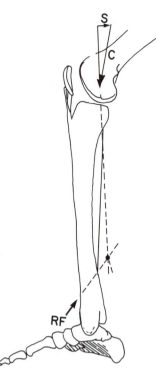

Figure 11-2 Mathematical model showing shear and compressive force vectors. S = shear, C = compressive.

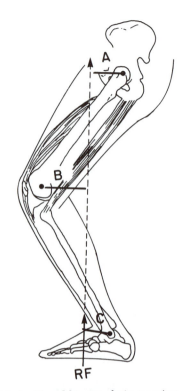

Figure 11-4 Closed-kinetic-chain exercises induce hamstring contraction by creating a flexion moment at **A,** hip; **B,** knee; and **C,** ankle.

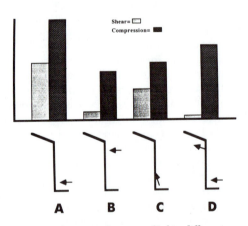

Figure 11-3 Resistive forces applied in different positions alter the magnitude of the shear and compressive forces. **A,** Resistive force applied distally. **B,** Resistive force applied proximally. **C,** Resistive force applied axially. **D,** Resistive force applied distally with hamstring co-contraction.

the knee, with the contracting hamstrings stabilizing the hip and the quadriceps stabilizing the knee. A **moment** is the product of force and distance from the axis of rotation. Also referred to as torque, it describes the turning effect produced when a force is exerted on the body that is pivoted about some fixed point (Figure 11-4). Co-contraction of the hamstring muscles helps to counteract the tendency of the quadriceps to cause anterior tibial translation. Co-contraction of the hamstrings is most efficient in reducing shear force when the resistive force is directed in an axial orientation relative to the tibia, as is the case in a weight-bearing exercise.[30] Several studies have shown that co-contraction is useful in stabilizing the knee joint and decreasing shear forces.[22,32,36]

The tension in the hamstrings can be further enhanced with slight anterior flexion of the trunk. Trunk flexion moves the center of gravity anteriorly, decreasing the knee flexion moment and thus reducing knee shear force and decreasing patellofemoral compression forces.[29] Closed-kinetic-chain exercises try to minimize the flexion moment at the knee while increasing the flexion moment at the hip.

A flexion moment is also created at the ankle when the resistive force is applied to the bottom of the foot. The soleus stabilizes ankle flexion and creates a knee extension moment, which again helps to neutralize anterior shear force (see Figure 11-4). Thus the entire lower-extremity kinetic chain is recruited by applying an axial force at the distal segment.

In an open-kinetic-chain exercise involving seated leg extensions, the resistive force is applied to the distal tibia, creating a flexion moment at the knee only. This negates the effects of a hamstring co-contraction and thus produces maximal shear force at the knee joint. Shear forces created by isometric open-kinetic-chain knee flexion and extension at 30 and 60 degrees of knee flexion are greater than with closed-kinetic-chain exercises.[26] Decreased anterior tibial displacement during isometric closed-kinetic-chain knee flexion at 30 degrees when measured by knee arthrometry has also been demonstrated.[43]

The Patellofemoral Joint. The effects of open- versus closed-kinetic-chain exercises on the patellofemoral joint must also be considered. In open-kinetic-chain knee extension exercise, the flexion moment increases as the knee extends from 90 degrees of flexion to full extension, increasing tension in the quadriceps and patellar tendon. Thus the patellofemoral joint reaction forces are increased, with peak force occurring at 36 degrees of joint flexion.[13] As the knee moves toward full extension, the patellofemoral contact area decreases, causing increased contact stress per unit area.[3,20]

In closed-kinetic-chain exercise, the flexion moment increases as the knee flexes, once again causing increased quadriceps and patellar tendon tension and thus an increase in patellofemoral joint reaction forces. However, the patella has a much larger surface contact area with the femur, and contact stress is minimized.[3,13,20] Closed-kinetic-chain exercises might be better tolerated in the patellofemoral joint, because contact stress is minimized.

CLOSED-KINETIC-CHAIN EXERCISES FOR REHABILITATION OF LOWER-EXTREMITY INJURIES

For many years, sports therapists have made use of open-kinetic-chain exercises for lower-extremity strengthening. This practice has been partly due to design constraints of existing resistive exercise machines. However, the current popularity of closed-kinetic-chain exercises can be attributed primarily to a better understanding of the kinesiology and biomechanics, along with the neuro-muscular control factors, involved in rehabilitation of lower-extremity injuries.

For example, the course of rehabilitation after injury to the anterior cruciate ligament (ACL) has changed drastically in recent years. (Specific rehabilitation protocols will be discussed in detail in Chapter 23.) Technological advances have created significant improvement in surgical techniques, and this has allowed sports therapists to change their philosophy of rehabilitation. The current literature provides a great deal of support for accelerated rehabilitation programs that recommend the extensive use of closed-kinetic-chain exercises.[4,8,12,13,27,35,41,47]

Because of the biomechanical and functional advantages of closed-kinetic-chain exercises described earlier, these activities are perhaps best suited to rehabilitation of the ACL. The majority of these studies also indicate that closed-kinetic-chain exercises can be safely incorporated into the rehabilitation protocols very early. Some sports therapists recommend beginning within the first few days after surgery.

SPECIFIC CLOSED-KINETIC-CHAIN STRENGTHENING EXERCISES FOR THE LOWER EXTREMITY

In the sports medicine setting, several different closed-kinetic-chain exercises have gained popularity and have been incorporated into rehabilitation protocols.[23] Among those exercises commonly used are the mini-squat, wall slides, lunges, leg press, stair-climbing machines, lateral step-up, terminal knee extension using tubing, and stationary bicycling, slide boards, BAPS boards, and the Fitter.

Minisquats, Wall Slides, and Lunges

The minisquat (Figure 11-5) or wall slide (Figure 11-6) involves simultaneous hip and knee extension and is performed in a 0 to 40 degree range.[47] As the hip extends, the rectus femoris contracts eccentrically while the hamstrings contract concentrically. Concurrently, as the knee extends, the hamstrings contract eccentrically while the rectus femoris contracts concentrically. Both concentric and eccentric contractions occur simultaneously at either end of both muscles, producing a concurrent shift contraction. This type of contraction is necessary during weight-bearing activities. It will be elicited with all closed-kinetic-chain exercises and is impossible with isolation exercises.[38]

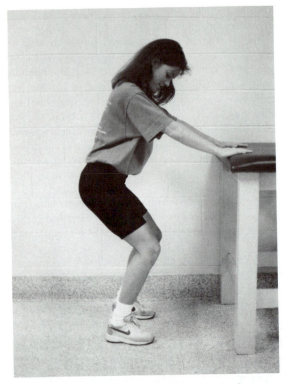

Figure 11-5 Minisquat performed in 0 to 40 degree range.

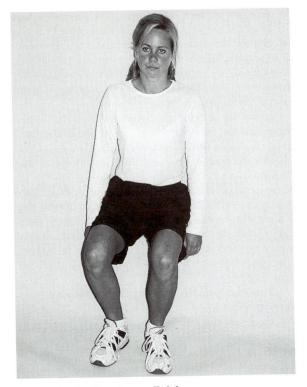

Figure 11-6 Standing wall slide.

These concurrent shift contractions minimize the flexion moment at the knee. The eccentric contraction of the hamstrings helps to neutralize the effects of a concentric quadriceps contraction in producing anterior translation of the tibia. Henning et al. found that the half squat produced significantly less anterior shear at the knee than did an open-chain exercise in full extension.[18] A full squat markedly increases the flexion moment at the knee and thus increases anterior shear of the tibia. As mentioned previously, slightly flexing the trunk anteriorly will also increase the hip flexion moment and decrease the knee moment.

Lunges should be used later in a rehabilitation program to facilitate eccentric strengthening of the quadriceps to act as a decelerator[46] (Figure 11-7). Like the minisquat and wall slide, it facilitates cocontraction of the hamstring muscles.

Leg Press

Theoretically the leg press takes full advantage of the kinetic chain and at the same time provides stability, which decreases strain on the low back.[24] It also allows exercise with resistance lower than body weight and the capabil-

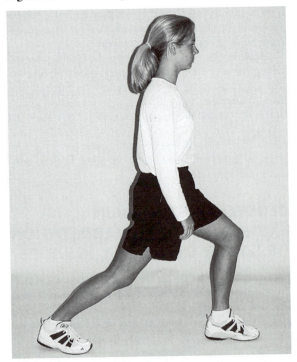

Figure 11-7 Lunges are done to strengthen quadriceps eccentrically.

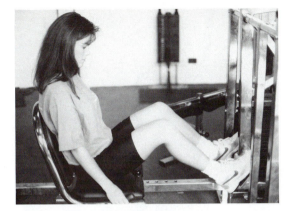

Figure 11-8 Leg-press exercise.

ity of exercising each leg independently[30] (Figure 11-8). It has been recommended that leg-press exercises be performed in a 0 to 60 degree range of knee flexion.[47]

It has also been recommended that leg-press machines allow full hip extension to take maximum advantage of the kinetic chain. Full hip extension can only be achieved in a supine position. In this position, full hip and knee flexion and extension can occur, thus reproducing the concurrent shift and ensuring appropriate hamstring recruitment.[30]

The foot plates should also be designed to move in an arc of motion rather than in a straight line. This movement would facilitate hamstring recruitment by increasing the hip flexion moment and decreasing the knee moment. Foot plates should be fixed perpendicular to the frontal plane of the hip to maximize the knee extension moment created by the soleus.

Stair Climbing

Stair-climbing machines have gained a great deal of popularity, not only as a closed-kinetic-chain exercise device useful in rehabilitation, but also as a means of improving cardiorespiratory endurance (Figure 11-9). Stair-climbing machines have two basic designs. One involves a series of rotating steps similar to a department store escalator; the other uses two foot plates that move up and down to simulate a stepping-type movement. With the latter type of stair climber, also sometimes referred to as a stepping machine, the foot never leaves the foot plate, making it a true closed-kinetic-chain exercise device.

Stair climbing involves many of the same biomechanical principles identified with the leg-press exercise. When exercising on the stair climber, the body should be held erect with only slight trunk flexion, thus maximizing hamstring recruitment through concurrent shift contrac-

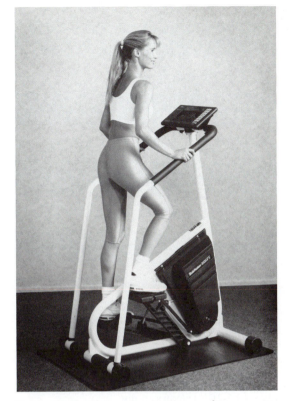

Figure 11-9 Stairmaster stepping machine.

tions while increasing the hip flexion moment and decreasing the knee flexion moment.

Exercise on a stepping machine produces increased electromyogram (EMG) activity in the gastrocnemius. Because the gastrocnemius attaches to the posterior aspect of the femoral condyles, increased activity of this muscle could produce a flexion moment of the femur on the tibia. This motion would cause posterior translation of the femur on the tibia, increasing strain on the ACL. Peak firing of the quadriceps might offset the effects of increased EMG activity in the gastrocnemius.[10]

Lateral Step-Ups

Lateral step-ups are another widely used closed-kinetic-chain exercise (Figure 11-10). Lateral step-ups seem to be used more often clinically than forward step-ups. Step height can be adjusted to patient capabilities and generally progresses up to about 8 inches. Heights greater than 8 inches create a large flexion moment at the knee, increasing anterior shear force and making hamstring co-contraction more difficult.[5,10]

Lateral step-ups elicit significantly greater mean quadriceps EMG activity than a stepping machine. When

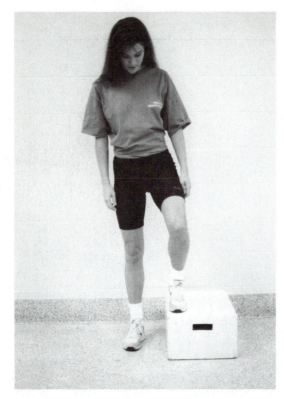

Figure 11-10 Lateral step-ups.

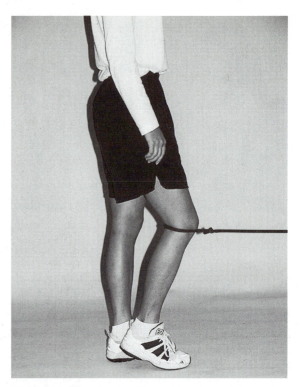

Figure 11-11 Terminal knee extensions using surgical tubing resistance.

performing a step-up, the entire body weight must be raised and lowered, while on the stepping machine the center of gravity is maintained at a relatively constant height. The lateral step-up can produce increased muscle and joint shear forces compared to stepping exercise.[10] Caution should be exercised by the sports therapist in using the lateral step-up in cases where minimizing anterior shear forces is essential. Contraction of the hamstrings appears to be of insufficient magnitude to neutralize the shear force produced by the quadriceps.[5] In situations where strengthening of the quadriceps is the goal, the lateral step-up has been recommended as a beneficial exercise. However, lateral stepping exercises have failed to increase isokinetic strength of the quadriceps muscle.

Terminal Knee Extensions Using Surgical Tubing

It has been reported in numerous studies that the greatest amount of anterior tibial translation occurs between 0 and 30 degrees of flexion during open-kinetic-chain exercise.[14,16,21,28,32,33,47] Avoiding terminal knee extension after surgery became a well-accepted rule among sports

therapists. Unfortunately, this practice led to quadriceps weakness, flexion contracture, and patellofemoral pain.[34]

Closed-kinetic-chain terminal knee extensions using surgical tubing resistance have created a means of safely strengthening terminal knee extension (Figure 11-11). Application of resistance anteriorly at the femur produces anterior shear of the femur, which eliminates any anterior translation of the tibia. This type of exercise performed in the 0 to 30 degree range also minimizes the knee flexion moment, further reducing anterior shear of the tibia. The use of rubber tubing produces an eccentric contraction of the quadriceps when moving into knee flexion.

Stationary Bicycling

The stationary bicycle has been routinely used in sports medicine, primarily for conditioning purposes when the injured athlete cannot engage in running activities (Figure 11-12). However, it also can be of significant value as a closed-kinetic-chain exercise device.

The advantage of stationary bicycling over other closed-kinetic-chain exercises for rehabilitation is that the amount of the weight-bearing force exerted by the in-

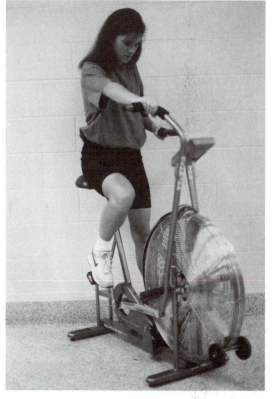

Figure 11-12 Stationary bicycle.

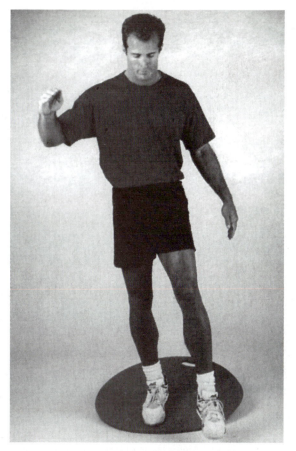

Figure 11-13 BAPS board exercise.

jured lower extremity can be adapted within patient limitations. The seat height should be carefully adjusted to minimize the knee flexion moment on the downstroke. However, if the stationary bike is being used to regain range of motion in flexion, the seat height should be adjusted to a lowered position using passive motion of the injured extremity. Toe clips will facilitate hamstring contractions on the upstroke.

BAPS Board and Minitramp

The BAPS board (Figure 11-13) and minitramp (Figure 11-14) both provide an unstable base of support that helps to facilitate reestablishing proprioception and joint position sense in addition to strengthening. Working on the BAPS board allows the sports therapist to provide stress to the lower extremity in a progressive and controlled manner.[6] It allows the athlete to work simultaneously on strengthening and range of motion, while trying to regain neuromuscular control and balance. The minitramp may be used to accomplish the same goals, but it can also be used for more advanced plyometric training.

Slide Boards and Fitter

Shifting the body weight from side to side during a more functional activity on either a slide board (Figure 11-15) or a Fitter (Figure 11-16) helps to reestablish dynamic control as well improving cardiorespiratory fitness.[6] These motions produce valgus and varus stresses and strains to the joint that are somewhat unique to these two pieces of equipment.

BIOMECHANICS OF OPEN- VERSUS CLOSED-KINETIC-CHAIN ACTIVITIES IN THE UPPER EXTREMITY

Although it is true that closed-kinetic-chain exercises are most often used in rehabilitation of lower-extremity injuries, there are many injury situations where closed-kinetic-chain exercises should be incorporated into

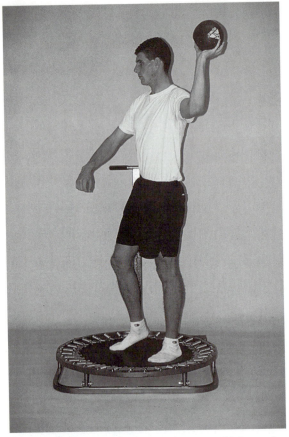

Figure 11-14 Minitramp provides a unstable base of support to which other functional plyometric activities may be added.

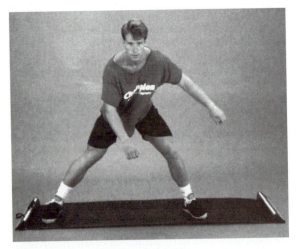

Figure 11-15 Slide board training.

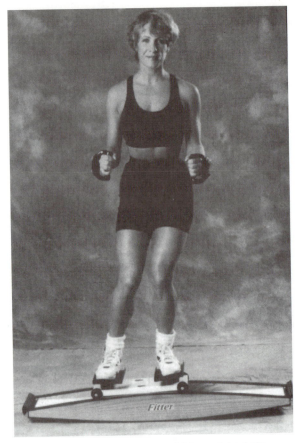

Figure 11-16 The Fitter is useful for weight shifting.

upper-extremity rehabilitation protocols. Unlike the lower extremity, the upper extremity is most functional as an open-kinetic-chain system. Most sport activities involve movement of the upper extremity in which the hand moves freely. These activities are generally dynamic movements, often occurring at high velocities, such as throwing a baseball, serving a tennis ball, or spiking a volleyball. In these movements, the proximal segments of the kinetic chain are used for stabilization while the distal segments have a high degree of mobility. Push-ups, chinning exercises, and handstands in gymnastics are all examples of closed-kinetic-chain activities in the upper extremity. In these cases, the hand is stabilized, and muscular contractions around the more proximal segments, the elbow and shoulder, function to raise and lower the body. Still other activities such as swimming and cross-country skiing involve rapid successions of alternating open- and closed-kinetic-chain movements, much in the same way as running does in the lower extremity.[48]

For the most part in rehabilitation, closed-kinetic-chain exercises are used primarily for strengthening and establishing neuromuscular control of those muscles that act to stabilize the shoulder girdle. In particular, the scapular stabilizers and the rotator cuff muscles function at one time or another to control movements about the shoulder. It is essential to develop both strength and neuromuscular control in these muscle groups, thus allowing them to provide a stable base for more mobile and dynamic movements that occur in the distal segments.

The Shoulder Complex Joint

Closed-kinetic-chain weight-bearing activities can be used to both promote and enhance dynamic joint stability. Most often closed-kinetic-chain exercises are used with the hand fixed and thus with no motion occurring. The resistance is then applied either axially or rotationally. These exercises produce both joint compression and approximation, which act to enhance muscular co-contraction about the joint producing dynamic stability.[48]

Two essential force couples must be reestablished around the glenohumeral joint; the anterior deltoid along with the infraspinatus and teres minor in the frontal plane, and the subscapularis counterbalanced by the infraspinatus and teres minor in the transverse plane. These opposing muscles act to stabilize the glenohumeral joint by compressing the humeral head within the glenoid via muscular co-contraction.

The scapular muscles function to dynamically position the glenoid relative to the position of the moving humerus, resulting in a normal scapulohumeral rhythm of movement. However, they must also provide a stable base on which the highly mobile humerus can function. If the scapula is hypermobile, the function of the entire upper extremity will be impaired. Thus force couples between the inferior trapezius counterbalanced by the upper trapezius and levator scapula—and the rhomboids and middle trapezius counterbalanced by the serratus anterior—are critical in maintaining scapular stability. Again, closed-kinetic-chain activities done with the hand fixed should be used to enhance scapular stability.

The Elbow

The elbow is a hinged joint that is capable of 145 degrees of flexion from a fully extended position. In some cases of joint hyperelasticity, the joint can hyperextend a few degrees beyond neutral. The elbow consists of the humeroulnar, humeroradial, and radioulnar articulations. The concave radial head articulates with the convex surface of the capitellum of the distal humerus and is connected to the proximal ulna via the annular ligament. The proximal radioulnar joint constitutes the forearm, which when working in conjunction with the elbow joint permits approximately 90 degrees of pronation and 80 degrees of supination.

In athletic activity, the elbow must perform several functions in an open kinetic chain. In throwing sports, the elbow helps to propel an object at a rapid velocity with accuracy. In power sports, such as hitting, the elbow must possess static stability and adequate dynamic strength to be able to transfer force to a hitting implement. In swimming, the elbow must be able to produce power and stability to propel the swimmer through the water. In gymnastics or wrestling, the elbow functions in a closed kinetic chain in both static and dynamic modes to provide stability and propulsive power.

OPEN- AND CLOSED-KINETIC-CHAIN EXERCISES FOR REHABILITATION OF UPPER-EXTREMITY INJURIES

Most typically, closed-kinetic-chain glenohumeral joint exercises are used during the early phases of a rehabilitation program, particularly in the case of an unstable shoulder to promote co-contraction and muscle recruitment, in addition to preventing shutdown of the rotator cuff secondary to pain and/or inflammation.[2] Likewise, closed-kinetic-chain exercise should be used during the late phases of a rehabilitation program to promote muscular endurance of muscles surrounding the glenohumeral and scapulothoracic joints. They may also be used during the later stages of rehabilitation in conjunction with open-kinetic-chain activities to enhance some degree of stability, on which highly dynamic and ballistic motions may be superimposed. At some point during the middle stages of the rehabilitation program, traditional open-kinetic-chain strengthening exercises for the rotator cuff, deltoid, and other glenohumeral and scapular muscles must be incorporated.[19,48]

In the elbow, exercises should also be designed to enhance muscular balance and neuromuscular control of the surrounding agonists and antagonists. Closed-kinetic-chain exercise should be used to improve dynamic stability of the more proximal muscles surrounding the elbow in those sports where the elbow must provide some degree of proximal stability, such as in the case of a football lineman blocking. Open-kinetic-chain exercises for strengthening flexion, extension, pronation, and supination are essential to regain high-velocity dynamic movements of the elbow that are necessary in throwing-type activities.

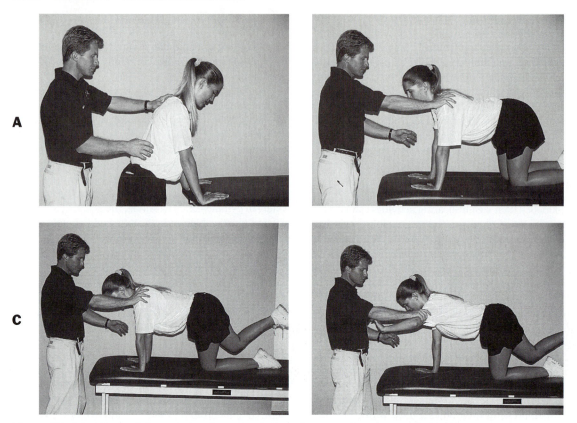

Figure 11-17 Weight shifting. **A**, Standing. **B**, Quadruped. **C**, Tripod. **D**, Opposite knee and arm.

Weight Shifting

A variety of weight-shifting exercises can be done to assist in facilitating glenohumeral and scapulothoracic dynamic stability through the use of axial compression.[9] Weight shifting can be done in standing, quadruped, tripod, or biped (opposite leg and arm), with weight supported on a stable surface such as the wall or a treatment table (Figure 11-17A–D), or on a movable, unstable surface such as a BAPS board, a wobble board, the KAT system, or a plyoball (Figure 11-18A–D). Shifting may be done side to side, forward and backward, or on a diagonal. Hand position may be adjusted from a wide base of support to one hand placed on top of the other to increase difficulty. The athlete can adjust the amount of weight being supported as tolerated. The sports therapist can provide manual force or resistance in a random manner to which the athlete must rhythmically stabilize and adapt. A D2 PNF pattern may be used in a tripod to force the contralateral support limb to produce a co-contraction and thus stabilization (Figure 11-19).[48] Rhythmic stabilization can also be used regain neuromuscular control of the scapular muscles with the hand in a closed kinetic chain and random pressure applied to the scapular borders (Figure 11-20).

Push-Ups, Push-Ups with a Plus, Press-Ups, Step-Ups

Push-ups and/or press-ups are also done to reestablish neuromuscular control. Push-ups done on an unstable surface such as on a plyoball require a good deal of strength in addition to providing an axial load that requires co-contraction of agonist and antagonist force couples around the glenohumeral and scapulothoracic joints while the distal part of the extremity has some limited movement (Figure 11-21). A variation of a standard push-up would be to have the athlete use reciprocating

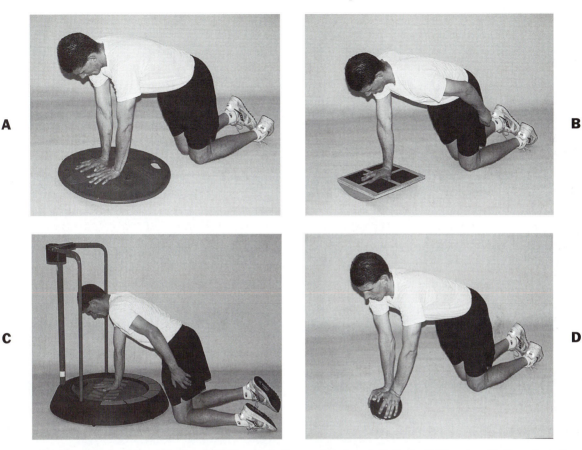

Figure 11-18   Weight shifting. **A,** On a BAPS board. **B,** On a wobble board. **C,** On the KAT system. **D,** On a plyoball.

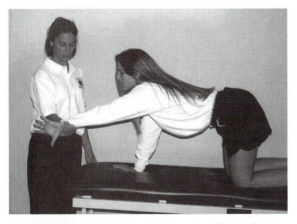

Figure 11-19   D2 PNF pattern in a tripod to produce stabilization in the contralateral support limb.

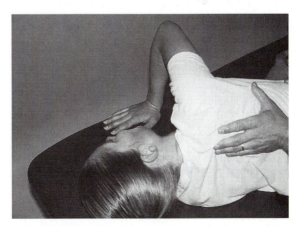

Figure 11-20   Rhythmic stabilization for the scapular muscles.

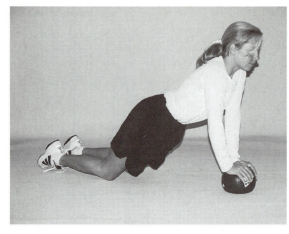

Figure 11-21   Push-ups done on a plyoball.

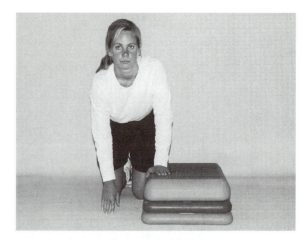

Figure 11-23   Single-arm lateral step-ups.

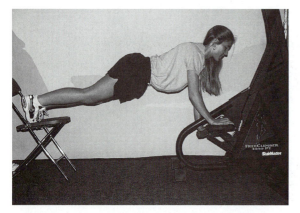

Figure 11-22   Push-ups done on a stair climber.

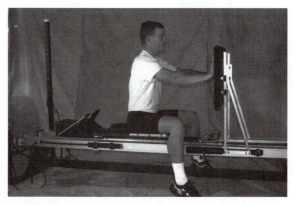

Figure 11-24   Push-ups can be done in a variety of positions on a Shuttle 2000.

contractions on a stair climber (Figure 11-22) or doing single-arm lateral step-ups onto a step (Figure 11-23). Also, the athlete may perform push-ups in a variety of positions, including to overhead position on the Shuttle 2000.[40] (Figure 11-24). Push-ups with a plus are done to strengthen the serratus anterior, which is critical for scapular dynamic stability in overhead activities (Figure 11-25). Press-ups involve an isometric contraction of the glenohumeral stabilizers (Figure 11-26).

Slide Board

Upper-extremity closed-kinetic-chain exercises performed on a slide board are useful not only for promoting strength and stability but also for improving muscular endurance.[40,48] In a kneeling position, the athlete uses a reciprocating motion, sliding the hands forward and backward, side to side, in a "wax on–wax off" circular pattern, or both hands laterally (Figure 11-27). It is also possible to do wall slides in a standing position.

Isokinetic Closed-Kinetic-Chain Exercise

Biodex manufactures an attachment for existing equipment that will allow for isokinetic conditioning and testing of the lower extremity in a closed-kinetic-chain seated position (Figure 11-28). Data on reliability, validity, and effectiveness of the particular piece of equipment are not yet available.

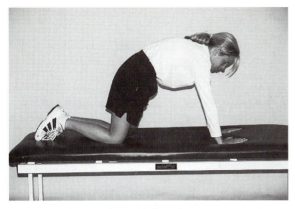

Figure 11-25   Push-ups with a plus.

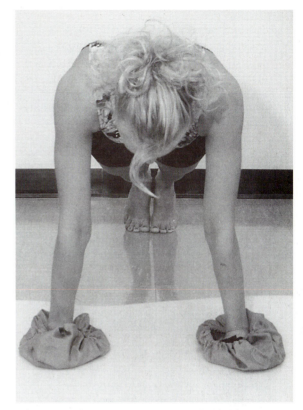

Figure 11-27   Slide board strengthening exercise.

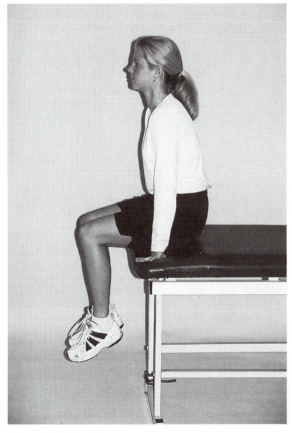

Figure 11-26   Press-ups

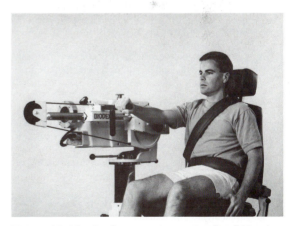

Figure 11-28   Biodex upper-extremity closed-kinetic-chain exercise system.

Summary

1. A closed-kinetic-chain exercise is one in which the distal segment of the extremity is fixed or stabilized. In an open kinetic chain, the distal segment is mobile and is not fixed.

2. Both open- and closed-kinetic-chain exercises have their place in the rehabilitative process.

3. The concepts of the reversibility of muscle actions and the concurrent shift are hallmarks of closed-kinetic-chain exercises.

4. Open- and closed-kinetic-chain exercises offer distinct advantages and disadvantages in the rehabilitation process. The choice to use one or the other depends on the desired treatment goal.

5. It has been suggested that closed-kinetic-chain exercises are safer due to muscle co-contraction and joint compression; that closed-kinetic-chain exercises tend to be more functional; and that they more effectively facilitate the integration of proprioceptive and joint position sense feedback than open-kinetic-chain exercises.

6. Open- and closed-kinetic-chain exercises have different biomechanical effects on the joints of the lower extremity.

7. Closed-kinetic-chain exercises in the lower extremity decrease the shear forces, reducing anterior tibial translation, and increase the compressive forces, which increases stability around the knee joint.

8. Minisquat, wall slides, lunges, leg press, stair-climbing machines, lateral step-up, terminal knee extension using tubing, stationary bicycling, slide boards, BAPS boards, and the Fitter are all examples of closed-kinetic-chain activities for the lower extremity.

9. Although it is true that closed-kinetic-chain exercises are most often used in rehabilitation of lower-extremity injuries, there are many injury situations where closed-kinetic-chain exercises should be incorporated into upper-extremity rehabilitation protocols.

10. Closed-kinetic-chain exercises in the upper extremity are used primarily for strengthening and establishing neuromuscular control of those muscles that act to stabilize the shoulder girdle.

11. Closed-kinetic-chain activities, such as push-ups, press-ups, weight-shifting, and slide board exercises, are strengthening exercises used primarily for improving shoulder stabilization in the upper extremity.

References

1. Andersen, S., D. Terwilliger, and C. Denegar. 1995. Comparison of open- versus closed-kinetic-chain test positions for measuring joint position sense, *Journal of Sport Rehabilitation* 4(3): 165–71.

2. Andrews, J., J. Dennison, and K. Wilk. 1995. The significance of closed-chain kinetics in upper extremity injuries from a physician's perspective. *Journal of Sport Rehabilitation* 5(1): 64–70.

3. Baratta, R., M. Solomonow, and B. Zhou. 1988. Muscular coactivation: The role of the antagonist musculature in maintaining knee stability. *American Journal of Sports Medicine* 16(2): 113–22.

4. Blair, D., and R. Willis. 1991. Rapid rehabilitation following anterior cruciate ligament reconstruction. *Ath Training* 26(1): 32–43.

5. Brask, B., R. Lueke, and G. Soderberg. 1984. Electromyographic analysis of selected muscles during the lateral step-up. *Physical Therapy* 64(3): 324–29.

6. Bunton, E., W. Pitney, and A. Kane. 1993. The role of limb torque, muscle action and proprioception during closed-kinetic-chain rehabilitation of the lower extremity. *Journal of Athletic Training* 28(1): 10–20.

7. Butler, D., F. Noyes, and E. Grood. 1980. Ligamentous restraints to anterior-posterior drawer in the human knee: a biomechanical study. *Journal of Bone and Joint Surgery* 62(A): 259–70.

8. Case, J., B. DePalma, and R. Zelko. 1991. Knee rehabilitation following anterior cruciate ligament repair/reconstruction: An update. *Ath Training* 26(1): 22–31.

9. Cipriani, D. 1994. Open- and closed-chain rehabilitation for the shoulder complex. In *The athlete's shoulder*, edited by J. Andrews and K. Wilk. New York: Churchill Livingston.

10. Cook, T., C. Zimmerman, K. Lux, et al. 1992. EMG comparison of lateral step-up and stepping machine exercise. *Journal of Orthopaedic and Sports Physical Therapy* 16(3): 108–13.

11. Davies, G. 1995. The need for critical thinking in rehabilitation. *Journal of Sport Rehabilitation* 4(1): 1–22.

12. DeCarlo, M., D. Shelbourne, J. McCarroll, et al. 1992. A traditional versus. accelerated rehabilitation following ACL reconstruction: A one-year follow-up. *Journal of Orthopaedic and Sports Physical Therapy* 15(6): 309–16.

13. Fu, F., S. Woo, and J. Irrgang. 1992. Current concepts for rehabilitation following anterior cruciate ligament reconstruction. *Journal of Orthopaedic and Sports Physical Therapy* 15(6): 270–78.

14. Fukubayashi, T., P. Torzilli, and M. Sherman. 1982. An in-vitro biomechanical evaluation of anterior/posterior motion of the knee: Tibial displacement, rotation, and torque. *Journal of Bone and Joint Surgery* 64[B]: 258–64.

15. Grahm, V., G. Gehlsen, and J. Edwards. 1993. Electromyographic evaluation of closed- and open-kinetic-chain knee rehabilitation exercises. *Journal of Athletic Training* 28(1): 23–33.

16. Grood, E., W. Suntag, F. Noyes, et al. 1984. Biomechanics of knee extension exercise. *Journal of Bone and Joint Surgery* 66[A]: 725–33.

17. Harter, R. 1995. Clinical rationale for closed-kinetic-chain activities in functional testing and rehabilitation of ankle pathologies. *Journal of Sport Rehabilitation* 5(1): 13–24.

18. Henning, S., M. Lench, and K. Glick. 1985. An in-vivo strain gauge study of elongation of the anterior cruciate ligament. *American Journal of Sports Medicine* 13:22–26.

19. Hillman, S. 1994. Principles and techniques of open-kinetic-chain rehabilitation: The upper extremity. *Journal of Sport Rehabilitation* 3(4): 319–30.

20. Hungerford, D., and M. Barry. 1979. Biomechanics of the patellofemoral joint. *Clin Orthop* 144:9–15.

21. Jurist, K., and V. Otis. 1985. Anteroposterior tibiofemoral displacements during isometric extension efforts. The roles of external load and knee flexion angle. *American Journal of Sports Medicine* 13:254–58.

22. Kaland, S., T. Sinkjaer, L. Arendt-Neilsen, et al. 1990. Altered timing of hamstring muscle action in anterior cruciate ligament deficient patients. *American Journal of Sports Medicine* 18(3): 245–48.

23. Kleiner, D., T. Drudge, and M. Ricard. 1994. An electromyographic comparison of popular open- and closed-kinetic-chain knee rehabilitation exercises. *Journal of Athletic Training* 29(2): 156–57.

24. LaFree, J., A. Mozingo, and T. Worrell. 1995. Comparison of open-kinetic-chain knee and hip extension to closed-kinetic-chain leg press performance. *Journal of Sport Rehabilitation* 3(2): 99–107.

25. Lepart, S., and T. Henry. 1995. The physiological basis for open- and closed-kinetic-chain rehabilitation for the upper extremity. *Journal of Sport Rehabilitation* 5(1): 71–87.

26. Lutz, G., M. Stuart, and H. Franklin. 1990. Rehabilitative techniques for athletes after reconstruction of the anterior cruciate ligament. *Mayo Clinic Proceedings* 65:1322–29.

27. Malone, T., and W. Garrett. 1992. Commentary and historical perspective of anterior cruciate ligament rehabilitation. *Journal of Orthopaedic and Sports Physical Therapy* 15(6): 265–69.

28. Nisell, R., M. Ericson, and G. Nemeth, et al. 1989. Tibiofemoral joint forces during isokinetic knee extension. *American Journal of Sports Medicine* 17:49–54.

29. Ohkoshi, Y., K. Yasuda, K. Kaneda, et al. 1991. Biomechanical analysis of rehabilitation in the standing position. *American Journal of Sports Medicine* 19(6): 605–11.

30. Palmitier, R., A. Kai-Nan, S. Scott, et al. 1991. Kinetic-chain exercise in knee rehabilitation. *Sports Medicine* 11(6): 402–13.

31. Rivera, J. 1994. Open- versus closed-kinetic-chain rehabilitation of the lower extremity: A functional and biomechanical analysis. *Journal of Sport Rehabilitation* 3(2): 154–67.

32. Renstrom, P, S. Arms, T. Stanwyck, et al. 1986. Strain within the anterior cruciate ligament during hamstring

33. Reynolds, N., T. Worrell, and D. Perrin. 1992. Effect of lateral step-up exercise protocol on quadriceps isokinetic peak torque values and thigh girth. *Journal of Orthopaedic and Sports Physical Therapy* 15(3): 151–156.

34. Sachs, R., D. Daniel, and M. Stone, et al. 1989. Patellofemoral problems after anterior cruciate ligament reconstruction. *American Journal of Sports Medicine* 17:760–65.

35. Shellbourne, D., and P. Nitz. 1990. Accelerated rehabilitation after anterior cruciate ligament reconstruction. *American Journal of Sports Medicine* 18:292–99.

36. Solomonow, M., R. Barata, B. Zhou, et al. 1987. The synergistic action of the anterior cruciate ligament and thigh muscles in maintaining joint stability. *American Journal of Sports Medicine* 15:207–13.

37. Snyder-Mackler, L. 1995. Scientific rationale and physiological basis for the use of closed-kinetic-chain exercise in the lower extremity. *Journal of Sport Rehabilitation* 5(1): 2–12.

38. Steindler, A. 1977. Kinesiology of the human body under normal and pathological conditions. Springfield, IL: Charles C. Thomas.

39. Stiene, H., T. Brosky, and M. Reinking. 1996. A comparison of closed-kinetic-chain and isokinetic joint isolation exercise in patients with patellofemoral dysfunction. *Journal of Orthopaedic and Sports Physical Therapy* 24(3): 136–41.

40. Stone, J., J. Lueken, and N. Partin. 1993. Closed-kinetic-chain rehabilitation of the glenohumeral joint. *Journal of Athletic Training* 28(1): 34–37.

41. Tovin, B., T. Tovin, and M. Tovin. 1992. Surgical and biomechanical considerations in rehabilitation of patients with intra-articular ACL reconstructions. *Journal of Orthopaedic and Sports Physical Therapy* 15(6): 317–22.

42. Valmassey, R. 1996. *Clinical biomechanics of the lower extremities.* St. Louis: Mosby.

43. Voight, M., S. Bell, and D. Rhodes. 1992. Instrumented testing of tibial translation during a positive Lachman's test and selected closed-chain activities in anterior cruciate deficient knees. *Journal of Orthopaedic and Sports Physical Therapy* 15:49.

44. Voight, M., and G. Cook. 1995. Clinical application of closed-chain exercise. *Journal of Sport Rehabilitation* 5(1): 25–44.

45. Voight, M., and S. Tippett. 1990. *Closed kinetic chain.* Paper presented at 41st Annual Clinical Symposium of the National Athletic Trainers Association, Indianapolis, June 12.

46. Wawrzyniak, J., J. Tracy, and P. Catizone. 1996. Effect of closed-chain exercise on quadriceps femoris peak torque and functional performance. *Journal of Athletic Training* 31(4): 335–45.

47. Wilk, K., and J. Andrews. 1992. Current concepts in the treatment of anterior cruciate ligament disruption. *Journal of Orthopaedic and Sports Physical Therapy* 15(6): 279–93.

48. Wilk, K., C. Arrigo, and J. Andrews. 1995. Closed- and open-kinetic-chain exercise for the upper extremity. *Journal of Sport Rehabilitation* 5(1): 88–102.

CHAPTER 12

Mobilization and Traction Techniques in Rehabilitation

William E. Prentice

After completion of this chapter, the student should be able to do the following:

- Differentiate between physiological movements and accessory motions.

- Discuss joint arthrokinematics.

- Discuss how specific joint positions can enhance the effectiveness of the treatment technique.

- Discuss the basic techniques of joint mobilization.

- Identify Maitland's five oscillation grades.

- Discuss indications and contraindications for mobilization.

- Discuss the use of various traction grades in treating pain and joint hypomobility.

- Explain why traction and mobilization techniques should be used simultaneously.

- Demonstrate specific techniques of mobilization and traction for various joints.

Following injury to a joint, there will almost always be some associated loss of motion. That loss of movement may be attributed to a number of pathological factors, including contracture of inert connective tissue (for example, ligaments and joint capsule); resistance of the contractile tissue or the musculotendinous unit (for example, muscle, tendon, and fascia) to stretch; or some combination of the two.[5,6] If left untreated, the joint will become hypomobile and will eventually begin to show signs of degeneration.[20]

Joint mobilization and traction are manual therapy techniques that involve slow, passive movements of articulating surfaces. They are used to regain normal active joint range of motion, to restore normal passive motions that occur about a joint, to reposition or realign a joint, to regain a normal distribution of forces and stresses about a joint, or to reduce pain, all of which will collectively improve joint function.[17] Joint mobilization and traction are two extremely effective and widely utilized techniques in the rehabilitation of sport-related injuries.

THE RELATIONSHIP BETWEEN PHYSIOLOGICAL AND ACCESSORY MOTIONS

For the sports therapist supervising a rehabilitation program, some understanding of the biomechanics of joint

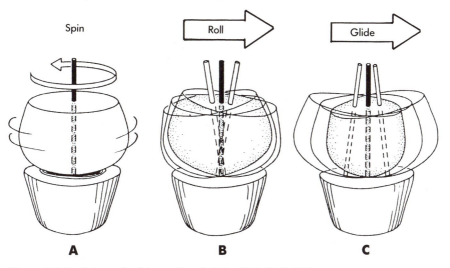

Figure 12-1   Joint arthrokinematics. **A**, Spin. **B**, Roll, **C**, Glide

movement is essential. There are basically two types of movement that govern motion about a joint. Perhaps the better known of the two types of movement are the **physiological movements** that result from either concentric or eccentric active muscle contractions that move a bone or a joint. This type of motion is referred to as **osteokinematic motion.** A bone can move about an axis of rotation or a joint into flexion, extension, abduction, adduction, and rotation. The second type of motion is **accessory motion.** Accessory motions involve the manner in which one articulating joint surface moves relative to another. Physiological movement is voluntary; accessory movements normally accompany physiological movement.[2] The two occur simultaneously. Although accessory movements cannot occur independently, they can be produced by some external force. Normal accessory component motions must occur for full-range physiological movement to take place. If any of the accessory component motions are restricted, normal physiological cardinal plane movements will not occur.[14,15] A muscle cannot be fully rehabilitated if the joint is not free to move, and vice versa.[20]

Traditionally in rehabilitation programs we have tended to concentrate more on passive physiological movements without paying much attention to accessory motions. The question is always being asked, "How much flexion or extension is this patient lacking?" Rarely will anyone ask, "How much is rolling or gliding restricted?"

It is critical for the sports therapist to closely evaluate the injured joint to determine whether motion is limited by physiological movement constraints involving muscu-

lotendinous units or by limitation in accessory motion involving the joint capsule and ligaments. If physiological movement is restricted, the athlete should engage in stretching activities designed to improve flexibility. Stretching exercises should be used whenever there is resistance of the contractile or musculotendinous elements to stretch. Stretching techniques are most effective at the end of physiological range of movement; they are limited to one direction, and they require some element of discomfort if additional range of motion is to be achieved. Stretching techniques make use of long lever arms to apply stretch to a given muscle.[9] Techniques of stretching have been discussed in Chapter 4, and PNF stretching techniques will be presented in Chapter 13.

If accessory motion is limited by some restriction of the joint capsule or the ligaments, the sports therapist should incorporate mobilization techniques into the treatment program. Mobilization techniques should be used whenever there are tight inert or noncontractile articular structures; they can be used effectively at any point in the range of motion, and they can be used in any direction in which movement is restricted. Mobilization techniques use a short lever arm to stretch ligaments and joint capsules, placing less stress on these structures, and consequently are somewhat safer to use than stretching techniques.[3]

JOINT ARTHROKINEMATICS

Accessory motions are also referred to as **joint arthrokinematics,** which include **spin, roll,** and **glide**[1,10,12] (Figure 12-1A–C).

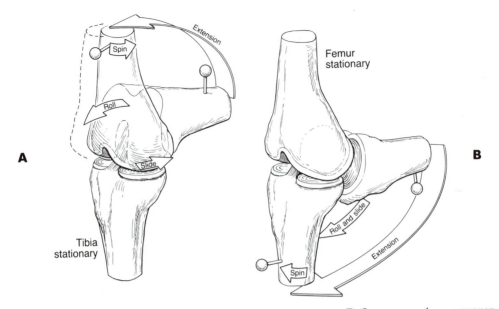

Figure 12-2 Convex-concave rule. **A,** Convex moving on concave. **B,** Concave moving on convex.

Spin occurs around some stationary longitudinal mechanical axis and can be in either a clockwise or a counterclockwise direction. An example of spinning is motion of the radial head at the humeroradial joint as occurs in forearm pronation/supination (Figure 12-1A).

Rolling occurs when a series of points on one articulating surface comes into contact with a series of points on another articulating surface. An analogy would be the rocker of a rocking chair rolling on the flat surface of the floor. An anatomical example would be the rounded femoral condyles rolling over a stationary flat tibial plateau (Figure 12-1B).

Gliding occurs when a specific point on one articulating surface comes into contact with a series of points on another surface. Returning to the rocking chair analogy, the rocker slides across the flat surface of the floor without any rocking at all. Gliding is sometimes referred to as *translation.* Anatomically, gliding or translation would occur during an anterior drawer test at the knee when the flat tibial plateau slides anteriorly relative to the fixed rounded femoral condyles (Figure 12-1C).

Pure gliding can occur only if the two articulating surfaces are congruent where either both are flat or both are curved. Virtually all articulating joint surfaces are incongruent, meaning that one is usually flat while the other is more curved, so it is more likely that gliding will occur simultaneously with a rolling motion. Rolling does not occur alone, because this would result in compression or perhaps dislocation of the joint.

Although rolling and gliding usually occur together, they are not necessarily in similar proportion, nor are they always in the same direction. If the articulating surfaces are more congruent, more gliding will occur, whereas if they are less congruent, more rolling will occur. Rolling will always occur in the same direction as the movement. For example, in the knee joint when the foot is fixed on the ground, the femur will always roll in an anterior direction when moving into knee extension and conversely will roll posteriorly when moving into flexion.

The direction of the gliding component of motion is determined by the shape of the articulating surface that is moving. If you consider the shape of two articulating surfaces, one joint surface can be determined to be convex in shape while the other may be considered to be concave in shape. In the knee, the femoral condyles would be considered the convex joint surface, while the tibial plateau would be the concave joint surface. In the glenohumeral joint, the humeral head would be the convex surface, while the glenoid fossa would be the concave surface.

This relationship between the shape of articulating joint surfaces and the direction of gliding is defined by the **convex-concave rule** (Figure 12-2). If the concave joint surface is moving on a stationary convex surface, gliding will occur in the same direction as the rolling motion. Conversely, if the convex surface is moving on a stationary concave surface, gliding will occur in an opposite direction to rolling. Hypomobile joints are treated by using a gliding technique. Thus it is critical to know the appropriate direction to use for gliding.

JOINT POSITIONS

Each joint in the body has a position in which the joint capsule and the ligaments are most relaxed, allowing for a maximum amount of **joint play.**[10,11] This position is called the **resting position.** It is essential to know specifically where the resting position is, because testing for joint play during an evaluation, and treatment of the hypomobile joint using either mobilization or traction, are both usually performed in this position. Table 12-1 summarizes the appropriate resting positions for many of the major joints.

Placing the joint capsule in the resting position allows the joint to assume a **loose-packed position** in which the articulating joint surfaces are maximally separated (Figure 12-3A). A **close-packed position** is one in which there is maximal contact of the articulating surfaces of bones with the capsule and ligaments tight or tense (Figure 12-3B). In a loose-packed position the joint will exhibit the greatest amount of joint play, whereas the close-packed position allows for no joint play. Thus the loose-packed position is most appropriate for mobilization and traction.

Both mobilization and traction techniques use a translational movement of one joint surface relative to the other. This translation can be in one of two directions: either perpendicular or parallel to the **treatment plane.** The treatment plane falls perpendicular to, or at a right angle to, a line running from the axis of rotation in the convex surface to the center of the concave articular surface[10,11] (Figure 12-4). Thus the treatment plane lies within the concave surface. If the convex segment moves, the treatment plane remains fixed. However, the treatment plane will move along with the concave segment. Mobilization techniques use glides that translate one articulating surface along a line parallel with the treatment plane. Traction techniques translate one of the articulating surfaces in a perpendicular direction to the treatment plane. Both techniques use a loose-packed joint position.[10]

JOINT MOBILIZATION TECHNIQUES

The techniques of joint mobilization are used to improve joint mobility or to decrease joint pain by restoring accessory movements to the joint and thus allowing full, nonrestricted, pain-free range of motion.[16,23]

Mobilization techniques may be used to attain a variety of either mechanical or neurophysiological treatment goals: reducing pain; decreasing muscle guarding; stretching or lengthening tissue surrounding a joint, in particular capsular and ligamentous tissue; reflexogenic effects that either inhibit or facilitate muscle tone or stretch reflex; and proprioceptive effects to improve postural and kinesthetic awareness.[1,8,15,18,20]

Movement throughout a range of motion can be quantified with various measurement techniques. Physiological movement is measured with a goniometer and composes the major portion of the range. Accessory motion is thought of in millimeters, although precise measurement is difficult.

Accessory movements can be hypomobile, normal, or hypermobile.[4] Each joint has a range of motion continuum with an anatomical limit (AL) to motion that is determined by both bony arrangement and surrounding soft tissue. In a hypomobile joint, motion stops at some point referred to as a pathological point of limitation (PL), short of the anatomical limit caused by pain, spasm, or tissue resistance. A hypermobile joint moves beyond its anatomical limit because of laxity of the surrounding structures. A hypomobile joint should respond well to techniques of mobilization and traction.[7] A hypermobile joint should be treated with strengthening exercises, stability exercises, and, if indicated, taping, splinting, or bracing.[19,20]

In a hypomobile joint, as mobilization techniques are used into the range of motion restriction, some deformation of soft tissue capsular or ligamentous structures occurs. If a tissue is stretched only into its elastic range, no permanent structural changes will occur. However, if that tissue is stretched into its plastic range, permanent structural changes will occur. Thus, mobilization and traction can be used to stretch tissue and break adhesions. If used inappropriately, they can also damage tissue and cause sprains of the joint.[20]

Treatment techniques designed to improve accessory movement are generally slow, small-amplitude movements, amplitude being the distance that the joint is moved passively within its total range. Mobilization techniques use these small-amplitude oscillating motions that glide or slide one of the articulating joint surfaces in an appropriate direction within a specific part of the range.[13]

Maitland has described various grades of oscillation for joint mobilization (Figure 12-5). The amplitude of each oscillation grade falls within the range-of-motion continuum between some beginning point (BP) and the AL.[14,15] Figure 12-5 shows the various grades of oscillation that are used in a joint with some limitation of motion. As the severity of the movement restriction increases, the PL will move to the left, away from the AL.

■ **TABLE 12-1** Shape, Resting Position, and Treatment Planes of Various Joints

Joint	Convex Surface	Concave Surface	Resting Position	Treatment Plane
Sternoclavicular	Clavicle*	Sternum*	Anatomical position	In sternum
Acromioclavicular	Clavicle	Acromion	Anatomical position, in horizontal plane at 60 degrees to sagittal plane	In acromion
Glenohumeral	Humerus	Glenoid	Shoulder abducted 55 degrees, horizontally adducted 30 degrees, rotated so forearm is in horizontal plane	In glenoid fossa in scapular plane
Humeroradial	Humerus	Radius	Elbow extended, forearm supinated	In radial head perpendicular to long axis of radius
Humeroulnar	Humerus	Ulna	Elbow flexed 70 degrees, forearm supinated 10 degrees	In olecranon fossa, 45 degrees to long axis of ulna
Radioulnar (Proximal)	Radius	Ulna	Elbow flexed 70 degrees, forearm supinated 35 degrees	In radial notch of ulna, parallel to long axis of ulna
Radioulnar (Distal)	Ulna	Radius	Supinated 10 degrees	In radius, parallel to long axis of radius
Radiocarpal	Proximal carpal bones	Radius Proximal phalanx	Line through radius and third metacarpal	In radius, perpendicular to long axis of radius
Metacarpophalangeal	Metacarpal	Distal phalanx	Slight flexion	In proximal phalanx
Interphalangeal	Proximal phalanx	Acetabulum	Slight flexion	In proximal phalanx
Hip	Femur		Hip flexed 30 degrees, abducted 30 degrees, slight external rotation	In acetabulum
Tibiofemoral	Femur	Tibia	Flexed 25 degrees	On surface of tibial plateau
Patellofemoral	Patella	Femur	Knee in full extension	Along femoral groove
Talocrural	Talus	Mortise	Plantarflexed 10 degrees	In the mortise in anterior/posterior direction
Subtalar	Calcaneus	Talus	Subtalar neutral between inversion/eversion	In talus, parallel to foot surface
Intertarsal	Proximal articulating surface	Distal articulating surface	Foot relaxed	In distal segment
Metatarsophalangeal	Tarsal bone	Proximal phalanx	Slight extension	In proximal phalanx
Interphalangeal	Proximal phalanx	Distal phalanx	Slight flexion	In distal phalanx

*In the sternoclavicular joint the clavicle surface is convex in a superior/inferior direction and concave in an anterior/posterior direction.

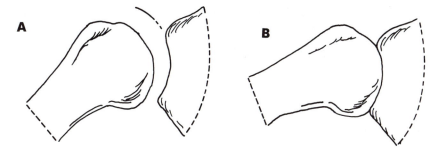

Figure 12-3   Joint capsule resting position. **A,** Loose-packed position. **B,** Close-packed position.

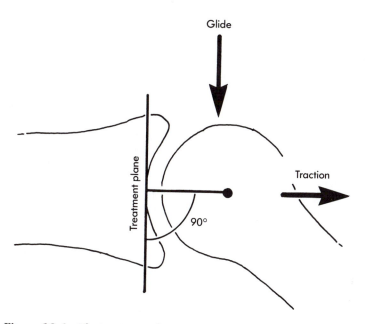

Figure 12-4   The treatment plane is perpendicular to a line drawn from the axis of rotation to the center of the articulating surface of the concave segment.

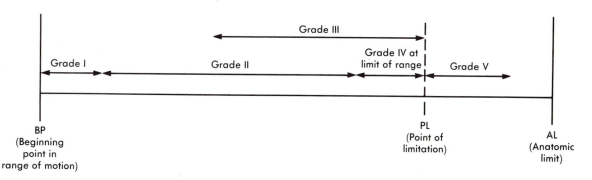

Figure 12-5   Maitland's five grades of motion. *PL* = point of limitation; *AL* = anatomical limit.

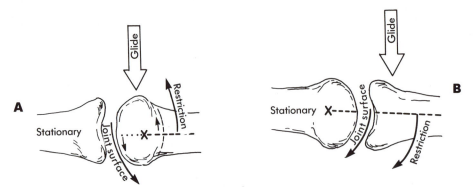

Figure 12-6 Gliding motions. **A,** Glides of the convex segment should be in the direction opposite to the restriction. **B,** Glides of the concave segment should be in the direction of the restriction.

However, the relationships that exist among the five grades in terms of their positions within the range of motion remain the same. The five mobilization grades are defined as follows:

Grade I. A small-amplitude movement at the beginning of the range of movement. Used when pain and spasm limit movement early in the range of motion.[25]

Grade II. A large-amplitude movement within the midrange of movement. Used when spasm limits movement sooner with a quick oscillation than with a slow one or when slowly increasing pain restricts movement halfway into the range.

Grade III. A large-amplitude movement up to the PL in the range of movement. Used when pain and resistance from spasm, inert tissue tension, or tissue compression limit movement near the end of the range.

Grade IV. A small-amplitude movement at the very end of the range of movement. Used when resistance limits movement in the absence of pain and spasm.

Grade V. A small-amplitude, quick thrust delivered at the end of the range of movement, usually accompanied by a popping sound, which is called a manipulation. Used when minimal resistance limits the end of the range. Manipulation is most effectively accomplished by the velocity of the thrust rather than by the force of the thrust.[21] Most authorities agree that manipulation should be used only by individuals trained specifically in these techniques, because a great deal of skill and judgment is necessary for safe and effective treatment.[22]

Joint mobilization uses these oscillating gliding motions of one articulating joint surface in whatever direction is appropriate for the existing restriction. The appropriate direction for these oscillating glides is determined by the convex-concave rule described previously. When

the concave surface is stationary and the convex surface is mobilized, a glide of the convex segment should be in the direction opposite to the restriction of joint movement.[10,11,24] (Figure 12-6A). If the convex articular surface is stationary and the concave surface is mobilized, gliding of the concave segment should be in the same direction as the restriction of joint movement (Figure 12-6B). For example, the glenohumeral joint would be considered to be a convex joint with the convex humeral head moving on the concave glenoid. If shoulder abduction is restricted, the humerus should be glided in an inferior direction relative to the glenoid to alleviate the motion restriction. When mobilizing the knee joint, the concave tibia should be glided anteriorly in cases where knee extension is restricted. If mobilization in the appropriate direction exacerbates complaints of pain or stiffness, the sports therapist should apply the technique in the opposite direction until the patient can tolerate the appropriate direction.[24]

Typical mobilization of a joint might involve a series of three to six sets of oscillations lasting between 20 and 60 seconds each, with one to three oscillations per second.[14,15]

Indications for Mobilization

In Maitland's system, grades I and II are used primarily for treatment of pain, and grades III and IV are used for treating stiffness. Pain must be treated first and stiffness second.[15] Painful conditions should be treated on a daily basis. The purpose of the small-amplitude oscillations is to stimulate mechanoreceptors within the joint that can limit the transmission of pain perception at the spinal cord or brain stem levels.

Joints that are stiff or hypomobile and have restricted movement should be treated 3 to 4 times per week on al-

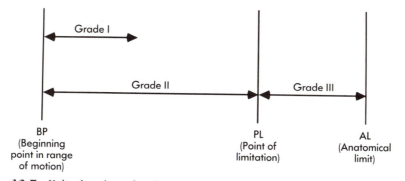

Figure 12-7 Kaltenborn's grades of traction. *PL* = point of limitation; *AL* = anatomical limit.

ternating days with active motion exercise. The sports therapist must continuously reevaluate the joint to determine appropriate progression from one oscillation grade to another.

Indications for specific mobilization grades are relatively straightforward. If the athlete complains of pain before the sports therapist can apply any resistance to movement, it is too early and all mobilization techniques should be avoided. If pain is elicited when resistance to motion is applied, mobilization using grades I and II is appropriate. If resistance can be applied before pain is elicited, mobilization can be progressed to grades III and IV. Mobilization should be done with both the athlete and the sports therapist positioned in a comfortable and relaxed manner. The sports therapist should mobilize one joint at a time. The joint should be stabilized as near one articulating surface as possible, while moving the other segment with a firm, confident grasp.

Contraindications for Mobilization

Techniques of mobilization and manipulation should not be used haphazardly. These techniques should generally not be used in cases of inflammatory arthritis, malignancy, bone disease, neurological involvement, bone fracture, congenital bone deformities, and vascular disorders of the vertebral artery. Again, manipulation should be performed only by those sports therapists specifically trained in the procedure, because some special knowledge and judgment are required for effective treatment.[24]

JOINT TRACTION TECHNIQUES

Traction is a technique involving pulling on one articulating segment to produce some separation of the two joint surfaces. Although mobilization glides are done parallel to the treatment plane, traction is performed perpendicular to the treatment plane (see Figure 12-4). Like mo-

bilization techniques, traction can be used either to decrease pain or to reduce joint hypomobility.[26]

Kaltenborn has proposed a system using traction combined with mobilization as a means of reducing pain or mobilizing hypomobile joints.[9] As discussed earlier, all joints have a certain amount of joint play or looseness. Kaltenborn referred to this looseness as *slack*. Some degree of slack is necessary for normal joint motion. Kaltenborn's three traction grades are defined as follows (Figure 12-7):

Grade I traction (loosen). Traction that neutralizes pressure in the joint without actual separation of the joint surfaces. The purpose is to produce pain relief by reducing the compressive forces of articular surfaces during mobilization and is used with all mobilization grades.

Grade II traction (tighten or "take up the slack"). Traction that effectively separates the articulating surfaces and takes up the slack or eliminates play in the joint capsule. Grade II is used in initial treatment to determine joint sensitivity.

Grade III traction (stretch). Traction that involves actual stretching of the soft tissue surrounding the joint to increase mobility in a hypomobile joint.

Grade I traction should be used in the initial treatment to reduce the chance of a painful reaction. It is recommended that 10-second intermittent grades I and II traction be used, distracting the joint surfaces up to a grade III traction and then releasing distraction until the joint returns to its resting position.

Kaltenborn emphasizes that grade III traction should be used in conjunction with mobilization glides to treat joint hypomobility[10] (Figure 12-8). Grade III traction stretches the joint capsule and increases the space between the articulating surfaces, placing the joint in a loose-packed position. Applying grade III and grade IV oscillations within the athlete's pain limitations should maximally improve joint mobility (Figure 12-9).

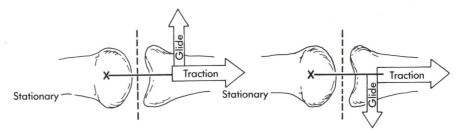

Figure 12-8   Traction vs. glides. Traction should be perpendicular to the treatment plane, while glides are parallel to the treatment plane.

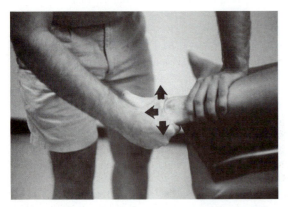

Figure 12-9   Traction and mobilization should be used together.

MOBILIZATION AND TRACTION TECHNIQUES

Throughout Chapters 19 to 26, photographs are used to show appropriate joint mobilization and traction techniques for each joint. These figures should be used to determine appropriate hand positioning, stabilization (S) and the correct direction for gliding (G), traction (T), and/or rotation (R). The information presented in this chapter should be used as a reference base for appropriately incorporating joint mobilization and traction techniques into the rehabilitation program.

Summary

1. Mobilization and traction techniques increase joint mobility or decrease pain by restoring accessory movements to the joint.
2. Physiological movements result from an active muscle contraction that moves an extremity through traditional cardinal planes.
3. Accessory motions are movements of one articulating joint surface relative to another.
4. Normal accessory component motions must occur for full-range physiological movement to take place.
5. Accessory motions are also referred to as joint arthrokinematics, which include spin, roll, and glide.
6. The convex-concave rule states that if the concave joint surface is moving on the stationary convex surface, gliding will occur in the same direction as the rolling motion, and that if the convex surface is

moving on a stationary concave surface, gliding will occur in an opposite direction to rolling.
7. The resting position is one in which the joint capsule and the ligaments are most relaxed, allowing for a maximum amount of joint play.
8. The treatment plane falls perpendicular to a line running from the axis of rotation in the convex surface to the center of the concave articular surface.
9. Maitland has proposed a series of five graded movements or oscillations in the range of motion to treat pain and stiffness.
10. Kaltenborn uses three grades of traction to reduce pain and stiffness.
11. Kaltenborn emphasizes that traction should be used in conjunction with mobilization glides to treat joint hypomobility.

References

1. Barak, T., E. Rosen, and R. Sofer. 1990. Mobility: Passive orthopedic manual therapy. In *Orthopedic and sports physical therapy*, edited by J. Gould and G. Davies. St. Louis: Mosby.

2. Basmajian, J. 1978. *Therapeutic exercise*. Baltimore: Williams & Wilkins.

3. Cookson, J. 1979. Orthopedic manual therapy: An overview: II. The spine. *Journal of the American Physical Therapy Association* 59:259.

4. Cookson, J., and B. Kent. 1979. Orthopedic manual therapy: An overview: I. The extremities. *Journal of the American Physical Therapy Association* 59:136.

5. Cyriax, J. 1974. *Textbook of orthopedic medicine: Treatment by manipulation, massage, and injection*. Vol. 2. Baltimore: Williams & Wilkins.

6. Donatelli, R., and H. Owens-Burkhart. 1981. Effects of immobilization on the extensibility of periarticular connective tissue. *Journal of Orthopaedic and Sports Physical Therapy* 3:67.

7. Edmond, S. 1993. *Manipulation and mobilization: Extremity and spinal techniques*. St. Louis: Mosby.

8. Grimsby, O. 1981. *Fundamentals of manual therapy: A course workbook*. Vagsbygd, Norway: Sorlandets Fysikalske Institutt.

9. Hollis, M. 1981. *Practical exercise*. Oxford: Blackwell Scientific.

10. Kaltenborn, F. 1980. *Mobilization of the extremity joints: Examination and basic treatment techniques*. Norway: Olaf Norlis Bokhandel.

11. Kisner, C., and L. Colby. 1997. *Therapeutic exercise: Foundations and techniques*. Philadelphia: F. A. Davis.

12. MacConaill, M., and J. Basmajian. 1969. *Muscles and movements: A basis for kinesiology*. Baltimore: Williams & Wilkins.

13. Maigne, R. 1976. *Orthopedic medicine*. Springfield, IL: Charles C. Thomas.

14. Maitland, G. 1977. *Extremity manipulation*. London: Butterworth.

15. Maitland, G. 1978. *Vertebral manipulation*. London: Butterworth.

16. Mennell, J. 1964. *Joint pain and diagnosis using manipulative techniques*. New York: Little, Brown.

17. Nygard, R. 1993. Manipulation: Definition, types, application. In *Rational manual therapies*, edited by J. Basmajian and R. Nyberg. Baltimore: Williams & Wilkins.

18. Paris, S. 1979. *The spine: Course notebook*. Atlanta: Institute Press.

19. Paris, S. 1979. Mobilization of the spine. *Physical Therapy* 59:988.

20. Saunders, D. 1985. *Evaluation, treatment and prevention of musculoskeletal disorders*. Bloomington, MN: Educational Opportunities.

21. Schiotz, E., and J. Cyriax. 1978. *Manipulation past and present*. London: Heinemann Medical Books.

22. Stoddard, A. 1969. *Manual of osteopathic practice*. London: Hutchinson Ross.

23. Taniqawa, M. 1972. Comparison of the hold-relax procedure and passive mobilization on increasing muscle length. *Physical Therapy* 52(7): 725–35.

24. Wadsworth, C. 1988. *Manual examination and treatment of the spine and extremities*. Baltimore: William & Wilkins.

25. Zohn, D., and J. Mennell. 1976. *Musculoskeletal pain: Diagnosis and physical treatment*. Boston: Little, Brown.

26. Zusman, M. 1985. Reappraisal of a proposed neurophysiological mechanism for the relief of joint pain with passive joint movements. *Physiother Pract* 1:61–70.

CHAPTER 13

Proprioceptive Neuromuscular Facilitation Techniques in Rehabilitation

William E. Prentice

After completion of this chapter, the student should be able to do the following:

• Explain the neurophysiological basis of PNF techniques.

• Discuss the rationale for use of the techniques.

• Discuss the basic principles of using PNF in rehabilitation.

• Identify the various PNF strengthening and stretching techniques.

• Describe PNF patterns for the upper and lower extremity, for the upper and lower trunk, and for the neck.

• Discuss the concept of muscle energy technique and explain how it is similar to PNF.

Proprioceptive neuromuscular facilitation (PNF) is an approach to therapeutic exercise based on the principles of functional human anatomy and neurophysiology. It uses proprioceptive, cutaneous, and auditory input to produce functional improvement in motor output and can be a vital element in the rehabilitation process of many sport-related injuries. These techniques have long been recommended for increasing strength, flexibility, and range of motion.[7,10,13,18,19,27] It is apparent that PNF techniques are also useful for enhancing neuromuscular control.[25] This discussion should guide the sports therapist using the principles and techniques of PNF as a component of a rehabilitation program.

THE NEUROPHYSIOLOGICAL BASIS OF PNF

The therapeutic techniques of PNF were first used in the treatment of patients with paralysis and neuromuscular disorders. Most of the principles underlying modern therapeutic exercise techniques can be attributed to the work of Sherrington,[24] who first defined the concepts of facilitation and inhibition.

An impulse traveling down the corticospinal tract or an afferent impulse traveling up from peripheral receptors in the muscle causes an impulse volley, which results in the discharge of a limited number of specific motor neurons, as well as the discharge of additional surrounding (anatomically close) motor neurons in the subliminal fringe area. An impulse causing the recruitment and discharge of additional motor neurons within the subliminal fringe is said to be facilitatory. Any stimulus that causes motor neurons to drop out of the discharge zone and away from the subliminal fringe is said to be inhibitory.[12]

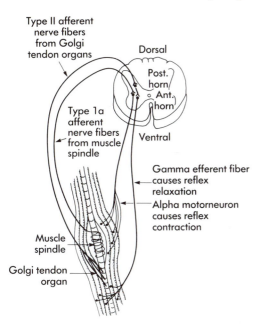

Figure 13-1   Diagrammatic representation of the stretch reflex.

(2) Golgi tendon organs, which detect changes in tension (Figure 13-1).

Stretching a given muscle causes an increase in the frequency of impulses transmitted to the spinal cord from the muscle spindle, which in turn produces an increase in the frequency of motor nerve impulses returning to that same muscle, thus reflexively resisting the stretch. However, the development of excessive tension within the muscle activates the Golgi tendon organs, whose sensory impulses are carried back to the spinal cord. These impulses have an inhibitory effect on the motor impulses returning to the muscles and cause that muscle to relax.

Two neurophysiological phenomena help to explain facilitation and inhibition of the neuromuscular systems. The first, **autogenic inhibition,** is defined as inhibition mediated by afferent fibers from a stretched muscle acting on the alpha motor neurons supplying that muscle, causing it to relax. When a muscle is stretched, motor neurons supplying that muscle receive both excitatory and inhibitory impulses from the receptors. If the stretch is continued for a slightly extended period of time, the inhibitory signals from the Golgi tendon organs eventually override the excitatory impulses and therefore cause relaxation. Because inhibitory motor neurons receive impulses from the Golgi tendon organs while the muscle spindle creates an initial reflex excitation leading to contraction, the Golgi tendon organs apparently send inhibitory impulses that last for the duration of increased tension (resulting from either passive stretch or active contraction) and eventually dominate the weaker impulses from the muscle spindle. This inhibition seems to protect the muscle against injury from reflex contractions resulting from excessive stretch.

The second mechanism, **reciprocal inhibition,** deals with the relationships of the agonist and antagonist muscles (Figure 13-2). The muscles that contract to produce joint motion are referred to as agonists, and the resulting movement is called an agonistic pattern. The muscles that stretch to allow the agonist pattern to occur are referred to as antagonists. Movement that occurs directly opposite to the agonist pattern is called the antagonist pattern.

When motor neurons of the agonist muscle receive excitatory impulses from afferent nerves, the motor neurons that supply the antagonist muscles are inhibited by afferent impulses.[2] Thus contraction or extended stretch of the agonist muscle must elicit relaxation or inhibit the antagonist. Likewise, a quick stretch of the antagonist muscle facilitates a contraction of the agonist. For facilitating or inhibiting motion, PNF relies heavily on the actions of these agonist and antagonist muscle groups.

Facilitation results in increased excitability, and inhibition results in decreased excitability of motor neurons.[29] Thus the function of weak muscles would be aided by facilitation, and muscle spasticity would be decreased by inhibition.[9]

Sherrington attributed the impulses transmitted from the peripheral stretch receptors via the afferent system as being the strongest influence on the alpha motor neurons.[24] Therefore the sports therapist should be able to modify the input from the peripheral receptors and thus influence the excitability of the alpha motor neurons. The discharge of motor neurons can be facilitated by peripheral stimulation, which causes afferent impulses to make contact with excitatory neurons and results in increased muscle tone or strength of voluntary contraction. Motor neurons can also be inhibited by peripheral stimulation, which causes afferent impulses to make contact with inhibitory neurons, resulting in muscle relaxation and allowing for stretching of the muscle.[24] To indicate any technique in which input from peripheral receptors is used to facilitate or inhibit, PNF should be used.[9]

The principles and techniques of PNF described here are based primarily on the neurophysiological mechanisms involving the stretch reflex. The stretch reflex involves two types of receptors: (1) muscle spindles, which are sensitive to a change in length, as well as the rate of change in length of the muscle fiber; and

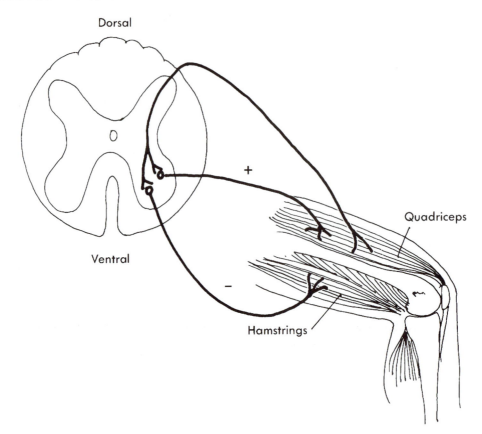

Figure 13-2 Diagrammatic representation of reciprocal inhibition.

A final point of clarification should be made regarding autogenic and reciprocal inhibition. The motor neurons of the spinal cord always receive a combination of inhibitory and excitatory impulses from the afferent nerves. Whether these motor neurons will be excited or inhibited depends on the ratio of these incoming impulses.

Several different approaches to therapeutic exercise based on the principles of facilitation and inhibition have been proposed. Among these are the Bobath method,[3] Brunnstrom method,[4] Rood method,[22] and the Knott and Voss method,[11] which they called proprioceptive neuromuscular facilitation. Although each of these techniques is important and useful, the PNF approach of Knott and Voss probably makes the most explicit use of proprioceptive stimulation.[11]

RATIONALE FOR USE

As a positive approach to injury rehabilitation, PNF is aimed at what the patient can do physically within the limitations of the injury. It is perhaps best used to de-

crease deficiencies in strength, flexibility, and coordination in response to demands that are placed on the neuromuscular system. The emphasis is on selective reeducation of individual motor elements through development of neuromuscular control, joint stability, and coordinated mobility. Each movement is learned and then reinforced through repetition in an appropriately demanding and intense rehabilitative program.[23]

The body tends to respond to the demands placed on it. The principles of PNF attempt to provide a maximal response for increasing strength, flexibility, and coordination. These principles should be applied with consideration of their appropriateness in achieving a particular goal. That continued activity during a rehabilitation program is essential for maintaining or improving strength or flexibility is well accepted. Therefore an intense program should offer the greatest potential for recovery.[21]

The PNF approach is holistic, integrating sensory, motor, and psychological aspects of a rehabilitation program. It incorporates reflex activities from the spinal levels and upward, either inhibiting or facilitating them as appropriate.

The brain recognizes only gross joint movement and not individual muscle action. Moreover, the strength of a muscle contraction is directly proportional to the activated motor units. Therefore, to increase the strength of a muscle, the maximum number of motor units must be stimulated to strengthen the remaining muscle fibers.[10,11] This "irradiation," or overflow effect, can occur when the stronger muscle groups help the weaker groups in completing a particular movement. This cooperation leads to the rehabilitation goal of return to optimal function.[2,11] The following principles of PNF should be applied to reach that ultimate goal.

BASIC PRINCIPLES OF PNF

Margret Knott, in her text on PNF,[11] emphasized the importance of the principles rather than specific techniques in a rehabilitation program. These principles are the basis of PNF that must be superimposed on any specific technique. The principles of PNF are based on sound neurophysiological and kinesiologic principles and clinical experience.[23] Application of the following principles can help promote a desired response in the patient being treated.

1. The patient must be taught the PNF patterns regarding the sequential movements from starting position to terminal position. The sports therapist has to keep instructions brief and simple. It is sometimes helpful for the sports therapist to passively move the patient through the desired movement pattern to demonstrate precisely what is to be done. The patterns should be used along with the techniques to increase the effects of the treatment.

2. When learning the patterns, the patient is often helped by looking at the moving limb. This visual stimulus offers the patient feedback for directional and positional control.

3. Verbal cues are used to coordinate voluntary effort with reflex responses. Commands should be firm and simple. Commands most commonly used with PNF techniques are "Push" and "Pull," which ask for an isotonic contraction; "Hold," which asks for an isometric or stabilizing contraction; and "Relax."

4. Manual contact with appropriate pressure is essential for influencing direction of motion and facilitating a maximal response, because reflex responses are greatly affected by pressure receptors. Manual contact should be firm and confident to give the patient a feeling of security.

The manner in which the sports therapist touches the athlete influences athlete confidence as well as the appropriateness of the motor response or relaxation.[23] A movement response may be facilitated by the hand over the muscle being contracted to facilitate a movement or a stabilizing contraction.

5. Proper mechanics and body positioning of the sports therapist are essential in applying pressure and resistance. The sports therapist should stand in a position that is in line with the direction of movement in the diagonal movement pattern. The knees should be bent and close to the patient such that the direction of resistance can easily be applied or altered appropriately throughout the range.

6. The amount of resistance given should facilitate a maximal response that allows smooth, coordinated motion. The appropriate resistance depends to a large extent on the capabilities of the patient. It may also change at different points throughout the range of motion. Maximal resistance may be applied with techniques that use isometric contractions to restrict motion to a specific point; it may also be used in isotonic contractions throughout a full range of movement.

7. Rotational movement is a critical component in all of the PNF patterns because maximal contraction is impossible without it.

8. Normal timing is the sequence of muscle contraction that occurs in any normal motor activity resulting in coordinated movement.[11] The distal movements of the patterns should occur first. The distal movement components should be completed no later than halfway through the total PNF pattern. To accomplish this, appropriate verbal commands should be timed with manual commands. Normal timing may be used with maximal resistance or without resistance from the sports therapist.

9. Timing for emphasis is used primarily with isotonic contractions. This principle superimposes maximal resistance, at specific points in the range, upon the patterns of facilitation, allowing overflow or irradiation to the weaker components of a movement pattern. The stronger components are emphasized to facilitate the weaker components of a movement pattern.

10. Specific joints may be facilitated by using traction or approximation. Traction spreads apart the joint articulations, and approximation

presses them together. Both techniques stimulate the joint proprioceptors. Traction increases the muscular response, promotes movement, assists isotonic contractions, and is used with most flexion antigravity movements. Traction must be maintained throughout the pattern. Approximation increases the muscular response, promotes stability, assists isometric contractions, and is used most with extension (gravity-assisted) movements. Approximation may be quick or gradual and may be repeated during a pattern.

11. Giving a quick stretch to the muscle before muscle contraction facilitates a muscle to respond with greater force through the mechanisms of the stretch reflex. It is most effective if all the components of a movement are stretched simultaneously. However, this quick stretch can be contraindicated in many orthopedic conditions because the extensibility limits of a damaged musculotendinous unit or joint structure might be exceeded, exacerbating the injury.

TECHNIQUES OF PNF

Each of the principles described above should be applied to the specific techniques of PNF. These techniques may be used in a rehabilitation program either to strengthen or facilitate a particular agonistic muscle group or to stretch or inhibit the antagonistic group. The choice of a specific technique depends on the deficits of a particular patient.[17] Specific techniques or combinations of techniques should be selected on the basis of the patient's problem.[1]

Strengthening Techniques

The following techniques are most appropriately used for the development of muscular strength, and endurance, as well as for reestablishing neuromuscular control.

The **rhythmic initiation** technique involves a progression of initial passive, then active-assistive, followed by active movement against resistance through the agonist pattern. Movement is slow, goes through the available range of motion, and avoids activation of a quick stretch. It is used for patients who are unable to initiate movement and who have a limited range of motion because of increased tone. It may also be used to teach the patient a movement pattern.

Repeated contraction is useful when a patient has weakness either at a specific point or throughout the en-

tire range. It is used to correct imbalances that occur within the range by repeating the weakest portion of the total range. The patient moves isotonically against maximal resistance repeatedly until fatigue is evidenced in the weaker components of the motion. When fatigue of the weak components becomes apparent, a stretch at that point in the range should facilitate the weaker muscles and result in a smoother, more coordinated motion. Again, quick stretch may be contraindicated with some musculoskeletal injuries. The amount of resistance to motion given by the sports therapist should be modified to accommodate the strength of the muscle group. The patient is commanded to push by using the agonist concentrically and eccentrically throughout the range.

Slow reversal involves an isotonic contraction of the agonist followed immediately by an isotonic contraction of the antagonist. The initial contraction of the agonist muscle group facilitates the succeeding contraction of the antagonist muscles. The slow-reversal technique can be used for developing active range of motion of the agonists and normal reciprocal timing between the antagonists and agonists, which is critical for normal coordinated motion.[20] The patient should be commanded to push against maximal resistance by using the antagonist and then to pull by using the agonist. The initial agonistic push facilitates the succeeding antagonist contraction.

Slow-reversal-hold is an isotonic contraction of the agonist followed immediately by an isometric contraction, with a hold command given at the end of each active movement. The direction of the pattern is reversed by using the same sequence of contraction with no relaxation before shifting to the antagonistic pattern. This technique can be especially useful in developing strength at a specific point in the range of motion.

Rhythmic stabilization uses an isometric contraction of the agonist, followed by an isometric contraction of the antagonist to produce co-contraction and stability of the two opposing muscle groups. The command given is always "Hold," and movement is resisted in each direction. Rhythmic stabilization results in an increase in the holding power to a point where the position cannot be broken. Holding should emphasize co-contraction of agonists and antagonists.

Stretching Techniques

The following techniques should be used to increase range of motion, relaxation, and inhibition.

Contract-relax is a stretching technique that moves the body part passively into the agonist pattern. The patient is instructed to push by contracting the antagonist (muscle that will be stretched) isotonically against the resistance of the sports therapist. The patient then relaxes the antagonist while the therapist moves the part passively through as much range as possible to the point where limitation is again felt. This contract-relax technique is beneficial when range of motion is limited by muscle tightness.

Hold-relax is very similar to the contract-relax technique. It begins with an isometric contraction of the antagonist (muscle that will be stretched) against resistance, followed by a concentric contraction of the agonist muscle combined with light pressure from the sports therapist to produce maximal stretch of the antagonist. This technique is appropriate when there is muscle tension on one side of a joint and may be used with either the agonist or antagonist.

Slow-reversal-hold-relax technique begins with an isotonic contraction of the agonist, which often limits range of motion in the agonist pattern, followed by an isometric contraction of the antagonist (muscle that will be stretched) during the push phase. During the relax phase, the antagonists are relaxed while the agonists are contracting, causing movement in the direction of the agonist pattern and thus stretching the antagonist. The technique, like the contract-relax and hold-relax, is useful for increasing range of motion when the primary limiting factor is the antagonistic muscle group.

Because the goal of rehabilitation in most sport-related injuries is restoration of strength through a full, nonrestricted range of motion, several of these techniques are sometimes combined in sequence to accomplish this goal.[15] Figure 13-3 shows a PNF stretching technique in which the sports therapist is stretching the injured athlete.

Treating Specific Problems with PNF Techniques

PNF strengthening and stretching techniques can be useful in a variety of different conditions. To some extent the choice of the most effective technique for a given situation will be dictated by the state of the existing condition and by the capabilities and limitations of the individual athlete.[28] There are some advantages to using PNF techniques in general.

Relative to strengthening, the PNF techniques are not encumbered by the design constraints of commercial exercise machines. With the PNF patterns, movement can occur in three planes simultaneously, thus more closely resembling a functional movement pattern. The amount of resistance applied by the sports therapist can be easily adjusted and altered at different points through the range of motion to meet patient capabilities. The

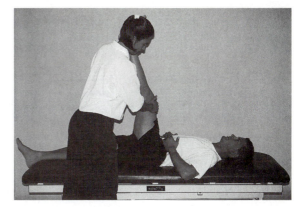

Figure 13-3 PNF stretching technique.

sports therapist can choose to concentrate on the strengthening through entire range of motion or through a very specific range. Combinations of several strengthening techniques can be used concurrently within the same PNF pattern.[16] Rhythmic initiation is useful in the early stages of rehabilitation when the athlete is having difficulty moving actively through a pain-free arc. Passive movement can allow the athlete to maintain a full range while using an active contraction to move through the available pain-free range. Slow reversal should be used to help improve muscular endurance. Slow-reversal-hold is used to correct existing weakness at specific points in the range of motion through isometric strengthening.

Rhythmic stabilization is used to achieve stability and neuromuscular control about a joint.[8] This technique requires co-contraction of opposing muscle groups and is useful in creating a balance in the existing force couples.

PNF PATTERNS

The PNF patterns are concerned with gross movement as opposed to specific muscle actions. The techniques identified previously can be superimposed on any of the PNF patterns. The techniques of PNF are composed of both rotational and diagonal exercise patterns that are similar to the motions required in most sports and in normal daily activities.

The exercise patterns have three component movements: flexion-extension, abduction-adduction, and internal-external rotation. Human movement is patterned and rarely involves straight motion because all muscles are spiral in nature and lie in diagonal directions.

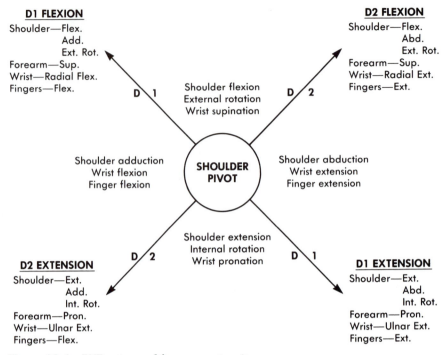

D1 FLEXION
Shoulder—Flex.
       Add.
       Ext. Rot.
Forearm—Sup.
Wrist—Radial Flex.
Fingers—Flex.

D2 FLEXION
Shoulder—Flex.
       Abd.
       Ext. Rot.
Forearm—Sup.
Wrist—Radial Ext.
Fingers—Ext.

D 1

Shoulder flexion
External rotation
Wrist supination

D 2

Shoulder adduction
Wrist flexion
Finger flexion

SHOULDER PIVOT

Shoulder abduction
Wrist extension
Finger extension

Shoulder extension
Internal rotation
Wrist pronation

D 2

D 1

D2 EXTENSION
Shoulder—Ext.
       Add.
       Int. Rot.
Forearm—Pron.
Wrist—Ulnar Ext.
Fingers—Flex.

D1 EXTENSION
Shoulder—Ext.
       Abd.
       Int. Rot.
Forearm—Pron.
Wrist—Ulnar Ext.
Fingers—Ext.

Figure 13-4   PNF patterns of the upper extremity.

The PNF patterns described by Knott and Voss[11] involve distinct diagonal and rotational movements of the upper extremity, lower extremity, upper trunk, lower trunk, and neck. The exercise pattern is initiated with the muscle groups in the lengthened or stretched position. The muscle group is then contracted, moving the body part through the range of motion to a shortened position.

The upper and lower extremities all have two separate patterns of diagonal movement for each part of the body, which are referred to as the diagonal 1 (D1) and diagonal 2 (D2) patterns. These diagonal patterns are subdivided into D1 moving into flexion, D1 moving into extension, D2 moving into flexion, and D2 moving into extension. Figures 13-4 and 13-5 diagram the PNF patterns for the upper and lower extremities respectively. The patterns are named according to the proximal pivots at either the shoulder or the hip (for example, the glenohumeral joint or femoralacetabular joint).

Tables 13-1 and 13-2 describe specific movements in the D1 and D2 patterns for the upper extremities. Figures 13-6 through 13-13 show starting and terminal positions for each of the diagonal patterns in the upper extremity.

Tables 13-3 and 13-4 describe specific movements in the D1 and D2 patterns for the lower extremities. Figures 13-14 through 13-21 show the starting and terminal positions for each of the diagonal patterns in the lower extremity.

Table 13-5 describes the rotational movement of the upper trunk moving into extension (also called chopping) and moving into flexion (also called lifting). Figures 13-22 and 13-23 show the starting and terminal positions of the upper-extremity chopping pattern moving into flexion to the right. Figures 13-24 and 13-25 show the starting and terminal positions for the upper-extremity lifting pattern moving into extension to the right.

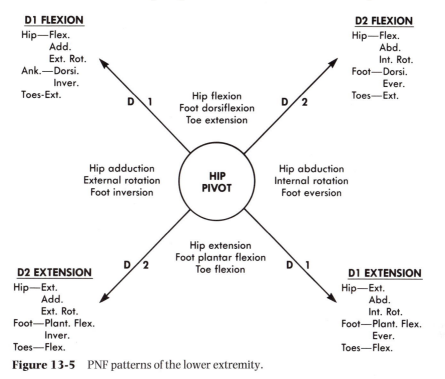

D1 FLEXION
Hip—Flex.
   Add.
   Ext. Rot.
Ank.—Dorsi.
   Inver.
Toes-Ext.

D2 FLEXION
Hip—Flex.
   Abd.
   Int. Rot.
Foot—Dorsi.
   Ever.
Toes—Ext.

Hip flexion
Foot dorsiflexion
Toe extension

Hip adduction
External rotation
Foot inversion

HIP PIVOT

Hip abduction
Internal rotation
Foot eversion

Hip extension
Foot plantar flexion
Toe flexion

D2 EXTENSION
Hip—Ext.
   Add.
   Ext. Rot.
Foot—Plant. Flex.
   Inver.
Toes—Flex.

D1 EXTENSION
Hip—Ext.
   Abd.
   Int. Rot.
Foot—Plant. Flex.
   Ever.
Toes—Flex.

Figure 13-5   PNF patterns of the lower extremity.

■ **TABLE 13-1**   D1 Upper-Extremity Movement Patterns

	Moving into Flexion		Moving into Extension	
Body Part	**Starting Position (Figure 13-6)**	**Terminal Position (Figure 13-7)**	**Starting Position (Figure 13-8)**	**Terminal Position (Figure 13-9)**
Shoulder	Extended	Flexed	Flexed	Extended
	Abducted	Adducted	Adducted	Abducted
	Internally rotated	Externally rotated	Externally rotated	Internally rotated
Scapula	Depressed	Flexed	Elevated	Depressed
	Retracted	Protracted	Protracted	Retracted
	Downwardly rotated	Upwardly rotated	Upwardly rotated	Downwardly rotated
Forearm	Pronated	Supinated	Supinated	Pronated
Wrist	Ulnar extended	Radially flexed	Radially flexed	Ulnar extended
Finger and thumb	Extended	Flexed	Flexed	Extended
	Abducted	Adducted	Adducted	Abducted
Hand position for sports therapist*	Left and inside of volar surface of hand		Left hand on back of elbow on humerus	
	Right hand underneath arm in cubital fossa of elbow		Right hand on dorsum of hand	
Verbal command	Pull		Push	

*For athlete's right arm.

■ **TABLE 13-2** D2 Upper-Extremity Movement Patterns

	Moving into Flexion		Moving into Extension	
Body Part	Starting Position (Figure 13-10)	Terminal Position (Figure 13-11)	Starting Position (Figure 13-12)	Terminal Position (Figure 13-13)
Shoulder	Extended	Flexed	Flexed	Extended
	Abducted	Adducted	Adducted	Abducted
	Internally rotated	Externally rotated	Externally rotated	Internally rotated
Scapula	Depressed	Flexed	Elevated	Depressed
	Retracted	Protracted	Protracted	Retracted
	Downwardly rotated	Upwardly rotated	Upwardly rotated	Downwardly rotated
Forearm	Pronated	Supinated	Supinated	Pronated
Wrist	Ulnar flexed	Radially extended	Radially flexed	Ulnar flexed
Finger and thumb	Flexed	Extended	Extended	Flexed
	Adducted	Abducted	Abducted	Adducted
Hand position for sports therapist*	Left hand on back of humerus		Left hand on volar surface of humerus	
	Right hand on dorsum of hand		Right hand on cubital fossa of elbow	
Verbal command	Push		Pull	

*For athlete's right arm.

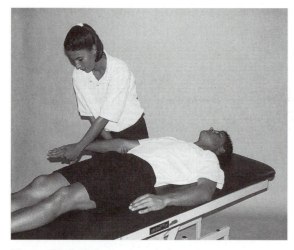

Figure 13-6 D1 upper-extremity movement pattern moving into flexion. Starting position.

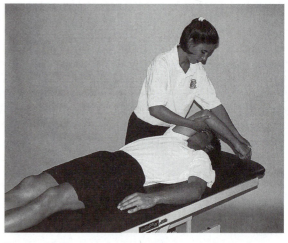

Figure 13-7 D1 upper-extremity movement pattern moving into flexion. Terminal position.

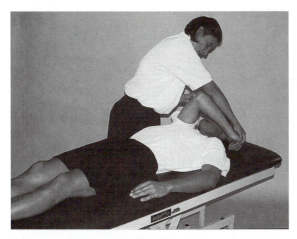

Figure 13-8 D1 upper-extremity movement pattern moving into extension. Starting position.

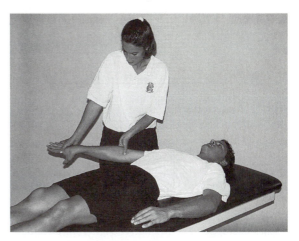

Figure 13-9 D1 upper-extremity movement pattern moving into extension. Terminal position.

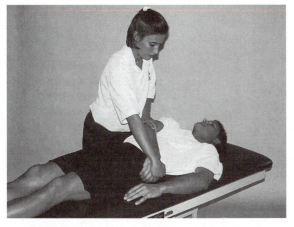

Figure 13-10 D2 upper-extremity movement pattern moving into flexion. Starting position.

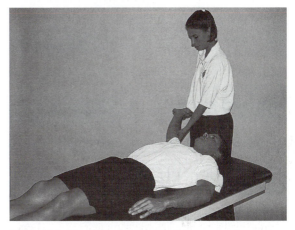

Figure 13-11 D2 upper-extremity movement pattern moving into flexion. Terminal position.

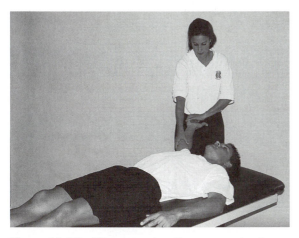

Figure 13-12 D2 upper-extremity movement pattern moving into extension. Starting position.

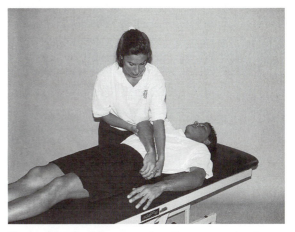

Figure 13-13 D2 upper-extremity movement pattern moving into extension. Terminal position.

■ **TABLE 13-3** D1 Lower-Extremity Movement Patterns

Body Part	Moving into Flexion		Moving into Extension	
	Starting Position (Figure 13-14)	Terminal Position (Figure 13-15)	Starting Position (Figure 13-16)	Terminal Position (Figure 13-17)
Hip	Extended	Flexed	Flexed	Extended
	Abducted	Adducted	Adducted	Abducted
	Internally rotated	Externally rotated	Externally rotated	Internally rotated
Knee	Extended	Flexed	Flexed	Extended
Position of tibia	Externally rotated	Internally rotated	Internally rotated	Externally rotated
Ankle and foot	Plantar flexed	Dorsiflexed	Dorsiflexed	Plantar flexed
	Everted	Inverted	Inverted	Everted
Toes	Flexed	Extended	Extended	Flexed
Hand position for sports therapist*	Right hand on dorsimedial surface of foot Left hand on anteromedial thigh near patella		Right hand on lateralplantar surface of foot Left hand on posteriolateral thigh near popliteal crease	
Verbal command	Pull		Push	

*For athlete's right leg.

■ **TABLE 13-4** D2 Lower-Extremity Movement Patterns

Body Part	Moving into Flexion		Moving into Extension	
	Starting Position (Figure 13-18)	Terminal Position (Figure 13-19)	Starting Position (Figure 13-20)	Terminal Position (Figure 13-21)
Hip	Extended	Flexed	Flexed	Extended
	Adducted	Abducted	Abducted	Adducted
	Externally rotated	Internally rotated	Internally rotated	Externally rotated
Knee	Extended	Flexed	Flexed	Extended
Position of tibia	Externally rotated	Internally rotated	Internally rotated	Externally rotated
Ankle and foot	Plantar flexed	Dorsiflexed	Dorsiflexed	Plantar flexed
	Inverted	Everted	Everted	Inverted
Toes	Flexed	Extended	Extended	Flexed
Hand position for sports therapist*	Right hand on dorsilateral surface of foot Left hand on anterolateral thigh near patella		Right hand on medialplantar surface of foot Left hand on posteriomedial thigh near popliteal crease	
Verbal command	Pull		Push	

*For athlete's right leg.

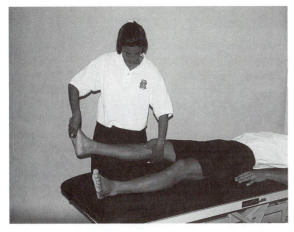

Figure 13-14 D1 lower-extremity movement pattern moving into flexion. Starting position.

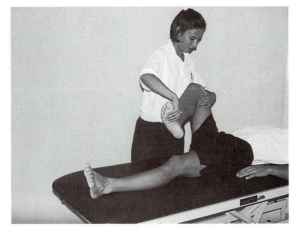

Figure 13-15 D1 lower-extremity movement pattern moving into flexion. Terminal position.

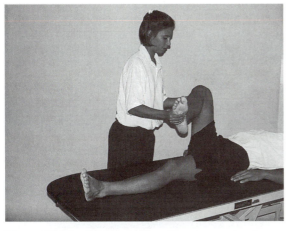

Figure 13-16 D1 lower-extremity movement pattern moving into extension. Starting position.

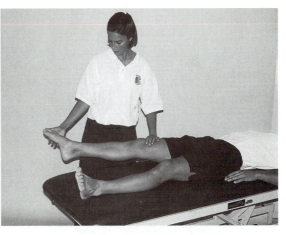

Figure 13-17 D1 lower-extremity movement pattern moving into extension. Terminal position.

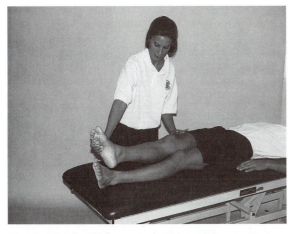

Figure 13-18 D2 lower-extremity movement pattern moving into flexion. Starting position.

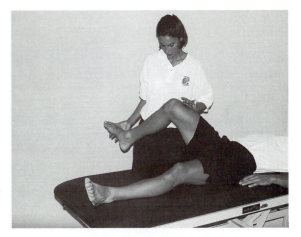

Figure 13-19 D2 lower-extremity movement pattern moving into flexion. Terminal position.

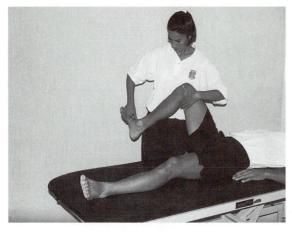

Figure 13-20 D2 lower-extremity movement pattern moving into extension. Starting position.

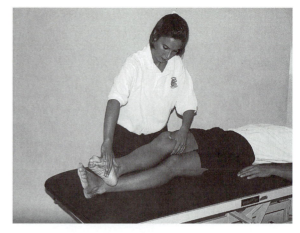

Figure 13-21 D2 lower-extremity movement pattern moving into extension. Terminal position.

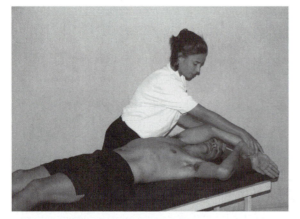

Figure 13-22 Upper-trunk pattern moving into extension or chopping. Starting position.

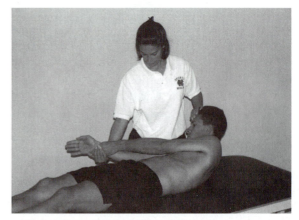

Figure 13-23 Upper-trunk pattern moving into extension or chopping. Terminal position.

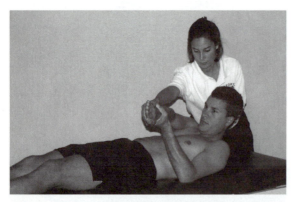

Figure 13-24 Upper-trunk pattern moving into flexion or lifting. Starting position.

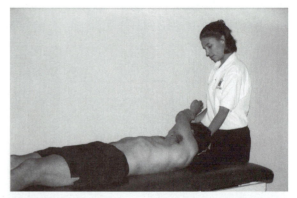

Figure 13-25 Upper-trunk pattern moving into flexion or lifting. Terminal position.

■ **TABLE 13-5** Upper-Trunk Movement Patterns

Body Part	Moving into Extension (Chopping)*		Moving into Flexion (Lifting)*	
	Starting Position (Figure 13-22)	Terminal Position (Figure 13-23)	Starting Position (Figure 13-24)	Terminal Position (Figure 13-25)
Right upper extremity	Flexed Adducted Internally rotated	Extended Abducted Externally rotated	Extended Adducted Internally rotated	Flexed Abducted Externally rotated
Left upper extremity (left hand grasps right forearm)	Flexed Abducted Externally rotated	Extended Adducted Internally rotated	Extended Abducted Externally rotated	Flexed Adducted Internally rotated
Trunk	Rotated and extended to left	Rotated and flexed to right	Rotated and flexed to left	Rotated and extended to right
Head	Rotated and extended to left	Rotated and flexed to right	Rotated and flexed to left	Rotated and extended to right
Hand position of sports therapist	Left hand on right anterolateral surface of forehead Right hand on dorsum of right hand		Right hand on dorsum of right hand Left hand on posteriolateral surface of head	
Verbal command	Pull down		Push up	

*Athlete's rotation is to the right.

■ **TABLE 13-6** Lower Trunk Movement Patterns

Body Part	Moving into Flexion*		Moving into Extension*	
	Starting Position (Figure 13-26)	Terminal Position (Figure 13-27)	Starting Position (Figure 13-28)	Terminal Position (Figure 13-29)
Right hip	Extended Abducted Externally rotated	Flexed Adducted Internally rotated	Flexed Adducted Internally rotated	Extended Abducted Externally rotated
Left hip	Extended Adducted Internally rotated	Flexed Abducted Externally rotated	Flexed Abducted Externally rotated	Extended Adducted Internally rotated
Ankles	Plantar flexed	Dorsiflexed	Dorsiflexed	Plantar flexed
Toes	Flexed	Extended	Extended	Flexed
Hand position of sports therapist	Right hand on dorsum of feet Left hand on anterolateral surface of left knee		Right hand on plantar surface of foot Left hand on posteriolateral surface of right knee	
Verbal command	Pull up and in		Push down and out	

*Athlete's rotation is to the left in flexion.
†Athlete's rotation is to the right in extension.

Table 13-6 describes rotational movement of the lower extremities moving into positions of flexion and extension. Figures 13-26 and 13-27 show the lower-extremity pattern moving into flexion to the left. Figures 13-28 and 13-29 show the lower-extremity pattern moving into extension to the left.

The neck patterns involve simply flexion and rotation to one side (Figures 13-30 and 13-31) with extension and rotation to the opposite side (Figures 13-32 and 13-33). The patient should follow the direction of the movement with their eyes.

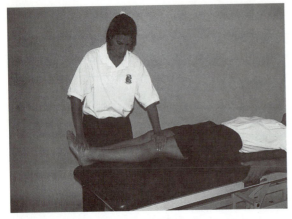

Figure 13-26 Lower-trunk pattern moving into flexion to the left. Starting position.

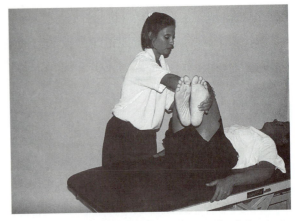

Figure 13-27 Lower-trunk pattern moving into flexion to the left. Terminal position.

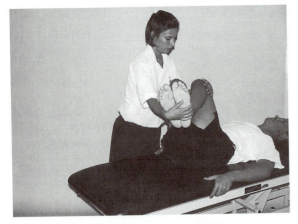

Figure 13-28 Lower-trunk pattern moving into extension to the left. Starting position.

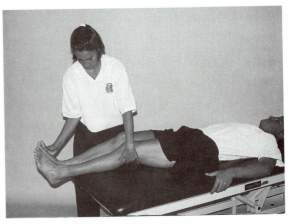

Figure 13-29 Lower-trunk pattern moving into extension to the left. Terminal position.

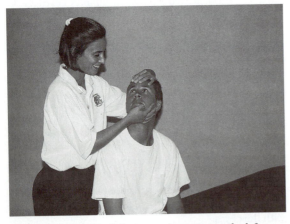

Figure 13-30 Neck flexion and rotation to the left. Starting position.

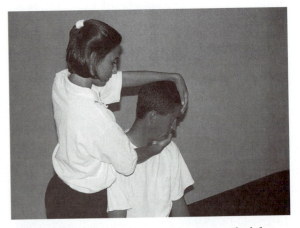

Figure 13-31 Neck flexion and rotation to the left. Terminal position.

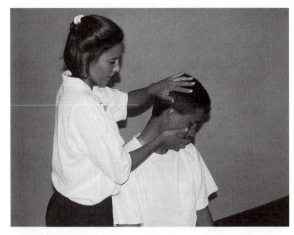

Figure 13-32 Neck extension and rotation to the right. Starting position.

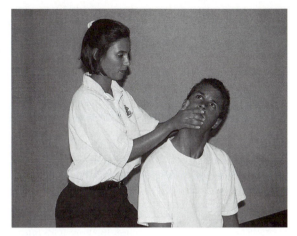

Figure 13-33 Neck extension and rotation to the right. Terminal position.

The principles and techniques of PNF, when used appropriately with specific patterns, can be an extremely effective tool for rehabilitation of sport-related injuries.[26] They can be used to strengthen weak muscles or muscle groups and to improve the range of motion about an injured joint. Specific techniques selected for use should depend on individual patient needs and may be modified accordingly.[5,6]

MUSCLE ENERGY TECHNIQUES

Muscle energy is a manual therapy technique that is a variation of the PNF contract-relax and hold-relax techniques. Like the PNF techniques, the muscle energy techniques are based on the same neurophysiological mechanisms involving the stretch reflex discussed earlier in this chapter. Muscle energy techniques involve a voluntary contraction of a muscle in a specifically controlled direction at varied levels of intensity against a distinctly executed counterforce applied by the sports therapist.[10] The patient provides the corrective *intrinsic* forces and controls the intensity of the muscular contractions while the sports therapist controls the precision and localization of the procedure.[14] The amount of patient effort can vary from a minimal muscle twitch to a maximal muscle contraction.[10]

Five components are necessary for muscle energy techniques to be effective:[10]

1. Active muscle contraction by the patient
2. A muscle contraction oriented in a specific direction
3. Some patient control of contraction intensity
4. Sports therapist control of joint position

5. Sports therapist application of appropriate counterforce

Clinical Applications

It has been proposed that muscles function not only as flexors, extenders, rotators, and side-benders of joints, but also as restrictors of joint motion. In situations where the muscle is restricting joint motion, muscle energy techniques use a specific muscle contraction to restore physiological movement to a joint.[14] Any articulation, whether in the spine or in the extremities, that can be moved by active muscle contraction can be treated using muscle energy techniques.

Muscle energy techniques can be used to accomplish a number of treatment goals:[10]

1. Lengthening of a shortened, contracted, or spastic muscle
2. Strengthening of a weak muscle or muscle group
3. Reduction of localized edema through muscle pumping
4. Mobilization of an articulation with restricted mobility
5. Stretching of fascia

Treatment Techniques

Muscle energy techniques can involve four types of muscle contraction: isometric, concentric isotonic, eccentric isotonic, and **isolytic.** An isolytic contraction involves a concentric contraction by the patient while the sports therapist applies an external force in the opposite direction, overpowering the contraction and lengthening that muscle.[14]

Isometric and concentric isotonic contractions are most frequently used in treatment. Isometric contractions are most often used in treating hypertonic muscles in the spinal vertebral column; isotonic contractions are most often used in the extremities. With both types of contraction the idea is to inhibit antagonistic muscles producing more symmetrical muscle tone and balance.

A concentric contraction can also be used to mobilize a joint against its *motion barrier* if there is motion restriction. For example, if a knee has a restriction due to tightness in the hamstrings that is limiting full extension, the following isometric muscle energy technique should be used (Figure 13-34):

1. The athlete should lie prone on the treatment table.
2. The sports therapist stabilizes the knee with one hand and grasps the ankle with the other.
3. The sports therapist fully extends the knee until an extension barrier is felt.
4. The athlete is instructed to actively flex the knee using a minimal sustained force.
5. The sports therapist provides an equal resistant counterforce for 3 to 7 seconds, after which the athlete completely relaxes.
6. The sports therapist once again extends the knee until a new extension barrier is felt.
7. This is repeated 3 to 5 times.

If a strength imbalance exists between the quadriceps and hamstrings, with weak quadriceps limiting knee extension, the following concentric isotonic muscle energy technique may be used:

1. The athlete should lie supine on the treatment table.
2. The sports therapist stabilizes the knee with one hand and grasps the ankle with the other.
3. The sports therapist fully flexes the knee.
4. The athlete is instructed to actively extend the knee, using as much force as possible.

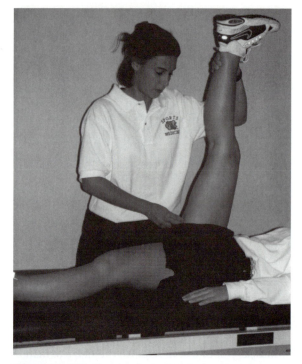

Figure 13-34   Position for isometric muscle energy technique for tightness of the hamstring muscle.

5. The sports therapist provides a resistant counterforce that allows slow knee extension throughout the available range.
6. Once the athlete has completely relaxed, the sports therapist moves the knee back to full flexion and the athlete repeats the contraction with additional resistance applied through the full range of extension. This is repeated 3 to 5 times with increasing resistance on each repetition.

Summary

1. The PNF techniques may be used to increase both strength and range of motion and are based on the neurophysiology of the stretch reflex.
2. The motor neurons of the spinal cord always receive a combination of inhibitory and excitatory impulses from the afferent nerves. Whether these motor neurons will be excited or inhibited depends on the ratio of the two types of incoming impulses.
3. The PNF techniques emphasize specific principles that may be superimposed on any of the specific techniques.
4. The PNF strengthening techniques include repeated contraction, slow-reversal, slow-reversal-hold, rhythmic stabilization, and rhythmic initiation.
5. The PNF stretching techniques include contract-relax, hold-relax, and slow-reversal-hold-relax.
6. The techniques of PNF are rotational and diagonal movements in the upper extremity, lower extremity, upper trunk, and the head and neck.
7. Muscle energy techniques involve a voluntary contraction of a muscle in a specifically controlled direction at varied levels of intensity against a distinctly executed counterforce applied by the sports therapist.

References

1. Barak, T., E. Rosen, and R. Sofer. 1985. Mobility: Passive orthopedic manual therapy. In *Orthopedic and sports physical therapy*, edited by J. Gould and G. Davies. St. Louis: Mosby.

2. Basmajian, J. 1978. *Therapeutic exercise*. Baltimore: Williams & Wilkins.

3. Bobath, B. 1955. The treatment of motor disorders of pyramidal and extrapyramidal tracts by reflex inhibition and by facilitation of movement. *Physiotherapy* 41:146.

4. Brunnstrom, S. 1970. *Movement therapy in hemiplegia*. New York: Harper & Row.

5. Cookson, J. 1979. Orthopedic manual therapy: An overview: II. The spine. *Journal of the American Physical Therapy Association* 59:259.

6. Cookson, J., and B. Kent. 1979. Orthopedic manual therapy: An overview: I. The extremities. *Journal of the American Physical Therapy Association* 59:136.

7. Cornelius, W., and A. Jackson. 1984. The effects of cryotherapy and PNF on hip extension flexibility. *Athletic Training* 19(3): 184.

8. Engle, R., and G. Canner. 1989. Proprioceptive neuromuscular facilitation (PNF) and modified procedures for anterior cruciate ligament (ACL) instability. *Journal of Orthopaedic and Sports Physical Therapy* 11(6): 230–6.

9. Greenman, P. 1993. *Principles of manual medicine*. Baltimore: Williams & Wilkins.

10. Hollis, M. 1981. *Practical exercise*. Oxford: Blackwell Scientific.

11. Knott, M., and D. Voss. 1968. *Proprioceptive neuromuscular facilitation: Patterns and techniques*. New York: Harper & Row.

12. Lloyd, D. 1946. Facilitation and inhibition of spinal motorneurons. *Journal of Neurophysiology* 9:421.

13. Markos, P. 1979. Ipsilateral and contralateral effects of proprioceptive neuromuscular facilitation techniques on hip motion and electromyographic activity. *Physical Therapy* 59(11)P: 1366–73.

14. Mitchell, F. 1993. Elements of muscle energy technique. In *Rational manual therapies*, edited by J. Basmajian and R. Nyberg. Baltimore: Williams & Wilkins.

15. Osternig, L., R. Robertson, R. Troxel, et al. 1990. Differential responses to proprioceptive neuromuscular facilitation stretch techniques. *Medicine and Science in Sports and Exercise* 22:106–11.

16. Osternig, L., R. Robertson, R. Troxel, and P. Hansen. 1987. Muscle activation during proprioceptive neuromuscular facilitation (PNF) stretching techniques . . . stretch-relax (SR), contract-relax (CR) and agonist contract-relax (ACR). *American Journal of Physical Medicine* 66(5): 298–307.

17. Prentice, W. 1993. *Proprioceptive neuromuscular facilitation* [Videotape]. St. Louis: Mosby.

18. Prentice, W. 1982. An electromyographic analysis of heat and cold and stretching for inducing muscular relaxation. *Journal of Orthopaedic and Sports Physical Therapy* 3:133–40.

19. Prentice, W. 1983. A comparison of static stretching and PNF stretching for improving hip joint flexibility. *Athletic Training* 18(1): 56–59.

20. Prentice, W. 1988. A manual resistance technique for strengthening tibial rotation. *Athletic Training* 23(3): 230–33.

21. Prentice, W., and E. Kooima. 1986. The use of proprioceptive neuromuscular facilitation techniques in the rehabilitation of sport-related injuries. *Athletic Training* 21:26–31.

22. Rood, M. 1954. Neurophysiologic reactions as a basis of physical therapy. *Physical Therapy Review* 34:444.

23. Saliba, V., G. Johnson, and C. Wardlaw. 1993. Proprioceptive neuromuscular facilitation. In *Rational manual therapies*, edited by J. Basmajian and R. Nyberg. Baltimore: Williams & Wilkins.

24. Sherrington, C. 1947. *The integrative action of the nervous system*. New Haven: Yale University Press.

25. Surburg, P., and J. Schrader. 1997. Proprioceptive neuromuscular facilitation techniques in sports medicine: A reassessment. *Journal of Athletic Training* 32(1): 34–39.

26. Surberg, P. 1954. Neuromuscular facilitation techniques in sportsmedicine. *Physical Therapy Review* 34:444.

27. Taniqawa, M. 1972. Comparison of the hold-relax procedure and passive mobilization on increasing muscle length. *Physical Therapy* 52(7): 725–35.

28. Worrell, T., T. Smith, and J. Winegardner. 1994. Effect of hamstring stretching on hamstring muscle performance. *Journal of Orthopaedic and Sports Physical Therapy* 20(3): 154–59.

29. Zohn, D., and J. Mennell. 1976. *Musculoskeletal pain: Diagnosis and physical treatment*. Boston: Little, Brown.

CHAPTER 14

Aquatic Therapy in Rehabilitation

Gina Selepak

After completion of this chapter, the student should be able to do the following:

- Explain the principles of buoyancy and specific gravity and the role they have in the aquatic environment.

- Identify and describe the three major resistive forces at work in the aquatic environment.

- Discuss the advantages and disadvantages of aquatic therapy in relation to traditional land exercises.

- Identify and describe the two prominent techniques of aquatic therapy.

In the past decade, widespread interest has developed in the area of aquatic therapy. It has rapidly become a popular rehabilitation technique among sports therapists. This newfound interest has sparked numerous research efforts to evaluate the effectiveness of aquatic therapy as a therapeutic modality. Current research shows aquatic therapy to be beneficial in the treatment of everything from orthopedic injuries to spinal cord damage, chronic pain, cerebral palsy, multiple sclerosis, and many other conditions, making it useful in a variety of settings.[23] It is also gaining acceptance as a preventative maintenance tool to facilitate overall fitness and sport-specific skills for healthy athletes.[19,21] Movement skills, conditioning, and strength can all be enhanced by aquatic therapy.[12]

Water healing techniques have been traced back through history as early as 2400 B.C., but it was not until the late nineteenth century that more traditional water exercise types of aquatic therapy came into existence. The development of the Hubbard tank in 1920 sparked the initiation of present-day therapeutic water exercise by allowing aquatic therapy to be conducted in a highly controlled, clinical setting.[6] Loeman and Roen took this a step farther in 1924 and stimulated interest in actual pool therapy. Only recently, however, has water come into its own as a therapeutic exercise medium.[25]

Aquatic therapy is believed to be successful because it lowers pain levels by decreasing joint compression forces. The perception of weightlessness experienced in the water seems to eliminate or drastically reduce the body's protective muscular guarding. This results in decreased muscular spasm and pain that can carry over into the patient's daily functional activities.[31] The primary goal of aquatic therapy is to teach the athlete how to use water as a modality for improving movement and fitness.[2] Then, along with other therapeutic modalities and treatments, aquatic therapy can become one more link in the athlete's recovery chain.[1]

PHYSICAL PROPERTIES AND RESISTIVE FORCES

The sports therapist must understand several physical properties of the water before designing an aquatic therapy program. Land exercise cannot always be converted to aquatic exercise, because buoyancy rather than gravity is the major force governing movement. A thorough understanding of buoyancy, specific gravity, the resistive forces of the water, and their relationships must be the groundwork of any aquatics program. The program must also be specific and individualized to the athlete's particular injury and sport if it is to be successful.

Buoyancy

Buoyancy is one of the primary forces involved in aquatic therapy. All objects, on land or in the water, are subjected to the downward pull of the earth's gravity. In the water, however, this force is counteracted to some degree by the upward buoyant force. According to Archimedes' Principle, any object submerged or floating in water is buoyed upward by a counterforce that helps support the submerged or partially submerged object against the downward pull of gravity. In other words, the buoyant force assists motion toward the water's surface and resists motion away from the surface.[15] Because of this buoyant force, a person entering the water experiences an apparent loss of weight.[10] The weight loss experienced is nearly equal to the weight of the liquid that is displaced when the object enters the water (Figure 14-1).

For example, a 100-pound individual, when almost completely submerged, displaces a volume of water that weighs nearly 95 pounds; therefore that person feels as though she or he weighs less than 5 pounds. This sensation occurs because, when partially submerged, the individual only bears the weight of the part of the body that is above the water. With immersion to the level of the seventh cervical vertebra, both males and females only bear approximately 6 to 10 percent of their total body weight (TBW). The percentages increase to 25 to 31 percent TBW for females and 30 to 37 percent TBW for males at the xiphisternal level and 40 to 51 percent TBW for females and 50 to 56 percent TBW for males at the anterosuperior iliac spine (ASIS) level[16] (Table 14-1). The percentages differ for males and females due to the

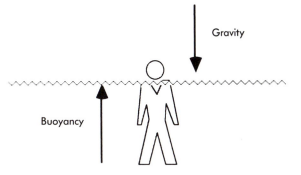

Figure 14-1   The buoyant force.

■ TABLE 14-1   Weight-Bearing Percentages

	Percentage of Weight Bearing	
Body Level	**Male**	**Female**
C7	8%	8%
Xiphisternal	28%	35%
ASIS	47%	54%

differences in centers of gravity. Males carry a higher percentage of their weight in the upper body, whereas females carry a higher percentage of their weight in the lower body. The center of gravity on land corresponds with a center of buoyancy in the water.[25] Also, variations of build and body type only minimally effect weight bearing values. Due to the decreased percentage of weight bearing each joint that is below the water is decompressed. This allows ambulation and vigorous exercise to be performed with little impact and drastically reduced friction between joint articular surfaces.

Specific Gravity

Buoyancy is partially dependent on body weight. However, the weight of different parts of the body is not a constant. Therefore, the buoyant values of different body parts will also vary. Buoyant values can be determined by several factors. The ratio of bone weight to muscle weight, the amount and distribution of fat, and the depth and expansion of the chest all play a role. Together, these factors determine the specific gravity of the individual body part. On the average, humans have a specific gravity slightly less than that of water. Any object with a specific gravity less than that of water will float. A specific

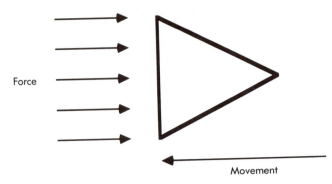

Figure 14-2 The bow force.

gravity greater than that of water will cause the object to sink. However, as with buoyant values, the specific gravity of all body parts is not uniform. Therefore, even with a total-body specific gravity of less than the specific gravity of water, the individual might not float horizontally in the water. Additionally, the lungs, when filled with air, can further decrease the specific gravity of the chest area. This allows the head and chest to float higher in the water than the heavier, denser extremities. Therefore, compensation with flotation devices at the extremities might be necessary for some treatments.

Resistive Forces

When an object moves in the water, just as on land, several resistive forces are at work that must be overcome. These forces include the cohesive force, the bow force, and the drag force.

Cohesive Force. There is a slight but easily overcome cohesive force that runs in a parallel direction to the water surface. This resistance is formed by the water molecules loosely binding together, creating a surface tension. Surface tension can be seen in still water, because the water remains motionless with the cohesive force intact unless disturbed.

Bow Force. A second force is the bow force, or the force that is generated at the front of the object during movement. When the object moves, the bow force causes an increase in the water pressure at the front of the object and a decrease in the water pressure at the rear of the object. This pressure change causes a movement of water from the high-pressure area in the front to the low-pressure area behind the object. As the water enters the low-pressure area, it swirls into the low-pressure zone and forms eddies, or small whirlpool turbulences.[9] These

eddies impede flow by creating a backward force, or drag force (Figure 14-2).

Drag Force. This third force, the drag force, is very important in aquatic therapy. The bow force, and therefore also the drag force, on an object can be controlled by changing the shape of the object or the speed of its movement (Figure 14-3).

Frictional resistance can be decreased by making the object more streamlined. This change minimizes the surface area at the front of the object. Less surface area causes less bow force and less of a change in pressure between the front and rear of the object, resulting in less drag force. In a streamlined flow, the resistance is proportional to the velocity of the object. Therefore, to assist a weak athlete, exercises should be performed slowly in the most streamlined position possible in order to decrease resistance to movement (Figure 14-4).

On the other hand, if the object is not streamlined, a turbulent situation exists. In a turbulent situation, drag is a function of the velocity squared. Therefore by increasing the speed of movement 2 times, the resistance the object must overcome is increased 4 times.[10] This provides a method to increase resistance progressively during aquatic rehabilitation. However, increases in speed also affect stability adversely. Single-limb movements are generally not as affected as trunk exercise by this loss of stability. Considerable turbulence can be generated when the speed of movement is increased, causing the muscles to work harder to keep the movement going. This is especially true when changes of direction take place. Therefore, by simply changing the shape of a limb through the addition of rehabilitation equipment or increasing the speed of movement, the sports therapist can modify the athlete's workout intensity to match strength increases (Figure 14-5).

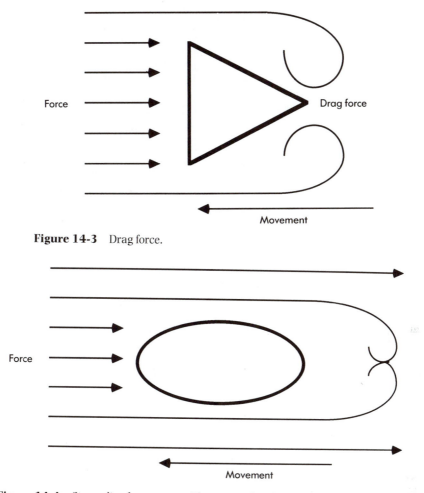

Figure 14-3 Drag force.

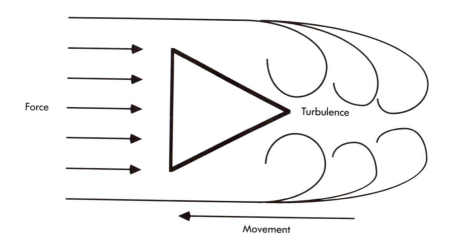

Figure 14-4 Streamlined movement. This creates less drag force and less turbulence.

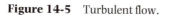

Figure 14-5 Turbulent flow.

ADVANTAGES OF AQUATIC REHABILITATION

The addition of an aquatic therapy program can offer many advantages to an athlete's therapy.[13] The buoyancy of the water allows active exercise while providing a sense of security and causing little discomfort.[28] Utilizing a combination of the water's buoyancy, resistance, and warmth, the athlete can typically achieve more in the aquatic environment than is possible on land.[21] Early in the rehabilitation process, aquatic therapy is useful in restoring range of motion and flexibility. As normal function is restored, resistance training and sport-specific activities can be added.

Following an injury, the aquatic experience provides a medium where early motion can be performed in a supportive environment. The slow-motion effect of moving through water provides extra time to control movement, which allows the athlete to experience multiple movement errors without severe consequences.[27] This is especially helpful in lower-extremity injuries where balance and proprioception are impaired. The increased amount of time to react, combined with a medium in which the fear of falling is removed, assists the athlete's ability to regain proprioception. Additionally, tactile stimulation from the turbulence generated during movement provides feedback that aids in the return of proprioception and balance. The warmth of the water also helps induce muscular relaxation. The stimulation from the aquatic environment can act as a gating mechanism, decreasing pain. This allows greater pain-free range of motion. There is also an often overlooked benefit of edema reduction due to hydrostatic pressure. This would benefit pain reduction and increase range of motion.

Using the buoyant principles, the aquatic environment can provide a gradual transition from non-weight-bearing to full-weight-bearing land exercises. This gradual increase in percentage of weight bearing helps provide a return to smooth, coordinated movements that are pain-free. By utilizing the buoyant force to decrease apparent weight and joint compressive forces, locomotor activities can begin much earlier following an injury to the lower extremity. This provides an enormous advantage to the athletic population. The ability to work out hard without the fear of reinjury provides a psychological boost to the athlete. This helps keep motivation high and can help speed the athlete's return to normal function.[21] Psychologically, aquatic therapy increases confidence, because the athlete experiences increased success at locomotor, stretching, or strengthening activities in the water. Tension and anxiety are decreased, and athlete morale increases, as does postexercise vigor.[9,10,25]

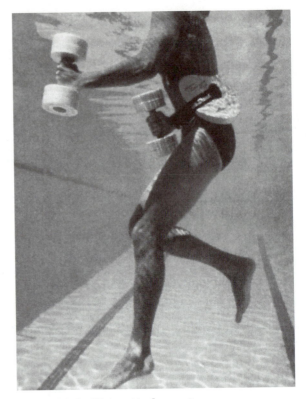

Figure 14-6   Wet vest in deep water.

Through careful use of Archimedes' Principle, a gradual increase in the percentage of weight bearing can be undertaken. Initially, the athlete would begin non-weight-bearing in the deep end of the pool. A wet vest or similar buoyant device might be used to help the athlete remain afloat for the desired exercises (Figure 14-6). If such a device is unavailable, empty plastic milk jugs held in each hand are also a quite effective and very inexpensive method of flotation (Figure 14-7).

Once therapy has progressed, the athlete could be moved to neck-deep water to begin light weight bearing. Gradual increases in the percentage of weight bearing are accomplished by systematically moving the athlete to shallower water. Even when in waist-deep water, both male and female athletes are only bearing approximately 50 percent of their TBW. By placing a sinkable bench or chair in the shallow water, step-ups can be initiated under partial-weight-bearing conditions long before the athlete is capable of performing the same exercise in full weight bearing on land. Thus the advantages of low weight bearing are coupled with the proprioceptive benefits of closed-kinetic-chain exercise, making aquatic therapy an excellent functional rehabilitation activity.

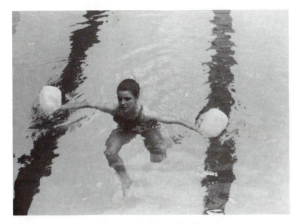

Figure 14-7 Milk jugs in water for flotation.

Muscular strengthening and reeducation can also be accomplished through aquatic therapy.[26] Progressive resistance exercises can be increased in extremely small increments by using combinations of different resistive forces. The intensity of exercise can be controlled by manipulating the body's position or through the addition of exercise equipment. This allows individuals with minimal muscle contraction capabilities to do work and see improvement. Yet the aquatic environment can still provide a challenging resistive workout to an athlete nearing full recovery. Additionally, the water serves as an accommodating resistance medium. This allows the muscles to be maximally stressed through the full range of motion available. One drawback to this, however, is that strength gains depend largely on the effort exerted by the athlete, which is not easily quantified. Strength gains through aquatic exercises are also brought about by the increased energy needs of the body working in an aquatic environment. Studies have shown that aquatic exercise requires a higher energy expenditure than the same exercise performed on land. The athlete not only has to perform the activity but must also maintain a level of buoyancy and overcome the resistive forces of the water. For example, the energy cost for water running is four times greater than the energy cost for running the same distance on land.[9,10,20]

A simulated run in either shallow or deep water assisted by a tether or flotation devices can be an effective means of alternate fitness training for the injured athlete. Not only does the athlete benefit from early intervention, but the aquatic exercise helps prevent cardiorespiratory deconditioning through alterations in cardiovascular dynamics as a result of hydrostatic forces.[5,17,29] The heart actually functions more efficiently in the water. Hydrostatic pressure enhances venous return, leading to a greater stroke volume and a reduction in the heart rate

needed to maintain cardiac output.[30] There is also a decrease in ventilations and an increase in central blood volume. This means that the injured athlete can maintain a near-normal $\dot{V}O_2$max with aquatic exercise.[11,24] Due to the hydrostatic effects on heart efficiency, it has been suggested that an environment-specific exercise prescription is necessary.[19,29,32] Some research suggests the use of perceived exertion as a method for controlling exercise intensity. Other research continues to use target heart rate values as with land exercise, but compensates for the hydrostatic changes by setting the target range 10 percent lower than would be expected for land exercise. Regardless of the method used, the keys to successful use of aquatic therapy are supervision and monitoring of the athlete during activity and good communication between athlete and sports therapist.

DISADVANTAGES OF AQUATIC REHABILITATION

As with any therapeutic modality, aquatic therapy has its disadvantages. The cost of building and maintaining a rehabilitation pool, if there is no access to an existing facility, can be very high. Also, qualified pool attendants must be present, and the sports therapist involved in the treatment must be trained in aquatic safety and therapy procedures.[7,20]

An athlete who requires high levels of stabilization will be more challenging to work with, because stabilization in the water is considerably more difficult than on land. Stabilization of the sports therapist is just as important as stabilization of the injured athlete. A wide stance in the water will help provide a solid base and better support of the athlete by the sports therapist. Flotation devices placed at the neck, hips, and extremities can also help support the athlete in the water (Figure 14-8).[4]

The presence of any open wounds or sores on the patient is a contraindication to aquatic therapy, as are contagious skin diseases. This restriction is obvious for health reasons to reduce the chance of infection of the patient or of others who use the pool.[18,23] Because of this risk, all surgical wounds must be completely healed before the athlete enters the pool. An excessive fear of the water would also be a reason to keep an athlete out of an aquatic exercise program. Fever, urinary tract infections, allergies to the pool chemicals, cardiac problems, and uncontrolled seizures are also contraindications.

FACILITIES AND EQUIPMENT

When considering an existing facility or when planning to build one, certain characteristics of the pool should be

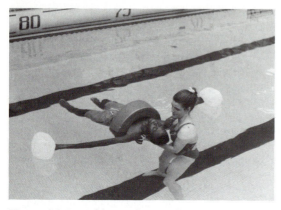

Figure 14-8 Athlete and sports therapist using shallow water with floats.

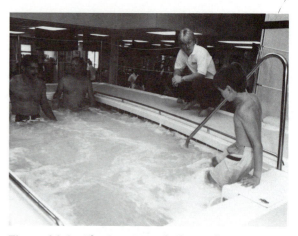

Figure 14-9 The SwimEx pool. This pool's even, controllable water flow allows for the application of individualized prescriptive exercise and therapeutic programs. As many as three patients can be treated simultaneously.

taken into consideration. The pool should not be smaller than 10 feet by 12 feet. It can be in-ground or above-ground as long as access for the athlete is well planned. Both a shallow area (2½ feet) and a deep area (5+ feet) should be present to allow standing exercise and swimming or nonstanding exercise.[8] The pool bottom should be flat and the depth gradations clearly marked. Water temperature will vary depending on the activity. For water exercise, 92 to 95° F is appropriate; however, lower temperatures of 85 to 90° F are more suitable for active swimming.[25] Temperature is an important factor, because water that is too warm can lead to fatigue or even heat exhaustion, and water that is too cool can cause shivering, increased muscular tension, or hypothermia.

Some prefabricated pools come with an in-water treadmill or current-producing device (Figure 14-9). These devices can be beneficial but are not essential to treatment. Rescue tubes, inner tubes, or wet vests can be purchased to assist in flotation activities such as deep-water running. Hand paddles and pull buoys are effective in strengthening the upper extremity, while kickboards and fins are useful for strengthening the lower extremity. Most of these products can be purchased from local sporting goods stores with no special ordering required. Equipment aids for aquatic therapy, or so called "pool toys," are limited only by the imagination of the sports therapist.[14] Plastic milk jugs, balls, and other common items can be substituted for the more expensive commercial equipment, with comparable results (Figure 14-10). What is important is to stimulate the athlete's interest in therapy and to keep in mind what goals are to be accomplished.

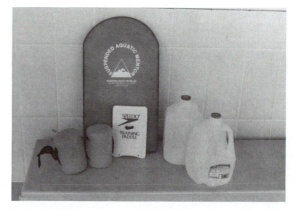

Figure 14-10 Aquatic exercise equipment. Kickboard, fins, pull buoys, paddles, wet vest, and rescue tube are common forms of exercise equipment.

TECHNIQUES

Designing an aquatic therapy program is very similar to designing a program for land exercises. A thorough history and evaluation of the injury is the first step. Once contraindications have been ruled out, the athlete's water safety skills, swimming ability, and general comfort level in the water should be evaluated. The athlete must be supervised at all times and should not be left unattended for any reason. From this point, an aquatic program that is specific and individualized can be developed using the principles of aquatic therapy techniques.[3]

Buoyancy Technique

Several popular aquatic therapy approaches are currently being used. The most common aquatic therapy technique seems to be the buoyancy technique. This technique is actually a three-part progression moving from buoyancy-assisted exercises to buoyancy-supported and finally to buoyancy-resisted exercises.[6] A rehabilitation progression would begin with the sports therapist assisting the athlete in the water through passive range of motion in any plane. Then the patient could move actively from below the water toward the surface in the buoyancy-assisted phase. The next phase would be to move parallel to the water surface while at the buoyant level. In this phase only the cohesive force is resisting motion. This would be a buoyancy-supported position. An intermediate stage would have movement start at the buoyant level and continue toward the surface. This stage is limited in use because some individuals' buoyant level is already at the surface. Therefore, no movement would be possible. In the buoyancy-resisted phase, the athlete would move downward from the buoyant level against the upward buoyant force. Finally, flotation devices could be used to increase the difficulty of moving against the buoyant force.[25] Thus, every joint could be moved either actively or passively and with or without resistance or assistance through its full range of motion. Increasing the speed of movement or decreasing the streamline by changing the body positioning or adding rehabilitation equipment increases the drag force resistance as the patient gets stronger, making workouts more challenging.[23]

An example of a shoulder progression for flexion using this approach would begin with the sports therapist and the athlete together in neck-deep water. Passive range of motion of the injured extremity would be initiated in the flexion pattern by the sports therapist. In the next stage, the sports therapist would place the extremity below the buoyant level and allow the buoyant force to assist the athlete's active shoulder flexion. To accomplish this stage, the athlete stands upright while the arm is passively moved to the athlete's side by the sports therapist. Then the athlete actively flexes the shoulder until the arm reaches the water surface. The flexion pattern for the next phase, the buoyancy-supported stage, begins with the athlete side-lying with the injured shoulder closest to the pool bottom. Support with floats would be needed at the feet, hips, and neck, as well as additional support from the sports therapist at the torso. In this position, the athlete could work both flexion and extension while encountering resistance only from the cohesive force, al-

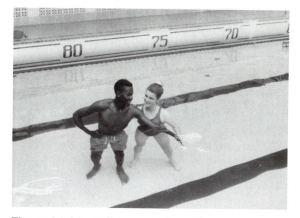

Figure 14-11 Milk jugs used for resistance.

lowing an excellent opportunity to increase active range of motion. Generally, two to three sets of 10 repetitions are appropriate, depending on the athlete's tolerance.

In the strengthening phase, the buoyancy-resisted stage, the athlete is standing once again. Active flexion and extension of the shoulder begins at a starting position parallel to the water surface and progresses to the side of the thigh. From the thigh, the assistance of the buoyant force is resisted while the arm is returned to the starting position. When two to three sets of 10 repetitions can be completed without pain, equipment may be added to increase the difficulty. Hand paddles provide a greater surface area and therefore more resistance and a higher intensity. Plastic milk jugs partially filled with water are another excellent way to increase resistance. By placing less water in the jug, its buoyancy is increased, and the resistance on the arm increases correspondingly (Figure 14-11). It is important to remember to keep the shoulder and upper arm under the water during upper extremity exercise. This is to avoid sudden shoulder overload and impingement, as the arm can weigh up to eight times its original weight at 90 degrees abduction or flexion. The forearm, however, may come above the water to allow full rotation range of motion.[28]

Bad Ragaz Technique

A second common technique in aquatic therapy is Bad Ragaz. In this method, buoyancy is used for flotation purposes only and not to assist or resist movement. The bow force ahead and drag force behind are the means for providing resistance. Three main positions apply in this method. The sports therapist should be in waist-deep water to maintain optimal stability. In the first position, the athlete actively moves while being fixated by the sports therapist (isokinetic). The athlete determines the resistance by controlling the speed of movement. For example, to work on knee flexion, the athlete could be stabilized side-lying with the involved leg closest to the surface. The buoyant force will act on that leg, and movement occurs, resulting in bow and drag forces. The bow force pushes the knee into flexion while the drag force pulls the knee in the same direction.

A second position has the athlete and sports therapist moving together in the direction of the desired motion (isotonic). To work on knee flexion in this position, the athlete is pushed forward, either side-lying or back-lying. This position facilitates movement of the knee into flexion, because the bow force helps the athlete's active contraction to push the knee into flexion. This position decreases the streamline of the leg and increases the drag force, which also assists by pulling the knee into flexion. In this situation, the sports therapist controls the speed and therefore the resistance.

The third position in this technique has the athlete holding a fixed position while being pushed by the sports therapist (isometric). In this position, the athlete holds an isometric contraction against the bow and drag forces (Figure 14-12).

Hold-relax, repeated contraction, and other PNF techniques can also be used in the water. They are very similar to those done on land but are performed in a

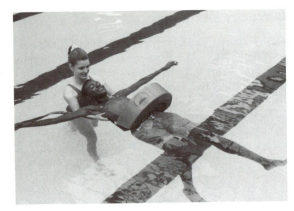

Figure 14-12 Bad Ragaz technique.

buoyancy-assisted position to enhance results.[6,9] PNF techniques should be done carefully, because research by Hurley and Turner[18] suggests the patient might have a reduced perception of stretch in the water. Once again, as the athlete's strength increases, resistive equipment should be added to make the workouts more challenging.

Aquatic therapist's are limited only by their imagination when utilizing aquatic therapy principles as a basis for workouts in the water. This additional method of therapy can help stimulate interest and motivation in the athlete, helping to supplement traditional exercise and return the athlete to normal function and competition.[22]

Summary

1. The buoyant force counteracts the force of gravity as it assists motion toward the water's surface and resists motion away from the surface.
2. Because of differences in the specific gravity of the body, the head and chest tend to float higher in the water than the heavier, denser extremities, making compensation with flotation devices necessary.
3. The three forces that oppose movement in the water are the cohesive force, the bow force, and the drag force.
4. Aquatic therapy allows for fine gradations of exercise, increased control over the percentage of weight bearing, increased range of motion and strength, decreased pain, and increased confidence.
5. Cost, decreased stabilization, and athlete contraindications are some disadvantages of aquatic therapy.
6. Pool size, water temperature, and equipment will vary depending on the population using the facility.
7. The buoyancy technique consists of buoyancy-assisted, buoyancy-supported, and buoyancy-resisted phases.
8. The Bad Ragaz technique uses isokinetic, isotonic, and isometric holding positions.
9. Aquatic therapy is meant to complement, not replace, traditional land exercise.

References

1. Arrigo, C. ed. 1992. Aquatic rehabilitation. *Sports Medicine Update* 7(2).
2. Arrigo, C., C. S. Fuller, and K. E. Wilk. 1992. Aquatic rehabilitation following ACL-PTG reconstruction. *Sports Medicine Update* 7(2): 22–27.
3. Bolton, F., and D. Goodwin. 1974. *Pool exercises.* Edinburgh and London: Churchill Livingstone.
4. Broach, E., D. Groff, R. Yaffe, J. Dattilo, and D. Gast. 1995. *Effects of aquatics therapy on physical behavior of adult with multiple sclerosis.* Paper presented at the 1995 Leisure

Research Symposium, San Antonio, TX. Available online at http://www.indiana.edu/~Irs/Irs95/ebroach95.html.

5. Butts, N. K., M. Tucker. and C. Greening. 1991. Physiologic responses to maximal treadmill and deep water running in men and women. *American Journal of Sports Medicine* 19(6): 612–14.

6. Campion, M. R. 1990. *Adult hydrotherapy: A practical approach.* Oxford: Heineman Medical.

7. Dioffenbach, L. 1991. Aquatic therapy services. *Clinical Management* 11(1): 14–19.

8. Dougherty, N. J. 1990. Risk management in aquatics. *JOHPERD* (May/June): 46–48.

9. Duffield, N. H. 1976. *Exercise in water.* London: Bailliere Tindall.

10. Edlich, R. F., M. A. Towler, R. J. Goitz, et al. 1987. Bioengineering principles of hydrotherapy. *Journal of Burn Care Rehabilitation* 8(6): 580–84.

11. Eyestone, E. D., G. Fellingham, J. George, and G. Fisher. 1993. Effect of water running and cycling on maximum oxygen consumption and 2 mile run performance. *American Journal of Sports Medicine* 21(1): 41–44.

12. Fawcett, C. W. 1992. Principles of aquatic rehab: A new look at hydrotherapy. *Sports Medicine Update* 7(2): 6–9.

13. Genuario, S. E., and J. J. Vegso. 1990. The use of a swimming pool in the rehabilitation and reconditioning of athletic injuries. *Contemp Orthop* 20(4): 381–87.

14. Golland, A. 1961. Basic hydrotherapy. *Physiotherapy* 67(9): 258–62.

15. Haralson, K. M. 1985. Therapeutic pool programs. *Clinical Management* 5(2): 10–13.

16. Harrison, R., and S. Bulstrode. 1987. Percentage weight bearing during partial immersion in the hydrotherapy pool. *Physiotherapy Practice* 3:60–63.

17. Hertler, L., M. Provost-Craig, D. Sestili, A. Hove, and M. Fees. 1992. Water running and the maintenance of maximal oxygen consumption and leg strength in runners. *Medicine and Science in Sports and Exercise* 24(5): S23.

18. Hurley, R., and C. Turner. 1991. Neurology and aquatic therapy. *Clinical Management* 11(1): 26–27.

19. Koszuta, L. E. 1989. From sweats to swimsuits: Is water exercise the wave of the future? *Physician and Sports Medicine* 17(4): 203–6.

20. Kolb, M. E. 1957. Principles of underwater exercise. *Physical Therapy Review* 27(6): 361–64.

21. Levin, S. 1991. Aquatic Therapy. *Physician and Sports Medicine* 19(10): 119–126.

22. McWaters, J. G. 1992. For faster recovery just add water. *Sports Medicine Update* 7(2): 4–5.

23. Meyer, R. I. 1990. Practice settings for kinesiotherapy-aquatics. *Clinical Kinesiology* 44(1): 12–13.

24. Michaud, T. L., D. K. Brennean, R. P. Wilder, and N. W. Sherman. 1992. Aquarun training and changes in treadmill running maximal oxygen consumption. *Medicine and Science in Sports and Exercise* 24(5): S23.

25. Moor, F. B., S. C. Peterson, E. M. Manueall, et al. 1964. *Manual of hydrotherapy and massage.* Mountain View, CA: Pacific Press.

26. Nolte-Heuritsch, I. 1979. *Aqua rhythmics: Exercises for the swimming pool.* New York: Sterling.

27. Simmons, V., and P. D. Hansen. 1996. Effectiveness of water exercise on postural mobility in the well elderly: An experimental study on balance enhancement. *Journal of Gerontology* 51A(5): M233–M238.

28. Speer, K., J. T. Cavanaugh, R. F. Warren, L. Day, and T. L. Wickiewicz. 1993. A role for hydrotherapy in shoulder rehabilitation. *American Journal of Sports Medicine* 21(6): 850–53.

29. Svendenhag, J., and J. Seger. 1992. Running on land and in water: Comparative exercise physiology. *Medicine and Science in Sports and Exercise* 24(10): 1155–60.

30. Town, G. P., and S. S. Bradley. 1991. Maximal metabolic responses of deep and shallow water running in trained runners. *Medicine and Science in Sports and Exercise* 23(2): 238–41.

31. Triggs, M. 1991. Orthopedic aquatic therapy. *Clinical Management* 11(1): 30–31.

32. Wilder, R. P., D. Brennan, and D. Schotte. 1993. A standard measure for exercise prescription and aqua running. *American Journal of Sports Medicine* 21(1): 45–48.

Suggested Readings

Berger, M. A., G. deGroot, and A. P. Hollander. 1995. Hydrodynamic drag and lift forces on human hand/arm models. *Journal of Biomechanics* 28(2): 125–33.

Bishop, P. A., S. Frazier, J. Smith, and D. Jacobs. 1989. Physiologic responses to treadmill and water running. *Physician and Sports Medicine* 17(2): 87–94.

Cassady, S. L., and O. H. Nielsen. 1992. Cardiorespiratory responses of healthy subjects to calisthenics performed on land versus in water. *Physical Therapy* 72(7): 532–38.

Christie, J. L., L. M. Sheldahl, and F. E. Tristani. 1990. Cardiovascular regulation during head-out water immersion exercise. *Journal of Applied Physiology* 69(2): 657–64.

Eckerson, J., and T. Anderson. 1992. Physiological response to water aerobics. *Journal of Sports Medicine and Physical Fitness* 32(3): 255–61.

Frangolias, D. D., and E. C. Rhodes. 1995. Maximal and ventilatory threshold responses to treadmill and water immersion running. *Medicine and Science in Sports and Exercise* 27(7): 1007–13.

Green, J. H., N. T. Cable, and N. Elms. 1990. Heart rate and oxygen consumption during walking on land and in deep water. *Journal of Sports Medicine and Physical Fitness* 30(1): 49–52.

Ritchie, S. E., and W. G. Hopkins. 1991. The intensity of exercise in deep-water running. *International Journal of Sports Medicine* 12(1): 27–29.

CHAPTER 15

Using Therapeutic Modalities in Rehabilitation

William E. Prentice

After completion of this chapter, the student should be able to do the following:

- Describe the approach of the sports therapist in using therapeutic modalities.

- Discuss the physiological effects of thermotherapy and cryotherapy techniques.

- Discuss the use of ultrasound as a deep-heating modality.

- Discuss the use of diathermy in rehabilitation.

- Discuss the potential physiological responses of biological tissue to electrical stimulating currents.

- Describe the possible uses for the low-power laser in sports medicine.

- Explain how intermittent compression can be used to decrease swelling.

- Discuss how the various massage techniques may be used clinically.

- Discuss the progression of modality use as the healing process progresses through the different phases of healing.

- List indications and contraindications for use of the various modalities.

- Discuss the physiological effects associated with the use of the different modalities.

Therapeutic modalities, when used appropriately, can be extremely useful tools in the rehabilitation of the injured athlete. Like any other tool, their effectiveness is limited by the knowledge, skill, and experience of the person using them.[14] For the sports therapist, decisions regarding how and when a modality can best be used should be based on a combination of theoretical knowledge and practical experience. Modalities should not be used at random, nor should their use be based on what has always been done before. Instead, consideration must always be given to what should work best in a specific clinical situation. In any program of rehabilitation, modalities should be used primarily as adjuncts to therapeutic exercise and certainly not at the exclusion of range-of-motion and strengthening exercises.[24]

There are many different approaches and ideas regarding the use of modalities in injury rehabilitation. Therefore no "cookbook" exists for modality use. Instead, sports therapists should make their own decision from the options in a given clinical situation about which modality will be most effective.

SUPERFICIAL HEATING AND COOLING MODALITIES (INFRARED)

The superficial heating and cooling modalities used in a sports medicine setting are all classified as **infrared** modalities.[27] Heating modalities are referred to as **thermotherapy.** Thermotherapy is used when a rise in tissue temperature is the goal of treatment. The use of cold, or **cryotherapy,** is most effective in the acute stages of the healing process immediately after injury when tissue temperature loss is the goal of therapy (Figure 15-1). Cold applications can be continued into the reconditioning state of athletic injury management. The term **hydrotherapy** can be applied to any cryotherapy or thermotherapy technique that uses water as the medium for heat transfer.[37]

Clinical Use of Heat and Cold

The physiological effects of heat and cold are rarely the result of direct absorption of infrared energy. There is general agreement that no form of infrared energy can have a depth of penetration greater than 1 centimeter. Thus the effects of the infrared modalities are primarily superficial and directly affect the cutaneous blood vessels and the cutaneous nerve receptors.[27]

Absorption of infrared energy cutaneously increases and decreases circulation subcutaneously in both the muscle and fat layers. If the energy is absorbed cutaneously over a period long enough to raise the temperature of the circulating blood, the hypothalamus will reflexively increase blood flow to the underlying tissue. Likewise, absorption of cold cutaneously can decrease blood flow via a similar mechanism in the area of treatment.[21]

If the primary treatment goal is a tissue temperature increase with corresponding increase in blood flow to the deeper tissues, a wiser choice is perhaps a modality, such as diathermy or ultrasound, that produces energy that can penetrate the cutaneous tissues and be directly absorbed by the deep tissues.[27] If the primary treatment goal is to reduce tissue temperature and decrease blood flow to an injured area, the superficial application of ice or cold is the only modality capable of producing such a response.

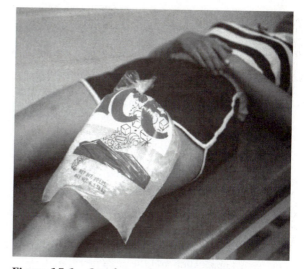

Figure 15-1 Cryotherapy is a superficial therapeutic technique used to decrease tissue temperature.

Perhaps the most effective use of the infrared modalities is for **analgesia,** that is, reducing the sensation of pain associated with injury. The infrared modalities primarily stimulate the cutaneous nerve receptors. Through one of the mechanisms of pain modulation, most likely gate control, hyperstimulation of these nerve receptors by heating or cooling reduces pain. Within the philosophy of an aggressive program of rehabilitation, as is standard in most sports medicine settings, the reduction of pain as a means of facilitating therapeutic exercise is a common practice. As emphasized earlier, therapeutic modalities are perhaps best used as an adjunct to therapeutic exercise. Certainly, this should be a prime consideration when selecting an infrared modality for use in any treatment program.[27]

Cryotherapy

Cryotherapy is the use of cold to treat acute trauma and subacute injury and to decrease discomfort after athletic reconditioning and rehabilitation.[22] Tools of cryotherapy include ice packs, cold whirlpool, ice whirlpool, ice massage, commercial chemical cold spray, and contrast baths. Application of cryotherapy produces a three- to four-stage sensation. The first sensation of cold is followed by a stinging, then a burning or aching feeling, and finally numbness. Each stage is related to the nerve endings as they temporarily cease to function as a result of decreased blood flow. The time required for this sequence varies from 5 to 15 minutes.[18] After 12 to 15 minutes, a reflex deep-tissue vasodilation called the

hunting response has been said to occur with intense cold (10° C or 50° F). However, this response appears to occur only in the distal extremities, and its value as a protective mechanism is debatable.[16] A minimum of 15 minutes is necessary to achieve extreme analgesic effects.

Application of ice is safe, simple, and inexpensive. Cryotherapy is contraindicated in patients with cold allergies (hives, joint pain, nausea), Raynaud's phenomenon (arterial spasm), and some rheumatoid conditions.[22]

Depth of penetration depends on the amount of cold and the length of the treatment time. The body is well equipped to maintain skin and subcutaneous tissue viability through the capillary bed by reflex vasodilation of up to four times normal blood flow. The body can decrease blood flow to the body segment that is supposedly losing too much body heat by shunting the blood flow. Depth of penetration is also related to intensity and duration of cold application and the circulatory response to the body segment exposed. If the person has normal circulatory responses, frostbite should not be a concern. Even so, caution should be exercised when applying intense cold directly to the skin. If deeper penetration is desired, ice therapy is most effective with ice towels, ice packs, ice massage, and whirlpools.[22] Patients should be advised of the four stages of cryotherapy and the discomfort they will experience. The sports therapist should explain this sequence and advise the athlete of the expected outcome, which might include a rapid decrease in pain.[27]

Thermotherapy

Heat is still used as a universal treatment for pain and discomfort.[19] Much of the benefit derives from the fact that the treatment simply feels good. In the early stages after injury, however, heat causes increased capillary blood pressure and increased cellular permeability, which results in additional swelling or edema accumulation.[27] No athlete with edema should be treated with any heat modality until the reasons for edema are determined. The best interest of the sports therapist is to use cryotherapy techniques or contrast baths to reduce the edema before heat applications. Superficial heat applications seem to feel more comfortable for complaints of the neck, back, low back, and pelvic areas and might be most appropriate for the athlete who exhibits some allergic response to cold application. However, the tissues in these areas are absolutely no different from those in the extremities. The same physiological responses to the use of heat or cold are elicited in all body areas.

Primary goals of thermotherapy include increased blood flow and muscle temperature to stimulate analgesia, increased nutrition to the cellular level, reduction of

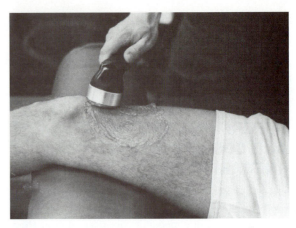

Figure 15-2 Technique for applying ultrasound.

edema, and removal of metabolites and other products of the inflammatory process.[27]

Continued investigation and research into the use of heat and cold is warranted to provide useful data for the sports medicine professional. Heat and cold applications, when used properly and efficiently, provide the sports therapist with tools to enhance recovery and provide the athlete with optimal health-care management. Thermotherapy and cryotherapy are only two of the tools available to assist in maintaining the well-being and reconditioning of the injured athlete.

ULTRASOUND

Ultrasound is defined as inaudible, acoustic vibrations of high frequency that can produce either thermal or nonthermal physiological effects.[26] It has been traditionally classified as a "deep-heating modality" and used primarily to elevate tissue temperatures[4] (Figure 15-2).

The main piece of equipment for delivering therapeutic ultrasound is a high-frequency generator, which provides an electrical current through a coaxial cable to a transducer contained within an applicator. Ultrasound is produced by a piezoelectric crystal within the transducer that converts electrical energy to acoustic energy through mechanical deformation via the piezoelectric effect.[35]

Ultrasound energy travels within the tissues as a highly focused collimated beam with a nonuniform intensity distribution. The intensity of the ultrasound beam is determined by the amount of energy delivered to the sound head (applicator). It is expressed in the number of watts per square centimeter (watts/cm^2). As a therapeutic modality used in sports medicine, it ranges from 0.1 to 3 watts/cm^2.[38]

As the ultrasound wave is transmitted through the various tissues, there will be **attenuation,** or a decrease in energy intensity due to either absorption of energy by the tissues or dispersion and scattering of the sound wave. Tissue penetration depends on impedance, or acoustical properties of the media that are proportional to tissue density. Therapeutic ultrasound has a frequency range between 0.75 and 3.0 MHz (Megahertz). Ultrasound energy generated at 1 MHz is transmitted through the more superficial tissues and absorbed primarily in the deeper tissues. A 1 MHz frequency is most useful in individuals with a high percent of cutaneous body fat, and whenever the desired effects are in the deeper structures.[26] At 3 MHz the energy is absorbed in the more superficial tissues.

Virtually all therapeutic ultrasound generators can emit either continuous or pulsed ultrasound waves. Continuous ultrasound is most commonly used when the desired effect is to produce thermal effects. The clinical effects of using ultrasound to heat the tissues are similar to other forms of superficial heat which have already been discussed. Whenever ultrasound is used to produce thermal changes, nonthermal changes will also occur simultaneously. However, if appropriate treatment parameters are selected, nonthermal effects can occur with minimal thermal effects. The use of pulsed ultrasound results in a reduced average heating of the tissues. Pulsed ultrasound or continuous ultrasound at a low intensity will produce nonthermal or mechanical effects that might be associated with soft tissue healing.[26]

The nonthermal effects of therapeutic ultrasound include cavitation and acoustic microstreaming. Cavitation is the formation of gas-filled bubbles that expand and compress due to ultrasonically induced pressure changes in tissue fluids.[7] Cavitation results in an increased flow in the fluid around these vibrating bubbles. Microstreaming is the unidirectional movement of fluids along the boundaries of cell membranes resulting from the mechanical pressure wave in an ultrasonic field.[26] Microstreaming can alter cell membrane structure and function due to changes in cell membrane permeability to sodium and calcium ions important in the healing process. As long as the cell membrane is not damaged, microstreaming can be of therapeutic value in accelerating the healing process.[26] The nonthermal effects of therapeutic ultrasound in the treatment of injured tissues might be as important as, if not more important than, the thermal effects. The nonthermal effects of cavitation and microstreaming can be maximized while minimizing the thermal effects by using an intensity of 0.1 to 0.2 watts/cm^2 with continuous ultrasound.

Application Technique

Therapeutic ultrasound is most effective when an appropriate coupling medium and technique using either direct contact, immersion, or a bladder is combined with a moving transducer. The purpose of a coupling medium is to provide an airtight contact with the skin and a slick, friction-proof surface for the ultrasound head to glide over. Coupling mediums for direct contact can include a variety of materials, some of which are mineral oil, water-soluble creams, or gels. Underwater administration of ultrasound is suggested for such irregular body parts as the wrist, hand, elbow, ankle, and foot. Another technique for treating irregular surfaces has been recommended in which a water-filled balloon is placed between the transducer and the treatment area with sufficient amounts of coupling gel to ensure good contact.[26]

Moving the transducer in a circular pattern or a stroking pattern during treatment leads to a more even distribution of energy within the treatment area and can reduce the likelihood of developing hot spots. The transducer should be moved slowly at approximately 4 cm per second. The transducer should be kept in maximum contact with the skin via some coupling agent throughout the treatment.

Dosage of ultrasound varies according to the depth of the tissue treated and the state of injury, such as subacute or chronic. Basically, 0.1 to 0.3 watts/cm^2 is regarded as low intensity, 0.4 to 1.5 watts/cm^2 is medium intensity, and 1.5 to 3 watts/cm^2 is high intensity. The duration of treatment time ranges from 5 to 10 minutes.[26]

Therapeutic Uses

Therapeutic ultrasound when applied to biological tissue can induce clinically significant responses in cells, tissues, and organs through both thermal effects, which produce a tissue temperature increase, and nonthermal effects, which include cavitation and microstreaming.[10] Even though there is relatively little documented evidence from the sports medicine community concerning the efficacy of ultrasound, it is most often used for soft tissue healing and repair; with scar tissue and joint contracture; for chronic inflammation; for bone healing; with plantar warts; and for placebo effects.

It is generally accepted that acute conditions require more frequent treatments over a shorter period of time, and that more chronic conditions require fewer treatments over a longer period of time.[26] Ultrasound treatments should begin as soon as possible following injury, ideally within hours but definitely within 48 hours to maximize effects on the healing process.[26] Acute conditions may be treated using low-intensity ultrasound once or even twice daily for 6 to 8 days until acute symptoms such as pain and swelling subside. In chronic conditions, when acute symptoms have subsided, treatment may be done on alternating days for a total of 10 to 12 treatments.[11]

In sports medicine, it is not uncommon to combine modalities to accomplish a specific treatment goal. Ultrasound is frequently used with other modalities, including hot packs, cold packs, and electrical stimulating currents.[6,11]

Phonophoresis

Phonophoresis is a technique in which ultrasound is used to drive molecules of a topically applied medication, usually either an anti-inflammatory or anagelsic, into the tissues.[30] Like iontophoresis, it is designed to move medication into injured tissues, but phonophoresis is not as likely to damage or burn skin and it produces a greater depth of penetration.

The most widespread use of the phonophoresis technique in sports medicine has been to deliver hydrocortisone, which has anti-inflammatory effects. This technique has been successful in treating painful trigger points, tendinitis, and bursitis.[38] Salicylates have also been used to evoke a number of pharmacological effects, including analgesia and decreased inflammation. Lidocaine is a commonly used local anesthetic drug. The use of phonophoresis with lidocaine was found to be effective in treating a series of trigger points.

In phonophoresis, coupling can be either direct or accomplished using immersion. The medication in preparation is rubbed directly into the surface of the skin over the treatment area. With the direct technique, transmission gel should be applied, and with immersion the treatment area with the preparation applied is simply treated underwater.

Both pulsed and continuous ultrasound have been used in phonophoresis. Continuous ultrasound at an intensity great enough to produce thermal effects can induce a pro-inflammatory response.[7]

DIATHERMY

Diathermy is the application of high-frequency electromagnetic energy that is primarily used to generate heat in body tissues (Figure 15-3). Diathermy as a therapeutic agent may be classified as two distinct modalities, **shortwave diathermy** and **microwave diathermy**. Shortwave diathermy can be continuous or pulsed. The physiological effects of continuous shortwave and microwave diathermy are primarily thermal, resulting from high-

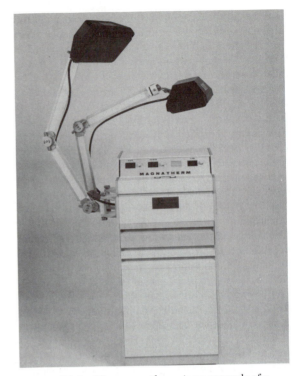

Figure 15-3 The magnatherm is an example of a shortwave diathermy unit.

frequency vibration of molecules. However, pulsed shortwave diathermy has been used for its nonthermal effects in the treatment of soft-tissue injuries and wounds.[28] Clinically the use of the diathermies, particularly shortwave pulsed diathermy, is once again on the rise.

A shortwave diathermy unit that generates a high-frequency electrical current will produce both an electrical field and a magnetic field in the tissues. The ratio of the electrical field to the magnetic field depends on the characteristics of the different units as well as on the characteristics of the electrodes or applicators. The capacitance technique, using capacitor electrodes (air space plates and pad electrodes), creates a strong electrical field that is essentially the lines of force exerted on charged ions by the electrodes, which cause charged particles to move from one pole to the other. The inductance technique, using induction electrodes (cable electrodes and drum electrodes), creates a strong magnetic field when current is passed through a coiled cable. It affects surrounding tissues by inducing localized secondary currents, called eddy currents, within the tissues.[28]

Pulsed diathermy is created by simply interrupting the output of continuous shortwave diathermy at consistent intervals. Generators that deliver pulsed shortwave diathermy typically use a drum-type electrode to induce energy in the treatment area via the production of a magnetic field. Pulsed diathermy is claimed to have therapeutic value and to produce nonthermal effects with minimal thermal physiological effects, depending on the intensity of the application.[15] When pulsed diathermy is used in intensities that create an increase in tissue temperature, its effects are no different from those of continuous shortwave diathermy. Successful treatments have largely resulted from the application of higher intensities and longer treatment times.

Microwave diathermy units generate a strong electrical field and relatively little magnetic field through either circular shaped and rectangular shaped applicators that beam energy to the treatment area. With microwave diathermy, the energy can be focused toward the body part to be treated. This focus allows for greater penetration because more of the energy strikes the skin perpendicularly. Scatter of the energy is minimized, and absorption is maximized. Because microwave energy can be focused, therapeutic tissue temperature increases can occur up to a depth of 5 centimeters, and microwave diathermy is probably as effective as shortwave diathermy in producing deep-tissue temperature rise.

The diathermies have been used in the treatment of a variety of musculoskeletal conditions, including muscle strains, contusions, ligament sprains, tendinitis, tenosynovitis, bursitis, joint contractures, and myofascial trigger points.[33] There are probably more treatment precautions and contraindications for the use of either shortwave or microwave diathermy than for any of the other physical agents used in a sports medicine setting. Effective treatments using the diathermies require practice in application and adjustment of techniques to the individual patient.

ELECTRICAL STIMULATING CURRENTS

Electrical stimulating currents are among the therapeutic modalities most often used by the sports therapist[12] (Figure 15-4). The effects of electrical current passing through biological tissues can be physiological, chemical, or thermal. All biological tissue has some response to this current flow. The type and extent of the response depends on (1) the type of tissue and physiological response characteristics and (2) the parameters of the electrical current applied, that is, its intensity, duration, waveform, modulation, and polarity. Biological tissue responds to electrical energy in a manner similar to how it normally functions and grows.

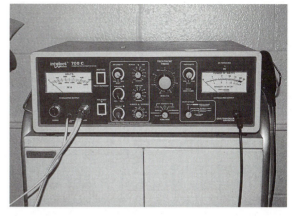

Figure 15-4 Electrical stimulating unit. Depending on the treatment parameters selected, the physiological effects may involve sensory or motor nerves, or chemical changes.

Clinically, the sports therapist uses electrical currents for several purposes: (1) to produce muscle contraction through stimulation of nerve muscle, (2) to stimulate sensory nerves to help treat pain, (3) to create an electrical field on the skin surface to drive ions into tissues (iontophoresis), and (4) to create an electrical field within the tissues to stimulate or alter the healing process (medical galvanism). In a sports medicine environment, the major therapeutic uses of electricity center on muscle contraction, sensory stimulation, or ion transfer.[12]

To produce any physiological response in the nerve and muscle fibers, an electrical current must be of sufficient intensity and duration to equal or exceed the nerve membrane's basic threshold for excitation. When this occurs, depolarization of the nerve fiber results in an action potential.[34]

Different types (sizes) of nerves have different thresholds for depolarization. The **strength-duration curves** in Figure 15-5 represent graphically the thresholds for depolarization of sensory (Aβ), motor (A), and pain (C) nerve fibers. If current intensity or duration is increased to a level great enough to reach the minimal threshold for depolarization of Aβ fibers, the electrical current can be felt. If current intensity or duration is increased further, a muscle contraction can be elicited by reaching the threshold for depolarization of the A fibers. If the intensity and/or duration continues to increase, eventually a level is reached that causes depolarization of the C fibers and pain. By simply changing current intensity, current duration, or some combination of the two, very different physiological responses can be achieved.[12]

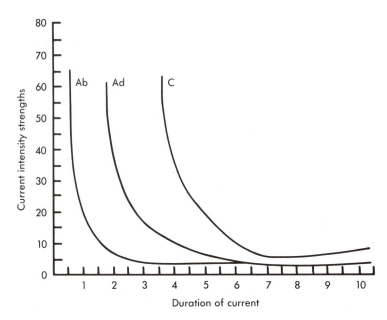

Figure 15-5 Strength-duration curves. Curves represent the thresholds for depolarization of the various types of nerve fibers. Ab, Sensory nerves; Ad, motor fibers, C, pain fibers.

Traditionally, various types of electric currents have been classified, such as high volt, low volt, alternating, direct, pulsed, interferential, Russian, and microamperage (MENS or LIS). Electrical stimulators that output any of these varieties of current (with the possible exception of some new LIS or MENS units in which the intensity is not great enough) can produce any of these physiological responses if the current parameters are adjusted appropriately.[25]

Electrical stimulators are designed to deliver pulses with a waveform that generally differs depending on the manufacturer. Electrical currents are either direct (DC), alternating (AC), or pulsed and can take on sine, square, or triangular waveforms.[25] Various claims concerning the effectiveness of specific waveforms have been made by manufacturers, and although one type of waveform might be more effective for a particular patient, generalizations are difficult to make. These waveforms refer to the waveform produced by the stimulator and delivered to the patient and not the waveform of the current used to drive the generator.

The electrical stimulating units are connected via electrodes placed on the skin surface, generally in or over the area of pain. Electrodes placed at the painful region may be within the dermatome, on a specific point, or over a peripheral nerve supplying the painful region. Spinal cord segments that give rise to a specific nerve root conveying nociceptive input provide another choice for electrode placement. Electrodes are often placed along vertebrae or between spinous processes in conjunction with electrodes placed over specific dermatomal regions.[12]

Stimulation of Sensory Nerves

Transcutaneous electrical nerve stimulation (TENS) has been traditionally defined as a technique used to stimulate sensory nerve fibers with electrodes placed on the skin specifically to relieve either chronic or acute pain. TENS is an effective, noninvasive, nonpharmacological method of pain modulation.[36]

Peripheral nerves are actually bundles of a large number of large- and small-diameter sensory and motor nerve fibers, innervating skin, muscle, and visceral structures. As previously mentioned, different sizes of nerve fibers have characteristic strength-duration curves. The large diameter sensory fibers (Aβ) are more easily excited by an electrical stimulus than smaller fibers are. As stimulus intensity (or duration) is increased, large-diameter afferent motor fibers (Aβ) are excited (or recruited) before smaller sensory fibers. If the intensity or duration of the stimulus is increased sufficiently, both motor (Aβ) and small-diameter sensory or pain fibers (C) are excited. With conventional TENS, the objective is to maximally stimulate the large-diameter afferent or Aβ fibers without concomitant motor nerve responses or pain.[12]

Mechanisms of Pain Relief. The mechanism by which TENS produces pain relief is a matter for debate. Currently several different models attempt to explain pain modulation. It must be stressed that these models of pain control are not mutually exclusive but rather are the result of overlapping processes.[5]

Gate control and ascending pain control. The first TENS units were designed and tried clinically on the basis of Melzack and Wall's gate-control theory of pain, originally proposed in 1965 with several subsequent modifications.[5] According to this theory, pain information is conveyed from the periphery to the spinal cord by small-diameter type C fibers. By stimulating large-diameter Aβ fibers coming from cutaneous receptors, synaptic transmission between the pain fibers and the ascending transmission cells is blocked or inhibited at the spinal cord level, and thus pain is not transmitted to higher conscious pain centers in the brain. This has been referred to as "closing the gate."

More recent theories expand on gate-control theory, maintaining that stimulation of large-diameter afferent (Aβ) fibers releases endogenously produced opiatelike substances called **enkephalins** from small enkephalin interneurons in the dorsal horn of the spinal cord. Enkephalins inhibit synaptic transmission of pain information to the brain through ascending spinal tracts, helping to "close the gate" and thus blocking the pain message before it reaches sensory levels.[5]

Many commercial TENS units have variable adjustments for pulse duration, amplitude or intensity, and frequency. At very short pulse durations (on an order of 10 microseconds), the difference between the stimulus intensity necessary to excite large-diameter type Aβ sensory fibers and that necessary to excite very-small-diameter type C pain fibers is maximized. Optimal stimulation of large-diameter Aβ fibers (and therefore maximal pain relief) is obtained if a short-duration pulse is chosen and the intensity is gradually increased until a tingling sensation is perceived. Although optimal frequency of stimulation has not been determined, it is recommended that frequency be set at the maximum allowed by the stimulator.[5]

Central biasing and descending pain control. A second mechanism of the pain-control system involves descending efferent pathways.[5] This so-called central bi-

asing mechanism is located in the brain stem and exerts a powerful inhibitory influence on transmission of impulses conveying pain information. Stimulation of the periaqueductal gray matter and the Raphe nucleus via ascending input from both A and C fibers activates this descending mechanism. Descending efferent fibers in the spinal cord synapse with enkephalin interneurons, releasing enkephalin within the dorsal horn of a specific spinal segment, once again inhibiting synaptic transmission of impulses to the ascending or afferent neurons. Through this system, it has been hypothesized, emotional influences, previous experiences, sensory perception, and other factors could influence the transmission of the pain message and the perception of pain.

This model provides an explanation for the analgesia that occurs with the use of brief, intense electrical stimulation of peripheral pain (C) fibers by low-frequency, high-intensity stimulation of acupuncture or trigger points. Whereas in conventional TENS, the duration of relief is generally short because of the relatively short half-life of enkephalins, relief after using high-intensity electrical stimulation generally lasts for several hours, and in some cases the relief might be permanent.[5]

Beta-endorphin and dynorphin release. Another effect of such intense electrical stimulation is the release of another endogenous opiate called **beta-endorphin,** along with ACTH. Beta-endorphin is released from within the brain and is active within the central nervous system. β-endorphin stimulates the Raphe nucleus, which increases the activity of the descending pain-control mechanisms discussed earlier. The release of ACTH results in corticosteroid release from the adrenal glands. These anti-inflammatory substances might affect pain reduction seen after high-intensity stimulation.[5]

This process is stimulated through low-frequency (1–5 pulses/sec), high-intensity stimulation of specific acupuncture or trigger points. This technique has been referred to as **acustim** or **electroacutherapy.**[12]

Stimulation of Motor Nerves

Electrical stimulation of motor nerve (A) fibers at sufficient intensity and duration to produce depolarization results in muscular contraction. Once a stimulus reaches the depolarizing threshold, an increase in the intensity of the stimulus does not alter the quality of the contraction. However, the frequency of stimulation is increased, the time for repolarization of the muscle fiber is decreased, and thus the contractions tend to summate. When the stimulation frequency reaches 50 pulses/second or greater, the muscle exhibits a tetanic contraction.

Several therapeutic gains can be accomplished by electrically stimulating muscle contraction. Electrically induced **muscle-pumping** contractions can facilitate circulation by pumping fluid and blood through the venous and lymphatic channels away from an area of swelling.[12]

Muscular inhibition after periods of immobilization or surgery or as a result of swelling is an indication for muscle reeducation. Electrically stimulating the muscle to contract produces an increase in the sensory input from the muscle and assists the patient in **relearning a muscular response** or pattern.[12]

Muscular strengthening can be accomplished using high-frequency AC current in conjunction with voluntary muscle contractions.[12] The exclusive use of electrical current does not appear to increase muscle strength. Electrically stimulating the muscle to contract during periods of immobilization retards muscle atrophy and might potentially reduce the time required for rehabilitation after immobilization.

Electrical currents might also assist in **increasing range of motion** about a joint where contractures are limiting motion. Repeated contraction over an extended time appears to make the contracted joint structures and muscle modify and lengthen.[34]

Interferential Currents

Interferential current is a nonmodulated sine waveform alternating current produced by two simultaneously applied electrical generators that each produce this current at different frequencies. When the two currents intersect, the pulse intensities combine, and the difference in frequency produces a low-frequency "beat" pattern. Individual beats produce a physiological response that is essentially identical to a single pulse produced by a conventional electrical stimulator.

Proponents of interferential currents claim that this beating pulse lowers skin resistance and produces a more comfortable stimulation with a greater depth of penetration than other stimulators. However, higher voltages also reduce tissue impedance; thus the relative comfort is no different than with high-volt stimulators. Interferential currents are simply a different electrical approach to achieve the same excitatory responses that traditional high-volt stimulators produce. The disadvantages of interferential units are that they are expensive and not as versatile as other high-volt generators. They can be used for pain modulation, edema reduction, and muscle relaxation. They are not suitable for muscle reeducation because there is no interrupt mode or modulation.[34]

Low-Intensity Stimulation (LIS)

Low-intensity stimulation (LIS) used to be referred to as microcurrent electrical neuromuscular stimulation (MENS).[12] LIS is one of the newer types of electrical stimulating currents currently being used by the sports therapist. Certainly, the type of current being produced by these LIS generators is no different from current produced by other electrical stimulator generators. The majority of other electrical stimulating devices are capable of producing microcurrent. The only difference is that with LIS treatment the intensity of the current is at subsensory levels (below 1,000 microamps) at a frequency of less than 1 pulse per second.[3]

Most literature dealing with microcurrents centers around research on stimulation of the healing process in fractures and skin wounds, and in pain modulation. The mechanism of their effectiveness is thought to be based on changes that occur at the cellular level rather than having to do with the effects of depolarization of sensory and motor nerve fibers.[12] Microcurrent treatments may well be a useful addition to the electrical therapies. However, to date they are untested clinically, and claims of their effectiveness are based primarily on empirical rather than experimental evidence.[12]

Russian Current

Russian current is another relatively new type of current used by sports therapists. It uses an AC current at a high frequency (2,500 to 10,000 PPS) produced in a series of "bursts." By putting the current in bursts, a greater intensity of current can be used, and the athlete will have a high tolerance to the current. As intensity of stimulation increases, more muscle fibers are stimulated and a stronger contraction occurs.[2]

When used for muscle strengthening, this current is most effective when combined with active muscle contraction against resistance.

Iontophoresis

Electrical stimulating currents may also be used to produce chemical changes. Electricity is used in the clinic to cause chemical change in two important ways. The first is **iontophoresis, or ion transfer,** defined as the introduction of chemical ions into superficial body tissues for medicinal purposes with the use of direct current. For iontophoresis to work, the chemical substance must be in an ionic form. Because like charges repel, chemical substances with a positive charge are introduced through the skin with the positive electrode, or anode, and substances with a negative charge must be introduced with the negative electrode, or cathode.[23]

The Phoresor is an electrical stimulating device designed specifically for iontophoresis. In recent years, this technique has gained significant popularity as a treatment modality. If the drug is in solution form, it is generally applied to a gauze pad that is placed directly over the area to be treated. The active electrode of the same polarity as the charge of the ion is then placed on top of the drug-soaked gauze and secured firmly in place. The dispersive or indifferent electrode is generally placed at a remote area of the same extremity. Drugs in paste form are usually rubbed onto the skin surface, and a moist electrode with the proper polarity is then secured. In general, intensity is adjusted to tolerance. Treatment time is generally indicated by the physician, but 10 to 15 minutes is a typical treatment time.

Some care must be taken with very potent drugs that could potentially have deleterious systemic effects. However, iontophoretically applied medicinal ions generally do not migrate far below the surface of the skin or mucous membranes.

Some of the more common substances that might be iontophoretically applied are the following:[23]

1. Heavy metal ions, such as zinc and copper, to fight certain types of skin infections
2. Chloride ions to loosen superficial scars
3. Local anesthetics
4. Vasodilating drugs
5. Magnesium ions for plantar warts

Medical Galvanism

The other major use of direct current that can be included under the general category of chemical effects has been termed **medical galvanism,** defined as the use of low-voltage galvanic or direct current for therapeutic purposes without the introduction of pharmacological substances. The therapeutic benefit is thought to result largely from local ionic changes that result in increased circulation to body parts between the electrodes. Presumably the improved circulation speeds up absorption of inflammatory products, such as accumulated metabolites, with subsequent pain relief. Low-volt electrical currents might speed wound healing, decrease edema, and help fight localized infection. Conditions for which galvanic current has been used effectively include contusions, sprains, myositis, acute edema, certain forms of arthritis, tenosynovitis, and neuritis.[25]

Some other effects of long-duration, low-volt current, which seem to be polarity-specific and result from local ionic and electrical changes, are as follows:

Positive pole	hardening	decreases nerve
(anode)	of tissues	excitability
Negative pole	softening of	increases nerve
(anode)	tissues	excitability

LOW-POWER LASER

Laser is an acronym that stands for *light amplification of stimulated emissions of radiation.*[32] Lasers are relatively new to the medical community and are certainly the newest of the modalities used by sports therapists. The principles of physics under which laser energy is produced are complex. Basically, an atom is excited when energy is applied and raises an orbiting electron to a higher orbit. When the electron returns to its original orbit, it releases energy (photons) through **spontaneous emission.** Stimulated emission occurs when the photon is released from the excited atom, and it promotes the release of an identical photon to be released from a similarly excited atom. For lasers to operate, a medium of excited atoms must be generated. This is termed **population inversion** and results when an external energy source or pumping device is applied to the medium.[32]

Laser light differs from conventional light in that laser light is monochromic (single color or wavelength), coherent (in phase), and collimated (minimal divergence). Laser can be thermal (hot) or nonthermal (low power, soft, cold). The categories include solid-state (glass or crystal), gas, semiconductor, dye, and chemical lasers.[32]

Helium-neon (HeNe gas) and gallium arsenide (GaAs semiconductor) lasers are two low-power lasers currently being investigated by the FDA for potential application in physical medicine. The HeNe lasers deliver a characteristic red beam with a wavelength of 632.8 nanometers. They are delivered in a continuous wave and have a direct penetration of 2 to 5 millimeters and an indirect penetration of 10 to 15 millimeters. The GaAs laser is invisible, with a wavelength of 904 nanometers. It is delivered in a pulse mode at a very low power output. It has a direct penetration of 1 to 2 centimeters and an indirect penetration of 5 centimeters.[8]

The proposed therapeutic applications of lasers in physical medicine include acceleration of collagen synthesis, decrease in microorganisms, increase in vascularization, and reduction of pain and inflammation.[32]

Laser application is ideally done with light contact to the surface and should be perpendicular to the target surface. Dosage appears to be the critical factor in eliciting a response, but exact dosages have not been determined. Dosage is altered by varying the pulse frequency and the treatment times. The treatment is applied by developing an imaginary grid over the target area. The grid comprises 1-centimeter squares, and the laser is applied to each square for a predetermined time. Trigger or acupuncture points are also treated for painful conditions.

The FDA considers low-power lasers to be low-risk devices. Although no deleterious effects have been reported, certain precautions and contraindications exist. For instance, one should avoid lasing over cancerous tissue, directly into the eyes, and during the first trimester of pregnancy. Initial pain increases and episodes of syncope have been reported but do not warrant treatment cessation.

INTERMITTENT COMPRESSION

Intermittent compression units are used to control or reduce swelling after acute injury or pitting edema, which tends to develop in the injured area several hours after injury. Intermittent compression uses a nylon pneumatic inflatable sleeve applied around the injured extremity (Figure 15-6). The sleeve can be inflated to a specific pressure that forces excessive fluid accumulated in the interstitial spaces into vascular and lymphatic channels, through which it is removed from the area of injury. Compression facilitates the movement of lymphatic fluid, which helps to eliminate the by-products of the injury process.[13]

Intermittent compression devices have essentially three parameters that can be adjusted: on-off time, inflation pressures, and treatment time. Recommended treatment protocols have been established through clinical trial and error; there is little experimental data currently available to support any protocol.[31] On-off times include 1 minute on and 2 minutes off, 2 minutes on and 1 minute off, and 4 minutes on and 1 minute off. These recommendations are not based on research. Patient comfort should be the primary guide. Recommended inflation pressures have been loosely correlated with blood pressures. The Jobst Institute recommends that pressure be set at 30 to 50 mm Hg for the upper extremity and at 30 to 60 mm Hg for the lower extremity. Because arterial capillary pressures are approximately 30 mm Hg, any pressure that exceeds this rate should encourage the absorption of edema and the flow of lymphatic fluid.[13] Clinical studies have demonstrated a significant reduction in limb volume after 30 minutes of compression. Thus a 30-minute treatment time seems to be efficient in reducing edema.

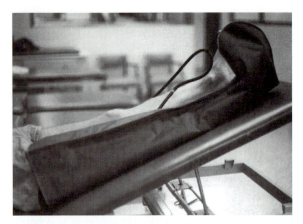

Figure 15-6 Jobst full-leg sleeve. Intermittent compression is generally used to reduce swelling.

Some intermittent compression units can combine cold along with compression. Electrical stimulating currents may also be used to produce muscle pumping and thus facilitate lymphatic flow.[1]

SPORTS MASSAGE

Massage is a mechanical stimulation of the tissues by means of rhythmically applied pressure and stretching[9] (Figure 15-7). Over the years many claims have been made relative to the therapeutic benefits of massage in the athletic population, but few are based on well-controlled, well-designed studies. Sports therapists have used massage to increase flexibility and coordination as well as to increase pain threshold; to decrease neuromuscular excitability in the muscle being massaged; to stimulate circulation, thus improving energy transport to the muscle; to facilitate healing and restore joint mobility; and to remove lactic acid, thus alleviating muscle cramps.[29] Conclusive evidence of the efficacy of massage as an ergogenic aid in the athletic population is lacking.

How these effects can be accomplished is determined by the specific approaches used with massage techniques and how they are applied. Generally the effects of massage are either *reflexive* or *mechanical*. The effect of massage on the nervous system will differ greatly according to the method employed, the pressure exerted, and the duration of applications. Through the reflex mechanism, sedation is induced. Slow, gentle, rhythmical, and superficial **effleurage** may relieve tension and soothe, rendering the muscles more relaxed. This indicates an effect on sensory and motor nerves locally and some central nervous system response. The mechanical approach seeks to

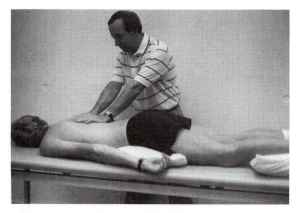

Figure 15-7 Therapeutic massage.

make mechanical or histological changes in myofascial structures through direct force applied superficially.[29]

Among the massage techniques used in sports medicine are the following:[29]

1. *Hoffa massage.* The classic form of massage. Strokes include effleurage, petrissage, percussion or tapotement, and vibration.
2. *Friction massage.* Used to increase the inflammatory response, particularly in cases of chronic tendinitis or tenosynovitis.
3. *Acupressure.* Massage of acupuncture and trigger points. Used to reduce pain and irritation in anatomical areas known to be associated with specific points.
4. *Connective tissue massage.* A stroking technique used on layers of connective tissue. A relatively new form of treatment in this country, primarily affecting circulatory pathologies.
5. *Myofascial release.* Used for the purpose of relieving soft tissue from the abnormal grip of tight fascia.
6. *Rolfing.* A system devised to correct inefficient structure by balancing the body within a gravitational field through a technique involving manual soft-tissue manipulation.
7. *Trager.* Attempts to establish neuromuscular control so that more normal movement patterns can be routinely performed.

INJURY MANAGEMENT USING MODALITIES

Traditionally in a sports medicine setting, injuries have been classified as being either acute injuries resulting from trauma or chronic injuries resulting primarily from overuse. This operational definition is not necessarily correct. If there is active inflammation, including the classic symptoms of tenderness, swelling, redness, and so on, the injury should be considered acute and must be treated accordingly using rest, compression, and elevation. Even if active inflammation persists for months after initial injury, it should still be considered acute. The point is that classification of an injury should be made according to the existing signs and symptoms that indicate the various stages of the healing process, and not according to time frames or mechanisms of injury. Once the signs of acute inflammation are no longer present, the injury may be considered to be chronic. As discussed in Chapter 2, inflammation may be considered chronic when the normal cellular response in the inflammatory process is altered by replacing leukocytes with macrophages and plasma cells, along with degeneration of the injured structure.

Based on these definitions of acute and chronic injury, the rehabilitation progression after injury may be loosely classified in four phases: initial acute injury, acute inflammatory response, fibroblastic-repair, and maturation-remodeling. These phases overlap, and the estimated time frame for each phase shows extreme variability between patients. Table 15-1 summarizes the various modalities that may be used in each of the four phases.

Initial Acute Injury Phase

Modality use in the initial treatment phase should be directed toward limiting the amount of swelling and reducing pain that occurs acutely. The acute phase is marked by swelling, pain when touched, and pain on both active and passive motion. In general, the less initial swelling, the less the time required for rehabilitation. Traditionally, the modality of choice has been and still is **ice.**

Cryotherapy produces vasoconstriction, at least superficially and perhaps indirectly in the deeper tissues, and thus limits the bleeding that always occurs with injury. Ice bags, cold packs, and ice massage may all be used effectively. Cold baths should be avoided because these place the foot in the gravity-dependent position. Cold whirlpools also place the foot in the gravity-dependent position and produce a massaging action that is likely to retard clotting. The importance of cryotherapy techniques for reducing acute swelling has probably been exaggerated. Cryotherapy is perhaps best used for producing analgesia, which most likely results from stimulation of sensory cutaneous nerves that, via the gating mechanism, blocks or reduces pain.

■ TABLE 15-1 Clinical Decision Making on the Use of Various Therapeutic Modalities in Treatment of Acute Injury

Phase	Approximate Time Frame	Clinical Picture	Possible Modalities Used	Rationale for Use
Initial acute	Injury–day 3	Swelling, pain to touch, pain on motion	CRYO ESC IC LPL Rest	↓ Swelling, ↓pain ↓ Pain ↓ Swelling ↓ Pain
Inflammatory response	Day 1–day 6	Swelling subsides, warm to touch, discoloration, pain to touch, pain on motion	CRYO ESC IC LPL Range of motion	↓ Swelling, ↓pain ↓ Pain ↓ Swelling ↓ Pain
Fibroblastic-repair	Day 4–day 10	Pain to touch, pain on motion, swollen	THERMO ESC LPL IC Range of motion Strengthening	Mildly ↑ circulation ↓ Pain-muscle pumping ↓ Pain Facilitate lymphatic flow
Maturation-remodeling	Day 7–recovery	Swollen, no more pain to touch, decreasing pain on motion	ULTRA ESC LPL SWD MWD Range of motion Strengthening Functional activities	Deep heating to ↑ circulation ↑ Range of motion, ↑ strength ↓ Pain ↓ Pain Deep heating to ↑ circulation Deep heating to ↑ circulation

CRYO, Cryotherapy; *ESC,* electrical stimulating currents; *IC,* intermittent compression; *LPL,* low-power laser; *MWD,* microwave diathermy; *SWD,* shortwave diathermy; *THERMO,* thermotherapy; *ULTRA,* ultrasound; ↓ decrease; ↑ increase.

Compression is perhaps the most critical element in controlling swelling initially. An intermittent compression device may be used to provide even pressure around an injured extremity. The pressurized sleeve mechanically reduces the amount of space available for swelling to accumulate. Units that combine both compression and cold are extremely useful in this phase. Regardless of the specific techniques selected, cold and compression should always be combined with elevation to avoid any additional pooling of blood in the injured area from the effects of gravity.

Electrical stimulating currents may also be used in the initial phase for pain reduction. Parameters should be adjusted to maximally stimulate sensory cutaneous nerve fibers, again to take advantage of the gate control mechanism of pain modulation. Intensities that produce muscle contraction should be avoided initially because they might increase clotting time.

Low-intensity ultrasound with a intensity of less than 0.1 watts/cm^2 may be used immediately following injury to take advantage of the nonthermal physiological effects that are thought to benefit the healing process. However, caution must be applied, because the moving transducer may tend to interfere with clotting, once again due to the massage effect. It is perhaps best to wait until at least 24 hours following injury until clotting is firmly established.

The low-power laser has also been demonstrated to be effective in pain modulation through the stimulation of trigger points and may be used acutely.

The injured part should be rested and protected for at least the first 24 to 48 hours to allow the inflammatory phase of the healing process to do what it is supposed to.

Inflammatory-Response Phase

The inflammatory-response phase begins immediately following injury and can last as long as day 6 after injury, depending on severity. Clinically, swelling begins to subside and eventually stops altogether. The injured area might feel warm to the touch, and some discoloration is usually apparent. The injury is still painful to the touch, and pain is elicited on movement of the injured part. As in the initial injury stage, modalities should be used to control pain and reduce swelling. Cryotherapy should still be used during the inflammatory stage. Ice bags, cold packs, and ice massages provide analgesic effects. The use of cold also reduces the likelihood of swelling, which might continue during this stage. The acute process of swelling will likely subside completely by the end of this phase.

It must be emphasized that heating an injury too soon is a bigger mistake than using ice on an injury for too long. Many sports therapists elect to stay with cryotherapy for weeks after injury; some never switch to the superficial heating techniques. This procedure is simply a matter of personal preference that should be dictated by experience. Once swelling has stopped, the sports therapist may elect to begin contrast baths with a longer cold-to-hot ratio.[20]

An intermittent compression device may be used to decrease swelling by facilitating resorption of the by-products of injury by the lymphatic system. Electrical stimulating currents and low-power laser can be used to help reduce pain. Low-intensity ultrasound is still useful for facilitating healing.

After the initial stage, the athlete should begin to work on active and passive range of motion. Decisions regarding how rapidly to progress exercise should be determined by the response of the injury to that exercise. If exercise produces additional swelling and markedly exacerbates pain, then the level or intensity of the exercise is too great and should be reduced. Sports therapists should be aggressive in their approach to rehabilitation, but the approach will always be limited by the healing process.

Fibroblastic-Repair Phase

Once the inflammatory response has subsided, the fibroblastic-repair phase begins. During this phase of the healing process, fibroblastic cells lay down a matrix of collagen fibers and form scar tissue. This stage might begin as early as 4 days after the injury and might last for several weeks. At this point, swelling has stopped completely. The injury is still tender to the touch but is not as painful as during the last stage. Pain is also less on active and passive motion.

Treatments may change during this stage from cold to heat, once again using increased swelling as a precautionary indicator. Thermotherapy techniques, including hydrocollator packs, paraffin, or eventually warm whirlpool, can safely be used. The purpose of thermotherapy is to increase circulation to the injured area to promote healing. These modalities can also produce some degree of analgesia.

Intermittent compression can once again be used to facilitate removal of injury by-products from the area. Electrical stimulating currents can be used to assist this process by eliciting a muscle contraction and thus inducing a muscle pumping action. This facilitates lymphatic flow. Electrical currents can once again be used for modulation of pain, as can stimulation of trigger points with the low-power laser.

The sports therapist must continue to stress the importance of range-of-motion and strengthening exercises and progress them appropriately during this phase.

Maturation-Remodeling Phase

The maturation-remodeling phase is the longest of the four phases and might last for several years, depending on the severity of the injury. The ultimate goal during the maturation stage of the healing process is the return to activity. The injury is no longer painful to the touch, although some progressively decreasing pain might still be felt on motion. The collagen fibers must be realigned according to tensile stresses and strains placed upon them. Virtually all modalities may safely be used during this stage; thus decisions should be based on what seems to work most effectively in a given situation.

At this point some type of heating modality is beneficial to the healing process. The deep-heating modalities, ultrasound, or shortwave and microwave diathermy should be used to increase circulation to the deeper tissues. Increased blood flow delivers the essential nutrients to the injured area to promote healing, and increased lymphatic flow assists in the breakdown and removal of waste products. The superficial heating modalities are certainly less effective at this point.

Electrical stimulating currents can be used for a number of purposes. As before, they may be used in pain modulation. They may also be used to assist in increasing range of motion or muscular strength. Low-power laser can also assist in modulating pain. If pain is reduced, therapeutic exercises may be progressed more quickly.

Range-of-motion and strengthening exercises can be increased relatively quickly and progress toward a full, pain-free return to levels required for successful participation in sport activities.

Other Considerations in Treating Injury

During the rehabilitation period after injury, athletes must alter their training and conditioning habits to allow the injury to heal sufficiently. The sports therapist must not neglect fitness training in designing a rehabilitation program. Consideration must be given to maintaining levels of strength, flexibility, and cardiorespiratory endurance.[17]

Modality use should be combined with anti-inflammatory medication, particularly during the initial acute and acute inflammatory phases of rehabilitation. A complete discussion of the effects of various medications on the rehabilitation process appears in Chapter 16.

INDICATIONS AND CONTRAINDICATIONS

Table 15-2 is a summary list of indications, contraindications, and precautions in using the various modalities. This list should help the sports therapist make decisions regarding the appropriate use of a therapeutic modality in a given clinical situation.

■ **TABLE 15-2**   Indications and Contraindications for Therapeutic Modalities

Therapeutic Modality	Physiological Responses (Indications for Use)	Contraindications and Precautions
Electrical stimulating currents—high voltage	Pain modulation Muscle reeducation Muscle pumping contractions Retard atrophy Muscle strengthening Increase range of motion Fracture healing Acute injury	Pacemakers Thrombophlebitis Superficial skin lesions
Electrical stimulating currents—low voltage	Wound healing Fracture healing Iontophoresis	Malignancy Skin hypersensitivities Allergies to certain drugs
Electrical stimulating currents—interferential	Pain modulation Muscle reeducation Muscle pumping contractions Fracture healing Increase range of motion	Same as high-voltage
Electrical stimulating currents—Russian	Muscle strengthening	Pacemakers

■ **TABLE 15-2** Indications and Contraindications for Therapeutic Modalities—Cont'd

Therapeutic Modality	Physiological Responses (Indications for Use)	Contraindications and Precautions
Electrical stimulating currents— MENS	Fracture healing Wound healing	Malignancy Infections
Shortwave diathermy and microwave diathermy	Increase deep circulation Increase metabolical activity Reduce muscle guarding/spasm Reduce inflammation Facilitate wound healing Analgesia Increase tissue temperatures over a large area	Metal implants Pacemakers Malignancy Wet dressings Anesthetized areas Pregnancy Acute injury and inflammation Eyes Areas of reduced blood flow Anesthetized areas
Cryotherapy—cold packs, ice massage	Acute injury Vasoconstriction—decreased blood flow Analgesia Reduce inflammation Reduce muscle guarding/spasm	Allergy to cold Circulatory impairments Wound healing Hypertension
Thermotherapy—hot whirlpool, paraffin, hydrocollator, infrared lamps	Vasodilation—increased blood flow Analgesia Reduce muscle guarding/spasm Reduce inflammation Increase metabolical activity Facilitate tissue healing	Acute and postacute trauma Poor circulation Circulatory impairments Malignancy
Low-power laser	Pain modulation (trigger points) Facilitate wound healing	Pregnancy Eyes
Ultraviolet	Acne Aseptic wounds Folliculitis Pityriasis rosea Tinea Septic wounds Sinusitis Increase calcium metabolism	Psoriasis Eczema Herpes Diabetes Pellagra Lupus erythematosus Hyperthyroidism Renal and hepatic insufficiency Generalized dermatitis Advanced atherosclerosis
Ultrasound	Increase connective tissue extensibility Deep heat Increased circulation Treatment of most soft tissue injuries Reduce inflammation Reduce muscle spasm	Infection Acute and postacute injury Epiphyseal areas Pregnancy Thrombophlebitis Impaired sensation Eyes
Intermittent compression	Decrease acute bleeding Decrease edema	Circulatory impairment

Summary

1. Modalities are best used by the sports therapist as adjuncts to other forms of therapeutic exercise. Decisions on how a particular modality can best be used should be based on both theoretical knowledge and practical experience.

2. The effects of thermotherapy and cryotherapy are primarily superficial. These modalities are perhaps most effectively used to produce analgesia. They also have an indirect effect on circulation in the deeper tissues.

3. Ultrasound is vibrational acoustic energy that causes a tissue temperature increase in addition to other physiological effects that aid healing.

4. Shortwave and microwave diathermy units use extremely high frequency electrical currents to produce a tissue temperature increase in the deeper tissues.

5. Electrical stimulating currents may be used to stimulate sensory nerves to modulate pain, stimulate motor nerves to elicit a muscle contraction, introduce chemical ions into superficial tissues for medicinal purposes, and create an electrical field in the tissues to stimulate or alter the healing process.

6. The physiological response of the biological tissues to electrical stimulating currents is to a great extent determined by the treatment parameters of the current selected by the sports therapist.

7. Low-power lasers are the newest modality used in sports medicine settings. They are used primarily to promote wound healing and modulate pain through stimulation of acupuncture and trigger points.

8. Massage is the mechanical stimulation of tissue by means of rhythmically applied pressure and stretching. It allows the therapist, as a health care provider, to help a patient overcome pain and relax through the application of the therapeutic massage techniques.

9. Modality use in the initial acute injury phase should be directed toward one goal: to reduce the amount of swelling. The less initial swelling, the less time will be required for rehabilitation.

10. During the inflammatory-response stage of healing, modalities should be used to reduce pain and limit the amount of swelling. The injured part should be rested to allow the healing process to work.

11. During the fibroblastic-repair phase, thermotherapy may be used to increase blood flow to the injured area. Also during this time, strengthening and range-of-motion exercises should begin.

12. The maturation-remodeling phase is a long-term process during which the athlete returns to activity. Deep-heating modalities that increase blood flow and assist in the breakdown and removal of the by-products of the healing process should be used. The quantity and intensity of therapeutic exercise should be progressively increased during this phase of healing.

References

1. Angus, J., W. Prentice, and D. Hooker. 1994. A comparison of two external intermittent compression devices and their effect on post acute ankle edema. *Journal of Athletic Training* 29(2): 178.

2. Baker, L., D. McNeal, and L. Benton. 1993. *Neuromuscular electrical stimulation.* Downey, CA: Rancho Los Amigos Medical Center.

3. Brown, S. 1994. The effect of microcurrent on edema, range of motion, and pain in treatment of lateral ankle sprains, [Abstract]. *Journal of Orthopaedic and Sports Physical Therapy* 19:55.

4. Castel, C., D. Draper, and D. Castel. 1994. Rate of temperature increase during ultrasound treatments: Are traditional times long enough? *Journal of Athletic Training* 29(2): 156.

5. DeVahl, J. 1992. Neuromuscular electrical stimulation (NMES) in rehabilitation. In *Electrotherapy in rehabilitation,* edited by M. Gersh. Philadelphia: F. A. Davis.

6. Draper, D., S. Schulthies, and P. Sorvisto. 1994. The effect of cooling the tissue prior to ultrasound treatment. *Journal of Athletic Training* 29(2): 154.

7. Dyson, M. 1989. The use of ultrasound in sports physiotherapy. In *Sports Injuries: International perspectives in physiotherapy,* edited by V. Grisogono. Edinburgh: Churchill Livingstone.

8. Enwemeka, C. 1988. Laser biostimulation of healing wounds: Specific effects and mechanisms of action. *Journal of Orthopaedic and Sports Physical Therapy* 9:333–38.

9. Fritz, S. 1995. *Fundamentals of therapeutic massage.* St. Louis: Mosby.

10. Geick, J., et al. 1984. Therapeutic ultrasound: Technology, performance standards, biological effect, and clinical application. HSH Publication No. FOA 84-0000 (August).

11. Harris, S., D. Draper, and S. Schulthies. 1995. The effect of ultrasound on temperature rise in preheated human muscle. *Journal of Athletic Training* 30(2): S-42.

12. Hooker, D. 1999. Electrical stimulating currents. In *Therapeutic modalities in sports medicine*, edited by W. Prentice. Dubuque, IA: WCB/McGraw-Hill.

13. Hooker, D. 1999. Intermittent compression devices. In *Therapeutic modalities in sports medicine*, edited by W. Prentice. Dubuque, IA: WCB/McGraw-Hill.

14. Hooker, D. 1999. Traction as a specialized modality. In *Therapeutic modalities in sports medicine*, edited by W. Prentice. Dubuque, IA: WCB/McGraw-Hill.

15. Kloth, L. 1996. Shortwave and microwave diathermy. In *Thermal agents in rehabilitation*, edited by S. L. Michlovitz. Philadelphia: F. A. Davis.

16. Knight, K. 1995. *Cryotherapy in sport injury management.* Champaign, IL: Human Kinetics.

17. Krumholz, A., B. Gelfand, and P. O'Conner. 1995. Therapeutic modalities. In *The lower extremity and spine in sports medicine*, vol. 1, edited by J. Nicholas and E. B. Hershman. St Louis: Mosby Yearbook.

18. Lehmann, J. F., and B. J. DeLateur. 1982. Cryotherapy. In *Therapeutic heat and cold*, 3d ed., edited by J. F. Lehmann. Baltimore: Williams & Wilkins.

19. Lehmann, J. F., and B. J. DeLateur. 1982. Therapeutic heat. In *Therapeutic heat and cold*, 3d ed., edited by J. F. Lehmann. Baltimore: Williams & Wilkins.

20. Meyer, J., D. Draper, and E. Durrant. 1994. Contrast therapy and intramuscular temperature in the leg. *Journal of Athletic Training* 29(4): 318–24.

21. Michlovitz, S. L. 1996. Biophysical principles of heating and superficial heat agents. In *Thermal agents in rehabilitation*, edited by S. L. Michlovitz. Philadelphia: F. A. Davis.

22. Michlovitz, S. L. 1996. Cryotherapy: The use of cold as a therapeutic agent. In *Thermal agents in rehabilitation*, edited by S. L. Michlovitz. Philadelphia: F. A. Davis.

23. Prentice, W. 1999. Iontophoresis. In *Therapeutic modalities in sports medicine*, edited by W. Prentice. Dubuque, IA: WCB/McGraw-Hill.

24. Prentice, W. 1999. Preface. In *Therapeutic modalities in sports medicine*, edited by W. Prentice. Dubuque, IA: WCB/McGraw-Hill.

25. Prentice, W. 1999. Basic principles of electricity. In *Therapeutic modalities in sports medicine*, edited by W. Prentice. Dubuque, IA: WCB/McGraw-Hill.

26. Prentice, W., and D. Draper. 1999. Therapeutic ultrasound. In *Therapeutic modalities in sports medicine*, edited by W. Prentice. Dubuque, IA: WCB/McGraw-Hill.

27. Prentice, W., and G. Bell. 1999. Infrared modalities. In *Therapeutic modalities in sports medicine*, edited by W. Prentice. Dubuque, IA: WCB/McGraw-Hill.

28. Prentice, W., and P. Donley. 1999. Shortwave and microwave diathermy. In *Therapeutic modalities in sports medicine*, edited by W. Prentice. Dubuque, IA: WCB/McGraw-Hill.

29. Prentice, W., and C. Lehn. 1999. Therapeutic massage. In *Therapeutic modalities in sports medicine*, edited by W. Prentice. Dubuque, IA: WCB/McGraw-Hill.

30. Quillin, W. S. 1982. Ultrasonic phonophoresis. *Physician and Sports Medicine* 10:211.

31. Rucinski, T., W. Prentice, D. Hooker, E. Shields, and D. Murray. 1991. The effects of intermittent compression on edema in postacute ankle sprains. *Journal of Orthopaedic and Sports Physical Therapy* 13(8): 65–69.

32. Saliba, E., and S. Foreman. 1999. Low-power laser. In *Therapeutic modalities in sports medicine*, edited by W. Prentice. Dubuque, IA: WCB/McGraw-Hill.

33. Schliephakle, E. 1966. Carrying out treatment. In *Introduction to shortwave and microwave therapy*, 3d ed., edited by H. Throm. Springfield, IL: Charles C. Thomas.

34. Snyder-Mackler, L., and A. Robinson. 1997. *Clinical electrophysiology: Electrotherapy and electrophysiology.* Baltimore: Williams & Wilkins.

35. ter Harr, C. 1987. Basic physics of therapeutic ultrasound. *Physiotherapy* 73(3): 110–13.

36. Thorsteinsson, G. 1983. Electrical stimulation for analgesia. In *Therapeutic electricity and ultraviolet radiation*, 7th ed., edited by G. K. Stillwell. Baltimore: Williams & Wilkins.

37. Walsh, M. 1997. Hydrotherapy: The use of water as a therapeutic agent. In *Thermal agents in rehabilitation*, edited by S. L. Michlovitz. Philadelphia: F. A. Davis.

38. Ziskin, M. C., and S. L. Michlovitz. 1997. Therapeutic ultrasound. In *Thermal agents in rehabilitation*, edited by S. L. Michlovitz. Philadelphia: F. A. Davis.

CHAPTER 16

Using Pharmacological Agents in a Rehabilitation Program

Patsy Huff
William E. Prentice

After completion of this chapter, the student should be able to do the following:

- Discuss the reasons for use of various analgesics, anti-inflammatories, and antipyretics as an adjunct form of treatment in a rehabilitation program.

- Identify the potential adverse effects and reactions of medications that act on the respiratory tract, medications that affect the gastrointestinal tract, and antibiotics.

- Discuss the importance of record keeping when administering medications in a sports medicine environment.

- Be aware of the legalities of dispensing versus administering medications by sports medicine personnel.

- Discuss the impact of drug-testing programs on the use of various medications in a rehabilitation setting.

The use of medications prescribed for various medical conditions by qualified physicians can be of great value to the athlete, as it can for any other person.[37] Under average circumstances an athlete would be expected to respond to medication just as anyone else would. However, because of the nature of physical activity, the athlete's situation is not average; with intense physical activity, special consideration should be given to the effects of certain types of medication.

For the sports therapist supervising a program of rehabilitation, some knowledge of the potential effects of certain types of drugs on performance during the rehabilitation program is essential. The sports therapist working under the direction of a team physician is responsible for keeping the athlete healthy and ready to train and compete under physically, mentally, and emotionally demanding circumstances. The sports therapist should be concerned not only with rehabilitation but also with evaluation, prevention, and acute management of sport-related injuries. On occasion, the sports therapist must make decisions regarding the appropriate use of medications based on knowledge of the indications for use and the possible side effects in athletes who are involved in rehabilitation programs.

The sports therapist must be cognizant of the potential effects and side effects of over-the-counter and prescription medications on the athlete during rehabilitation, as well as during competition.

This chapter concentrates on special considerations regarding those medications most commonly used in a sports medicine environment.

COMMON MEDICATIONS

This section provides the sports therapist with some special considerations regarding medications most commonly prescribed for and used by individuals involved in a sport-related activity. The classifications of medication discussed include (1) analgesics, antipyretics, and anti-inflammatories; (2) drugs that affect the respiratory tract; (3) drugs that affect the gastrointestinal tract; and (4) antibiotic medications (Table 16-1).

Analgesics, Antipyretics, and Anti-inflammatories

Medications are most commonly used in a sport-medicine environment for pain relief. The athlete is continuously in situations where injuries are very likely. Fortunately, most of the injuries that occur are not serious and lend themselves to rapid rehabilitation. However, pain can be associated with even minor injury.

The over-the-counter nonnarcotic analgesics often used include aspirin (salicylate), acetaminophen, naproxen sodium ketoprofen, and ibuprofen. These belong to the group of drugs called **nonsteroidal anti-inflammatory drugs (NSAIDs).** Aspirin is one of the most commonly used drugs in the world.[34] Because of its easy availability, it is also likely the most misused drug. Aspirin is a derivative of salicylic acid and is used for its analgesic, anti-inflammatory, and antipyretic capabilities.

Analgesia can result from several mechanisms. Aspirin can interfere with the transmission of painful impulses in the thalamus.[26] Soft-tissue injury leads to tissue necrosis. This tissue injury causes the release of arachidonic acid from phospholipid cell walls. Oxygenation of arachidonic acid by cyclooxygenase produces a variety of prostaglandins, thromboxane, and prostacyclin that mediate the subsequent inflammatory reaction.[1] The predominant mechanism of action of aspirin and other NSAIDs is the inhibition of prostaglandin synthesis by blocking the cyclooxygenase pathway.[41] Pain and inflammation are reduced by the blockage of accumulation of proinflammatory prostaglandins in the synovium or cartilage.

Stabilization of the lysosomal membrane also occurs, preventing the efflux of destructive lysosomal enzymes into the joints.[19] Aspirin is the only NSAID that irreversibly inhibits cyclooxygenase; the other NSAIDs provide reversible inhibition. Aspirin also can reduce fever by altering sympathetic outflow from the hypothalamus, which produces increased vasodilation and heat loss through sweating.[26,38] Among the side effects of aspirin usage are gastric distress, heartburn, some nausea, tinni-

tus, headache, and diarrhea. More serious consequences can develop with prolonged use or high dosages.[3]

An athlete should be very cautious about selecting aspirin as a pain reliever, for a number of reasons.[36] Aspirin inhibits aggregation of platelets and thus impairs the clotting mechanism should injury occur.[30] Aspirin's irreversible inhibition of cyclooxygenase, which leads to reduced production of clotting factors, creates a bleeding risk not present with the other NSAIDs.[40] Prolonged bleeding at an injured site will increase the amount of swelling, which has a direct effect on the time required for rehabilitation.

Use of aspirin as an anti-inflammatory should be recommended with caution. Other anti-inflammatory medications do not produce many of the undesirable side effects of aspirin. Generally, prescription anti-inflammatories are considered to be equally effective.

Aspirin sometimes produces gastric discomfort. An athlete's intense physical activity can exacerbate this side effect. Buffered aspirin is no less irritating to the stomach than regular aspirin, but enteric-coated tablets resist aspirin breakdown in the stomach and might minimize gastric discomfort. Regardless of the form of aspirin ingested, it should be taken with meals or with large quantities of water (8 to 10 ounces/tablet) to reduce the likelihood of gastric irritation.

Ibuprofen is classified as a NSAID; however, it also has analgesic and antipyretic effects. Like aspirin, ibuprofen has a number of side effects, including the potential for gastric irritation. It does not affect platelet aggregation as aspirin does. Ibuprofen administered at a dose of 200 mg does not require a prescription and at that dosage may be used for analgesia. At a dose of 400 mg, the effects are both analgesic and anti-inflammatory. Dosage forms greater than 200 mg require a prescription. For names and recommended doses of prescription NSAIDs, refer to Table 16-2.

Acetaminophen, like aspirin, has both analgesic and antipyretic effects, but it does not have significant anti-inflammatory capabilities.[3] Acetaminophen is indicated for relief of mild somatic pain and fever reduction through mechanisms similar to those of aspirin.[17]

The primary advantage of acetaminophen for the athlete is that it does not produce gastritis, irritation, or gastrointestinal bleeding. Likewise, it does not affect platelet aggregation and thus does not increase clotting time after an injury.

For the athlete who is not in need of an anti-inflammatory medication but who requires some pain-relieving medication or an antipyretic, acetaminophen should be the drug of choice. If inflammation is a consideration, the team physician may elect to use a type of

■ TABLE 16-1   Athletic Trainer's Guide to Medications Frequently Used in Sports Medicine

Generic Name	Trade Name	Primary Use of Drug/Precautions	Sports Medicine Considerations
Analgesics, Antipyretics, and Anti-inflammatories (NSAIDs)			
Aspirin	Many trade names	Analgesic, antipyretic, anti-inflammatory.	Gastric irritation, nausea, tinnitus, prolonged bleeding if injured in contact sports.
Acetaminophen	Tylenol, Datril, others	Analgesic, antipyretic.	None.
Flurbiprofen	Ansaid*	All are analgesic, antipyretic, anti-inflammatory (NSAIDs).	Gastric irritation less common than with aspirin except for indomethacin. These should be used
Ketoprofen	Orudis*	Notify MD immediately for skin rash, itching,	for reducing pain and inflammation; should not
Indomethacin	Indocin*	visual disturbances, weight gain, edema, black	be substituted for acetaminophen in cases of
Ibuprofen	Advil, Motrin*, Nuprin	stools, dark urine or persistent headache.	mild headache or low fever. Adequate
Naproxen	Naprosyn*, Anaprox*	*Drug Interactions:* salicylates, other NSAIDs,	hydration reduce the risk of adverse effects in
Diflunisal	Dolobid*	probenecid, cimetidine, phenylpropanolamine,	the renal system.
Piroxicam	Feldene*	diuretics, lithium, phenytoin, beta-blockers,	*NSAID Hypersensitivity:* Because of cross
Tolmectin	Tolectin*	ACE inhibitors, anticoagulants, digoxin.	sensitivity to aspirin and all other NSAIDS, do
Fenoprofen	Nalfon*		not give these agents to athletes in whom
Meclofenamate	Meclomen*		aspirin, iodides, or other NSAIDs have caused
Diclofenac	Voltaren*		symptoms of asthma, rhinitis, rash, nasal
Ketoralac	Toradol*		polyps, bronchospasm, or other symptoms of
Etodolac	Lodine*		allergic reactions.
Bromphenac	Duract*		
Mefenamic acid	Ponstel*		
Antifungal Agents			
Ketaconazole	Nizoral*	Systemic (oral) antifungal drug. Drug has been associated with hepatic toxicity including fatalities. Notify MD immediately for unusual fatigue, anorexia, nausea, jaundice, dark urine, pale stools, abdominal pain, fever or diarrhea.	Should not be taken within 2 hours of antacids. May cause dizziness or drowsiness. *Hypersensitivity:* Anaphylaxis has been reported.
Griseofulvin	Fulvicin P/G*, Gris-Peg*	Oral antifungal agent. Notify MD immediately for fever, sore throat, or skin rash. Reduces the effectiveness of oral contraceptives.	Photosensitivity may occur: Patient should avoid prolonged exposure to sunlight or sunlamps.

continued

■ TABLE 16-1   Athletic Trainer's Guide to Medications Frequently Used in Sports Medicine—Cont'd

Generic Name	Trade Name	Primary Use of Drug/Precautions	Sports Medicine Considerations
Fluconazole	Diflucan*	Oral antifungal agent. Warnings: hepatic injury, anaphylaxis, dermatologic changes have been reported. Notify MD immediately for skin rash. *Drug Interactions:* cimetidine, rifampin, nonsedating antihistamines, phenytoin, theophylline, zidovudine.	
Terbinafine	Lamisil*	Oral antifungal agent for treatment of toenails or fingernails, scalp, body, groin, or feet. Notify MD immediately for skin rash, itching, aching joints, dark urine, difficulty swallowing, fever, chills, pale skin, pale stool, redness, blistering, peeling or loosening of skin, unusual tiredness, and yellowing of skin or eyes. *Drug Interactions:* cimetidine, rifampin, terfenadine, caffeine.	Weeks to months may be required to resolve infection. Alcohol consumption during treatment increases risk of liver toxicity.
Antibiotics			
Penicillins	V-Cillin-K*, Pen Vee K Trimox*	*Drug Interactions:* beta-blockers, oral contraceptives, erythromycin, tetracycline.	If diarrhea occurs, do not give Imodium AD.
Cephalosporins	Keflex*, Ceftin*	*Drug Interactions:* oral contraceptives, alcohol, probenecid.	Patients allergic to penicillin may have cross sensitivity to cephalosporins.
Macrolides	Ery-Tab*, Zithromax*, Biaxin*, Dynabac*	*Drug Interactions:* fluconazole, zidovudine, theophylline, nonsedating antihistamines, oral contraceptives, carbamazepine, ergot alkaloids, penicillins.	
Fluoroquinolones	Cipro*, Noroxin*, Floxin*, Penetrex*, Maxaquin*, Zagam*, Levaquin*	Notify MD immediately for agitation, confusion, tremors, fever, skin rash. *Drug Interactions:* antacids, sucralfate, Pepto-Bismol, cimetidine, caffeine, probenecid, phenytoin, theophylline, oral contraceptives. Photosensitivity: avoid overexposure to sunlight or sunlamps.	May cause dizziness. Rarely associated with pain, inflammation, or rupture of a tendon.
Tetracyclines	Sumycin*, Vibramycin*	*Drug Interactions:* antacids, anticoagulants, cimetidine, insulin, lithium, oral contraceptives, penicillins, sodium bicarbonate.	Should not be taken with milk, antacids, or minerals because of reduced absorption. Photosensitivity may occur.

continued

■ **TABLE 16-1**   Athletic Trainer's Guide to Medications Frequently Used in Sports Medicine—Cont'd

Generic Name	Trade Name	Primary Use of Drug/Precautions	Sports Medicine Considerations
Drugs That Affect The Respiratory Tract			
Chlorpheniramine	Chlor-Trimeton	Antihistamine for allergies.	Used primarily for treatment of allergic rhinitis. Causes drowsiness, decreased coordination.
Cromolyn	Nasalcrom	Nasal allergy symptom controller, prevents and relieves nasal allergy symptoms.	Allergic rhinitis, seasonal allergies.
Oxymetazoline	Afrin, Dristan Long Lasting, Neosynephrine 12 Hour, Allerest	Adrenergic decongestant applied topically as spray or nose drops.	Do not exceed recommended duration of treatment because of rebound congestion; may cause sneezing, dryness of nasal mucosa, and headache.
Pseudoephedrine	Sudafed, Cenafed, Oranyl, others	Adrenergic decongestant used orally.	Produces stimulation of the central nervous system; topically applied decongestants work faster, but oral decongestants are preferred for long-term use.
Diphenhydramine	Benadryl, Benylin cough syrup	Antihistamine used primarily for allergic reaction; also used for sleep.	Produces drowsiness and dry mouth; found in over-the-counter sleeping medications.
Dextromethorphan	Robitussin DM, Benylin DMO, Sucrets Lozenges	Nonnarcotic antitussive used for cough suppression. *Drug Interaction:* newer antidepressants.	Very effective in cases of unproductive cough; rarely produces drowsiness and other side effects.
Terfenadine	Seldane*	Antihistamine.	Nonsedating. Watch for cardiotoxic drug interactions with erythromycin, grapefruit juice, oral antifungals and other drugs.
Cetirizine	Zyrtec	Antihistamine: Effective for some allergic reactions.	May cause some sedation but less than traditional antihistamines.
Fexofenadine Loratidine Astemizole	Allegra Claritin Hismanyl	Antihistamines.	Nonsedating.
Benzonatate	Tessalon*	Peripherally acting antitussive that acts as an anesthetic.	May cause dizziness; should not be chewed.
Codeine	Robitussin AC	Narcotic antitussive that depresses the central cough mechanism.	Used in combination with expectorant; can produce sedation, dizziness, constipation, or nausea.
Guaifenesin	Robitussin, Glyate	Expectorant used for symptomatic relief of unproductive cough.	Used for treating a dry or sore throat; good hydration maximizes effects.

continued

■ TABLE 16-1 Athletic Trainer's Guide to Medications Frequently Used in Sports Medicine—Cont'd

Generic Name	Trade Name	Primary Use of Drug/Precautions	Sports Medicine Considerations
Drugs That Affect The Gastrointestinal Tract			
Sodium bicarbonate	Soda Mint	Antacid used for quick relief of upset stomach.	Produces gas, belching; overuse may cause systemic alkalinity.
Aluminum hydroxide	Amphogel, Dialume	Antacid used for upset stomach.	May produce constipation; moderate acid neutralizer.
Calcium carbonate	Titralac, Mallamint	Antacid used for upset stomach and for calcium supplementation.	May produce constipation and acid rebound; high acid neutralizing capacity.
Magnesium hydroxide	Milk of Magnesia	Laxative used for constipation.	May cause diarrhea.
Cimetidine	Tagamet HB	Histamine 2 antagonist used for relief of upset stomach, heartburn, acid indigestion.	Numerous drug interactions.
Nizatidine Ranitidine Famotidine	Axid AR Zantac 75 Pepcid AC	Histamine 2 antagonist used for relief of upset stomach, heartburn, acid indigestion.	
Combination antacids	Alka-Seltzer, Digel, Gaviscon, Gelusil, Maalox, Mylanta, Wingel, others	Combination drugs for controlling gastric upset.	May produce either diarrhea or constipation.
Promethazine	Phenergan*	Antiemetic used for preventing motion sickness, nausea, and vomiting.	Produces sedation and drowsiness.
Diphenoxylate HCL Loperamide	Lomotil, Uni-Lom Imodium AD	Narcotic antidiarrheal. Nonnarcotic systemic antidiarrheal.	Causes dry mouth, nausea, drowsiness. Abdominal discomfort, drowsiness with large doses.
Combination antidiarrheals	Donnagel, Kaopectate	Relief of diarrhea.	All are relative safe with few side effects; effectiveness is questionable.
	Pepto-Bismol		Effective for traveler's diarrhea.

*Requires a prescription

■ **TABLE 16-2** NSAIDs Frequently Used Among Athletes: Prescription Required

Drug	Dosage Range (mg) and Frequency	Maximum Daily Dose (mg)
Aspirin	325–650 mg every 4 hours	4,000
Duract	25 mg every 6 to 8 hours	150
Voltaren	50–75 mg twice a day	200
Cataflam	50–75 mg twice a day	200
Dolobid	500–1,000 mg followed by 250–500 mg 2 to 3 times a day	1,500
Nalfon	300–600 mg 3 to 4 times a day	3,200
Motrin, Rufin	400–800 mg 3 to 4 times a day	3,200
Indocin	5–150 mg a day in 3 to 4 divided doses	200
Orudis	75 mg 3 times a day or 50 mg 4 times a day	300
Ponstel	500 mg followed by 250 mg every 6 hours	1,000
Naprosyn	250–500 mg twice a day	1,250
Anaprox	550 mg followed by 275 mg every 6 to 8 hours	1,375
Feldene	20 mg per day	20
Clinoril	200 mg twice a day	400
Tolectin	400 mg 3 to 4 times a day	1,800
Ansaid	50–100 mg 2 to 3 times a day	300
Toradol	10 mg every 4 to 6 hours for pain: Not to be used for more than 5 days	40
Lodine	200–400 mg every 6 to 8 hours for pain	1,200

NSAID. Most NSAIDs are prescription medications that, like aspirin, have not only anti-inflammatory but also analgesic and antipyretic effects.[19] They are effective for patients who cannot tolerate aspirin because of associated gastrointestinal distress. Patients who have the aspirin allergy triad of (1) nasal polyps, (2) associated bronchospasm/asthma, and (3) history of anaphylaxis should not receive any NSAID. Caution is advised when using NSAIDs in persons who might be predisposed to dehydration during training and competition. NSAIDs inhibit prostaglandin synthesis and therefore can compromise the elaboration of prostaglandins within the kidney during salt and/or water deficits. This can lead to ischemia within the kidney.[8,21] Adequate hydration is essential to reduce the risk of renal toxicity in athletes taking NSAIDs.

NSAID anti-inflammatory capabilities are thought to be equal to those of aspirin, their advantages being that NSAIDs have fewer side effects and relatively longer duration of action. NSAIDs have analgesic and antipyretic capabilities; the short-acting over-the-counter NSAIDs may be used in cases of mild headache or increased body temperature in place of aspirin or acetaminophen. They can be used to relieve many other mildly to moderately painful somatic conditions like menstrual cramps and soft-tissue injury.[22]

It has been recommended that patients receiving long-acting NSAIDs have monitoring of liver function enzymes during the course of therapy because of case reports of hepatic failure associated with the use of long-acting NSAIDs.[29]

The NSAIDs are used primarily for reducing the pain, stiffness, swelling, redness, and fever associated with localized inflammation, most likely by inhibiting the synthesis of prostaglandins.[11] The sports therapist must be aware that inflammation is simply a response to some underlying trauma or condition and that the source of irritation must be corrected or eliminated for these anti-inflammatory medications to be effective. Both naproxen and ketoprofen (now available without a prescription) have been shown to provide additional benefit when administered concomitantly with physical therapy.[21]

Muscle spasm and guarding accompany many musculoskeletal injuries. Elimination of this spasm and guarding should facilitate programs of rehabilitation. In many situations, centrally acting oral muscle relaxants are used to reduce spasm and guarding. However, to date the efficacy of using muscle relaxants has not been substantiated, and they do not appear to be superior to analgesics or sedatives in either acute or chronic conditions.[15]

Many analgesics and anti-inflammatory products are available over the counter in combination products (i.e., those containing two or more nonnarcotic analgesics with or without caffeine). Chronic use of analgesics containing aspirin and phenacetin or acetaminophen contributes to the development of papillary necrosis and

■ **TABLE 16-3** Selected Combination Analgesics Available in the United States

BC (Tablets)	Saleto (Tablets)
BC (Powder)	Buffets II (Tablets)
Goody's	Goody's
(Extra Strength Tablets)	(Headache Powder)
Excedrin (Extra Strength)	

analgesic-associated nephropathy. The presence of caffeine plays a role in dependency on these products leading to chronic use. Table 16-3 identifies selected available combination analgesics. It has been suggested that because of the higher risk for renal injury with combination analgesics, that these products should be withdrawn from the market.[23]

Drugs That Affect the Respiratory Tract

Antihistamines. Antihistamines reduce the effects of the chemical histamine on various tissues by selectively blocking receptor sites to which histamines attach. Histamine is abundant in the mast cells of the skin and lungs and in the basophils of blood. It is also found in the gastrointestinal tract and in the brain, where it acts as a neurotransmitter.[9] Histamine is released in response to some toxin, physical or chemical agent, drug, or antigen that has been introduced into the system. Thus it has a major function in many allergic or hypersensitivity reactions.[28]

Antihistamines are most typically used in the treatment of allergic reactions but may also be used as an antiemetic in the prevention of nausea and vomiting.[16] Histamine produces a number of systemic responses: (1) swelling and inflammation in the skin or mucous membranes (angioedema), (2) spasm of smooth bronchial muscle (asthma), (3) inflammation of nasal membranes (rhinitis), and (4) the possibility of anaphylaxis. These responses in varying degrees are typical of allergic reactions to insect stings, food, drugs, and anything else that might facilitate the release of histamine.

Histamine produces these reactions by binding with the cells that compose the various tissues at specific receptor sites. An antihistamine medication can competitively block these receptor sites and thus prevent the typical histamine response. Antihistamines are classified as either H1 or H2 receptor blockers. The so-called true antihistamines affect the H1 receptors only; H2 blockers affect cells in the stomach that secrete hydrochloric acid. Antihistamines do not reverse the effects of histamine;

they simply block the receptor sites. Newer nonsedating antihistamines, such as fexophenadine (Allegra) and loratidine (Claritin), require a prescription. Because of the potential risk of drug interactions, these newer antihistamines should be used only under the supervision of a physician. An athlete would benefit from different types of antihistamine medications for (1) relief from various types of allergic reactions, (2) prevention of motion sickness, or (3) relief of rhinitis from allergies.

Athletes, particularly those involved with fall and spring sports, practice outdoors where they are exposed to a number of allergens (such as pollen and insects) that potentially can produce a histamine response. Most cases are mild allergic reactions that may be treated by the sports therapist with an over-the-counter antihistamine. These medications are most effective in reducing the effects of histamine on the vascular system, which symptomatically include urticaria, rhinitis, and angioedema. These medications are effective in approximately 70 percent of patients treated.[9] Chlorpheniramine and diphenhydramine are over-the-counter antihistamines commonly used to treat mild allergic reactions.

A competitive schedule can require the athlete to do a great deal of traveling. People riding in a bus, car, or airplane often develop nausea and discomfort in response to motion. This motion sickness may be treated with a number of antihistamine medications. Dimenhydrinate and meclizine are the most commonly used drugs for the prevention of motion sickness. They are best used prophylactically before motion sickness occurs. Like other over-the-counter antihistamines, the major side effect is drowsiness and sedation.[6]

In the case of the athlete, antihistamines should be used with caution. The most common side effects of antihistamines are drowsiness and in some cases decreased coordination. Both of these side effects can adversely affect athletic performance and potentially predispose the athlete to unnecessary injury. Thus, use of antihistamine medication immediately before athletic competition is not recommended. The athlete should also be reminded that use of any sedating antihistamine along with consumption of alcohol will markedly increase drowsiness.

Decongestants. Nasal congestion can have a number of causes, including pollinosis or hay fever; perennial rhinitis, a chronic inflammatory condition that occurs with constant exposure to an allergen; and infectious rhinitis, which is symptomatic of the common cold.[34] Antihistamines also have anticholinergic effects and can often help dry up a runny nose. In addition, nasal congestion may be treated with sympathomimetic or decongestant medications, which may be used topically or orally. Oxymetazoline is an adrenergic topical nasal decongestant that, when sprayed on the nasal mucosa, produces prolonged vasoconstriction and reduces edema and fluid exudation. Pseudoephedrine is also an adrenergic decongestant taken orally. Nose drops and sprays act more rapidly than the oral decongestants, and oral medications cause more side effects such as stimulation of the central nervous system. However, oral medications are preferred in long-term use.[22]

Some medications combine both antihistamines and decongestants into a single tablet taken orally. Product selection should be based on symptoms (i.e., a decongestant for congestion, an antihistamine for rhinitis).

Drugs that can increase the rate of heat exhaustion. Heatstroke is a medical emergency with a mortality rate of 17 to 70 percent.[25] Patients of all ages can experience heatstroke. When the ambient temperature approaches body temperature and humidity approaches 100 percent, loss of heat from the body ceases. Physical exertion and stress, dehydration, drug therapy, lack of nutrition, lack of acclimatization, alcohol intoxication, age, obesity, and other disease states can contribute to the precipitation of heatstroke.[25] Thermoregulation involves the central and peripheral nervous system and circulatory mechanisms. Drugs that affect neurotransmitters in these systems could affect temperature regulation. Table 16-4 lists drugs that can predispose to heatstroke. Anticholinergics and antihistamines can decrease the peripheral mechanism of sweating and therefore eliminate the body's ability to lose heat from this mechanism. Sympathomimetic amines, including decongestants, are vasoconstrictors that can predispose an athlete to heatstroke. Phenothiazines affect both hot and cold temperature regulation. Tricyclic antidepressants have been shown to affect hypothalamic heat control and to have anticholinergic activity. Diuretics can prevent volume expansion and limit cutaneous vasodilation.[25]

Lithium carbonate can increase the risk of heatstroke by its effects on potassium levels. It is important that the sports therapist recognize medications that can increase the risk of heatstroke, especially when athletes are taking any of these medications and exercising in a warm climate.

Antitussives and expectorants. Drugs that suppress coughing are antitussives. Coughing is a reflex response to some irritation of the throat or airway. A cough is productive if some material is brought up. This type of cough is beneficial in clearing excessive mucus or sputum. An unproductive cough might be caused by postnasal drip, dry air, a sore throat, or anything else that irritates the throat. An unproductive cough is of no benefit and should be treated with medication. If the cause of the cough is a dry or a sore throat, an expecto-

■ **TABLE 16-4** Drugs That Might Predispose an Athlete to Heat Illness

Category	Examples of Specific Drug(s)
Neuroleptics	Thorazine, Haldol, Mellaril, others
Antidepressants	Elavil, Nardil, others
Anticholinergics	Atropine, Donnagel, Bentyl, Belladonna
Antihistamines	Chlor-Trimeton
Anti-Parkinson Drugs	Cogentin
Decongestants	Sudafed, Entex LA
Diuretics	Oretic

rant medication can be used to increase production of fluid in the respiratory system to coat the dry and irritated mucosal linings.[22]

Antitussive drugs are divided into those that depress the central cough center in the medulla (these can be either narcotic or nonnarcotic) and those that act peripherally to reduce irritation in the throat or trachea. Codeine is one of the more common narcotic antitussives that also has analgesic effects. In small doses, it is an effective antitussant and is considered safe. Codeine is found primarily in liquid form and is often combined with a decongestant, an analgesic, an expectorant, or an antihistamine. In most states, any liquid preparation that contains codeine is a prescription medication. The side effects of codeine include sedation, dizziness, constipation, and nausea.[9]

The most common nonnarcotic antitussives are diphenhydramine, dextromethorphan, and benzonatate. Perhaps their biggest advantage is that they have no analgesic effects and do not produce dependence. Diphenhydramine is an antihistamine-antitussive that produces both drowsiness and a drying effect. Dextromethorphan is the most widely used antitussive. It is as effective as codeine in medicating an unproductive cough but does not cause severe side effects. Benzonatate causes a local anesthetic action on the stretch receptors in the throat and thus dampens the cough reflex. Its side effects include drowsiness and a chilled sensation.[9] The peripherally acting antitussives are primarily expectorants. Although expectorants are thought to increase production of fluid in the throat, little experimental evidence suggests that the use of an expectorant is any more effective than drinking water or sucking a piece of hard candy. Expectorants are often combined with some other medication such as an antihistamine or a decongestant.[8]

■ **TABLE 16-5**   Medications Recommended for the Management of Asthma

Long-Term Control Medications	Quick Relief Medications
Inhaled corticosteroids	Short-acting beta-2-agonists
Beclomethasone (Beclovent, Vanceril)	Albuterol (Proventil, Ventolin)
Fluticasone propionate (Flovent)	Bitolterol mesylate (Tornalate)
Flunisolide (Aero-Bid)	Pirbuterol (Maxair)
Triamcinolone acetonide (Azmacort)	Terbutaline (Brethaire)
Cromolyn (Intal)	Anticholinergics
Nedocromil (Tilade)	Ipratropium bromide (Atrovent)
Long-acting beta-2-agonists	Oral Corticosteroids
Salmeterol (Serevent)	Methylprednisolone (Medrol)
Albuterol sustained-release (Proventil Repetabs)	Prednisolone (Various generics)
	Prednisone (Various generics)
Theophyllin (Theodur, Theolair-SR)	
Leukotriene modifiers	
Zafirlukast (Accolate)	
Zileuton (Zyflo)	

The athlete who is in need of antitussive or expectorant medication can benefit greatly from it. Physical activity tends to exacerbate the problem of a dry sore throat that may be responsible for an unproductive cough. The biggest consideration for the sports therapist would be the effects of other medications (that is, antihistamines or decongestants) that are contained in these fluids or lozenges. The drowsiness, gastric irritability, and lack of coordination that might occur will detract from athletic performance.

Drugs for Asthma.   Asthma is a chronic inflammatory lung disorder that is characterized by obstruction of the airways as a result of complex inflammatory processes, smooth muscle spasm, and hyperresponsiveness to a variety of stimuli.[27] Asthma triggers include exercise, viral infection, animal exposure, dust mites, mold, air pollutants, weather, and NSAIDS, as well as other drugs. The National Asthma Education and Prevention Program (NAEPP) has established international guidelines for the diagnosis and management of asthma.[27,35] The goals of asthma therapy are to prevent chronic and troublesome symptoms, maintain normal lung function and activity levels, prevent asthma exacerbations, provide optimal pharmacotherapy with minimal adverse effects, and meet patients' and families' expectations for, and satisfaction with, asthma care.

Exercise-induced bronchospasm (EIB) is a limiting and disruptive experience. Any asthma patient may be subject to EIB. A bronchospastic event caused by loss of heat, water, or both from lungs during exercise or exertion, EIB results from hyperventilation of air that is cooler and dryer than that in the respiratory tract.[2] EIB can occur during or minutes after physical activity, reaches its peak in 5 to 10 minutes after stopping the activity, and usually resolves in 20 to 30 minutes. In some asthma patients, exercise might be the only precipitating factor.

It is important that the athlete who has asthma be monitored carefully. The NAEPP recommends measurements of the following: asthma signs and symptoms, pulmonary function (peak flow or spirometry), quality of life/functional status, history of asthma exacerbations, and pharmacotherapy. Table 16-5 identifies medications recommended for asthma management.

Drugs That Affect the Gastrointestinal Tract

Dyspepsia is a vague, poorly defined disorder. Symptoms include indigestion, heartburn, bloating, nausea, diarrhea, and constipation problems that virtually everyone has experienced at one time or another. Because of factors such as the stress associated with competition, inconsistent travel schedules, eating patterns on road trips, and even motion sickness during travel, the athlete is likely to experience gastric upset.

Antacids.   The primary function of an antacid is to neutralize acidity in the upper GI tract by raising the pH, inhibiting the activity of the digestive enzyme pepsin, and thus reducing its action on the gastric mucosal nerve endings.[13,39] Antacids are effective not only for relief of acid indigestion and heartburn but also in the treatment of peptic ulcer. Antacids available in the market possess a wide range of acid neutralizing capabilities and side effects. The sports therapist has to be aware of these side effects when selecting a specific antacid preparation.

Sodium bicarbonate or baking soda is an antacid that quickly neutralizes hydrochloric acid and yields carbon dioxide gas and water. Sodium bicarbonate is rapidly absorbed by the blood to produce systemic alkalinity. In patients with normal renal function, excess bicarbonate is rapidly excreted by the kidney. In patients with poor renal function, however, sodium bicarbonate can accumulate, leading to metabolic alkalosis. Belching is usually associated with sodium bicarbonate ingestion, and ingestion of excess sodium bicarbonate often produces a rebound effect in which gastric acid secretion increases in response to an alkaline environment.[24] It is contraindicated for chronic therapy and should be used only for short-term relief of overeating or indigestion.

Some antacids can slow absorption of other medications from the GI tract. Ingestion of antacids containing magnesium tends to have a laxative effect; those containing aluminum or calcium can cause constipation. Consequently, many antacid liquids or tablets are combinations of magnesium and either aluminum or calcium hydroxides.[9] If use of a specific antacid produces diarrhea, for example, it can be replaced by another antacid that is higher in aluminum or calcium content to counteract the effects of the magnesium. An antacid high in magnesium content can reduce constipation. Simethicone is a silicone added to many of these preparations to reduce gas trapped in the upper GI tract through its antifoaming action, but evidence to support its benefit is limited.[34]

Selection of specific antacids should be based on consideration of their potential side effects, such as tendency to produce diarrhea or constipation, and on how well the patient tolerates their use in terms of taste, side effects, and cost.[22]

Calcium supplementation to increase calcium uptake by bone, and hence increase bone density as a means of reducing the incidence of fractures, is being recommended by some sports medicine specialists. Caution should be exercised in ingesting large amounts of calcium carbonate from antacids because of the potential constipation that can accompany prolonged use.

Another medication used for relief of gastric discomfort is an antihistamine that is an H2 receptor blocker. Histamine2 receptor blockers (i.e., cimetidine, ranitidine) inhibit the action of histamine on cells in the stomach that secrete hydrochloric acid and are most typically used to treat ulcers. H2 blockers are thought to be no more effective in the treatment of indigestion than antacid preparations.[33]

Reduced doses of H2 blockers are available without a prescription and are FDA approved for the treatment and/or prevention of heartburn, acid indigestion, and sour stomach brought on by consuming food and beverages. Numerous drug-drug interactions have been reported with cimetidine. Although significant drug interactions at low over-the-counter doses of cimetidine are not likely, patients receiving medications that interact with cimetidine should instead be given famotidine, ranitidine, or nizatidine.

Antiemetics. This group of drugs is used to treat the nausea and vomiting that can result from a variety of causes. Vomiting serves as a means of eliminating irritants from the stomach before they can be absorbed. Most of the time, however, purging the stomach is not necessary, and vomiting serves only to make the athlete uncomfortable. Frequently, nausea can be treated by giving the individual carbonated soda, tea, or ice to suck. If nausea and vomiting persist, some medication might be beneficial.

Antiemetics are classified as acting either locally or centrally. The locally acting drugs, such as most over-the-counter medications (for example, Pepto-Bismol and Alka-Seltzer) are topical anesthetics that reportedly affect the mucosal lining of the stomach. However, the effects of soothing an upset stomach can be more of a placebo effect.[34] The centrally acting drugs affect the chemoreceptor trigger zone in the medulla by making it less sensitive to irritating nerve impulses from the inner ear or stomach.

A variety of prescription antiemetics can be used for controlling nausea and vomiting, including phenothiazines, antihistamines, anticholinergic drugs for preventing motion sickness, and sedative drugs. The primary side effect of these medications is again extreme drowsiness. The sports therapist should deal with nausea and vomiting first by using fluids, which have a calming effect on the stomach, followed by the administration of one of the locally acting medications. If vomiting persists, the athlete will become drowsy and might be unable to perform at competitive levels, and dehydration and the problems that accompany it are important considerations for an athlete who has been nauseated and vomiting. Antiemetics can also potentiate central nervous system depressants.

Antidiarrheals. Diarrhea can result from many causes, but it is generally considered to be a symptom rather than a disease. It can occur as a result of emotional stress, allergies to food or drugs, or many different types of intestinal problems. Diarrhea can be acute or chronic. Acute diarrhea, the most common, comes on suddenly and can be accompanied by nausea, vomiting, chills, and intense abdominal pain. It typically runs its course very rapidly, and symptoms subside once the irritating agent is removed from the system. Chronic diarrhea, which can last for weeks, might result from more serious disease states.

The athlete suffering from acute diarrhea can be totally incapacitated in terms of athletic performance. The major problem of diarrhea is potential dehydration. An athlete, particularly when exercising in a hot environment, depends on body fluids to maintain normal temperature. An individual who becomes dehydrated has difficulty with regulation of temperature and might experience some heat-related problem. The sports therapist's primary concern should be replacing lost body fluids and electrolytes. Medication may be used on a short-term basis for relief of the symptoms, but it is also important to identify and treat the cause of the problem.

Medications used for control of diarrhea are either locally acting or systemic. The locally acting medications most typically contain kaolin, which absorbs other chemicals, and pectin, which soothes the irritated bowel. Some contain substances that add bulk to the stool. The effectiveness of locally acting medications is questionable, but they are considered safe and inexpensive.[12]

The systemic agents, which are generally antiperistaltic or antispasmodic medications, are considered to be much more effective in relieving symptoms of diarrhea, but most, except loperamide, are prescription drugs. The systemic medications are either opiate derivatives or anticholinergic agents, both of which reduce peristalsis. Common side effects of the systemic antidiarrheals include drowsiness, nausea, dry mouth, and constipation. Long-term use of the opiate drugs can lead to dependence.[5]

If the cause of diarrhea is a noninvasive bacteria, a physician might choose to administer multispectrum antibiotics along with an antiperistaltic agent.

Cathartics.   Laxatives can be used to empty the GI tract and eliminate constipation. In most cases, constipation can be relieved by proper diet, sufficient fluid intake, and exercise.[22] A cathartic medication is generally not necessary.

An athlete who complains of constipation should first be advised to consume the foods and juices that cause bulk in the feces and stimulate gastrointestinal peristalsis, such as bran cereals, fresh fruits, coffee, and chocolate. Increased fluid intake also facilitates peristalsis in the bowel.

Generally speaking, athletes seem to suffer less from constipation than from diarrhea. This tendency may be attributed as much to activity levels as to any other single factor. If a laxative medication is necessary, the bulk-forming laxatives are among the safest but should be used only for short periods, and dietary modifications should also be encouraged.

Antibiotic Medications

Many of the medications discussed have been over-the-counter medications that may be selected and adminis-tered by the sports therapist following strict guidelines and protocols for administration established by the team physician. In the case of infectious diseases, the team physician must be directly involved in the selection of specific antimicrobial agents. The sports therapist is often the individual who first recognizes an athlete's signs of developing infection, such as fever, redness, swelling, tenderness, purulent drainage, and swollen lymph nodes. The sports therapist should have the responsibility of referring the athlete with a suspected infection to the physician for a total assessment, including physical examination and laboratory tests. The team physician will then prescribe for the athlete an appropriate antibiotic medication that is selectively capable of destroying the invading microorganism without affecting the patient.[26] The sports therapist may be asked to provide adjunctive therapy, such as applying hot compresses or soaks in antiseptic solutions in open infections.

In the case of an athlete who is using an antibiotic medication, the sports therapist's role should be to monitor the patient for signs and symptoms of allergic response or drug-induced toxicity. Many individuals exhibit hypersensitivity reactions to antimicrobial agents. Perhaps the most common reaction occurs with the use of penicillin. Antibiotics are also capable of damaging the tissues they contact. They can damage the mucosa of the stomach and cause diarrhea, nausea, and vomiting. They can also affect kidney function and interfere with nervous system function. Should these reactions occur, the athlete should be sent back to the physician, who might elect to change to another type of antibiotic medication.[42]

An athlete who has an infection, be it localized or systemic, that requires use of an antibiotic will usually be advised not to train or compete until the infection is under control. The sports therapist should be certain that the athlete adheres to this recommendation, both to benefit the infected athlete and to limit the possibility of the infection spreading or being transmitted to other athletes.

ADMINISTERING VERSUS DISPENSING MEDICATION

The methods by which drugs may be administered and dispensed vary according to individual state laws. Sports medicine settings are subject to those laws. *Administration* of a drug is giving the athlete a single dose of a particular medication. *Dispensing* of medication is giving the athlete a drug in a quantity greater than would be used in a single dose. In most cases, the team physician is the individual ultimately responsible for prescribing medications. These prescription medications are then dispensed by either the physician, the physician extender licensed to dispense, or the pharmacist. **The sports therapist may not dispense medication. However, in most states they may legally administer a single dose of a nonprescription medication.** The sports therapist typically does not possess the background or the experience to make decisions about the appropriate use of medication and should be subject to strict protocols if and when administering medication.

On occasion, over-the-counter medications are placed on a countertop in the sports -medicine clinic for use as the athlete sees fit. Although this method of administering medication saves time for the clinician, this somewhat indiscriminate use of even over-the-counter drugs by an athlete should be discouraged. The sports therapist who is administering over-the-counter medication of any variety should be knowledgeable about the possible effects of various drugs during exercise. Likewise, sports therapists should be subject to strict protocols established by the team physician for administering medication. Table 16-6 and the Administration Protocols for common over-the-counter drugs used in sports medicine on pages 262–63 present the guidelines used for the administration of over-the-counter medications by the sports therapist for a number of minor illnesses or conditions seen commonly in the athletic population. Failure to follow these guidelines or protocols can make the sports therapist legally liable, should something happen to the athlete that can be attributed to use or misuse of a particular drug.

Labeling Requirements

Over-the-counter drugs are required to have adequate directions for use, precautions, and adequate readability. Table 16-7 identifies the requirements of the Federal 7-Point Label for nonprescription drugs. Nonprescription drugs may not be repackaged without meeting labeling criteria. All drugs dispensed from the training room must be properly labeled. Legal violations can occur if a portion of a nonprescription drug is removed from an original properly labeled package and dispensed to an athlete. This practice carries the same liability as dispensing prescription drugs, because the athlete is not given the opportunity to review the label for name, contents, precautions, directions, and other information considered essential for the safe use of the product. Liability for any averse patient outcome is therefore transferred to the dispenser of the improperly labeled over-the-counter drug.

Record Keeping

Those involved in any health-care profession are acutely aware of the necessity of maintaining complete up-to-date medical records. Again the sports medicine setting is no exception. If medications are administered by a sports therapist, maintaining accurate records of the types of medications administered is just as important as recording progress notes, treatments given, and rehabilitation plans. The sports therapist might be dealing with a number of different patients simultaneously while trying to get a team ready for practice or competition. At times things become hectic, and stopping to record each time a medication is administered is difficult. Nevertheless, the sports therapist should include the following information on a type of medication administration log: (1) name of the athlete, (2) complaint or symptoms, (3) type of medication given, (4) quantity of medication given, and (5) time of administration.

DRUG TESTING

Perhaps no topic related to pharmacology has received more attention from the media during recent years than the use and abuse of drugs by athletes. Much has been written and discussed regarding the use of performance-enhancing drugs among Olympic athletes, the widespread use of "street drugs" by professional athletes, and the use of pain-relieving drugs by athletes at all levels.[10,14,16]

Although much of the information being disseminated to the public by the media might be based on hearsay and innuendo, the use and abuse of many different types of drugs can have a profound impact on athletic performance.

To say that many experts in the field of sports medicine regard drug abuse among athletes with growing concern is a gross understatement. Drug testing of athletes at all levels for the purpose of identifying individuals who might be abusing drugs is becoming commonplace. Both the NCAA and the International Olympic Committee have established lists of substances that are banned from use by athletes. The lists include performance-enhancing drugs and "street" or "recreational" drugs, as well as many over-the-counter and prescription drugs. The legality and ethics of testing only those individuals involved with sports are still open to debate. The pattern of drug usage among athletes might simply reflect that of our society in general.

The sports therapist who is working with an athlete who might be tested for drugs at the NCAA level or with world-class or Olympic athletes should be very familiar with the list of banned drugs. Having an athlete disqualified because of the indiscriminate use of some over-the-counter drug during a rehabilitation program would be most unfortunate.

■ **TABLE 16-6** Protocols for the Use of Over-the-Counter Drugs for Sports Therapists

The sports therapist is often responsible for initial screening of athletes who present with various illnesses/injuries. Frequently, sports therapists must make decisions regarding the appropriate use of over-the-counter medications for their athletes. Subjective findings such as onset, duration, medication taken, and known allergies must be included in the screening evaluation.

The following protocols should be viewed as guidelines to the disposition of the athlete. The protocols are aimed at clarifying the use of over-the-counter drugs in the treatment of common problems encountered by the sports therapist while covering or traveling with a particular team. These guidelines do not cover every situation the sports therapist encounters in assessing and managing the athlete's physical problems. Therefore, physician consultation is recommended wherever there is uncertainty in making a decision regarding the appropriate care of the athlete.

Existing Illness/Injury	Appropriate Treatment Protocol
Temperature	
Greater than or equal to 102° F orally	(1) Consult physician ASAP
Less than 102° F but more than 99.5° F orally	(1) Patient may be given acetaminophen. See acetaminophen administration protocol.
	(2) Limit exercise of athlete. Do not allow participation in practice.
	(3) If fever decreases to less than 99.5° F, the athlete may participate in practice.
	(4) If athlete is to be involved in an intercollegiate event, consult with a physician concerning participation.
Less than or equal to 99.5° F orally	(1) Follow management guidelines for fever less than 102° F but allow athlete to practice and/or compete.
Throat	

History
  Sore throat
  No fever
  No chills
	(1) Advise saline gargles (1/2 tsp. salt in a glass of warm water).

	(2) Patient may also be given Cepastat/Chloraseptic throat lozenges. Before administering determine:
	a. Is the patient allergic to Cepastat/Chloraseptic (phenol containing) lozenges?[a] [a]If yes, do not administer. Refer to physician.
Sore throat Fever	b. Determine temperature. If fever, manage as outlined in temperature protocol and consult physician ASAP.
Sore throat and/or fever and/or swollen glands	(1) Consult physician ASAP.
Nose	
Watery discharge	Patient may be given pseudoephedrine (Sudafed) tablets. *See pseudoephedrine administration protocol.*
Nasal congestion	Patient may be given oxymetazoline HCl (Afrin) nasal spray. *See oxymetazoline administration protocol.*
Chest	
Cough Dry hacking or Clear mucoid sputum	You may administer Robitussin DMR (generic or guaifenesin with dextromethorphan). Before administering determine: Is the patient going to be involved in practice or game within 4 hours from administration of medication?[b] [b]If yes, do not give Robitussin DMR.

continued

■ **TABLE 16-6** Protocols for the Use of Over-the-Counter Drugs for Sports Therapists —Cont'd

Existing Illness/Injury	Appropriate Treatment Protocol
	If indicated, you may administer one dose, 10 ml (2 tsp.). Inform the patient that drowsiness may occur. Repeat doses may be administered every 6 hours. Push fluids, encourage patient to drink as much as possible.
Green or rusty sputum	(1) Consult physician ASAP.
Severe, persistent cough	(1) Consult physician ASAP.
Ears	
Discomfort due to ears popping	Patient may be given pseudoephedrine (Sudafed) tablets and/or oxymetazoline HCL (Afrin) nasal spray. *See pseudoephedrine administration protocol and/or oxymetazoline protocol.*
Earache (or external otitis)	Patient may be given acetaminophen. Consult physician ASAP. *See acetaminophen administration protocol.*
Recurrent earache	(1) Consult physician ASAP.
Prevention of Motion Sickness	
Complaint: History of nausea, dizziness, and/or vomiting associated with travel	Patient may be given dimenhydrinate (Dramamine) or diphenhydramine (Benadryl)
	Before administering, determine:
	(a) Is the patient sensitive or allergic to Dramamine, Benadryl, or any other antihistamine?*
	(b) Has the patient taken any other antihistamines (e.g. Actifed, Chlor-Trimeton, various cold medications) or other medications that cause sedation, within the last 6 hours?[a]
	(c) Does the patient have asthma, glaucoma, or enlargement of the prostate gland?[a]
	(d) Is the patient going to be involved in practice or game within 4 hours from administration of medication?[a,c]
	Administer Dramamine or Benadryl dose based on body weight, 30 to 60 minutes before departure time: Under 125 lb: one Dramamine 50 mg tablet. Over 125 lbs: two Dramamine 50 mg tablets
	Benadryl dose:
	Under 125 lb: one 25 mg capsule
	Over 125 lb: two 25 mg capsules
	[c]Inform the patient that drowsiness may occur for 4–6 hours after taking this medication. Avoid alcoholic beverages. Avoid driving for 6 hours after taking. If traveling time is extended, another dose may be administered 6 hours after the first dose.
Nausea, Vomiting	
Prolonged, severe nausea and vomiting	(1) Consult physician ASAP.
Nausea, Gastric Upset, Heartburn, Butterflies In The Stomach, Acid Indigestion	
Associated with dietary indiscretion or tension.	You may administer an antacid as a single dose, as defined by label of particular antacid (e.g., Riopan, Gelusil, Maalox, Pepto-Bismol, Titralac), or a histamine (H2) antagonist (Pepcid AC, Tagamet HB, Axid A, Zantac 75) *See histamine H2 antagonist protocol.*

continued

■ TABLE 16-6   Protocols for the Use of Over-the-Counter Drugs for Sports Therapists —Cont'd

Existing Illness/Injury	Appropriate Treatment Protocol
Associated with abdominal or chest pain	(1) Consult physician ASAP.
Vomiting, nausea—no severe distress	Monitor symptoms. Patient may be given dimenhydrinate (Dramamine) or diphenhydramine (Benadryl) orally. Same as instructions and precautions under motion sickness.
Vomiting: projectile, coffee ground, febrile	(1) Consult physician ASAP.

Diarrhea

Associated with abdominal pain or tenderness and/or dehydration, bloody stools, febrile, recurrent diarrhea	(1) Consult physician ASAP.
Frequent loose stools not associated with any of the above signs or symptoms.	Encourage clear liquid diet. Encourage avoidance of dairy products and high-fat foods for 24 hours. If it persists, consult physician ASAP. Patient may be given loperamide (Imodium AD). Before administering, determine: (a) How long has patient had diarrhea? If longer than 24 hours, see physician. You may administer one dose (2 caplets) of loperamide (Imodium AD 2 mg per caplet). One caplet may be administered after each loose stool, not to exceed 8 mg (4 caplets) per 24 hours. Inform the patient that dizziness or drowsiness may occur within 12 hours after taking this medication. Avoid alcoholic beverages. Use caution while driving or performing tasks requiring alertness.

Constipation

Prolonged or severe abdominal pain or tenderness, nausea or vomiting	(1) Consult physician ASAP.
Discomfort associated with dietary change or decreased fluid intake	You may administer milk of magnesia 30 ml as a single dose. Before administering determine: (a) Does the patient have chronic renal disease?[a] Recommend increased fluid intake, increased intake of fruits, bulk vegetables, or cereals.

Headache

Pain associated with elevated BP, temperature elevation, blurred vision, nausea, vomiting, or history of migraine.	(1) Consult physician ASAP.
Pain across forehead (mild headache)	Patient may be given acetaminophen or patient may be given NSAID. *See Acetaminophen Administration or NSAID Administration Protocol.*
Tension headache, occipital pain	Patient may be given acetaminophen. *See acetaminophen administration protocol.*
Pain in antrum or forehead associated with sinus or nasal congestion.	Patient may be given pseudoephedrine (Sudafed) tablets and acetaminophen. *See protocols for Pseudoephedrine and acetaminophen administration.*

Musculoskeletal Injuries

Deformity	Consult physician ASAP.
Localized pain and tenderness, impaired range of motion	First aid to part as soon as possible.

continued

■ **TABLE 16-6** Protocols for the Use of Over-the-Counter Drugs for Sports Therapists —Cont'd

Existing Illness/Injury	Appropriate Treatment Protocol
	Ice
	Compression—Ace bandage.
	Elevation.
	Protection—crutches or sling and/or splint.
Pain with swelling discoloration, no impaired movement or localized tenderness	If this injury interferes with patient's normal activities, consult physician within 24 hours.
	Patient may be given acetaminophen or NSAID. *See acetaminophen administration or NSAID administration protocol.*

Skin

Localized or generalized rash accompanied by elevated temperature, enlarged lymph nodes, sore throat, stiff neck, infected skin lesion, dyspnea, wheezing	(1) Consult physician ASAP.
Mild, localized, nonvesicular skin eruptions accompanied by pruritis	Hydrocortisone 1.0% cream may be applied.
	Before administering, determine:
	(a) Is the patient taking any medication?[a]
	(b) Are eyes or any large area of the body involved?[a]
	(c) Is there any evidence of lice infestation?
	The cream may be repeated every 6 hours if needed. Do not use more than 3 times daily.
Abrasions	Control bleeding. Clean with antibacterial soap and water. Apply appropriate dressing and antibiotic ointment. Monitor for signs of infection. Dressing may be changed 2–3 times a day if needed.
Localized erythema due to ultraviolet rays	Advise application of compresses soaked in a solution of cold water.
Jock itch or athlete's foot	Advise 10–15 minute application of compresses soaked in cool water to relieve intense itching.
	Patient may be given miconazole (Micatin) cream topically. Before administering determine:
	(a) Is the patient sensitive or allergic to miconazole?[d]
	(b) Is the patient receiving other types of treatment for rash in same area?[d]
	[d]If yes, do not administer. Consult physician ASAP.
	Instruct patient to wash and dry area of rash, and then apply 1/4–1/2 inch ribbon of cream (give patient the cream on a clean gauze pad) and rub gently on the infected area. Spread evenly and thinly over rash. The dose may be repeated in 8–12 hours (twice a day). Consult physician within 24 hours.

Skin Wounds

Lacerations	Control bleeding. Cleanse area with antibacterial soap and water. Apply steristrips. Consult physician immediately if there is any question about the necessity of suturing.
Extensive lacerations or other severe skin wounds	Control bleeding. Protect area with dressing. Refer to physician immediately.

Wound Infection

Febrile, marked cellulitis, red streaks, tender or enlarged nodes	(1) Consult physician ASAP.

continued

■ **TABLE 16-6**   Protocols for the Use of Over-the-Counter Drugs for Sports Therapists —Cont'd

Existing Illness/Injury	Appropriate Treatment Protocol
Localized inflammation, afebrile, absence of nodes and streaks	Warm soaks to affected area. Consult physician ASAP.

Burns

1st degree—erythema of skin, limited area	Apply cold compresses to affected area. Dressing is not necessary on 1st-degree burns. If less than 45 minutes have elapsed since burn injury, clean gently with soap and water. Patient may be given acetaminophen. *See acetaminophen administration protocol.*
1st degree with extensive involvement over body	(1) Consult physician ASAP.
2nd degree—erythema with blistering	(1) Consult physician ASAP.
3rd degree—pearly white appearance of affected area, no pain	(1) Consult physician ASAP.

Allergies

Athlete with known seasonal allergies who forgot to bring own medication	Patient may be given chlorpheniramine (Chlor-Trimeton) 4 mg tablets. Before administering determine: (a) Is the patient sensitive to chlorpheniramine?[d] (b) Does the patient have urinary retention, or glaucoma?[d] (c) Is patient going to be involved in training or game within 4 hours of administration of medication?[d] (d) Has the patient taken any other antihistamines (e.g., Actifed, Dramamine, various cold medications) or other medications that cause drowsiness within the last 6 hours?[d] You may administer 1 dose of chlorpheniramine 4 mg, 1/2 or 1 tablet. Repeat doses may be administered every 6 hours. Inform the patient that drowsiness may occur for 4–6 hours after taking this medication. Avoid alcoholic beverages. Avoid driving or operation of machinery for 6 hours after taking. Contact physician if symptoms do not abate.

Contact Lens Care

	Note: There are 3 types of contact lenses: (a) hard (b) gas permeable (c) soft Solutions are labeled for use with a particular type of lens and should not be used for any other type of lens. Do not use solutions preserved with thimersol or chlorhexidine because of possible allergy or irritation.
Lens needs rinsing/wetting before insertion	(a) Hard lens: use all-purpose wetting/soaking solution (e.g., Wet-N-Soak). (b) Gas permeable lens: use all-purpose wetting/soaking solution (e.g., Wet-N-Soak). (c) Soft lens: use rinsing/soaking solution (e.g., Soft Mate ps).
Lens needs soaking/storage	(a) Hard lens: use all-purpose wetting/soaking solution (e.g., Wet-N-Soak). (b) Gas permeable lens: use all-purpose wetting/soaking solution (e.g., Wet-N-Soak). (c) Soft lens: use rinsing/soaking solution (e.g., Soft Mate ps).

continued

■ **TABLE 16-6** Protocols for the Use of Over-the-Counter Drugs for Sports Therapists —Cont'd

Existing Illness/Injury	Appropriate Treatment Protocol
Lens needs cleaning	(a) Hard lens: use cleaning solution (e.g., EasyClean).
	(b) Gas permeable lens: use cleaning solution (e.g., EasyClean).
	(c) Soft lens: use cleaning solution (e.g., Lens Plus Daily Cleaner).
Eye Care	
Foreign body—Minor: sand, eye lash etc.	Use eye wash irrigation solution (Dacriose).
Irritation—Minor	Use artificial tears. Do not use with contact lens in eye.
Severe irritation, foreign body not easily removed, trauma	(1) Consult physician ASAP.

Administration protocols for common over-the-counter drugs used in sports medicine

Acetaminophen Protocol (Tylenol)

Before *administering,* determine:
   (a) Is the patient allergic to acetominophen?[a]
You may *administer* acetaminophen 325 mg, two tablets. Repeat doses may be *administered* every 4 hours if needed. If *dispensing* occurs, use labeled 2/pack only. Patient instructions must accompany *dispensing.*

Pseudoephedrine Protocol (Sudafed)

Before *administering,* determine:
   (a) Is the patient allergic or sensitive to pseudoephedrine?[b]
   (b) Does the patient have high blood pressure, heart disease, diabetes, urinary retention, glaucoma or thyroid disease?[b]
   (c) Does the patient have problems with sweating?[*]
   (d) Do not administer 4 hours before practice or game.
   (e) Do not administer if patient is involved in postseason play.
You may *administer* pseudoephedrine (Sudafed) 30 mg, two tablets. Repeat doses may be *administered* every 6 hours up to 4 times a day. If *dispensing* occurs, use labeled 2/pack only. Patient instructions must accompany *dispensing.*

Oxymetazoline Protocol (Afrin)

Before administering, determine:
   (a) Is the patient allergic or sensitive to Afrin or Otrivin?[c]
   (b) Does the patient react unusually to nose sprays or drops?[c]
You may administer 2–3 sprays of oxymetazoline (Afrin) 0.05% nasal spray into each nostril. Repeat doses may be administered every 12 hours. (The container can be marked with the patient's name and maintained by the trainer for repeat administration or *dispensed* to the patient. Patient instructions must accompany *dispensing.*)
Do not use the same container for different patients.
Do not use for more than 3 days without MD supervision.
Use small package sizes to reduce risk of overuse/rebound congestion.

[a]If yes, do not give acetaminophen.
[*]If yes, do not give pseudoephedrine.
[c]If yes, do not administer.
[d]If yes, do not give ibuprofen, because even though ibuprofen contains no aspirin or saliculates, cross reactions can occur in patients allergic to aspirin.

Administration protocols for common over-the-counter drugs used in sports medicine—Cont'd

NSAID Protocol (ibuprofen: Advil; naproxen sodium: Aleve; ketoprofen: Orudis KT, Actron)

Before *administering*, determine:
    (a) Is the patient allergic to aspirin (e.g., asthma, swelling, shock or hives associated with aspirin use?)[d]
    (b) Does the patient have renal disease or gastrointestinal ulcerations?[e]
You may *administer* ibuprofen 200 mg (Advil) one or two tablets. Repeat doses may be *administered* every 6 hours if
    needed. Do not exceed 6 tablets in a 24 hour period without consulting an MD. Do not administer if patient is less than
    12 years of age.
Or
You may administer naproxen sodium 220 mg (Aleve), one tablet every 8 to 12 hours or two tablets to start followed by
    1 tablet 12 hours later. Do not exceed 3 tablets in a 24-hour period without consulting a physician. Do not administer
    if patient is less than 12 years of age.
Or
You may administer ketoprofen 12.5 mg (Orutis KT, Actron) one tablet or caplet every 4 to 6 hours if needed. If pain or
    fever persists after 1 hour, one more 12.5 mg tablet or caplet may be given. Do not exceed 6 tablets or caplets in a 24-
    hour period without consulting a physician. Do not administer if the patient is less than 16 years of age.
The patient should take the NSAID with a full glass of water and food if occasional and mild heartburn, upset stomach,
    or mild stomach pain occurs. Consult MD if these symptoms are more than mild or persist. Discontinue drug if patient
    experiences skin rash, itching, dark, tarry stools, visual disturbances, dark urine, or persistent headache. Instruct
    patient to avoid concurrent aspirin or alcoholic beverages.

Histamine H$_2$ Antagonist Protocol (ranitidine: Zantac 75; nizatidine: Axid AR; famotidine: Pepsid AC; cimetidine: Tagamet-HB)

Before *administering*, determine:
    a. Is the patient less than 12 years of age[f]?
    b. Does the patient have difficulty swallowing or persistent abdominal pain[f]?
You may *administer* ranitidine (Zantac 75) one 5 mg tablet with water up to two times a day. Do not administer more
    than 2 tablets in a 24-hour period.
Or
You may administer nizatidine (Axid AR) one 75 mg tablet with water up to two times a day. Do not administer more
    than two tablets in a 24-hour period.
Or
You may administer famotidine (Pepsid AC) one 10 mg tablet with water up to two times a day. Do not administer more
    than 2 tablets in a 24-hour period.
Or
You may administer cimetidine (Tagamet-HB) one 10 mg tablet with water up to two times a day. Do not administer
    more than two tablets in a 24-hour period. Do not administer cimetidine if the patient is taking phenytoin (Dilantin) or
    theophyllin (Theodur).

[e]If yes, do not administer ibuprofen.
[f]If yes, do not give H$_2$ antagonist.

■ **TABLE 16-7** Federal 7-Point Label

The label of a nonprescription drug is required to contain the following information:
1. The name of the product
2. The name and address of the manufacturer, packer, or distributor
3. The net contents of the package
4. The established name of all active ingredients and the quantity of certain other ingredients whether active or not.
5. The name of any habit-forming drug contained in the preparation
6. Cautions and warnings needed to protect the consumer
7. Adequate directions for safe and effective use

Summary

1. An athlete who requires an analgesic for pain relief should be given acetaminophen, because aspirin can produce gastric upset and slow clotting time.

2. For treating inflammation, NSAIDs are recommended because they do not produce many of the side effects associated with aspirin use.

3. Antihistamines are used primarily in the treatment of allergic reactions and can produce drowsiness and sedation.

4. Decongestants are used to reduce nasal congestion and can be used orally or topically.

5. Antitussives and expectorants are used to suppress coughing and keep the throat moist. They generally produce drowsiness, gastric irritability, and some lack of coordination.

6. Antacids neutralize acidity in the upper GI tract and can produce diarrhea or constipation.

7. Antiemetics are used to treat nausea and vomiting and should be used with large quantities of fluid to prevent dehydration.

8. Antidiarrheals act to reduce peristaltic action in the lower GI tract and can produce drowsiness, nausea, dry mouth, and constipation.

9. Cathartics are used to empty the GI tract and reduce constipation.

10. Antibiotics are used to treat various infections and can produce hypersensitivity reactions in the athlete. Generally an athlete who is using an antibiotic should avoid training and competition until the infection subsides.

11. The use of medication in a sports medicine setting should be subject to strict preestablished guidelines and protocols and monitored closely by the sports therapist supervising a rehabilitation program.

12. The sports therapist should maintain a log that documents all medications administered during a rehabilitation program.

13. The sports therapist must be aware of medications commonly used in treatment of various disorders that might be detected in a drug test as banned substances.

References

1. Almekinders, L. 1990. The efficacy of nonsteroidal anti-inflammatory drugs in the treatment of ligament injuries. *Sports Medicine* 9(3): 137–42.

2. Barnes, P. 1981. Is immunotherapy for asthma worthwhile? *New England Journal of Medicine* 334:531–32.

3. Beaver, W. 1981. Aspirin and acetaminophen as constituents of analgesic combinations. *Archives of Internal Medicine* 141:293–300.

4. Beaver, W., T. Kantor, and G. Levy. 1975. On guard for aspirin's harmful side effects. *Patient Care* 13:48.

5. Bertholf, C. 1980. Protocol, acute diarrhea. *Nurse Pract* 3:8.

6. Black, F., M. Correia, and F. Stucker. 1980. Easing proneness to motion sickness. *Patient Care* 14(6): 114.

7. Boyd, E. 1970. A review of expectorants and inhalants. *Int J Clin Pharmacol Ther Toxicol* 3:55.

8. Calabrese, L., and T. Rooney. 1986. The use of nonsteroidal antiinflammatory drugs in sports. *Physician and Sports Medicine* 14:89–97.

9. Clark, J., S. Queener, and V. Karb. 1992. *Pharmacologic basis of nursing practice.* St Louis: Mosby.

10. Clarke, K. S. 1984. Sports medicine and drug control programs of the US Olympic Committee. *J Allergy Clin Immunol* 73:740–44.

11. Clyman, B. 1986. Role of the non-steroidal anti-inflammatory drugs in sports medicine. *Sports Medicine* 3:212–46.

12. Dahr, G., and K. Soergel. 1979. Principles of diarrhea therapy. *Am Fam Physician* 19(1): 165.

13. Dretchen, K., D. Hollander, and J. Kirsner. 1975. Roundup on antacids and anticholinergics. *Patient Care* 9(6): 94.

14. Drugs in the Olympics. 1984. *Med Lett Drugs Ther* 26:66.

15. Elenbaas, J. K. 1980. Centrally acting skeletal muscle relaxants. *Am J Hosp Pharm* 37:1313–23.

16. Hill, J. 1983. The athletic polydrug abuse phenomenon. *American Journal of Sports Medicine* 11:269–71.

17. Koch-Weser, J. 1976. Acetaminophen. *New England Journal of Medicine* 255:1297.

18. Krausen, A. 1979. Antihistamines: Guidelines and implications. *Ann Otol Rhinol Laryngol* 85:686.

19. Levy, G. 1981. Comparative pharmacokinetics of aspirin and acetaminophen. *Archives of Internal Medicine* 141:279–81.

20. Levy, J., and D. Smith. 1989. Clinical differences among nonsteroidal anti-inflammatory drugs: Implications for therapeutic substitution in ambulatory patients. *DICP, Ann Pharmacotherapy* 23:76–85.

21. McCormack, K., and K. Brune. 1993. Toward defining the analgesic role of non-steroidal anti-inflammatory drugs in the management of acute and soft tissue injuries. *Clin J Sports Medicine* 3:106–17.

22. Malseed, R. 1985. *Pharmacology: Drug therapy and nursing considerations.* Philadelphia: Lippincott.

23. Matzke, G. 1997. Clinical consequences of non-narcotic analgesic use. *Ann Pharmacotherapy* 31:245–48.

24. Mehlisch, D. R. 1983. Review of the comparative analgesic efficacy of salicylates, acetaminophen and pyrazolones. *American Journal of Medicine* 75[A]:47–52.

25. Mirtallo, J. 1978. Drug induced heat stroke. *Drug Intell Clin Pharm* 12:652–57.

26. Moncada, S., and J. Vane. 1979. Mode of action of aspirin-like drugs. *Adv Int Med* 24:1.

27. National Asthma Education and Prevention Coordinating Committee, National Heart Lung and Blood Institute, and World Health Organization. 1995. *Global initiative for asthma.* Publication No. NIH-95-3659. Bethesda, MD: National Institutes of Health.

28. Pearlman, D. 1976. Antihistamines: Pharmacology and clinical use. Drugs 12:258.

29. Purdum, P., S. Shelden, and J. Boyd. 1994. Oxaprozin-induced hepatitis. *Ann Pharmacotherapy* 28:1159–61.

30. Quick, A. 1966. Salicylates and bleeding: The aspirin tolerance test. *Am J Med Sci* 252:265–69.

31. Reynolds, R. C., P. Floetz, and T. S. Thielke. 1984. Comparative analysis of drug distribution costs for controlled versus noncontrolled oral analgesics. *Am J Hosp Pharm* 41:1558–63.

32. Rodman, M. 1977. Antiinfectives you administer: Choosing the right drug for every job. *RN* 40:73.

33. Rodman, M. 1981. A fresh look at OTC drug interactions: Antacid preparations. *RN* 46:84.

34. Rodman, M., and D. Smith. 1984. Clinical pharmacology in nursing. Philadelphia: Lippincott.

35. Second Expert Panel on the Management of Asthma, National Heart, Lung, and Blood Institute. 1997. *Highlights of expert panel report 2: Guidelines for the diagnosis and management of asthma.* Publication No. NIH 97-4051A. Bethesda, MD: National Institutes of Health.

36. Settipane, G. A. 1981. Adverse reactions to aspirin and related drugs. *Archives of Internal Medicine* 141:328–32.

37. Strauss, R. 1984. *Sports medicine.* Philadelphia: W. B. Saunders.

38. Szczeklik, A. 1983. Antipyretic analgesics and the allergic patient. *American Journal of Medicine* 75[A]:82–84.

39. Texter, E., D. Smart, and R. Butler. 1975. Antacids. *Am Fam Physician* 11(4): 111.

40. Vane, J. 1971. Inhibition of prostaglandin synthesis as a mechanism of action for aspirin like drugs. *Nature (New Biol)* 231:232–35.

41. Vane, J. 1987. The evolution of nonsteroidal antiinflammatory drugs and their mechanism of action. *Drugs* 33(1): 18–27.

42. Weinstein, L. 1977. Some principles of antibiotic therapy. *Ration Drug Ther* 11(3): 1.

CHAPTER 17

Functional Progressions and Functional Testing in Rehabilitation

Michael McGee

After completion of this chapter, the student should be able to do the following:

• Define the concept of a functional progression.

• Discuss how and when functional progressions should be used in the rehabilitation process.

• Identify and describe the physical benefits associated with a functional progression.

• Identify and describe the psychological benefits associated with a functional progression.

• Identify and describe the disadvantages associated with a functional progression.

• Describe the components of a functional progression.

• Develop a functional progression for an athlete.

• Identify and describe various functional tests.

• Develop a functional test for an athlete.

I n the athletic community, injuries and subsequent disability frequently occur. Disabilities can be described as restrictive influences that "disease and injury exert upon neuromotor performances."[11] Thus, in an effort to reduce the lasting effects of injury, the sports therapist should direct rehabilitation toward improving neuromuscular coordination and agility, and not simply toward increasing strength and endurance. If rehabilitation is directed toward regaining range of motion, flexibility, strength, and endurance, and perhaps primarily toward increasing neuromuscular coordination and agility, a full return to activity is possible. However, if the program simply provides a means for reducing signs and symptoms associated with the injury, the athlete will not return to a safe and effective level of activity.[24] As a result, rehabilitation of athletic injuries needs to focus on return to preinjury fitness levels.[18]

THE ROLE OF FUNCTIONAL PROGRESSIONS IN REHABILITATION

Sports therapists must adapt rehabilitation to the sport-specific demands of each individual sport and playing position. But rehabilitation programs in a clinical setting cannot predict the ability of the injured part to endure the demands of full competition on the playing field. For example, the complex factors surrounding a solid tackle in competition play cannot be produced in the clinical setting.

The role of the functional progression is to improve and complete the clinical rehabilitation process.[22] **A functional progression is a succession of activities that simulate actual motor and sport skills, enabling the athlete to acquire or reacquire the skills needed to perform athletic endeavors safely and effectively.** The sports therapist takes the activities involved in a given sport and breaks them down into individual components. In this way the athlete concentrates on individual parts of the game or activity in a controlled environment before combining them together in an uncontrolled environment as would exist during full competition. The functional progression places stresses and forces on each body system in a well-planned, positive, and progressive fashion, ultimately improving the athlete's overall ability to meet the demands of daily activities as well as sport competition. The functional progression is essential in the rehabilitation process, because tissues not placed under performance-level stresses do not adapt to the sudden return of such stresses with the resumption of full activity. Thus, the functional progression is integrated into the normal rehabilitation scheme, as one component of exercise therapy, rather than replacing traditional rehabilitation altogether.[12]

Generally, rehabilitation has two goals: The first is to prevent athletic injuries and to safely and quickly return injured athletes to their prior levels of competition. The second is divided into three main stages: immediate, short-term, and long-term. The immediate goal stage begins at the time of injury and involves the treatment or management of the injury. This includes minimizing pain and swelling, protection from further injury, and restricted activity. The short-term goal stage deals with the healing process, allowing the symptoms to subside and decreasing the level of dysfunction. Also during this stage, uninvolved body parts can be exercised to maintain normal function and fitness levels. The long-term goal stage overlaps the short-term goal stage and progresses to a point of full return to activity. Once the athlete meets criteria to return to controlled activity, exercise therapy may begin. The functional progression serves as a component of exercise therapy to assist the athlete in meeting the preestablished criteria for return to play.

BENEFITS OF USING FUNCTIONAL PROGRESSIONS

Functional progressions provide both physical and psychological benefits to the injured athlete. The physical benefits include improvements in muscular strength and endurance, mobility and flexibility, cardiorespiratory endurance, and neuromuscular coordination, along with an increase in the functional stability of an injured joint. Psychologically, the progression can reduce the feelings of anxiety, apprehension, and deprivation commonly observed in the injured athlete.

Improving Functional Stability

Functional stability is provided by (1) passive restraints on the ligaments, (2) joint geometry, (3) active restraints generated by muscles, and (4) joint compressive forces that occur with activity and force the joint together.[20] Stability is maintained by the neuromuscular control mechanisms involved in proprioception and kinesthesia (as discussed in Chapter 6). Functional stability cannot always be determined by examining the athlete in the clinic. Therefore, the functional progression can be used to evaluate functional stability both objectively and subjectively. Can the athlete complete all tasks with no adverse affects? Does the athlete appear to perform at the same level, or close to the same level, as prior to injury? Performance during a functional task can be evaluated for improvement, and functional testing can be incorporated to provide an objective measure of ability.[12]

Muscular Strength

Increased strength is a physical benefit of the functional progression. Strength is the ability of the muscle to produce tension or apply force maximally against resistance. This occurs statically or dynamically, in relation to the imposed demands. Strength increases are possible if the load imposed on a muscle exceeds that muscle's anatomic capabilities during exercise. This is commonly referred to as the overload principle and is possible due to increased efficiency in motor unit recruitment and muscle fiber hypertrophy.[14] To see these improvements, the muscle must be worked to the point of fatigue with either high or low resistance. The functional progression will develop strength using the SAID (*specific adaptation to imposed demands*) principle. The muscles involved will be strengthened dynamically, under stresses similar to those encountered in competition.

Endurance

Muscular and cardiorespiratory endurance can both be enhanced with a functional progression. Endurance is necessary for long-duration activity, whether in daily living or in the repeated motor functions found with sport participation. The functional progression will enhance muscular endurance through the repetition of the individual activities and their combination into one general activity. The progression provides an environment for improving muscular strength and endurance without using more than one program. Cardiorespiratory endurance can be improved through the repetition of movements involved in the progression in the same way as regular fitness levels improve with continuous exercise.

Flexibility

With injury, tissues will shorten or tighten in response to immobilization. This can inhibit proper function. With a functional progression, the injured area is stressed within a controlled range. This stress should be significant enough to allow the tissue to elongate and return to proper length. This improved mobility and flexibility is crucial to the athlete. Strength and endurance do not mean much if the injured body part cannot move through a full range of motion. Tissues also become stronger with consistent stresses, so tissues other than muscle can also be improved with the functional progression.[14]

Muscle Relaxation

Relaxation involves the concerted effort to reduce muscle tension. The functional progression can teach an individual to recognize this tension and eventually control or remove it by consciously relaxing the muscles after exercise. The total body relaxation that can ensue relaxes the injured area, helping to relieve the muscle guarding that can inhibit the joint's full range of motion.[14]

Motor Skills

Coordination, agility, and motor skills are complex aspects of normal function defined as appropriate contractions at the most opportune time and with the appropriate intensity.[14] An athlete needs coordination, agility, and motor skills to transform strength, flexibility, and endurance into full-speed performance. This is especially important for an injured athlete. If the athlete does not regain or improve their coordination and agility, their performance is hampered and can in itself lead to further injury. Repetition and practice are important to learning motor skills. Regular motions that are consciously controlled develop into automatic reactions via motor learning. This is possible due to the constant repetition and reinforcement of a particular skill.[11] In order to acquire these "automatic reactions," one needs an intact and

functional neuromuscular system. Because this system is disturbed by injury, decreases in performance will occur, increasing the potential for injury. The functional progression can be used to minimize the loss of normal neuromuscular control by providing exercises that stress proprioception, motor-skill integration, and proper timing. The functional progression is indicated for improvement in agility and skill because of the constant repetition of sport-specific motor skills, use of sensory cues, and progressive increases in activity levels. Proprioception can be enhanced by stimulating the intra-articular and intramuscular mechanoreceptors. These are all components of, or general principles for, enhancing neuromuscular coordination.[14] The practice variations used with functional progressions allow the athlete to relearn the various aspects of their sport that they might encounter in competition.

Rehabilitative exercise programs must stress neuromuscular coordination and agility. Increases in strength, endurance, and flexibility are unquestionably necessary for a safe and effective return to play, but without the neuromuscular coordination to integrate these aspects into proper function, little performance enhancement can occur. For this reason, functional progressions should become an integral part of the long-term rehabilitation stage so that injured athletes can maximize their ability to return to competition at their preinjury level.

PSYCHOLOGICAL AND SOCIAL CONSIDERATIONS

Functional progressions can also provide psychological benefits to the athlete. Anxiety, apprehension, and feelings of deprivation are all common emotions found with injuries. The functional progression can aid the rehabilitation process and facilitate the return to play by diminishing these emotions. Chapter 3 discusses the psychological aspects of the rehabilitative process.

Anxiety

Uncertainty about the future is a reason many athletes give for their feelings of anxiety. Athletes experience this insecurity because they have only a vague understanding of the severity of their injury and the length of time it will take for them to fully recover.[12] The progression can lessen anxiety because the athlete is gradually placed into more demanding situations that allow the athlete to experience success and not be concerned as much with failure in the future.

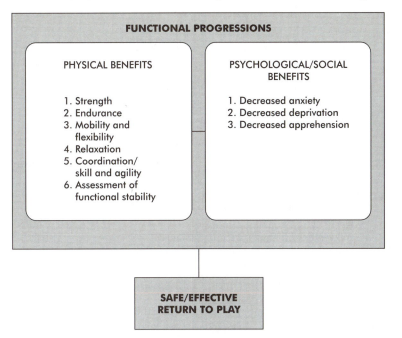

Figure 17-1   Physical and psychological benefits of using functional progressions.

Deprivation

The athlete might experience feelings of deprivation after losing direct contact with his team and coaches for an extended period of time. The functional progression can limit such feelings of deprivation, because the athlete can exercise during regular team practice times at the practice site. By engaging in an activity that can be completed during practice, the athlete remains close in proximity and socially and feels little loss in team cohesion.[12]

Apprehension

Apprehension is often listed as an obstacle to performance and many times serves as a precursor to reinjury.[12] Functional progressions enable athletes to adapt to the imposed demands of their sports in a controlled environment, helping to restore confidence, thus decreasing apprehension. Each success builds on past success, allowing the athlete to feel in control as they return to full activity.

Figure 17-1 provides a list of the physical and psychological benefits of functional progressions.

COMPONENTS OF A FUNCTIONAL PROGRESSION: EXTERNAL CONSIDERATIONS

To provide a safe and effective return to play with the use of functional progressions, several considerations should be addressed. First, what are the physician's expectations for the athlete's return to activity? Second, what are the athlete's expectations for his or her return to activity? Third, what is the total disability of the athlete? And fourth, what are the parameters of physical fitness for this athlete? Keeping the total well-being of the injured athlete in perspective is a significant factor.[24]

Activity Considerations

Exercise can be viewed from two perspectives. From one perspective, exercise is a single activity involving simple motor skills. From the second perspective, exercise involves the training and conditioning effect of repetitive activity.[11] It is well accepted that preinjury status can be regained only if appropriate activities of sufficient intensity are used

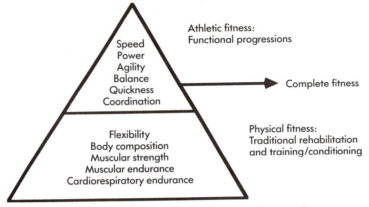

Figure 17-2 Combining components of physical fitness with components of athletic fitness in functional progressions.

to train and condition the athlete. To provide the athlete with these activities, four principles must be observed. First, the individuality of the athlete, the sport, and the injury must be addressed. Second, the activities should be positive, not negative; no increased signs and symptoms should occur. Third, an orderly progressive program should be utilized. And fourth, the program should be varied to avoid monotony.[14] Steps to minimize monotony include these:

1. Vary exercise techniques used.
2. Alter the program at regular intervals.
3. Maintain fitness base to avoid reinjury with return to play.
4. Set achievable goals, reevaluate, and modify regularly.
5. Use clinical, home, and on-field programs to vary the activity.[11]

Athletes are continually exposed to situations that make reinjury likely, so every effort should be made to understand and incorporate the inherent demands of the sport into the rehabilitation program. The sport therapist can emphasize the importance of sport-specific activities to enhance the athlete's return to activity rather than simply concentrating on traditional rehabilitation methods involving only weight machines and analgesics.

The components of fitness are listed in Figure 17-2. There are two distinct components in this model. The physical fitness items used in more traditional rehabilitation programs should be merged with the athletic fitness items of functional progressions to maximize the athlete's chance to regain preinjury fitness levels.

The components of a functional progression should aim to incorporate all the factors listed in Figure 17-2 under athletic fitness items.

Demand of Sport

Before the rehabilitation program is implemented, there should be a complete analysis of the demands that will be placed on the athlete and the injured body part once return to play is achieved. Second, all tasks involved in the activity should be ranked on a continuum from easy to difficult. Primary concerns should include the intention of the activity, what activities should be included, and the order in which the activities should occur.[8] For example, if throwing a baseball is the purpose, the progression can be broken into an ordered sequence like this:

1. Grip the ball
2. Stance
3. Backswing of the upper limb
4. Forward swing of the upper limb
5. Release of the ball
6. Follow-through[8]

Next, the sports therapist makes regular evaluations of the injured body part. Assessment of present functional status of the injury should serve as a guide to safe progression.[14]

Factors Influencing Rehabilitation Goals

Several factors can influence rehabilitation goals. In formulating goals, the sports therapist should ask these questions:

1. What is the type of sport, and what position will be played? What demands will these place on the injury?
2. How much time remains in the season? An athlete at the end of the season has less time to

recover fully and return to play. A decision must be made as to whether the athlete realistically will return that season. All postseason play must be taken into account.

3. What other sports is the athlete involved in, and are they more important? For example, a sports therapist should not risk reinjury by hurrying a mediocre football player's rehabilitation and take a chance on him missing basketball season when he excels in basketball.

4. The sports therapist needs to know about injury rules pertaining to that sport. Can the athlete play with a splint, or is padding needed?

5. What is the psyche of the athlete? The sports therapist needs to measure the athlete's motivation, cooperation, compliance, competitiveness, and, especially, pain threshold.

6. Most importantly, what is the individuals' specific injury, and what type of rehabilitation will be best? The sports therapist must concentrate on these. There is no "cookbook program" that is going to work well for every athlete. General treatment goals might be similar for a given injury type, but the specific program has to be based on the goals of the individual athlete, the healing constraints, the level of irritation, progress to date, and the athlete's tolerance of the program and readiness to progress. These factors not only affect rehabilitation, but should also be used to choose appropriate activities for the progression.

Program Reevaluation

The progression itself should also be reevaluated at regular intervals. This will allow the sports therapist to curtail any activity that results in immediate pain, swelling, or patient anxiety in favor of less aggressive activities. The sports therapist can also use this reevaluation to gauge the progress of the individual. Achieving a certain skill level in a functional progression occurs when the skill can be completed at functional speed with high repetitions with no associated increase in pain or swelling or decrease in range of motion. The sports therapist and athlete should realize, however, that setbacks will occur and are common. Sometimes it takes two steps forward and one step back to achieve the needed level of improvement.

Full Return to Play

Deciding whether an athlete is ready to return to play at full participation is a difficult task. The decision requires a complete evaluation of the athlete's condition, including objective observations and subjective evaluation. The sports therapist should feel that the athlete is ready both physically and mentally before allowing a return to play.[7] Return to activity should not be attempted too soon, in order to avoid added stress to the injury, which can slow healing and result in a long, painful recovery or reinjury.[6] The following are criteria for allowing a full return to activity:

1. Physician's release
2. Free of pain
3. No swelling
4. Normal ROM
5. Normal strength (in reference to opposite extremity)
6. Appropriate functional testing completed with no adverse reactions

EXAMPLES OF FUNCTIONAL PROGRESSIONS

The Upper Extremity

Now that the benefits and components of a functional progression have been addressed, some examples of functional progression activities are warranted. Functional activities that will enhance the healing and performance of the upper extremity might include PNF patterns, swimming on land or in water, and using pulley machines or rubber tubing to simulate sport activity.[7]

A functional progression for the throwing shoulder should include the following steps. First the athlete must be instructed in and complete a proper warm-up. During the warm-up, the athlete should practice the throwing motion at a slow velocity and with low stress. The activity can then progress through increasingly difficult stages as indicated in Table 17-1. Table 17-2 provides an example of a functional progression for hitting a golf ball, and Table 17-3 provides a program for return to hitting a tennis ball. Any upper-extremity injury can benefit from one of these programs or can be exercised in similar fashion using any sport equipment needed for that sport.[3]

The Lower Extremity

The lower extremity follows the same basic pattern, with different exercises. The activities used should provide functional stress to the injured limb. An example of a functional progression for the lower extremity is found in Table 17-4.

■ **TABLE 17-1**   Upper-Extremity Progression for Throwing

1. Functional activity can begin early with assisted PNF techniques
2. Rubber tubing exercises simulating PNF patterns and/or sport motions
3. Swimming
4. Push-ups
5. Sport drills:
   - Interval throwing program
     45 ft phase

	Step 1:		Step 2:	
	1. Warm-up throwing		1. Warm-up throwing
	2. 25 throws		2. 25 throws
	3. Rest 10 minutes		3. 15 minute rest
	4. Warm-up throwing		4. Warm-up throwing
	5. 25 throws		5. 25 throws
			6. Rest 10 minutes
			7. Warm-up throwing
			8. 25 throws

Repeat steps 1 and 2 for 60, 90, 120, 150, and 180 feet, until full throwing from the mound or respective position is achieved.

■ **TABLE 17-2**   Interval Golf Rehabilitation Program

	Day 1	Day 2	Day 3
Week 1			
	5 min chipping/putting	5 min chipping/putting	5 min chipping/putting
	5 min rest	5 min rest	5 min rest
	5 min chipping	5 min chipping	5 min chipping
		5 min rest	5 min rest
		5 min chipping	5 min chipping
Week 2			
	10 min chipping	10 min chipping	10 min short iron
	10 min rest	10 min rest	10 min rest
	10 min short iron	10 min short iron	10 min short iron
		10 min rest	10 min rest
		10 min short iron	10 min short iron
Week 3			
	10 min short iron	10 min short iron	10 min short iron
	10 min rest	10 min rest	10 min rest
	10 min long iron	10 min long iron	10 min long iron
	10 min rest	10 min rest	10 min rest
	10 min long iron	10 min long iron	10 min long iron
Week 4			
	Repeat week 3, day 2	Play 9 holes	Play 18 holes

■ **TABLE 17-3** Interval Tennis Program

	Day 1	Day 2	Day 3
Week 1			
	12 FH	15 FH	15 FH
	8 BH	8 BH	10 BH
	10 min rest	10 min rest	10 min rest
	13 FH	15 FH	15 FH
	7 BH	7 BH	10 BH
Week 2			
	25 FH	30 FH	30 FH
	15 BH	20 BH	25 BH
	10 min rest	10 min rest	10 min rest
	25 FH	30 FH	30 FH
	15 BH	20 BH	15 BH
			10 Overheads (OH)
Week 3			
	30 FH	30 FH	30 FH
	25 BH	25 BH	30 BH
	10 OH	15 OH	15 OH
	10 min rest	10 min rest	10 min rest
	30 FH	30 FH	30 FH
	25 BH	25 BH	15 OH
	10 OH	15 OH	10 min rest
			30 FH
			30 BH
			15 OH
Week 4			
	30 FH	30 FH	30 FH
	30 BH	30 BH	30 BH
	10 OH	10 OH	10 OH
	10 min rest	10 min rest	10 min rest
	Play 3 games	Play set	Play 1.5 sets
	10 FH	10 FH	10 FH
	10 BH	10 BH	10 BH
	5 OH	5 OH	3 OH

FH = Forehand
BH = Backhand
OH = Overhead

■ **TABLE 17-4** Lower-Extremity Functional Progression

1. Functional activity can begin early in the rehabilitation process with:
   - Assisted proprioceptive neuromuscular facilitation (PNF) techniques
   - Cycling
   - Non-weight-bearing (NWB) BAPS board or tilt board exercises
   - Partial-weight-bearing (PWB) BAPS board or tilt board exercises
   - Full-weight-bearing (FWB) BAPS board or tilt board exercise (Figure 17-3)
   - Walking
     Normal
     Heel
     Toe
     Sidestep/shuffle slides (Figure 17-4)
2. Lunges:
   - 90° Pivot (Figure 17-5)
   - 180° Pivot (Figure 17-6)
3. Step-ups:
   - Forward step-up, 50–75% max speed (Figure 17-7A)
   - Lateral step-up, 50–75% max speed (Figure 17-7B)
4. Jogging:
   - Straight-aways on track; jog in turns (goal=2 miles)
   - Complete oval of track (goal=2–4 miles)
   - 100 yd—"S" course 75–100% max speed with gradual increase in number of curves (Figure 17-8)
   - 100 yd—"8" course 75–100% max speed with gradual decrease in size of "8" to fit 5–10 yd (Figure 17-9)
   - 100 yd—"Z" course 75–100% max speed with gradual increase in number of "Zs" (Figure 17-10)
   - Sidestep/shuffle slides
5. Lunges:
   - 90° Pivot with weight or increased speed
   - 180° Pivot with weight or increased speed
6. Sprints:
   - 10 yd × 10
   - 20 yd × 10
   - 40 yd × 10
   - Acceleration/deceleration; 50 yd × 10 (Figure 17-11)
   - "W" sprints × 10 (Figure 17-12)
7. Box runs: (Figure 17-13)
   - 5 yd clockwise/counterclockwise × 10
8. Carioca: (Figure 17-14)
   - 30 yd × 5 right lead-off; 30 yd × 5 left lead-off
9. Jumping: (Figure 17-15)
   - Rope
   - Lines
   - Boxes, balls, etc.
10. Hopping: (Figure 17-18)
    - Two feet
    - One foot
    - Alternate
11. Cutting, jumping, hopping on command
12. Sport drills used for preseason or inseason practice

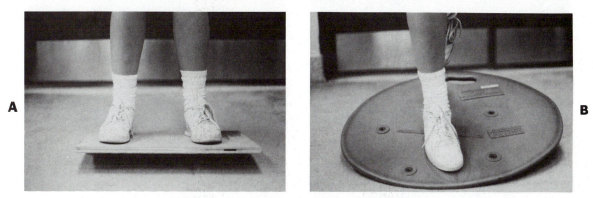

Figure 17-3 Board exercises. **A,** Tilt board exercise. **B,** BAPS board exercise.

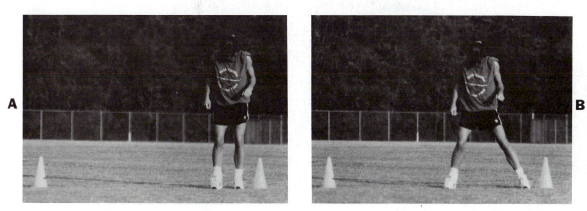

Figure 17-4 Shuffle slides. **A,** Starting position. **B,** Finish position.

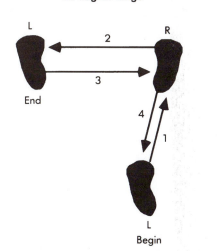

Figure 17-5 90-degree pivot. The athlete pushes off with the left foot, landing on the right foot directly in front, then steps immediately laterally landing on the left foot, then back laterally in the opposite direction landing on the right foot, then backward onto the left foot.

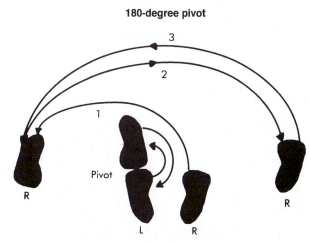

Figure 17-6 180-degree pivot. The athlete pushes off the right foot, pivoting on the left, thus rotating the body 180 degrees, landing on the right foot. Then pushing off the right foot, the body pivots on the left foot 180 degrees in the other direction, landing on the right foot.

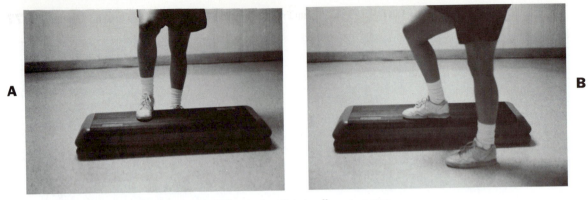

Figure 17-7 Step-ups. The athlete steps **A,** forward or **B,** laterally onto a step.

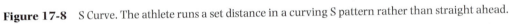

"S" curve course

Figure 17-8 S Curve. The athlete runs a set distance in a curving S pattern rather than straight ahead.

Figure "8" course

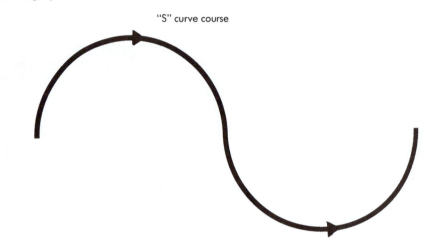

"Z" course (zigzag)

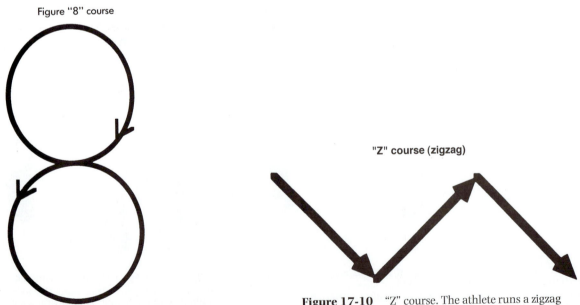

Figure 17-9 Figure 8. The athlete walks, jogs, or runs a figure 8 pattern around cones or markers.

Figure 17-10 "Z" course. The athlete runs a zigzag course to emphasize sharp cutting motions and quick controlled directional changes.

Acceleration/deceleration course

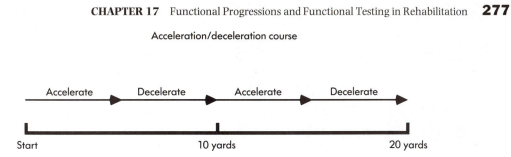

Figure 17-11 Acceleration/deceleration. The athlete accelerates to a maximum, then decelerates almost to a stop, then repeats this within a relatively short distance.

"W" sprint course

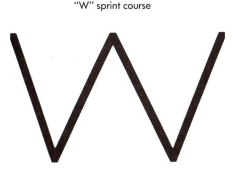

Figure 17-12 "W" sprints. The athlete sprints forward to the first marker, then backpedals to the second, then sprints forward to the third, and so on.

Box run course

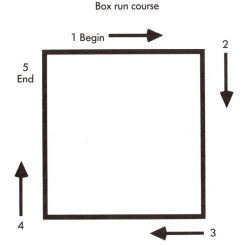

Figure 17-13 Box runs. Running both clockwise and counterclockwise, the athlete runs around four markers set in a box shape, concentrating on abrupt directional changes at each corner.

Carioca step

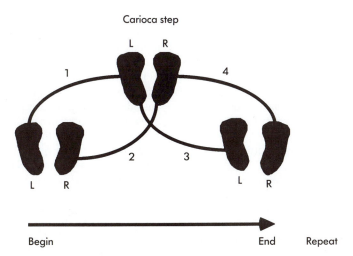

Figure 17-14 Carioca. The athlete sidesteps onto the right foot, then steps across with the left foot in front of the right, then steps back onto the right foot, then the left foot steps across in back of the right, then back onto the right, and so on.

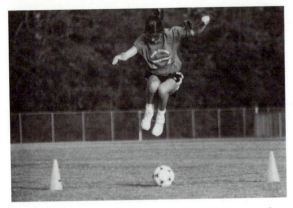

Figure 17-15 Timed exercise. The athlete jumps side to side over a ball or other obstacle in a timed exercise.

Applying Functional Progressions to a Specific Sport Case

The following is an example of how a functional progression may be applied to a specific sport-related injury:

Subject: 20-year-old female soccer player

History: Sustained anterior cruciate ligament (ACL) rupture of left knee while performing a cutting motion in practice. ACL reconstruction using an intra-articular patellar tendon graft was performed.

Rehabilitation for first 2 months was conducted both at home and in clinical setting. Emphasis of program concentrated on increasing range of motion (ROM) and decreasing pain and swelling, with some minor considerations to improving strength.

At 2 months postsurgery, the rehabilitation protocol consisted of emphasizing general physical fitness, strengthening via traditional rehabilitation means and strength testing, as well as improving ROM.

At approximately 3 months postsurgery a functional progression was initiated. The progression included the following activities an average of three times per week:

- Walking
- Proprioceptive neuromuscular facilitation techniques—using lower extremity D1, D2 patterns
- Jogging on track with walking of curves
- Jogging full track
- Running on track with jogging of curves
- Running full track

This progression occupied the majority of the next 2 months, coupled with traditional rehabilitation techniques to increase strength and maintain ROM. At 4 months the progression intensified to a 5-day-a-week program including the following:

- Running for fitness—2/3 miles three times per week
- Lunges—90 degree, pivot, 180 degree
- Sprints—"W," triangle, 6 second, 20 yd, 40 yd, 120 yd
- Acceleration/deceleration runs (see Figure 17-11)
- Shuffle slides progressing to shuffle run
- Carioca
- Ball work—Turn/stop the pass; turn/mark opponent; mark/steal/shoot the ball; two-touch and shoot; one-touch and shoot; volley and shoot; passing; pass/knock/move; coerver drills; light drill work at practice; one-on-one; scrimmage (begin with short period, progress to full game); full active participation.

FUNCTIONAL TESTING

According to Harter, functional testing is an indirect measure of muscular strength and power. Function is "quantified" using maximal performance of an activity.[10] Harter describes three purposes of functional testing as follows:

1. Determine risk of injury due to limb asymmetry
2. Provide objective measure of progress during a treatment or rehabilitation program
3. Measure the ability of the individual to tolerate forces.[10]

Functional testing can provide the sports therapist with objective data for review. Traditional rehabilitation programs and improvements in strength and range of motion do not always correlate with functional ability.[13] Functional testing should have a better correlation with functional ability.

When contemplating the use of a functional test or battery of tests, the sports therapist must evaluate the test(s) chosen. Validity and reliability must be considered. A test should measure what it intends to measure (validity) and should consistently provide similar results (reliability) regardless of the evaluator. Other factors must be considered before releasing an athlete to full activity. These include subjective evaluation of the injury, performance on functional tests, presence or absence of signs and symptoms, other recognized clinical tests (isokinetic testing, special tests, etc), and physician's approval.

Functional testing might be limited if the sports therapist does not have normative values or preinjury baseline values for comparison. Obviously, an athlete who cannot complete the test(s) is not ready for a return to play. However, what happens to the athlete who can complete the test(s), but has no preinjury data available for comparison? The sports therapist has to make a subjective decision based on the test result. If the normative data or preinjury data is available, the sports therapist can make an objective decision. If a soccer player is able to complete a sprint test with a mean of 20 seconds but her preinjury time was 17 seconds, then she is only 85 percent functional. Without the preinjury data, the sports therapist might be unable to determine the functional level. Of course, the sports therapist can always compare to the mean functional level of the uninjured team members to aid in the decision making.

Upper Extremity

There are many ways to functionally test an athlete. The most common and often the simplest ways include timed performance. For the upper extremity, a throwing velocity test is often used. This can be accomplished two ways, depending on the sports therapist's budget and the availability of complex testing tools.

1. Test velocity in a controlled environment, preferably indoors to decrease effects of the weather.
2. Set up a standard pitching distance (60 ft 6 in).
3. Have the athlete use a windup motion.
4. Measure a maximum of five throws—measured in mph with calibrated Magnum X ban radar gun (CMI corporation, Owensburg, KY) placed 36 inches high and to the right of the catcher.
5. Compute the mean of the five throws and compare to pretest value.

Many sports therapists do not have access to such equipment. A second way to test the upper extremity using velocity would be to use a similar setup but minus the radar gun. In this situation the sports therapist needs a stopwatch to time the flight of the ball. The sports therapist begins timing as the athlete releases the ball and stops when the catcher receives the ball. Again, a mean of five throws should be computed to help decrease testing error. As one can see, the first method will be the most accurate, but the second method can be used as an effective testing tool.[24]

To functionally test for the upper extremity, the key concept is to focus on the sport demand for the athlete. Careful attention should be focused on the skill involved with the sport. Does the athlete perform a primarily open-kinetic-chain skill, or is the skill performed in a closed kinetic chain? A gymnast might need more closed-kinetic-chain testing than a tennis player. Similarly, the sports therapist will not test a volleyball player using the pitching test above. The sports therapist will have to consult with the coach and determine what the athlete needs to do, and from this devise a test battery. For the volleyball player, it might be a serving test rather than the pitching test. Again, sports therapists are limited only by their creativity.

Lower Extremity

The lower extremity can be tested in many different ways, including sprint times, agility run times, jumping or hopping heights/distances, co-contraction tests, carioca runs, and shuttle runs. In-depth coverage of these tests is beyond the scope of this text, but we give an introduction to a variety of these tests.

Sprint Tests. The sprint test is exactly what the name implies.

1. A set distance is measured.
2. The athlete then runs the distance with a time per run recorded.
3. 3 to 5 sprints should be completed and the mean computed.
4. Pretest and posttest means are compared.

Agility Tests. Agility runs involve the same premise. The run is timed, and a mean is taken for five runs. The difference is the course. Rather than concentrating on straight-ahead motion, the agility run incorporates changes of direction, acceleration/deceleration, and quick starts and stops. For example, a simple figure eight can be set up with cones and the athlete is instructed to travel the cones as fast as possible while being timed for performance. Gross et al. described a figure eight course that was 5 by 10 meters. Each subject in their study was instructed to complete three trips around the eight while being timed. Two trials were conducted and the best time recorded.[9] Anderson and Foreman point out that there is no standard found in the literature that dictates testing procedures for the figure eight.[2] A standard procedure should be developed by each sports therapist or each institution to ensure the validity and reliability of the test.

Box runs are also beneficial as agility runs, because they emphasize pivoting and change of direction. The athlete is instructed to travel around four cones arranged in a box formation. The time to complete the box is recorded. Again, variations are prominent, with single laps versus multiple laps. The Barrow Zigzag Run is a variation of the box run using five cones. The four cones of the box are set as usual with the fifth cone in the center of the box. The box is a 16 by 10 ft course. The athlete travels around the cones as shown in Figure 17-16.[2]

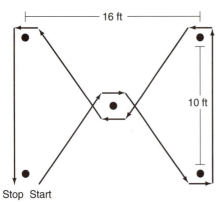

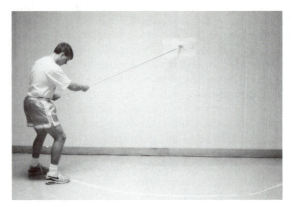

Figure 17-16 Barrow Zigzag Run test. The athlete essentially runs a figure 8 with sharp turns at the corners.

Figure 17-17 Co-contraction test. The athlete moves in a sidestep or shuffle fashion around the periphery of a semicircle, using surgical tubing for resistance.

It is beneficial to use agility runs because the level of difficulty can be changed. Early in the rehabilitation process, large figure eights that are more circular in shape can be used to provide functional data with low stress to the injury. As the injury heals the figure eight can be tighter to provide greater stresses to the injured body part.

Vertical Jump. The vertical jump test can also be used to evaluate the lower extremity.[4] In this test, the athlete has chalked fingertips and jumps to touch a piece of paper (of a different color than the chalk). Three to five jumps should be attempted and the mean height recorded (measured from fingertips standing to the chalk mark).[2,5,23] Variations in this test also exist. Anderson and Foreman mention alterations that include "bilateral vs. single leg jump, countermovement vs. static squat start, approach steps vs. stationary start, and use of the upper extremities for propulsion vs. restricted use of the upper extremities."[2] Many more expensive testing devices are available that can measure time differentials, force, and height.

Co-contraction Semicircular Test. The co-contraction semicircular test involves securing the athlete to a 48-inch resistance strap (TheraBand) that is attached to the wall 60 inches above the floor (see Figure 17-17). The strap is then stretched to twice its recoil length and the athlete completes five 180-degree semicircles, with a radius of 96 inches, around a tape line. The athlete is instructed to use a forward-facing lateral shuffle step. If the athlete starts on the left, she or he will travel around the semicircle until reaching the right boundary. This semicircle counts as one repetition. The athlete must complete five repetitions in the shortest amount of time possible. Three trials can be used, and the mean time is

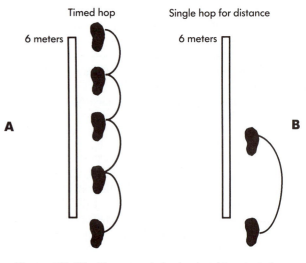

Figure 17-18 Hop tests. **A,** In the timed hop test, time required to cover a 6-meter distance is measured in seconds. **B,** The single hop for distance test measures the distance covered in a single hop. Both tests use a percentage of the injured leg compared to the uninjured leg.

calculated. This test is designed to provide a dynamic pivot shift for the ACL-insufficient knee.[15,16,17,19]

Hopping Tests. Hopping tests are also found in the literature (Figure 17-18) Booher et al. and Worrell et al. report that hopping tests might not be sensitive enough to evaluate the functional abilities of athletes.[5,26] However, hopping tests are noted in the literature and are used for clinical determination of function. Noyes et al. used a variety of hop tests to determine lower-extremity limb symmetry.[2,19,20] The more common hopping tests are the single-leg hop for distance, the timed hop test, the triple hop for distance, and the crossover hop for distance. The single-leg hop for distance requires the athlete to attempt to hop as far as possible while landing on the same limb. The timed hopping test measures the amount of time it takes the athlete to hop a distance of 6 meters. The triple hop for distance measures the distance traveled by the athlete with three consecutive hops. And finally the crossover hop for distance measures the distance traveled using three consecutive hops while crossing over a 15-cm-wide strip.[2,5,13,19,20,26]

Carioca Test. Carioca runs can be timed to measure improvement in function (see Figure 17-14). The carioca run involves a lateral grapevine or crossover step over a total distance of 80 feet. The athlete should choose which direction to face and maintain the stance. The athlete will then carioca 40 feet, change direction without turning around, and return to the starting position. The time to complete the 80-foot course is recorded. Three trials should be used and the mean time calculated.[15,16,17,19]

Shuttle Runs. Shuttle runs can involve many different drills. The most common requires the athlete to complete four 20-foot sprints, for a total of 80 feet, incorporating three direction changes. It is common to take three trials, and the mean should be calculated.[15,16,17,19] Another common shuttle run is the line drill, sometimes called "suicide sprints" or "death warmed over." The course is set with markers at various distances from the starting line. The athlete is instructed to sprint and touch the first marker and then return to the starting position. The athlete then continues the course, touching each marker and returning to the starting position. A total time is recorded.[2] This test is very flexible and can be used on the basketball, volleyball, or tennis courts, as well as football, soccer, or other playing fields.

Balance Tests. Balance is an important component of any motor skill activity. Following injury many athletes exhibit deficits in proprioception, which translate into a loss of balance. Anderson and Foreman[2] report that there is a "paucity" of research in balance testing with the athletic population. What is available might use expensive equipment unavailable to many sports therapists. They describe a simple single-leg balance test as a valid alternative to expensive testing. The athlete is instructed to stand on one leg, and timing begins. Timing stops when the athlete alters his or her position in order to maintain balance. This test can be modified to include eyes opened or closed to eliminate visual cues. Also, changes in surface can be made that require greater balance. Instead of testing on a floor surface, the sports therapist might choose to use a foam surface or a minitrampoline.[2] The sports therapist can also incorporate sport skills into a balance test.

Subjective Evaluation. Subjective evaluations of performance have been correlated with functional performance testing to determine predictive capabilities. Wilk et al. found strong correlations between subjective scores and knee extension peak torque, knee extension acceleration, and functional testing; however, no significant relationship was noted with hamstring function.[25] This is in contrast to Shelbourne's research, which showed a poor relationship between subjective evaluation, functional tests, and knee strength; Shelbourne concluded that only knee strength was a good measure of ability.[21] Subjective questionnaires or numeric scales might or might not be beneficial in the functional assessment of athletes, based on these correlations. If the subjective score is low, it could indicate an apprehension on the part of the athlete, which should serve as a warning sign of psychological unreadiness to return to play. The sports therapist should determine whether subjective evaluation is useful with respect to the given athlete.

Obviously, budget considerations and availability of equipment will determine the type of tests that the sports therapist can use, but simple timed sprints can indicate improved performance just as well as the more complicated tests that involve expensive equipment.[1,15,16,17]

CAROLINA FUNCTIONAL PERFORMANCE INDEX (CFPI)

The CFPI has been developed to help the sports therapist evaluate lower-extremity functional performance. The CFPI evaluates the athlete's existing functional performance capability. McGee and Futtrell evaluated 200 collegiate athletes and nonathletes using a battery of tests that included the co-contraction test, carioca test, shuttle run test, and one-legged timed hopping test. Table 17-5 shows the mean and standard deviation for each of these tests for males and for females. From this series of tests, a normative CFPI index was determined for males and females that can be used in accurately assessing functional performance based on the results of only two of the tests—the carioca test and the co-contraction test.[19]

Using stepwise regression techniques, the following prediction equations were established:

$$\text{Males: } 1.09(x_1) + 1.415(x_2) + 8.305 = \text{CFPI}$$
$$\text{Females: } 1.26(x_1) + 1.303(x_2) + 8.158 = \text{CFPI}$$
$$\text{(Where } x_1 = \text{co-contraction score in seconds,}$$
$$\text{and } x_2 = \text{carioca score in seconds)}$$

■ **TABLE 17-5** CFPI Mean Index and Performance Test Means

	Males Mean/standard deviation	Females Mean/standard deviation
CFPI	31.551/2.867	36.402/3.489
Carioca	7.812/1.188	8.899/1.124
Co-contraction test	11.188/1.391	13.218/1.736
One-legged hop test	4.953/0.53	5.746/0.63
Shuttle run	7.596/0.654	8.539/0.69

The sports therapist can test any individual using these two tests (co-contraction and carioca) and determine their individual CFPI. The CFPI value for that individual can be compared to the mean normative CFPI indices of 31.551 for males and 36.402 for females. If baseline preinjury testing was done, then the preinjury CFPI can be compared to the postinjury CFPI to determine how the athlete is progressing in their rehabilitation program. The CFPI provides a reliable objective criteria for functional performance testing.

CONCLUSION

Once the athletes can safely and effectively perform all specific tasks leading up to the motor skill, they can return to activity. For example, an athlete might progress from cycling, to walking, to jogging, to running, before returning to sprinting activities and competition in the 4 × 400 relay.

The sports therapist must note that these are only examples. No one program will benefit every athlete and every condition. Sports therapists should use these activities, along with others they develop, to help maximize the athlete's recovery. By providing athletes with every option available in rehabilitation, the sports therapist can return the athlete to participation at preinjury status. The preinjury status achieved with the functional progression not only can return the athlete to competition, but also can ensure a safer, more effective return to play.

Summary

1. Complete rehabilitation should strive to improve neuromuscular coordination and agility, strength, endurance, and flexibility.
2. The role of the functional progressions is to improve and complete the traditional rehabilitation process by providing sport-specific exercise.
3. The functional progression is a sequence of activities that simulate sport activity. The progression will begin easy and progress to full sport participation.
4. Each sport activity can be divided into smaller components, allowing the athlete to progress from easy to difficult.
5. Functional progressions are highly effective exercise therapy techniques that should be incorporated in the long-term rehabilitation stage.
6. Functional progressions allow for improvements in strength, endurance, mobility/flexibility, relaxation, coordination/agility/skill, and assessment of functional stability.
7. Functional progression can benefit the athlete psychologically and socially by decreasing the athlete's feelings of anxiety, deprivation, and apprehension.
8. Components of a functional progression that should be addressed include development, choice of activity, implementation, and termination.
9. Many functional tests exist and should be administered when deciding whether to return an athlete to competition.

References

1. Anderson, M. 1991. The relationships among isometric, isotonic, and isokinetic concentric and eccentric quadriceps and hamstring force and three components of athletic performance. *Journal of Orthopaedic and Sports Physical Therapy* 14:3.
2. Anderson, M. A., T. L. Foreman. 1996. Return to competition: Functional rehabilitation. In Athletic injuries and rehabilitation, edited by J. E. Zachazewski, D. J. Magee & W. S. Quillen. Philadelphia: W. B. Saunders.
3. Andrews, J. R. 1990. *Preventive and rehabilitative exercises for the shoulder and elbow.* Birmingham: American Sports Medicine Institute.
4. Bangerter, B. L. 1968. Contributive components in the vertical jump. *Research Quarterly* 39:432–36.
5. Booher, L. D., K. M. Hench, T. W. Worrell, and J. Stikeleather. 1993. Reliability of three single-leg hop tests. *Journal of Sport Rehabilitation* 2:165–70.

6. Croce, P., and J. Greg. 1991. Keeping fit when injured. In *Clinics in sports medicine*, edited by A. Nicholas, and D. Noble. Philadelphia: W. B. Saunders/Harcourt Brace Jovanovich.

7. Davis, J. M. 1986. Rehabilitation: A practical approach. In *Sports physical therapy*, edited by D. Bernhardt. Philadelphia: Churchhill Livingstone.

8. Galley, J. 1991. *Human movement: An introductory text for physiotherapists.* London: UK Limited.

9. Gross, M. T., J. R. Everts, and S. E. Roberson. 1994. Effect of DonJoy ankle ligament protector and Aircast Sport-Stirrup orthoses on functional performance. *Journal of Orthopaedic and Sports Physical Therapy* 19(3): 150–56.

10. Harter, R. 1996. Clinical rationale for closed kinetic chain activities in functional testing and rehabilitation of ankle pathologies. *Journal of Sport Rehabilitation* 5(1): 13–24.

11. Jokl, E. 1964. *The scope of exercise in rehabilitation.* Lexington, MA: Charles C. Thomas.

12. Kegerreis, S. 1983. The construction and implementation of functional progressions as a component of athletic rehabilitation. *Journal of Orthopaedic and Sports Physical Therapy* 63(4): 14–19.

13. Keskula, D. R., J. B. Duncan, and V. L. Davis. 1996. Functional outcome measures for knee dysfunction assessment. *Journal of Athletic Training* 31(2): 105–10.

14. Kisner, C., and L. Colby. 1985. *Therapeutic exercise foundations and techniques.* Philadelphia: F. A. Davis.

15. Lephart, S. 1992. Relationship between selected physical characteristics and functional capacity in the anterior cruciate ligament-insufficient athlete. *Journal of Orthopaedic and Sports Physical Therapy* 16(4): 174–81.

16. Lephart, S. M., and T. Henry. 1995. Functional rehabilitation for the upper and lower extremity. *Ortho Clinics of North America* 26(3): 579–92.

17. Lephart, S., D. Perrin, K. Minger, et al. 1991. Functional performance tests for the anterior cruciate ligament-insufficient athlete. *Journal of Athletic Training* 26:44–50.

18. Melliam, M. 1988. *Office management of sports injuries and athletic problems.* Philadelphia: Handy & Belfus.

19. McGee, M. R., and M. D. Futrell. *Functional testing of athletes and Non-athletes using the Carolina Functional Performance Index.* Unpublished master's thesis, University of North Carolina, Chapel Hill.

20. Noyes, F., S. Barber, and R. Mangine. 1991. Abnormal limb symmetry determined by function hop tests after anterior cruciate ligament rupture. *American Journal of Sports Medicine* 19(5): 513–18.

21. Shelbourne, D. 1987. Functional ability in athletes with anterior cruciate ligament deficiency. *American Journal of Sports Medicine* 15:628.

22. Tegner, Y., J. Lysholm, and M. Lysholm, et al. 1986. A performance test to monitor rehabilitation and evaluate anterior cruciate ligament injuries. *American Journal of Sports Medicine* 14:156–59.

23. Tibone, J. M., M. S. Antich, G. S. Fanton, et al. 1986. Functional analysis of anterior cruciate ligament instability. *American Journal of Sports Medicine* 13:34–39.

24. Torg, J., J. Vegso, and E. Torg. 1987. *Rehabilitation of athletic injuries: An atlas of therapeutic exercise.* Chicago: Year Book.

25. Wilk, K. E., W. T. Romaniello, S. M. Soscia, and C. A. Arrigo. 1994. The relationship between subjective knee scores, isokinetic testing, and functional testing in the ACL-reconstructed knee. *Journal of Orthopaedic and Sports Physical Therapy* 20(2): 60–71.

26. Worrell, T. W., L. D. Booher, and K. M. Hench. 1994. Closed kinetic chain assessment following inversion ankle sprain. *Journal of Sport Rehabilitation* 3(3): 197–203.

PART THREE

Rehabilitation Techniques for Specific Injuries

CHAPTER **18**

The Evaluation Process in Rehabilitation

David H. Perrin

After completion of this chapter, the student should be able to do the following:

- Discuss the important components of a preparticipation physical examination.

- Explain the differences between an on-field and an off-field injury evaluation.

- Outline the protocol to be followed for an on-field injury evaluation.

- Describe the usefulness of upper- and lower-quarter screening in the off-field evaluation.

- Describe the components and appropriate sequence for a comprehensive off-field evaluation.

- Discuss the importance of, and provide a format for, documentation of injury evaluation findings.

To be effective in supervising programs of rehabilitation, the sports therapist must be skillful in evaluating the status of the athlete. In a sports medicine setting, several different types of evaluations exist.[1,31]

Injuries can be prevented to some extent by including a preparticipation examination, which must be done long before injury occurs. Information gathered during the preparticipation examination will allow the sports therapist to incorporate intervention strategies to correct existing deficits. The examination not only is helpful for injury prevention but also establishes baseline information that can be useful in determining the severity of an injury.

After acute injury, the sports therapist typically performs an initial evaluation either on the field or court of competition or later in the athletic training room. In the first case, the sports therapist is at a distinct advantage over other health-care providers. First, the sports therapist may have viewed the mechanism of injury, a component of injury evaluation that lends a great deal of insight into the anatomical structures involved. Second, the sports therapist is able to assess the nature of the injury before the onset of muscle spasm and swelling; both factors can confound the accurate assessment of severity. In either the on- or the off-field setting, the examiner frequently has the advantage of knowing the athlete's personality, injury history, and pain threshold. Effective management of acute on-field injuries necessitates establishing an emergency plan that clarifies the roles and responsibilities of the personnel involved.[5]

The sports therapist cannot design an effective program of rehabilitation without conducting a thorough, detailed, sequential injury evaluation in the clinic or the training room. Throughout the rehabilitation process, the sports therapist must continuously reevaluate the status of the injured athlete and modify or adjust the program as necessary based on an understanding of the healing process.

Finally, accurate documentation of significant findings, both during initial evaluation and throughout the rehabilitation program, is critical.

PREPARTICIPATION EXAMINATION

Preparticipation examinations are an essential component of a comprehensive sports medicine health-care plan. The National Collegiate Athletic Association (NCAA) lists it as the first component of a safe athletic program and recommends a thorough evaluation upon a student athlete's initial entrance into an institution's intercollegiate athletic program.[23] A survey of the 50 states and the District of Columbia conducted to assess the requirements for scholastic preparticipation physical examinations showed that 35 states require a yearly examination of some type.[11]

The ideal preparticipation examination incorporates the expertise of medical doctors and sports therapists.[1] The role of the physician is to assess the status of the cardiorespiratory and musculoskeletal systems and review potential contraindications to participation. The team physician ultimately authorizes the athlete's participation in competitive sports.

The role of the sports therapist is to assess the strength, flexibility, and fitness of an athlete relative to the specific demands of the sport. The examination should be designed to screen for potential problem areas. A more definitive evaluation of problem areas should be conducted and referral made to appropriate medical specialists if necessary.

History

The preparticipation examination should begin with a complete medical history that includes questions pertaining to prior illnesses, injuries, surgery, allergies, and immunizations, as well as any current medication therapy. An accurate family history should also be obtained, including any cardiovascular disease, diabetes, allergies, sudden death, or orthopedic problems experienced by members of the athlete's immediate family.[3,13,26] Details about affirmative responses on the medical history form frequently need to be confirmed or explored through personal interview.

Flexibility

In determining normal flexibility, the requirements of the sport in question must be considered. For example, a person who is inflexible by the standards for a gymnast might be very flexible for an offensive lineman.

Assessment of flexibility should begin at the cervical region, include the trunk and all extremities, and focus especially on muscles frequently injured during athletic participation.[21] Normal cervical motion should permit the athlete to place the chin on the chest, look at the ceiling, nearly align the chin with the shoulder on right and left sides, and form a 45-degree angle while laterally flexing to the right and left (Figures 18-1 to 18-4). Shoulder motion can be screened with Apley's range-of-motion tests, which assess abduction and external rotation (Figure 18-5*A, B*) and adduction and internal rotation (Figure 18-6*A, B*). Inability to perform these tests would necessitate careful evaluation of each motion inherent to the shoulder girdle–joint complex. Elbow, forearm, and wrist range of motion can quickly be assessed by actively performing the motions inherent to these joints.

Evaluation of lower-extremity flexibility should include motions about the hip, knee, and ankle joints.[22] Figures 18-7 and 18-8 illustrate simple tests for evaluating flexibility of the hip flexors and adductor muscle groups. Hamstring flexibility can be assessed from a supine position with the hip stabilized at a 90-degree angle (Figure 18-9). Normal flexibility of the hamstring muscle group should permit the athlete to completely extend the knee. Low back and hamstring flexibility can be assessed by the sit-and-reach test (Figure 18-10). Tautness of the iliotibial band is frequently a cause of disability and can be assessed through use of the Ober test, as illustrated in Figure 18-11. Finally, flexibility of the triceps surae complex should be assessed with the knee first extended (gastrocnemius) and then flexed to a 90-degree angle (soleus).

Any limitations in flexibility detected by the examiner should be confirmed and documented through the use of standard goniometry.[24] Only in this way can limitations in motion be confirmed and the usefulness of prescribed stretching programs be ascertained.

Strength

Manual muscle testing should be performed to assess strength of the cervical spine muscles and the major muscle groups of the extremities. Several resources describe the technique of manual muscle testing for all major muscle groups of the body.[6,9,18]

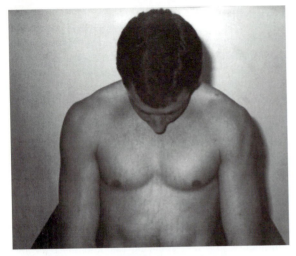

Figure 18-1 Cervical flexion range of motion.

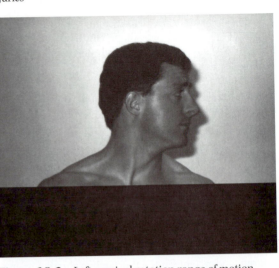

Figure 18-3 Left cervical rotation range of motion.

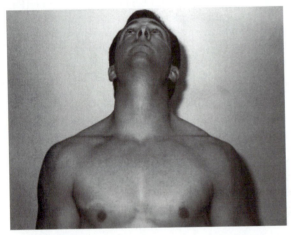

Figure 18-2 Cervical extension range of motion.

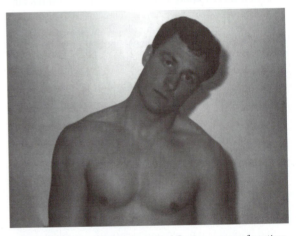

Figure 18-4 Left lateral cervical flexion range of motion.

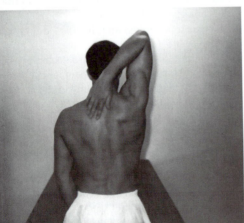

Figure 18-5 Apley's range-of-motion test—**A**, abduction and **B**, external rotation.

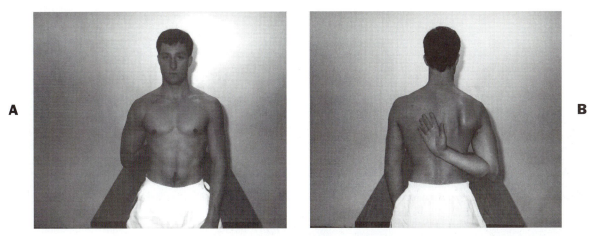

A   B

Figure 18-6   Apley's range-of-motion test—**A,** adduction and **B,** internal rotation.

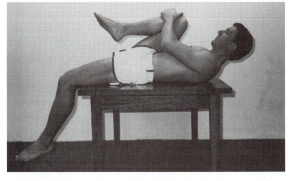

Figure 18-7   Negative Thomas test for tightness of the left hip flexors.

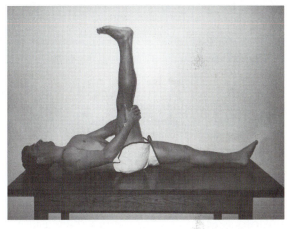

Figure 18-9   Test for hamstring flexibility. Inability to completely extend the knee indicates a positive test.

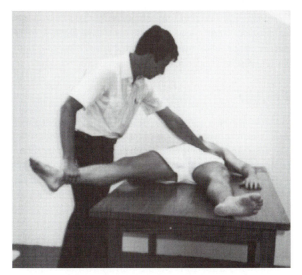

Figure 18-8   Test for tightness of the adductors.

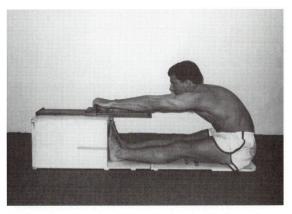

Figure 18-10   Sit-and-reach test for low back and hamstring flexibility.

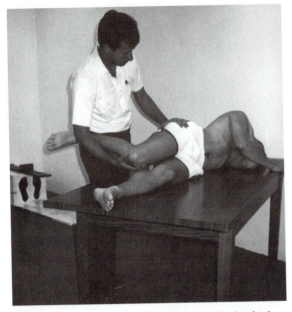

Figure 18-11 Ober test for tightness in the iliotibial band.

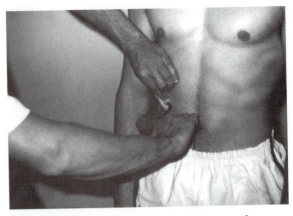

Figure 18-12 Measurement of subcutaneous fat.

Athletes presenting with obvious deficiencies in strength or with a history of musculoskeletal injury should be evaluated by any one of several commercially available strength dynamometers. Isokinetic testing enables the accurate evaluation of single muscle group performance and their relationship to bilateral and reciprocal muscle groups.[25] As with flexibility, the neuromuscular demands of a sport might dramatically influence the strength capacity of single muscle groups. This influence must be considered when establishing normal bilateral and reciprocal muscle group values for athletes in different sports. An extensive listing of normative isokinetic data for a variety of athletic and sedentary populations in both males and females can be found elsewhere.[25]

Body Composition

Assessment of body composition involves prediction of body density, from which the amount of body fat can be determined. The most accurate method for measuring body composition is hydrostatic weighing. Anthropometric techniques, which include a combination of height-weight indexes, skinfold fat, body circumference, and body diameters, are also available.[16]

When many athletes must be assessed, skinfold measurement of subcutaneous fat provides a rapid and reliable predictor of body density[16] (Figure 18-12). Jackson and Pollock[16] have recommended using the sum of three skin-

fold measurements to evaluate body composition in adults ranging from 18 to 61 years of age. Subcutaneous fat is distributed differently in men and women, so different sites are used for each group. For men, the sum of chest, abdomen, and thigh skinfolds are used, and for women the triceps, suprailium, and thigh skinfolds are recommended.

The generalized approach for determination of body composition proposed by Jackson and Pollock is appropriate for a large, heterogeneous population (18 to 61 years of age) but might not be appropriate for the high school athlete. Sports therapists dealing with prepubescent and pubescent athletes are encouraged to read the work of Slaughter et al.[30]

The purpose of determining body composition during the preparticipation examination is to provide the athlete with guidelines relative to desirable levels of body fat. Optimal levels of body fat vary considerably between sports. In general, highly trained athletes range from 4 to 10 percent body fat for men and from 13 to 18 percent body fat for women.[16]

Fitness

Aerobic fitness is a measure of the long-term energy system's efficiency and is most accurately determined through measurement of oxygen consumption during exhaustive work. However, this measurement also requires expensive laboratory equipment and is impractical for determining fitness of many athletes during the preparticipation examination. Several techniques have been used that predict fitness from recovery heart rates after vigorous stepping or cycling exercise. However, perhaps the most practical method for preparticipation screening of many athletes is the 12-minute run developed by Cooper[7] or a 2-mile run. These techniques predict maximal oxygen consumption from distance covered during a 12-minute run or time required to run 2 miles. From this information, athletes are categorized as having fitness levels falling somewhere between very poor and excellent. Based on test results and determined by the specific physiological demands of the sport, a conditioning program can be prescribed.

Anaerobic fitness assesses the immediate and short-term energy system's efficiency and can be assessed through a Wingate bicycle test, the Margaria stair-climbing test, a vertical jump, or 40-yard dash. Most exercise physiology textbooks provide the details of these anaerobic power tests. A review of the work of Wilmore[34] will be helpful in designing conditioning programs appropriate for athletes in many different sports.

ON-FIELD EVALUATION

Although most on-field injuries in athletics are not of a life-threatening nature, the first responsibility of a sports therapist is to establish an emergency plan in the event that a life-threatening injury does occur.[12] The important components of such a plan include the acquisition of appropriate emergency care supplies and equipment, such as airway devices, stretchers, spine board, and splints.[29] Accessibility to a telephone, whether competition is occurring indoors or outdoors, is essential. A mechanism for unlocking doors and gates along the path to the injured athlete is also a must. Finally, the lines of authority should be established early with regard to staff and student sports therapists, physicians, and coaches.

Prior knowledge of community rescue squad and hospital emergency room facilities and personnel can be very useful in ensuring the appropriate disposition of the injured athlete. Voluntary in-service training on athletic injuries for the community emergency medical technicians (EMT) and paramedics can be invaluable in establishing the expertise of the sports therapist. During on-field management of a suspected cervical spine injury on Saturday afternoon is not the time to debate removal of a football helmet with an EMT.[7]

Another responsibility of the sports therapist is to be aware of the rules of each sport as they pertain to injury management. For example, intercollegiate wrestling permits only 2 minutes for evaluation of an athletic injury before a decision to either continue wrestling or forfeit must be made. Stepping onto a basketball court to evaluate an injured player necessitates either removing the player from the game or taking a team time-out. The implication of these rules to the sports therapist, especially in the final moments of a close contest, make injury evaluation an even greater challenge.

Primary Injury Evaluation

The first responsibility during an on-field evaluation is to rule out serious and life-threatening injury via a primary survey.[28] Such injuries on the athletic field are generally those in which the athlete is not breathing or has sustained trauma to the vital organs (central nervous system or internal organs). The components of a primary survey include the *ABCs* of emergency care: ensuring that there is an open *Airway*, *Breathing* is taking place, and *Circulation* is present. Once the ABCs have been established, injury to the cervical spine must be ruled out before the athlete is moved in any way. Should injury to the cervical spine be suspected, extreme care must be taken to avoid further injury from inappropriate movement. Several excellent sources have outlined the proper immobilization technique for an athlete with an injured spinal cord.[10,32]

Injuries to the chest and abdomen can also pose a threat to the athlete's life. Signs of serious injury to the chest can include pain at the site, difficulty breathing, coughing up of blood, cyanosis of the lips, and a rapid, weak pulse and low blood pressure.

Signs of injury to the abdomen can include tenderness when palpated, pain within the abdomen, difficulty in moving, low blood pressure, rapid pulse, and shallow respiration. Occasionally pain from injury to an internal structure is referred elsewhere, such as with pain in the left shoulder from injury to the spleen (Kehr's sign).[1]

If injury to the chest or abdomen is suspected, the examiner should monitor the athlete's pulse, blood pressure, and respiration. Treatment should be directed toward the prevention of shock until emergency medical personnel arrive.

Secondary Injury Evaluation

The first task of the sports therapist in an on-field evaluation of an athlete is to gain access to the athlete and establish control of the situation. Fellow teammates should be instructed never to touch or move an injured teammate; a nondisplaced cervical spine fracture could become crippling or fatal by the act of a well-intentioned teammate. Also, the sports therapist must never feel pressured by game officials or coaches to hasten the evaluation process.

The very early phase of acute injury evaluation may very well be simply to comfort the athlete and wait for the initial surge of pain to subside. Attempts to evaluate an injured athlete writhing in pain generally prove useless. Athletes usually gain control of their faculties within a few moments, at which time the evaluation can continue.

The next phase of the evaluation is to determine the mechanism of injury. Athletes can frequently describe the position of the body part or the point of contact by another player at the time of injury. Occasionally fellow teammates, game officials, or a coach can provide useful information about the mechanism of injury.

The athlete should next be asked to identify the site of pain as precisely as possible. Occasionally the site of pain is quite diffuse immediately after injury but tends to become more circumscribed within a few minutes. Early in the on-field situation, the sports therapist should palpate the site of injury to rule out gross and obvious deformity and to determine the anatomical structures involved. The athlete's willingness to move the injured part can also be indicative of the severity of the injury.

Should the injury be determined to be ligamentous, stress tests should be used immediately. Transporting an athlete even to the sideline can often lead to muscle spasm and guarding, which can confound the accurate assessment of joint laxity.

At this point in the evaluation, a determination should be made about transporting the athlete from the field of play. In most cases of upper-extremity injury and with some lower-extremity injuries, the athlete is capable of ambulating to the sideline. If any question exists, however, the athlete should be transported without bearing weight until a more definitive sideline evaluation can be conducted.

Once the athlete is on the sideline, the injury evaluation should follow the guidelines described for the off-field evaluation. The sports therapist should note several important features of the injury that might become useful in determining severity. In particular, the degree and onset of swelling are noteworthy. For example, a knee joint that swells rapidly and substantially usually indicates significant ligamentous injury. Conversely, swelling that occurs slowly and overnight might suggest injury to a meniscal structure.

The amount of motion of the part after injury should also be noted. A knee injury possessing full range of motion after injury but lacking complete extension the next day is probably from muscle spasm or joint effusion rather than from a displaced intra-articular structure.

Finally, the degree of laxity about a joint immediately after injury can be far more revealing than that observed the next day. Such information can be essential to the team physician's evaluation even several hours later and especially the next day.

Perhaps the most difficult questions the sports therapist must answer immediately after many injuries concern classifying the severity and predicting the length of disability. For the reasons stated earlier, the course an injury follows over a 24-hour period can be very revealing relative to its severity and to the period of time before full

return to competition can be expected. Thus sports therapists should resist the attempts of others (coaches and press) to predict the period of disability associated with an injury immediately after its occurrence.

OFF-FIELD EVALUATION

Off-field evaluations are usually conducted in the athletic training room and allow the sports therapist the opportunity to perform a detailed and uninterrupted assessment of the injury. Two scenarios seem prevalent in athletics. The first is that of the injured athlete who knows exactly what hurts and can vividly describe the mechanism of injury. The second situation is the athlete who reports pain of an insidious onset and who has difficulty localizing the site of pain. In the first case, the evaluation may be more focused to the region where mechanism of injury and site of pain are known. In the latter situation, the injury evaluation protocol should begin with a series of range-of-motion, muscle, and neurological tests known as *upper-* or *lower-quarter screening.*

Quarter Screening

The purpose of upper- or lower-quarter screening is to isolate the site of pain and to establish that the site of pain and location of injury are the same.[4] Embryology of the human body occurs in a longitudinal manner through development of dermatomes and myotomes. Dermatomes are areas of sensation on the skin supplied by a single spinal segment, and myotomes are groups of muscles innervated by a single spinal segment. This formation is especially true in the extremities. The implication to the clinician is that pain from injury within a particular dermatome can be experienced at a point other than the actual site of injury. Also, injury to a nerve might manifest itself through sensory or motor deficit distally along the distribution of the nerve. This phenomenon of referred pain can confound the accurate assessment of injury to either an upper or a lower extremity.[15]

Deficits in strength, sensation, or tendon reflexes of specific spinal segments can also indicate pathology at the corresponding nerve root or spinal cord level. For example, impingement of a nerve root from a protruding disk can produce deficits in strength and loss of sensation at the myotome and dermatome that correspond to the spinal segment where the lesion exists. Table 18-1 summarizes the dermatomes, myotomes, and deep tendon reflexes for the upper and lower extremities.

Upper-quarter screening involves the quick assessment of the neck, shoulder girdle region, and arm. Lower-quarter screening involves similar assessment of the low back, hip region, and leg.

■ **TABLE   18-1**   Upper- and Lower-Extremity Dermatomes, Myotomes, and Deep Tendon Reflexes.

Spinal Level	Muscle Testing	Sensation	Deep Tendon Reflex
C5	Deltoid and biceps	Lateral arm	Biceps
C6	Wrist extensors	Lateral forearm	Brachioradialis
C7	Wrist flexors	Middle finger	Triceps
C8	Finger flexors	Medial forearm	None
T1	Finger abductors	Medial arm	None
L4	Anterior tibial	Medial foot	Patellar tendon
L5	Extensor muscle of toes	Dorsum of foot	None
S1	Long and short peroneal	Lateral foot	Achilles tendon

Upper-Quarter Screening. Upper-quarter screening should begin with the athlete in a seated position. Visual inspection to assess posture of the head and shoulder girdle complex should precede the evaluation. The evaluation includes a series of range-of-motion and manual muscle tests of the cervical region and proceeds distally along the upper extremity. Cervical spine motion is first assessed actively (see Figures 18-1 to 18-4) and then with slight overpressure, should active range-of-motion produce no pain or limitation of motion (Figure 18-13). (**Note:** In no instance should a suspected neck injury in the on-field situation include this assessment.) The muscles surrounding the cervical spine are then assessed with isometric resistance to examine for either neurological involvement or injury to a muscle (Figures 18-14 to 18-17). During assessment of the cervical region, the sports therapist should look for locally produced signs and symptoms and for pain that might emanate from the cervical region but refer distally elsewhere in the upper extremity.

Next the screening proceeds to the shoulder region and begins with range-of-motion tests (see Figures 18-5 and 18-6) for active motion of the shoulder girdle and glenohumeral joints. Resisted shoulder elevation (Figure 18-18) and abduction (Figure 18-19) are then tested to assess the C2 to C5 neurological levels. The screening continues along the upper extremity with testing in a similar manner at the elbow, wrist, and hand, as illustrated in Figures 18-20 to 18-27.

As the upper-quarter screening proceeds distally from the cervical spine, the sports therapist should note pain or weakness. Should none be encountered, the site of injury is suspected elsewhere, and the procedure continues until the entire upper extremity has been examined. Should pain, weakness, or asymmetry be found, a more detailed evaluation should be performed focusing on the region of pain.

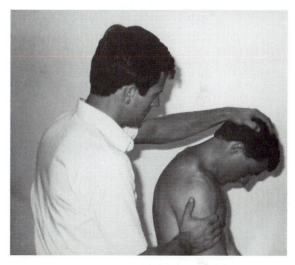

Figure 18-13   Cervical flexion with overpressure.

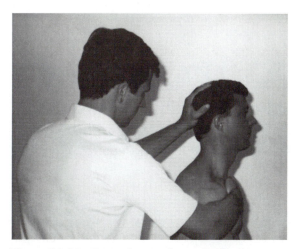

Figure 18-14   Resisted cervical extension.

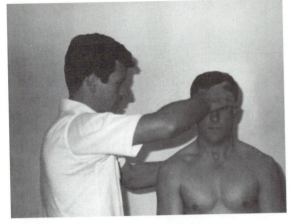

Figure 18-15   Resisted cervical flexion.

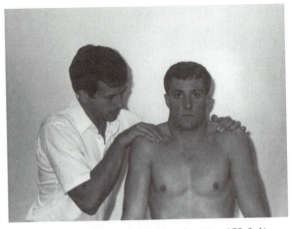

Figure 18-18   Resisted shoulder elevation (C2,3,4).

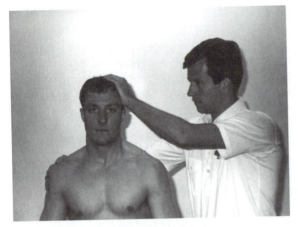

Figure 18-16   Resisted left lateral flexion.

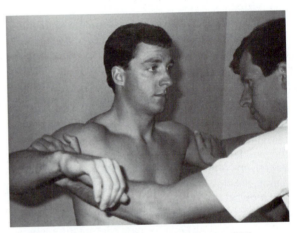

Figure 18-19   Resisted shoulder abduction (C5).

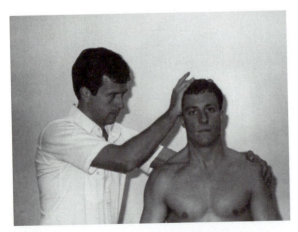

Figure 18-17   Resisted right lateral flexion.

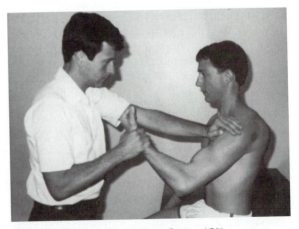

Figure 18-20   Resisted elbow flexion (C6).

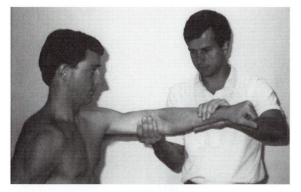

Figure 18-21   Resisted elbow extension (C7).

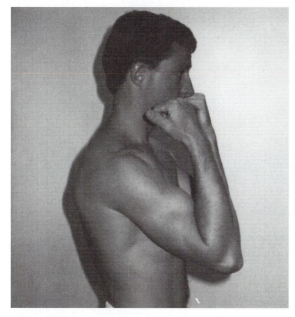

Figure 18-22   Elbow flexion range of motion.

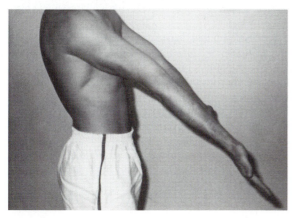

Figure 18-23   Elbow extension range of motion.

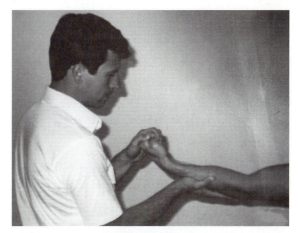

Figure 18-24   Resisted wrist flexion (C7).

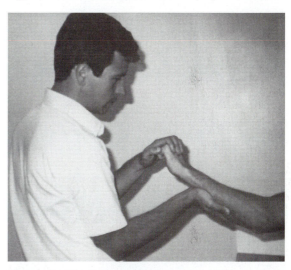

Figure 18-25   Resisted wrist extension (C6).

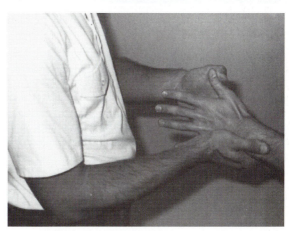

Figure 18-26   Resisted thumb extension (C8).

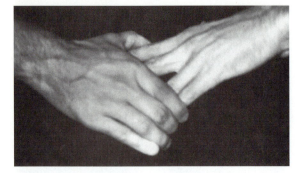

Figure 18-27 Resisted finger abduction (T1).

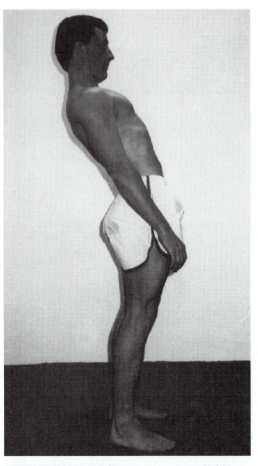

Figure 18-29 Lumbar extension range of motion.

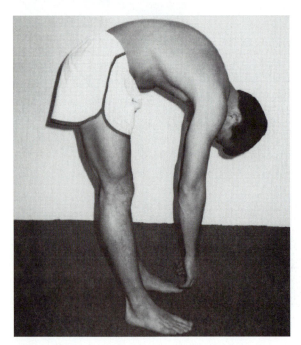

Figure 18-28 Lumbar flexion range of motion.

Lower-Quarter Screening. Lower-quarter screening involves a series of range-of-motion and manual muscle tests, beginning at the lumbar region and proceeding distally to include the entire lower extremity. As with the upper-quarter screening, the evaluation is preceded by a visual assessment of posture. The evaluation is conducted first while the athlete is standing and then from the sitting, supine, and prone positions.

While standing, the athlete is asked to perform active motion of the lumbar spine (Figures 18-28 to 18-31). Lo-

cally or distally produced pain or limitation of lumbar motion should be noted. Heel and toe walking should also be performed to assess neurological levels L4 and L5 (anterior tibial and long extensor of great toe; Figure 18-32) and S1 (gastrocnemius and soleus; Figure 18-33). Additional range-of-motion and manual muscle tests are performed while the athlete is sitting, supine, and prone (Figures 18-34 to 18-42).

As with the upper-quarter screening, pain or weakness should be noted. A region free from pain, weakness, or asymmetry is considered screened and thus not the site of injury. Should pain or weakness be found, a more detailed evaluation that focuses on the region of injury should follow.

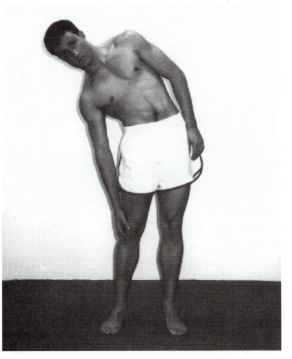

Figure 18-30   Lumbar right lateral flexion.

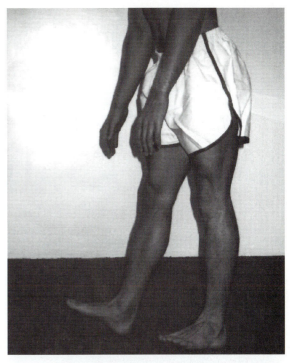

Figure 18-32   Heel walking (L4, L5).

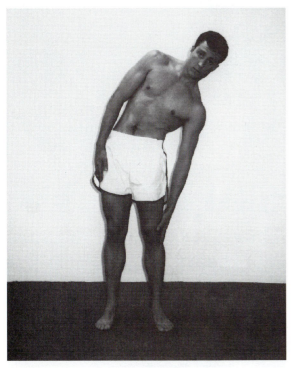

Figure 18-31   Lumbar left lateral flexion.

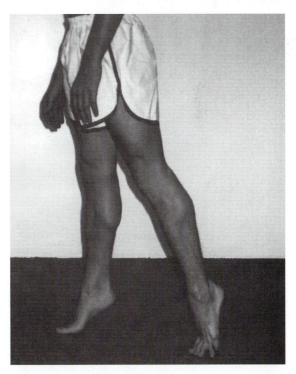

Figure 18-33   Toe walking (S1).

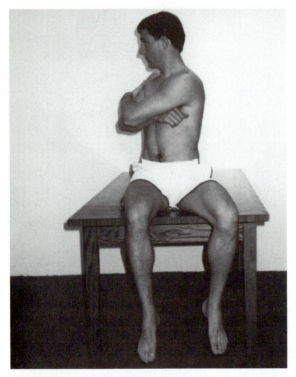

Figure 18-34 Trunk right rotation.

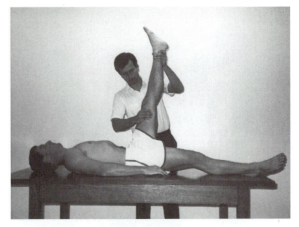

Figure 18-36 Straight leg raise for sciatic nerve involvement.

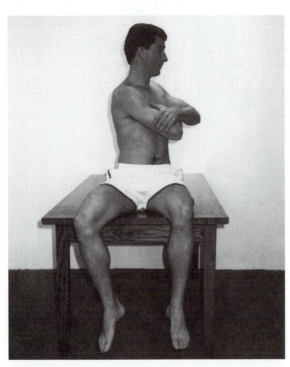

Figure 18-35 Trunk left rotation.

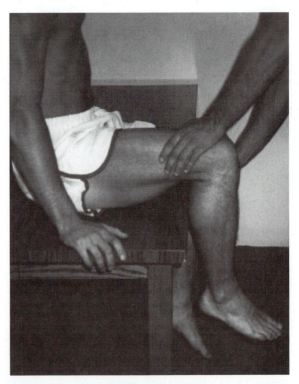

Figure 18-37 Resisted hip flexion (L1, L2).

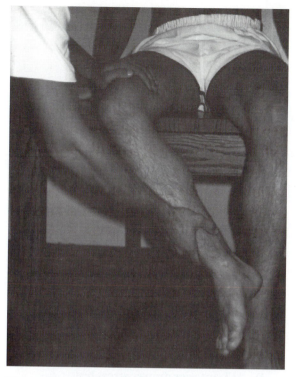

Figure 18-38 Hip internal rotation range of motion.

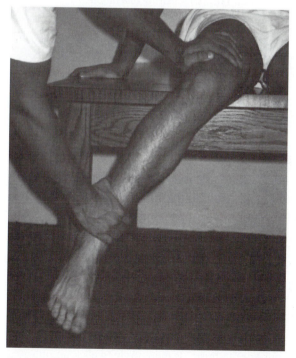

Figure 18-39 Hip external rotation range of motion.

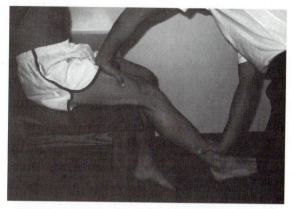

Figure 18-40 Resisted knee extension (L3, L4).

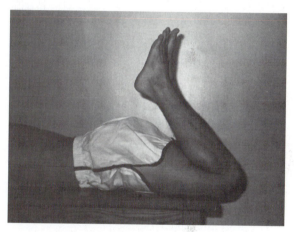

Figure 18-41 Knee flexion range of motion.

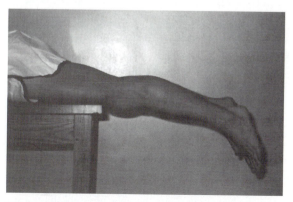

Figure 18-42 Knee extension range of motion.

Knee Injury Evaluation Checksheet

I. History
1. Ask what happened ____
2. Ask for description of mechanism ____
3. Ask for site of pain ____
4. Ask if any previous history ____

II. Inspection
1. Look for obvious deformity ____
2. Look for swelling and effusion ____
3. Compare bilaterally ____

III. Palpation
   A. Medial aspect
   1. MCL—femoral attachment ____
   2. MCL—tibial attachment ____
   3. Joint line ____
   B. Lateral aspect
   1. LCL—femoral attachment ____
   2. LCL—fibular attachment ____
   3. Joint line ____
   4. Fibular head ____
   C. Anterior aspect
   1. Suprapatellar pouch ____
   2. Quadriceps tendon ____
   3. Patella (superior pole) ____
   4. Patella (inferior pole) ____
   5. Patellar tendon ____
   6. Tibial tuberosity ____
   D. Posterior aspect
   1. Popliteal fossa ____
   2. Hamstring tendons ____

IV. Active Range of Motion
1. Knee flexion ____
2. Knee extension ____
3. Compare bilaterally ____

V. Passive Range of Motion
1. Knee flexion ____
2. Knee extension ____
3. Compare bilaterally ____

VI. Resistive Range of Motion
1. Knee extension ____
2. Knee flexion ____
3. Ankle plantar flexion ____

VII. Special Tests
   A. Menisci
   1. Check for terminal extension ____
   2. McMurray test ____
   B. MCL valgus stress test
   1. Correct hand placement ____
   2. Ensure muscular relaxation ____
   3. Stressed with terminal extension ____
   4. Stressed with slight flexion ____
   5. Compare bilaterally ____
   C. LCL varus stress test
   1. Correct hand placement ____
   2. Ensure muscular relaxation ____
   3. Stressed with slight flexion ____
   4. Compare bilaterally ____
   D. ACL anterior drawer stress test
   1. Correct hand placement ____
   2. Ensure hamstring relaxation ____
   3. Stressed at 90 degree flexion ____
   4. Compares bilaterally ____
   E. ACL Lachman stress test
   1. Correct hand placement ____
   2. Ensure muscular relaxation ____
   3. Stressed at 20 degree flexion ____
   4. Compare bilaterally ____

CLINICAL EVALUATION SCHEME

The key to successful injury evaluation is to establish a sequential and systematic approach that is followed in every case. Only through a systematic approach can the sports therapist be confident that an important component of evaluation will not be forgotten. However, every injury is also different and can present with unique signs and symptoms. Thus, although a systematic approach is important, the sports therapist must take care not to become robotized during the evaluation process. With this in mind, Knee Injury Evaluation Checksheet (above) and Shoulder Evaluation Checksheet (p. 301) show examples of injury evaluation formats for the knee and shoulder to assist the beginning sports therapist in establishing a sequential injury evaluation plan.

History

Perhaps the single most revealing component of injury evaluation is the history. The primary goals of the history are to determine the mechanism and site of injury. History taking includes recounting recent events leading to the injury and detailing previous injuries to the body part in question. The sports therapist should also refer to the injury profile obtained from the athlete during the preparticipation examination.

The role of the sports therapist in obtaining an accurate and pertinent history is to ask the right questions and listen carefully. Questions must be asked in a nonleading manner. For example, "What activities cause your knee to hurt?" is more likely to elicit an unbiased response than "Your knee probably hurts when you sit at

Shoulder Injury Evaluation Checksheet

I. History
1. Ask what happened ____
2. Ask for description of mechanism ____
3. Ask for site of pain ____
4. Ask if any previous history ____

II. Inspection
1. Gain visual access to region while maintaining athlete's modesty ____
2. Look for obvious deformity ____
3. Look for swelling ____
4. Compare bilaterally ____

III. Palpation
   A. Anterior aspect
   1. Sternoclavicular joint ____
   2. Clavicle ____
   3. Subacromial bursa ____
   4. Coracoid process ____
   B. Posterior aspect
   1. Scapula and scapular spine ____
   2. Supraspinatus muscle ____
   3. Infraspinatus muscle ____
   4. Teres minor muscle ____
   5. Rhomboid muscle ____
   C. Lateral aspect
   1. Deltoid muscle ____
   2. Biceps tendon ____
   3. Greater tuberosity ____
   4. Lesser tuberosity ____
   D. Superior aspect
   1. Acromioclavicular joint ____
   2. Trapezius muscle ____
   E. Inferior aspect
   1. Axilla ____
   2. Pectoralis major muscle ____
   3. Latissimus dorsi muscle ____

IV. Active Range of Motion
1. Cervical flexion ____
2. Cervical extension ____
3. Cervical right and left lateral flexion ____
4. Cervical right and left rotation ____
5. Shoulder flexion ____
6. Shoulder extension ____
7. Shoulder abduction ____
8. Shoulder adduction ____
9. Shoulder internal rotation ____
10. Shoulder external rotation ____
11. Shoulder horizontal flexion ____
12. Shoulder horizontal extension ____
13. Shoulder girdle elevation ____
14. Shoulder girdle depression ____
15. Check for normal glenohumeral/ scapular motion ____
16. Compare bilaterally ____

V. Passive Range of Motion
1. Shoulder flexion ____
2. Shoulder extension ____
3. Shoulder abduction ____
4. Shoulder adduction ____
5. Shoulder internal rotation ____
6. Shoulder external rotation ____
7. Shoulder horizontal flexion ____
8. Shoulder horizontal extension ____
9. Compare bilaterally ____

VI. Resistive Range of Motion
1. Shoulder flexion ____
2. Shoulder extension ____
3. Shoulder abduction ____
4. Shoulder adduction ____
5. Shoulder internal rotation ____
6. Shoulder external rotation ____
7. Shoulder horizontal flexion ____
8. Shoulder horizontal extension ____
9. Shoulder girdle elevation ____
10. Shoulder girdle depression ____

VII. Special Tests
   A. Yergason's bicipital tendinitis and subluxing biceps tendon test
   1. Correct hand placement ____
   2. Maintain elbow at 90 degrees ____
   3. Ask patient to supinate against resistance ____
   B. Drop-arm test for rotator cuff involvement
   1. Passively place patient's shoulder at 90 degrees ____
   2. Ask patient to hold position or lower slowly ____
   C. Empty-can test for supraspinatus strain
   1. Places shoulder at 90-degree abduction and 30-degree horizontal flexion ____
   2. Has patient internally rotate shoulder ____
   3. Attempts to adduct patient's shoulder ____
   D. Apprehension test for anterior dislocation/subluxation
   1. Ensures muscular relaxation ____
   2. Slowly abducts and externally rotates patient's shoulder ____
   E. Adson maneuver for thoracic outlet syndrome
   1. Has patient hold fully inspired breath ____
   2. Has patience extend and turn head toward side being examined ____

the movies, right?" From the athlete's responses, the evaluator must note the pertinent and disregard the irrelevant. Each response provides a key to the nature of the next question.

From the history, the sports therapist should determine whether the injury episode is acute or recurrent. If acute, knowledge of the athlete's posture at the moment of injury is important in determining the mechanism of injury. If swelling is present, the sports therapist should determine whether the onset was immediate or slow. The athlete's ability to continue playing or need to stop immediately after the injury can be indicative of severity.

If chronic, the course of the injury should be ascertained relative to an increase or decrease of symptoms and the efficacy of previous treatment regimens. Asking whether the injury is getting better, getting worse, or staying the same provides the evaluator with information relative to the anatomical structures involved and the usefulness of previous or current treatments. From the history, the evaluator should have a visual image of the injury mechanism and a general impression of the injury. With this information the evaluator is ready to proceed with a specific injury evaluation plan.

Inspection

Visual inspection of the injury begins as the athlete enters the training room. Of special interest is the athlete's gait in the case of lower-extremity injury. If an upper extremity is involved, the carrying position of the part should be noted.

A bilateral comparison of the anatomical region in question must be made.[27] This comparison will necessitate removal of clothing in many cases. In all instances, the modesty of the athlete must be protected. Shorts alone may be worn by the male athlete; females should wear sleeveless shirts or halter tops for evaluation of upper-extremity injury. As the athlete removes clothing, limitations in motion and weight bearing should be observed.

The primary purpose of the visual inspection is to first rule out the presence of gross or obvious deformity. Articular dislocations, such as those of the finger or shoulder, are easily visualized with careful inspection. Fractures of superficially located bones may also be noted in some cases, although nondisplaced fractures of a bone, such as the clavicle, might be impossible to ascertain from physical examination. Swelling at the injury site should also be noted, as should the nature of its onset (rapid and immediate, or gradual and slow). Finally, in the case of chronic injury, the presence of atrophy of muscles surrounding the region should be noted. For ex-

ample, an athlete experiencing patellofemoral pain over an extended period might present with a substantial deficit in thigh girth.

Palpation

Palpation of the injury site should occur early in the on-field evaluation for reasons previously described. During the more detailed off-field evaluation, palpating later in the injury evaluation process might be better. The disadvantage of palpating the injury site early is that such manual probing can elicit a pain response that will detract from the findings of the active, passive, and resistive motions that follow. Furthermore, the phenomenon of referred pain can make localization of the injury site difficult until other components of the evaluation have been performed.

The purpose of palpation is to identify as closely as possible the exact anatomical structures involved with the injury.[33] Palpation can be quite revealing at some regions (ankle, knee, or elbow) but might be far less helpful at others (shoulder or hip). From palpation, the presence of excessive heat from infection or inflammation should be noted. The volume and consistency of swelling might indicate effusion or hemarthrosis at a joint, and calcification might be identified in the residual hematoma from a soft tissue contusion. Rupture of a muscle or tendon might present as a gap at the point of separation. Some sports therapists believe malalignment of a skeletal structure, such as a vertebrae, can be ascertained through careful palpation.

Assessment of Motion

The goal of testing the motion of the injured part is to determine the nature of the anatomical structures involved. Cyriax has developed a method for locating and identifying a lesion by applying tension selectively to each of the structures that might potentially produce this pain.[8] Tissues are classified as being either contractile or inert. Contractile tissues include muscles and their tendons; inert tissues include bones, ligaments, joint capsules, fascia, bursae, nerve roots, and dura mater.

If a lesion is present in contractile tissue, pain occurs with active motion in one direction and with passive motion in the opposite direction. Thus a muscle strain would cause pain on both active contraction and passive stretch. Contractile tissues are tested through the midrange by an isometric contraction against maximum resistance. The specific location of the lesion within the musculotendinous unit cannot be specifically identified by the isometric contraction.

Categorization of End-Point "Feels"

Normal Endpoints

Soft tissue approximation	Soft and spongy, a gradual painless stop (for example, knee flexion)
Capsular feel	An abrupt, hard, firm end-point with only a little give (for example, end-point in hip rotation)
Bone-to-Bone	A distinct and abrupt end-point where two hard surfaces come in contact with one another (for example, elbow extension)
Muscular	Springy feel with some associated discomfort (for example, end of shoulder abduction)

Abnormal Endpoints

Empty feel	Movement is definitely beyond the anatomical limit, and pain occurs before the end of the range (for example, a complete ligament rupture)
Spasm	Involuntary muscle contraction that prevents motion because of pain; should also be called *guarding* (for example, back spasms)
Loose	Occurs in extreme hypermobility (for example, previously sprained ankle)
Springy block	A rebound at the end-point (for example, meniscus tear)

A lesion of inert tissue elicits pain on active and passive movement in the same direction.[2] A sprain of a ligament results in pain whenever that ligament is stretched, through either active contraction or passive stretching. Again, a specific lesion of inert tissue cannot be identified by looking at movement patterns alone.[17] Other special tests must be done to differentiate injured structures.

Active Range of Motion.   Movement assessment should begin with active motion. The sports therapist should evaluate the quality of movement, range of movement, motion in other planes, movement at varying speeds, and strength throughout the range but in particular at the end point. A complaint of pain on active motion does not distinguish contractile pain from inert pain.[14] Thus the sports therapist must proceed with an evaluation of both passive and resistive motion. An athlete who seems to be free of pain in each of these tests throughout a full range of motion should be tested by applying passive pressure at the endpoint.

Passive Range of Motion.   When passive range of motion is being assessed, the athlete must relax completely and allow the sports therapist to move the extremity to reduce the influence of the contractile elements. Particular attention should be directed toward the sensation of the athlete at the end of the passive range of motion. The sports therapist should categorize the "feel" of the end points as indicated in Categorization of End-Point "Feels" (above).[8] Figures 18-43 to 18-45 illustrate normal end-feels typically encountered during assessment of passive motion at the elbow. Common abnormal end-feels experienced during passive motion are the resistance encountered from a muscle in spasm or the springy block sensation resulting from a displaced intra-articular cartilage.

End-feel can also be quite revealing in assessment of ligamentous integrity. For example, the sensation of end-feel is probably more revealing than the amount of instability when performing the Lachman test to assess integrity of the anterior cruciate ligament of the knee.

Also of significance during passive motion is the presence of crepitus or clicking. Crepitus can indicate roughening of one or more articular surfaces such as found in advanced patellofemoral disease. Clicking might result from a subluxing tendon or displaced intra-articular cartilage. A biceps tendon subluxing from the intertubercular groove of the humerus and a torn meniscus catching between tibia and femur during knee motion are two forms of clicking.

Throughout the passive range of motion, the sports therapist is looking for limitation in movement and the presence of pain. Occasionally the sports therapist might encounter a phenomenon during passive motion known as a painful arc. A painful arc is pain that occurs at some point in the midrange but disappears as the limb passes this point in either direction. It occurs from pinching or impingement of sensitive structures between two surfaces, which can be caused either by a biomechanical fault in the articulating bones or by swollen tissue pinched between two normally aligned bony surfaces. Painful arcs are most typically associated with active motion but can also occur in passive motions in which a tissue is being stretched. A classic example of a painful arc is an impingement of the supraspinatus muscle. A painful arc is frequently found at the shoulder region as the subacromial bursa or supraspinatus tendon is pinched during movements inherent to activities such as swimming and throwing.

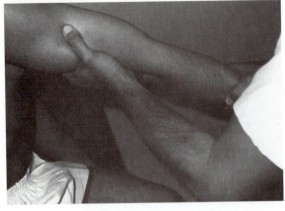

Figure 18-43 Passive elbow extension illustrating bone-to-bone end feel.

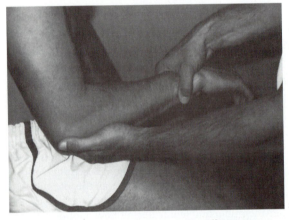

Figure 18-44 Passive elbow pronation illustrating capsular end feel.

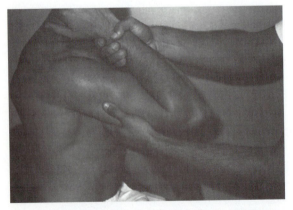

Figure 18-45 Passive elbow flexion illustrating tissue approximation end feel.

■ **TABLE 18-2** Capsular Patterns for Major Joints

Joint	Capsular Pattern
Neck	Equal limitation side bending and rotation, full range flexion painful, extension limited
Glenohumeral	Limited external rotation greater than abduction greater than internal rotation
Elbow	Greater limitation of flexion than extension
Hip	Gross limitation of flexion, abduction, and internal rotation, slight limitation of extension, little or no limitation of external rotation
Knee	Gross limitation of flexion, slight limitation of extension, rotation unlimited
Talocrural	More limitation of plantarflexion than dorsiflexion
Subtalar	Inversion progressively limited

Pain that occurs at the end point in the range of motion is usually caused by shortening or contracture of the capsule and ligaments. This tightness in the capsule places the joint in a close-packed position that abnormally compresses structures surrounding the joint. This problem might be eliminated by stretching the capsule in a neutral pain-free position. If the athlete reports pain before the end of the available range of motion, acute inflammation is likely indicated, in which stretching and manipulation are both contraindicated as treatments. Pain occurring synchronous with the end of the range of motion indicates that the condition is subacute and has progressed to some inert tissue fibrosis. During this stage, gentle stretching may be started. If no pain occurs at the end of the range of motion, the condition is chronic, and contractures have replaced inflammation. At this point, mobilization, stretching, and exercise are all indicated.[8]

Capsular patterns of motion. A lesion that exists in the joint capsule or the synovial lining limits active movement in proportion to the extent of the various motions possible about that joint. This capsular pattern manifests as a characteristic pattern of decreased movements at a joint and occurs only in synovial joints. Each joint exhibits its own capsular pattern (Table 18-2). When identifying a capsular pattern, movement restrictions are listed in sequence, with the first being the most limited. For example, the hip exhibits gross limitation of flexion, abduction, and internal rotation; slight limitation of extension; and little or no limitation of external rotation.[8] These capsular patterns exist whenever the entire capsule is affected. However, there are many situations where only one part of the capsule may be affected by trauma. In this case, limitation of motion will be evident only when that part of the capsule is stretched.

Noncapsular patterns of motion. In a noncapsular pattern, the limitation of motion does not follow the normal capsular pattern. It generally indicates the presence of a lesion outside the capsule. Cyriax has classified the following lesions as noncapsular.[8]

- A *ligamentous adhesion* occurs after injury and can result in a movement restriction in one plane, with a full pain-free range in other planes.
- *Internal derangement* involves a sudden onset of localized pain resulting from the displacement of a loose body within the joint. The mechanical block restricts motion in one plane while allowing normal, pain-free motion in the opposite direction. Movement restrictions can change as the loose body shifts its position in the joint space.
- An *extra-articular lesion* results from adhesions occurring outside the joint. Movement in a plane that stretches that adhesion results in pain, whereas motion in the opposite direction is pain-free and nonrestricted.

Resistive Motion. Resistive motion is movement performed by the athlete but against the opposite and equal resistance of the examiner. The goal of resistive motion is to assess the state of the contractile unit. Injury to any component of the muscle-tendon unit can result in pain or weakness during resistive motion. Also, injury to a component of the nervous system can manifest itself through muscular weakness, a situation that can confound the injury evaluation. Only through an integration of findings during active, passive, and resistive motion can the injured structure accurately be identified. Cyriax has designed a system for differentiating lesions through assessment of muscular contraction as indicated in Table 18-3.[8]

Resistive motion must be performed from a stationary joint position and while in the midrange of motion. Resistive motion assessed dynamically and allowed to progress to an extreme in the range of motion not only tests contractile capacity of the muscle in question but also stretches the antagonist muscle and inert tissue. Several excellent resources are available that illustrate manual muscle examination.[6,9] Table 18-4 indicates a numerical isometric grading system for rating the quality of the resisted movement.

Figures 18-20 and 18-40 illustrate the resistance, counterpressure, and joint positions for an upper- and lower-extremity muscle group.

■ TABLE 18-3 Results of Resistive Motion

Interpretation	Possible Pathology
Strong and painless	Healthy muscle-tendon unit
Strong and painful	Muscle-tendon unit injury
Weak and painful	Fracture or tendon avulsion
Weak and painless	Muscle rupture or nerve palsy
Pain on repetition	Single contraction is strong and painless, but repetition produces pain as in some vascular disorders
All muscles painful	May indicate serious emotional or psychological problem

■ TABLE 18-4 Numerical Isometric Grading System[1]

Numeral	Description
5	Maintains the test position against gravity and maximal resistance
4	Maintains the test position against gravity and moderate resistance
4−	Maintains the test position against gravity and less-than-moderate resistance
3+	Maintains the test position against gravity and minimal resistance
3	Maintains the test position against gravity

Special Tests

At this point in the evaluation, the examiner should have identified the structures involved in the injury. Depending on the examiner's findings, special tests are used to confirm suspicions or to assess severity of injury. For example, suspicion of recurrent anterior shoulder dislocation can be confirmed through use of an apprehension test designed to reproduce the typical mechanism of injury (Figure 18-46). Stress testing of knee ligaments is performed to confirm the structures involved and to determine the degree of laxity and thus severity of injury (Figure 18-47).

In some cases it might be appropriate to have the athlete perform a series of sport-specific functional drills to help determine readiness to return to competition.[20] A progression of functional tests might include straight-ahead running, large-to-small circles and figure-eights, carioca running, and other agility drills specific to the sport in question.

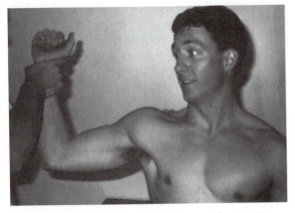

Figure 18-46 Apley's apprehension test for anterior shoulder dislocation.

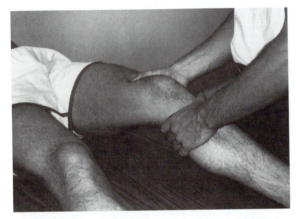

Figure 18-47 Lachman's test for anterior cruciate ligament insufficiency.

ARRIVING AT AN IMPRESSION

Only through a complete and systematic evaluation can a valid impression of an injury be made. One component of the evaluation alone usually provides insufficient information. Only through an integration of findings from the history and physical examination can the examiner arrive at a reasonable impression of injury. With this information, an appropriate treatment and rehabilitation plan can be implemented.

DOCUMENTATION OF FINDINGS

The final phase of the injury evaluation format is the documentation of findings. The medicolegal climate of sports necessitates careful and systematic documentation of injuries. Of no less importance is the role documentation of injury plays in the establishment of a bona fide profession. An effective system of documentation should include gathering and recording of specific information about an injury with respect to subjective and objective information, clinician assessment, and plan of treatment (SOAP notes).[19]

SOAP Notes

Documentation of acute athletic injury can be effectively accomplished through a system designed to record both subjective and objective findings and to document the immediate and future treatment plan for the athlete. This method combines information provided by the athlete and the observations of the examiner.

The Injury Report Form (p. 307) presents a recommended injury report form that includes the components of documentation discussed above. This form also includes a provision to document findings arising from more definitive evaluation or from the examiner's subsequent day evaluation.

S (Subjective). This component includes the subjective statements provided by the injured athlete. History taking is designed to elicit the subjective impressions of the athlete relative to time, mechanism, and site of injury. The type and course of the pain and the degree of disability experienced by the athlete are also noteworthy.

O (Objective). Objective findings result from the sports therapist's visual inspection, palpation, and assessment of active, passive, and resistive motion. Findings of special testing should also be noted here. Thus the objective report would include assessment of posture, presence of deformity or swelling, and location of point tenderness. Also, limitations of active motion and pain arising or disappearing during passive and resistive motion should be noted. Finally, the results of special tests relative to joint stability or apprehension are also included.

A (Assessment). Assessment of the injury is the sports therapist's professional judgment with regard to impression and nature of injury. Although the exact nature of the injury will not always be known initially, information pertaining to suspected site and anatomical structures involved is appropriate. A judgment of severity may be included but is not essential at the time of acute injury evaluation.

P (Plan). The plan should include the first aid treatment rendered to the athlete and the sports therapist's intentions relative to disposition. Disposition may include referral for more definitive evaluation or simply application of splint, wrap, or crutches and a request to report for reevaluation the next day. If the injury is of a more chronic nature, the examiner's plan for treatment and therapeutic exercise would be appropriate.

Injury Report Form

ATHLETE'S NAME _____   DATE OF INJURY _____

INJURY SITE: R L _____   TODAY'S DATE _____

                                                        SPORT _____

Subjective findings (history):

Objective findings (inspection, palpation, mobility, and special tests):

Assessment (impression):

Plan (treatment administered and disposition):

Follow-up notes: Date _____

EVALUATED BY _____

RECORDED BY _____

Summary

1. The components of the preparticipation examination include a medical history and evaluation of flexibility, strength, body composition, and fitness.
2. On-field evaluation requires the establishment of an emergency plan and early recognition of life-threatening injury.
3. Off-field evaluation permits a more detailed assessment of injury and may begin with upper- or lower-quarter screening.
4. The important components of off-field evaluation include history; inspection; palpation; assessment of active, passive, and resistive motion; and special tests.
5. The final phase of injury evaluation is effective record keeping, which includes documentation of subjective and objective findings, the evaluator's assessment, and the plan for injury management and treatment.

References

1. Arnheim, D., and W. Prentice. 1997. *Principles of athletic training.* Madison, WI: Brown & Benchmark.
2. Barak, T., E. Rosen, and R. Sofer. 1994. Mobility: Passive orthopedic manual therapy. In *Orthopedic and sports physical therapy,* edited by J. Gould and G. Davies. St. Louis: Mosby Year Book.
3. Bates, B. 1991. *A guide to physical examination and history taking.* Philadelphia: Lippincott.
4. Birnbaum, J. S. 1986. *The musculoskeletal manual.* Orlando: Grune & Stratton.
5. Booher, J. M., and G. A. Thibodeau. 1994. *Athletic injury assessment.* 3d ed. St. Louis: Mosby/Year Book.
6. Clarkson, H. M., and G. B. Gilewich. 1989. *Musculoskeletal assessment: Joint range of motion and manual muscle strength.* Baltimore: Williams & Wilkins.
7. Cooper, K. 1968. A means of assessing maximal oxygen uptake. *Journal of the American Medical Association* 203:135–38.
8. Cyriax, J. 1982. *Textbook of orthopaedic medicine: Diagnosis of soft tissue lesions.* Vol. 1. London: Bailliere Tindall.

9. Daniels, L., and C. Worthingham. 1996. *Muscle testing: Techniques of manual examination.* Philadelphia: W. B. Saunders.

10. Denegar, C. R., and E. N. Saliba. 1989. On the field management of the potentially cervical spine injured football player. *Athletic Training* 24:108–11.

11. Feinstein, R. A., E. J. Soileau, and W. A. Daniel. 1988. A national survey of preparticipation requirements. *Physician and Sports Medicine* 16:51–59.

12. Feld, F., and R. Blanc. 1988. Immobilizing the spine-injured football player. *J Emerg Med Serv* 12:38–40.

13. Gehring, P. 1991. Physical assessment begins with a history. *RN* 54(11): 27–31.

14. Hartley, A. 1991. *Practical joint assessment.* St. Louis: Mosby.

15. Hoppenfeld, S. 1976. *Physical examination of the spine and extremities.* New York: Appleton-Century-Crofts.

16. Jackson, A. S., and M. L. Pollock. 1985. Practical assessment of body composition. *Physician and Sports Medicine* 13:76–90.

17. Kaltenborn, F. M. 1980. *Mobilization of the extremity joints: Examination and basic treatments.* Oslo: Olaf Norlis Bokhandel.

18. Kendall, F., and E. Kendall. 1983. *Muscle testing and function.* Baltimore: Williams & Wilkins.

19. Kettenbach, G. 1990. *Writing SOAP notes.* Philadelphia: F. A. Davis.

20. Lephart, S. M., D. H. Perrin, K. Minger, et al. 1991. Sports specific functional tests for the anterior cruciate ligament insufficient athlete. *Athletic Training* 26:44–50.

21. Magee, D. J. 1997. *Orthopedic physical assessment.* Philadelphia: W. B. Saunders.

22. Moore, M. L. 1978. Clinical assessment of joint motion. In *Therapeutic exercise,* 3d ed., edited by J. F. Basmajian. Baltimore: Williams & Wilkins.

23. National Collegiate Athletic Association. 1987. *NCAA Sports medicine handbook.* Mission, KS: NCAA.

24. Nockin, C. C., and J. D. White. 1985. *Measurement of joint motion: A guide to goniometry.* Philadelphia: F. A. Davis.

25. Perrin, D. H. 1993. *Isokinetic exercise and assessment.* Champaign, IL: Human Kinetics.

26. Peterson, M., J. Holbrook, and D. Von-Hales. 1992. Contributions of the history, physical examination, and laboratory investigation in making medical diagnosis. *West J Med* 156(2): 163–65.

27. Post, M. 1987. *Physical examination of the musculoskeletal system.* Chicago: Year Book.

28. Powell, J. 1987. 635,000 injuries annually in high school football. *Athletic Training* 22:19–22.

29. Ray, R. L., and F. X. Feld. 1989. The team physician's medical bag in emergency treatment of the injured athlete. *Clinical Sports Medicine* 8:139–46.

30. Slaughter, M. H., T. Lowman, R. Blileau, et al. 1988. Skinfold equations for estimation of body fatness in children and youth. *Human Biology* 60:709–23.

31. Starkey, C., and J. Ryan. 1996. *Evaluation of orthopedic and athletic injuries.* Philadelphia: F. A.Davis.

32. Vegso, J. J., M. H. Bryant, and J. S. Torg. 1982. Field evaluation of head and neck injuries. In *Injuries to the head, neck, and face,* edited by J. S. Torg. Philadelphia: Lea & Febiger.

33. Wadsworth, C. 1988. *Manual examination and treatment of the spine and extremities.* Baltimore: Williams & Wilkins.

34. Wilmore, J. H. 1982. *Training for sport and activity: The physiological basis of the conditioning process.* 2d ed. Boston: Allyn & Bacon.

CHAPTER 19

Rehabilitation of Shoulder Injuries

Rob Schneider
William E. Prentice

After completion of this chapter, the student should be able to do the following:

• Discuss the functional anatomy and biomechanics associated with normal function of the shoulder joint complex.

• Discuss the various rehabilitative strengthening techniques for the shoulder, including both open- and closed-kinetic-chain isotonic, plyometric, isokinetic, and PNF exercises.

• Identify the various techniques for regaining range of motion including stretching exercises and joint mobilizations.

• Discuss exercises that may be used to reestablish neuromuscular control.

• Relate biomechanical principles to the rehabilitation of various shoulder injuries/pathologies.

• Discuss criteria for progression of the rehabilitation program for different shoulder injuries/pathologies.

• Describe and explain the rationale for various treatment techniques in the management of shoulder injuries.

FUNCTIONAL ANATOMY AND BIOMECHANICS

The anatomy of the shoulder joint complex allows for tremendous range of motion. This wide range of motion of the shoulder complex proximally permits precise positioning of the hand distally, creating both gross and skilled movements. However, the high degree of mobility requires some compromise in stability, which in turn increases the vulnerability of the shoulder joint to injury, particularly in dynamic overhead athletic activities.

The shoulder girdle complex is composed of three bones—the scapula, the clavicle, and the humerus—which are connected either to one another or to the axial skeleton or trunk via the glenohumeral joint, the acromioclavicular joint, the sternoclavicular joint, and the scapulothorasic joint (Figure 19-1). Dynamic movement and stabilization of the shoulder complex require integrated function of all four articulations if normal motion is to occur.

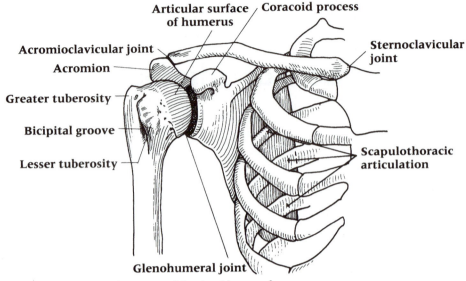

Figure 19-1 Skeletal anatomy of the shoulder complex.

Sternoclavicular Joint (SC joint)

The clavicle articulates with the manubrium of the sternum to form the sternoclavicular joint, the only direct skeletal connection between the upper extremity and the trunk. The sternal articulating surface is larger than the sternum, causing the clavicle to rise much higher than the sternum. A fibrocartilaginous disk is interposed between the two articulating surfaces. It functions as a shock absorber against the medial forces and also helps to prevent any displacement upward. The articular disk is placed so that the clavicle moves on the disk, and the disk, in turn, moves separately on the sternum. The clavicle is permitted to move up and down, forward and backward, in combination, and in rotation.

The sternoclavicular joint is extremely weak because of its bony arrangement, but it is held securely by strong ligaments that tend to pull the sternal end of the clavicle downward and toward the sternum, in effect anchoring it. The main ligaments are the anterior sternoclavicular, which prevents upward displacement of the clavicle; the posterior sternoclavicular, which also prevents upward displacement of the clavicle; the interclavicular, which prevents lateral displacement of the clavicle; and the costoclavicular, which prevents lateral and upward displacement of the clavicle.[3]

It should also be noted that for the scapula to abduct and upward rotate throughout 180 degrees of humeral abduction, clavicular movement must occur at both the sternoclavicular and acromioclavicular joints. The clavi-

cle must elevate approximately 40 degrees to allow upward scapular rotation.[51]

Acromioclavicular Joint (AC joint)

The acromioclavicular joint is a gliding articulation of the lateral end of the clavicle with the acromion process. This is a rather weak joint. A fibrocartilaginous disk separates the two articulating surfaces. A thin, fibrous capsule surrounds the joint.

The acromioclavicular ligament consists of anterior, posterior, superior, and inferior portions. In addition to the acromioclavicular ligament, the coracoclavicular ligament joins the coracoid process and the clavicle and helps to maintain the position of the clavicle relative to the acromion. The coracoclavicular ligament is further divided into the trapezoid ligament, which prevents overriding of the clavicle on the acromion, and the conoid ligament, which limits upward movement of the clavicle on the acromion. As the arm moves into an elevated position, there is a posterior rotation of the clavicle on its long axis, which permits the scapula to continue rotating thus allowing full elevation. The clavicle must rotate approximately 50 degrees for full elevation to occur; otherwise elevation would be limited to approximately 110 degrees.[51]

Coracoacromial Arch. The coracoacromial ligament connects the coracoid to the acromion. This ligament, along with the acromion and the coracoid, forms the coracoacromial arch over the glenohumeral joint. In the subacromial space between the coracoacromial arch superiorly and the humeral head inferiorly, lies the supraspinatus tendon, the long head of the biceps tendon, and the subacromial bursa. Each of these structures is subject to irritation and inflammation resulting either from excessive humeral head translation or from impingement during repeated overhead activities. In asymptomatic individuals the optimal subacromial space appears to be about 9 to 10 mm.[52]

Glenohumeral Joint

The glenohumeral joint is an enarthrodial, or ball-and-socket, synovial joint in which the round head of the humerus articulates with the shallow glenoid cavity of the scapula. The cavity is deepened slightly by a fibrocartilaginous rim called the glenoid labrum. The humeral head is larger than the glenoid, and at any point during elevation only 25 to 30 percent of the humeral head is in contact with the glenoid.[25] The glenohumeral joint is maintained by both static and dynamic restraints. Position is maintained statically by the glenoid labrum and the capsular ligaments, and dynamically by the deltoid and rotator cuff muscles.

Surrounding the articulation is a loose, articular capsule that is attached to the labrum. This capsule is strongly reinforced by the superior, middle, and inferior glenohumeral ligaments and by the tough coracohumeral ligament, which attaches to the coracoid process and to the greater tuberosity of the humerus.[47]

The long tendon of the biceps muscle passes superiorly across the head of the humerus and then through the bicipital groove. In the anatomical position the long head of the biceps moves in close relationship with the humerus. The transverse humeral ligament maintains the long head of the biceps tendon within the bicipital groove by passing over it from the lesser and the greater tuberosities, converting the bicipital groove into a canal.

Scapulothoracic Joint

The scapulothoracic joint is not a true joint, but the movement of the scapula on the wall of the thoracic cage is critical to shoulder joint motion. Contraction of the scapular muscles that attach the scapula to the axial skeleton is essential in stabilizing the scapula, thus providing a base on which a highly mobile joint can function.

Stability in the Shoulder Joint

Maintaining stability, while the four articulations of the shoulder complex collectively allow for a high degree of mobility, is critical in normal function of the shoulder

joint. Instability is very often the cause of many of the specific injuries to the shoulder that will be discussed later in this chapter. In the glenohumeral joint, the rounded humeral head articulates with a relatively flat glenoid on the scapula. During movement of the shoulder joint, it is essential to maintain the positioning of the humeral head relative to the glenoid. Likewise it is also critical for the glenoid to adjust its position relative to the moving humeral head while simultaneously maintaining a stable base. The glenohumeral joint is inherently unstable, and stability depends on the coordinated and synchronous function of both dynamic and static stabilizers.[41]

The Dynamic Stabilizers of the Glenohumeral Joint.   The muscles that cross the glenohumeral joint produce motion and function to establish dynamic stability to compensate for a bony and ligamentous arrangement that allows for a great deal of mobility. Movements at the glenohumeral joint include flexion, extension, abduction, adduction, circumduction, and rotation.

The muscles acting on the glenohumeral joint may be classified into two groups. The first group consists of muscles that originate on the axial skeleton and attach to the humerus; these include the latissimus dorsi and the pectoralis major. The second group originates on the scapula and attaches to the humerus; these include the deltoid, the teres major, the coracobrachialis, the subscapularis, the supraspinatus, the infraspinatus, and the teres minor. These muscles constitute the short rotator muscles whose tendons insert into the articular capsule and serve as reinforcing structures. The biceps and triceps muscles attach on the glenoid and affect elbow motion.

The muscles of the rotator cuff, the subscapularis, infraspinatus, supraspinatus, and teres minor along with the long head of the biceps function to provide dynamic stability to control the position and prevent excessive displacement or translation of the humeral head relative to the position of the glenoid.[8]

Stabilization of the humeral head occurs through co-contraction of the rotator cuff muscles. This creates a series of force couples that act to compress the humeral head into the glenoid, minimizing humeral head translation. A force couple involves the action of two opposing forces acting in opposite directions to impose rotation about an axis. These force couples can establish dynamic equilibrium of the glenohumeral joint regardless of the position of the humerus. If an imbalance exists between the muscular components that create these force couples, abnormal glenohumeral mechanics occur.

In the transverse plan a force couple exists between the subscapularis anteriorly and the infraspinatus and teres minor posteriorly (Figure 19-2). Co-contraction of the infraspinatus, teres minor, and subscapularis muscles

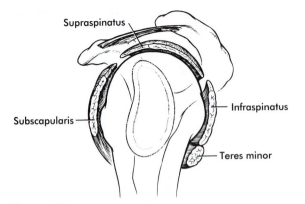

Figure 19-2 Transverse plane force couples.

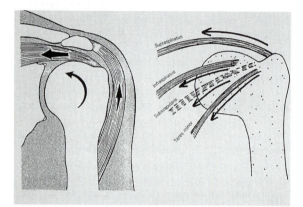

Figure 19-3 Coronal plane force couples.

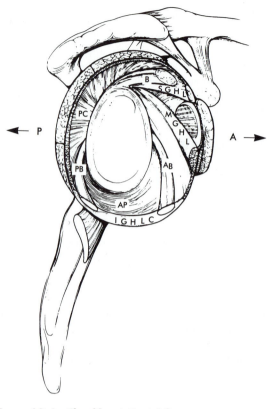

Figure 19-4 Shoulder static stabilizers.

both depresses and compresses the humeral head during overhead movements.

In the coronal plane, there is a critical force couple between the deltoid and the inferior rotator cuff muscles (Figure 19-3). With the arm fully adducted, contraction of the deltoid produces a vertical force in a superior direction causing an upward translation of the humeral head relative to the glenoid. Co-contraction of the inferior rotator cuff muscles produces both a compressive force and a downward translation of the humerus that counterbalances the force of the deltoid, stabilizing the humeral head. The supraspinatus compresses the humeral head into the glenoid and along with the deltoid initiates abduction on this stable base. Dynamic stability is created by an increase in joint compression forces from contraction of the supraspinatus and by humeral head depression from contraction of the inferior rotator cuff muscles.[14]

The long head of the biceps tendon also contributes to dynamic stability by limiting superior translation of the humerus during elbow flexion and supination.

Static Stabilizers. The primary static stabilizers of the glenohumeral joint are the glenohumeral ligaments, the posterior capsule, and the glenoid labrum (Figure 19-4).

The glenohumeral ligaments appear to produce a major restraint in shoulder flexion, extension, and rotation. The anterior glenohumeral ligament is tight when the shoulder is in extension, abduction, and/or external rotation. The posterior glenohumeral ligament is tight in extension with external rotation. The inferior glenohumeral ligament is tight when the shoulder is abducted, extended, and/or externally rotated. The middle glenohumeral ligament is tight when in flexion and external rotation. Additionally, the middle glenohumeral ligament and the subscapularis tendon limit lateral rotation from 45 to 75 degrees of abduction and are important anterior stabilizers of the glenohumeral joint.[3] The inferior gleno-

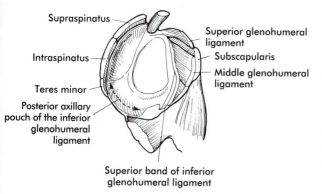

Figure 19-5   Rotator cuff tendons blend into the joint capsule.

humeral ligament is a primary check against both anterior and posterior dislocation of the humeral head and is the most important stabilizing structure of the shoulder in the overhead athlete.[3]

The tendons of the rotator cuff muscles blend into the glenohumeral joint capsule at their insertions about the humeral head (Figure 19-5). As these muscles contract, tension is produced, dynamically tightening the capsule and helping to center the humeral head in the glenoid fossa. This creates both static and dynamic control of humeral head movement.

The posterior capsule is tight when the shoulder is in flexion, abduction, internal rotation, or in any combination of these. The superior and middle segment of the posterior capsule has the greatest tension while the shoulder is internally rotated.

The bones and articular surfaces within the shoulder are positioned to contribute to static stability. The glenoid labrum, which is tightly attached to the bottom half of the glenoid and loosely attached at the top, increases the glenoid depth approximately two times, enhancing glenohumeral stability.[37] The scapula faces 30 degrees anteriorly to the chest wall and is tilted upward 3 degrees to enable easier movement on the anterior frontal plane and movements above the shoulder.[25] The glenoid is tilted upward 5 degrees to help control inferior instability.[39]

Scapular Stability and Mobility.   Like the glenohumeral muscles, the scapular muscles play a critical role in normal function of the shoulder. The scapular muscles produce movement of the scapula on the thorax and help to dynamically position the glenoid relative to the moving humerus. They include the levator scapula and upper trapezius, which elevate the scapula; the middle trapezius and rhomboids, which adduct the scapula; the lower trapezius, which adducts and depresses the scapula; the pectoralis minor, which depresses the scapula; and the serratus anterior, which abducts and upward rotates the scapula. Collectively they function to maintain a consistent length-tension relationship with the glenohumeral muscles.[43]

The only attachment of the scapula to the thorax is through these muscles. The muscle stabilizers must fix the position of the scapula on the thorax, providing a stable base for the rotator cuff to perform its intended function on the humerus. It has been suggested that the serratus anterior moves the scapula while the other scapular muscles function to provide scapular stability.[34] The scapular muscles act isometrically, concentrically, or eccentrically, depending on the movement desired and whether the movement is speeding up or slowing down.[39]

Scapulohumeral rhythm.   Scapulohumeral rhythm is the movement of the scapula relative to the movement of the humerus throughout a full range of abduction. As the humerus elevates to 30 degrees, there is no movement of the scapula. This is referred to as the setting phase during which a stable base is being established on the thoracic wall. From 30 to 90 degrees, the scapula abducts and upward rotates 1 degree for every 2 degrees of humeral elevation. From 90 degrees to full abduction, the scapula abducts and upward rotates 1 degree for each 1 degree of humeral elevation. If normal scapulohumeral rhythm is compromised, normal shoulder joint function in moving to a fully elevated position cannot occur, and adaptive compensatory motions can predispose the athlete to injury.[50]

Plane of the scapula.   The concept of the plane of the scapula refers to the angle of the scapula in its resting position, usually 35 to 45 degrees anterior to the frontal plane toward the sagittal plane. When the limb is positioned in the plane of the scapula, the mechanical axis of the glenohumeral joint is in line with the mechanical axis of the scapula. The glenohumeral joint capsule is lax, and the deltoid and supraspinatus muscles are optimally positioned to elevate the humerus. Movement of the humerus in this plane is less restricted than in the frontal or sagittal planes, because the glenohumeral capsule is not twisted.[19] Because the rotator cuff muscles originate on the scapula and attach to the humerus, repositioning the humerus into the plane of the scapula increases the length of those muscles, improving the length-tension relationship. This is likely to increase muscle force.[19] It has been recommended that many strengthening exercises for the shoulder joint complex be done in the scapular plane.[19,71,72]

REHABILITATION TECHNIQUES FOR THE SHOULDER

Strengthening Techniques

Isometric and Isotonic Open-Kinetic-Chain Exercises.

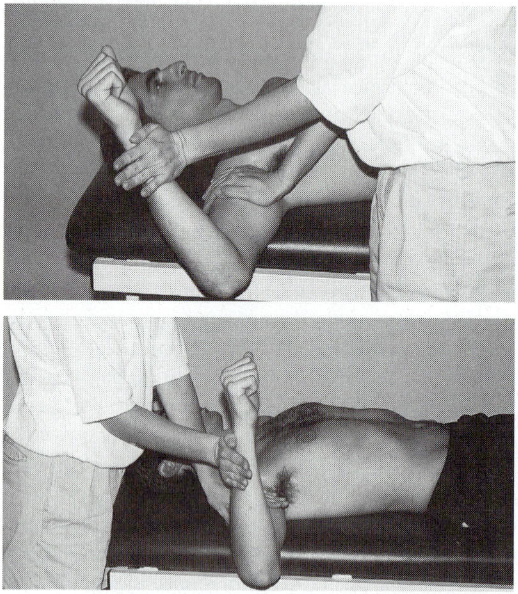

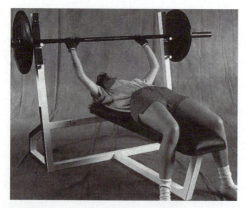

Figure 19-6   **A,** Isometric medial rotation; and **B,** isometric lateral rotation are useful in the early stages of a shoulder rehabilitation program when full ROM isotonic exercise is likely to exacerbate a problem. The towel under the arm is used to help establish neuromuscular control and help facilitate scapular stability.

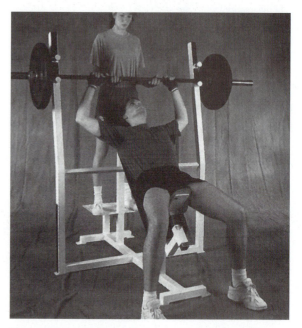

Figure 19-8   Incline bench press. Used to strengthen the pectoralis major (upper fibers), triceps, middle and anterior deltoid; and secondarily the coracobrachialis, upper trapezius and levator scapula muscles.

Figure 19-7   Bench press. Used to strengthen the pectoralis major, anterior deltoid, and triceps; and secondarily the coracobrachialis muscles. Performing this exercise with the feet on the bench serves to flatten the low back and helps to isolate these muscles.

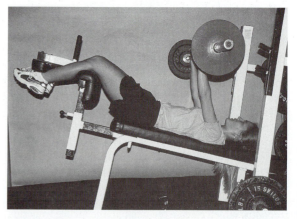

Figure 19-9   Decline bench press. Used to strengthen the pectoralis major (lower fibers), triceps, anterior deltoid, coracobrachialis, and latissimus dorsi muscles.

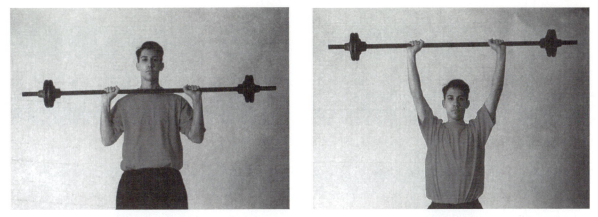

Figure 19-10 Military press. Used to strengthen the middle deltoid, upper trapezius, levator scapula, and triceps.

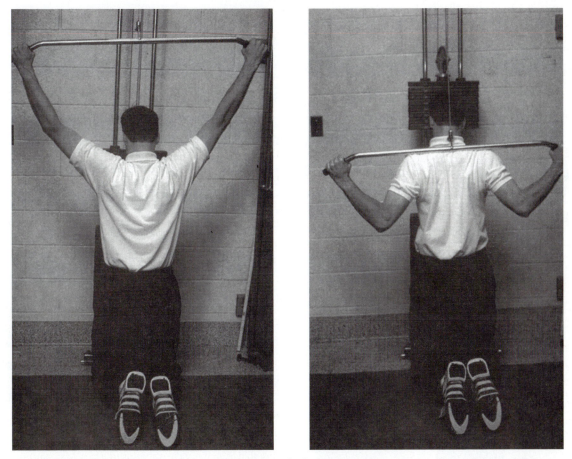

Figure 19-11 Lat pull-downs. Used to strengthen primarily the latissimus dorsi, teres major, and pectoralis minor; and secondarily the biceps muscles. This exercise may be done by pulling the bar down in front of the head or behind the neck. Pulling the bar down behind the neck requires contraction of the rhomboids and middle trapezius. Pull-ups done on a chinning bar can also be used as an alternative strengthening technique.

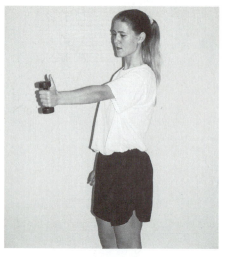

Figure 19-12 Shoulder flexion. Used to strengthen primarily the anterior deltoid, and coracobrachialis; and secondarily the middle deltoid, pectoralis major, and biceps brachii muscles. Note that the thumb should point upward.

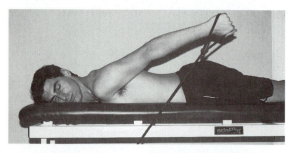

Figure 19-13 Shoulder extension. Used to strengthen primarily the latissimus dorsi, teres major, and posterior deltoid; and secondarily the teres minor and the long head of the triceps muscles. Note that the thumb should point downward. May be done standing using a dumbbell or lying prone using surgical tubing.

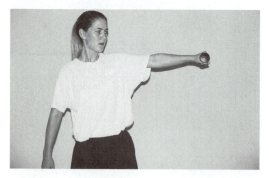

Figure 19-14 Shoulder abduction to 90 degrees. Used to strengthen primarily the middle deltoid and supraspinatus; and secondarily the anterior and posterior deltoid and serratus anterior muscles. Note that the thumb is in a neutral position.

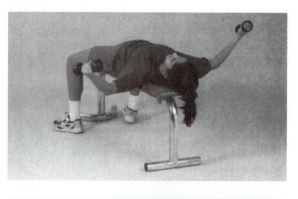

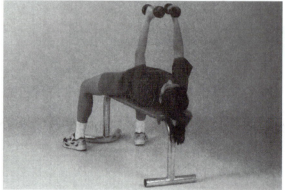

Figure 19-15 Flys (shoulder horizontal adduction). Used to strengthen primarily the pectoralis major; and secondarily the anterior deltoid. Note that the elbow may be slightly flexed. May be done in a supine position or standing with surgical tubing or wall pulleys behind.

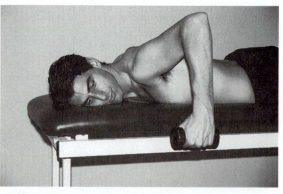

Figure 19-16 Reverse flys (shoulder horizontal abduction). Used to strengthen primarily the posterior deltoid; and secondarily the infraspinatus, teres minor, rhomboids, and middle trapezius muscles. May be done lying prone using either dumbbells or tubing. Note that with the thumb pointed upward the middle trapezius is more active, and with the thumb pointed downward the rhomboids are more active.

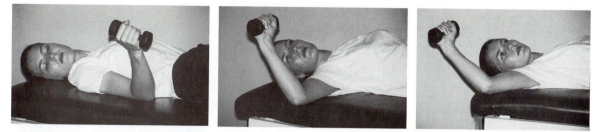

Figure 19-17   Shoulder medial rotation. Used to strengthen primarily the subscapularis, pectoralis major, latissimus dorsi, and teres major; and secondarily the anterior deltoid. This exercise may be done isometrically or isotonically, either lying supine using a dumbbell or standing using tubing. Strengthening should be done with the arm fully adducted at 0 degrees, and also in 90 degrees and 135 degrees of abduction.

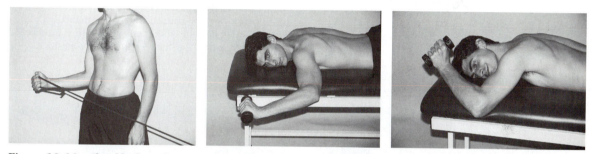

Figure 19-18   Shoulder lateral rotation. Used to strengthen primarily the infraspinatus and teres minor; and secondarily the posterior deltoid muscles. This exercise may be done isometrically or isotonically, either lying prone using a dumbbell or standing using tubing. Strengthening should be done with the arm fully adducted at 0 degrees, and also in 90 degrees and 135 degrees of abduction.

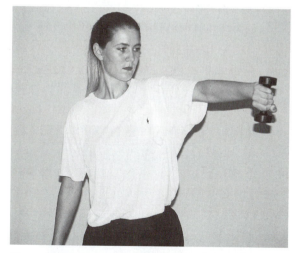

Figure 19-19   Scaption. Used to strengthen primarily the supraspinatus in the plane of the scapula; and secondarily the anterior and middle deltoid muscles. This exercise should be done standing with the arm horizontally adducted to 45 degrees and the thumb pointing downward.

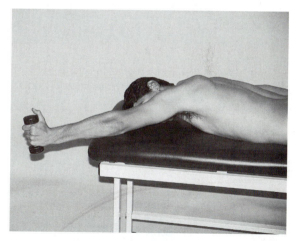

Figure 19-20   Alternative supraspinatus exercise. Used to strengthen primarily the supraspinatus; and secondarily the posterior deltoid. In the prone position with the arm abducted to 100 degrees, the arm is horizontally abducted in extreme lateral rotation. Note that the thumb should point upward.

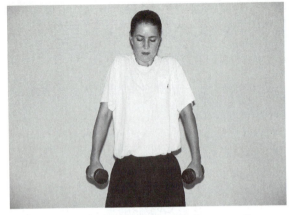

Figure 19-21 Shoulder shrugs. Used to strengthen primarily the upper trapezius and the levator scapula; and secondarily the rhomboids.

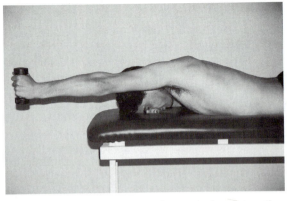

Figure 19-22 Superman. Used to strengthen primarily the inferior trapezius; and secondarily the middle trapezius. May be done lying prone using either dumbbells or tubing. Note that the thumb is in a neutral position.

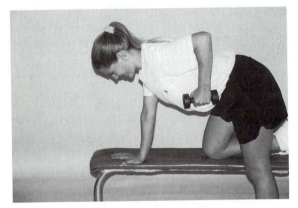

Figure 19-23 Bent-over rows. Used to strengthen primarily the middle trapezius and rhomboids. Done standing in a bent-over position with one knee supported on a bench.

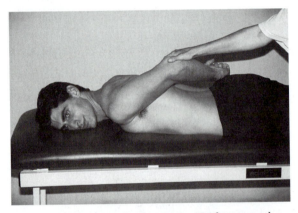

Figure 19-24 Rhomboids exercise. Used to strengthen primarily the rhomboids; and secondarily the inferior trapezius. Should be done lying prone with manual resistance applied at the elbow.

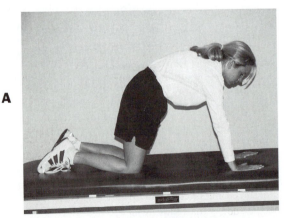

Figure 19-25 Push-ups with a plus. Used to strengthen the serratus anterior. There are several variations to this exercise, including **A**, regular push-ups, **B**, Weight-loaded push-ups.

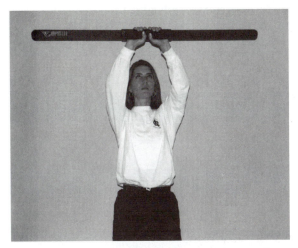

Figure 19-26 Scapular strengthening using a Body Blade. Holding an oscillating Body Blade with both hands, the athlete moves from a fully adducted position in front of the body to a fully elevated overhead position.

Closed-Kinetic-Chain Exercises.

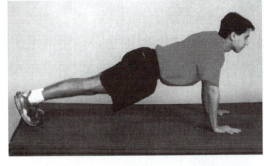

A

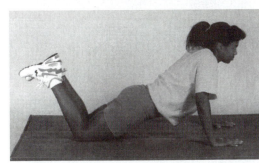

B

Figure 19-27 Push-ups. May be done with **A,** weight supported on feet, or **B,** modified to support weight on the knees.

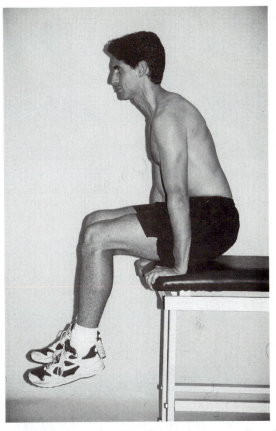

Figure 19-28 Seated push-up. Done sitting on the end of a table. Place hands on the table and lift weight upward off of the table isotonically.

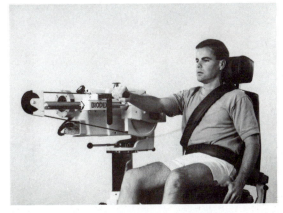

Figure 19-29 Biodex upper-extremity closed-chain device. One of the only isokinetic closed-kinetic-chain exercise devices currently available.

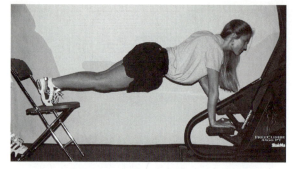

Figure 19-30 Stair Climber with feet on chair. An advanced closed-kinetic-chain strengthening exercise that places the hands on the footplates of a Stair Climber with the feet supported on a chair. Requires substantial upper-body strength.

Plyometric Strengthening Exercises.

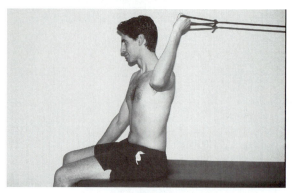

Figure 19-31 Surgical tubing. For example, to strengthen the medial rotators, use a quick eccentric stretch of the medial rotators to facilitate a concentric contraction of those muscles.

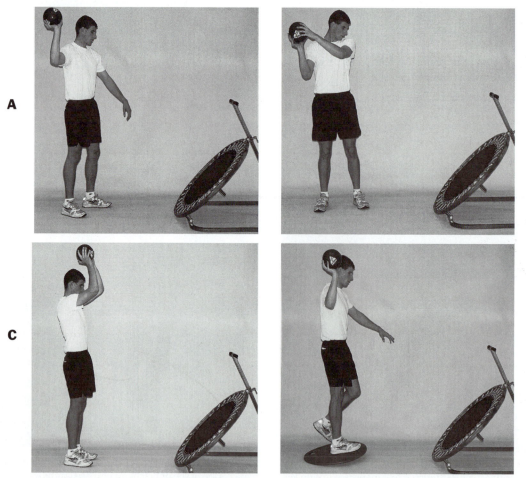

Figure 19-32 Plyoback. The athlete should catch the ball, decelerate it, then immediately accelerate in the opposite direction. **A,** single-arm toss; **B,** two-arm toss with trunk rotation; **C,** two-arm overhead toss; **D,** single-arm toss on unstable surface.

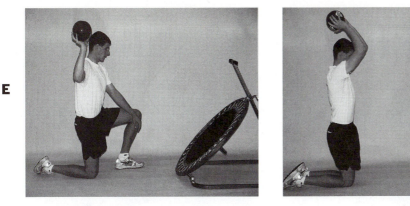

E **F**

Figure 19-32 *continued* **E,** kneeling single-arm toss; **F,** kneeling two-arm toss. The weight of the plyoball should be increased as rapidly as can be tolerated.[73]

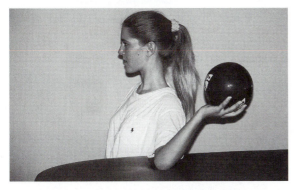

Figure 19-33 Seated single-arm weighted-ball throw. The athlete should be seated with the arm abducted to 90 degrees and the elbow supported on a table. The sports therapist tosses the ball to the hand, creating an overload in lateral rotation that forces the athlete to dynamically stabilize in that position.

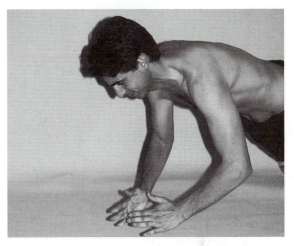

Figure 19-34 Push-ups with a clap. The athlete pushes off the ground, claps his hands, and catches his weight as he decelerates.

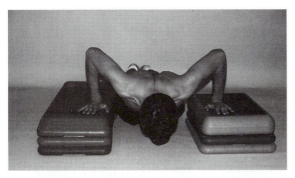

Figure 19-35 Push-ups on boxes. When performing a plyometric push-up on boxes, the athlete can stretch the anterior muscles, which facilitates a concentric contraction.

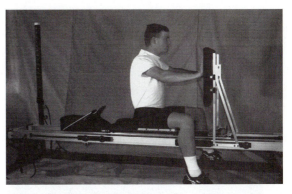

Figure 19-36 Shuttle 1900-1. The exercise machine can be used for plyometric exercises in either the upper or the lower extremity.

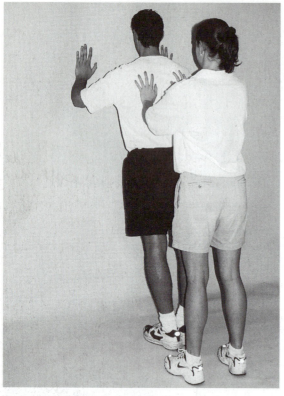

Figure 19-37 Push into wall. The sports therapist stands behind the athlete and pushes him toward the wall. The athlete decelerates the forces and then pushes off the wall immediately.

Isokinetic Strengthening Exercises.

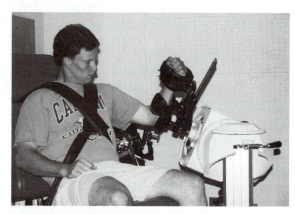

Figure 19-38 Isokinetic medial/lateral rotation. When using an isokinetic device for strengthening the shoulder, the athlete should be set up such that strengthening can be done in a scapular plane.[21]

PNF Strengthening Techniques.

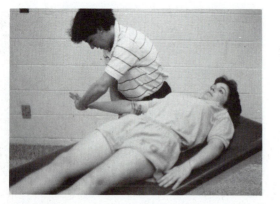

A

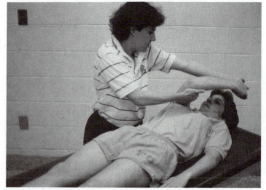

B

Figure 19-39 D1 upper-extremity movement pattern moving into flexion. **A,** Starting position. **B,** Terminal position.

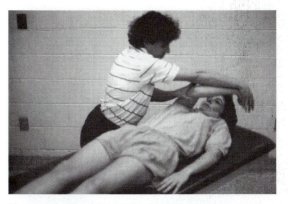

Figure 19-40 D1 upper-extremity movement pattern moving into extension. Starting position.

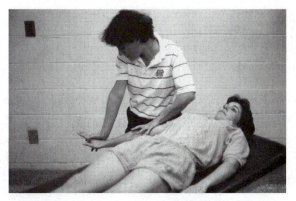

Figure 19-41 D1 upper-extremity movement pattern moving into extension.Terminal position.

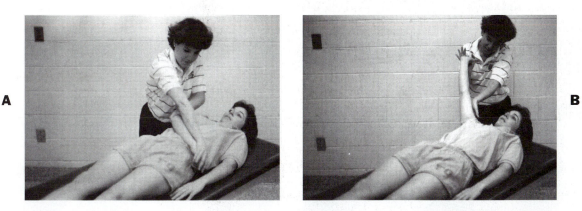

Figure 19-42 D2 upper-extremity movement pattern moving into flexion. **A,** Starting position. **B,** Terminal position.

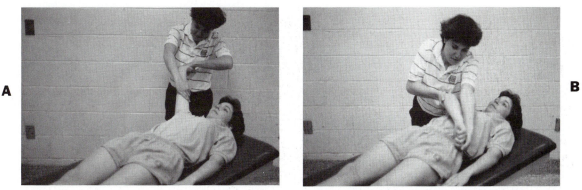

Figure 19-43 D2 upper-extremity movement pattern moving into extension. **A,** Starting position. **B,** Terminal position.

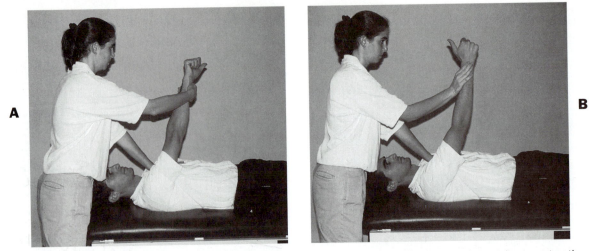

Figure 19-44 Rhythmic contraction. Using either a D1 or D2 pattern. **A,** the athlete uses an isometric co-contraction to maintain a specific position within the ROM; **B,** the sports therapist repeatedly changes the direction of passive pressure.

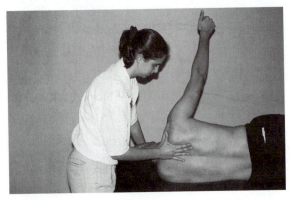

Figure 19-45 PNF technique for scapula. As the athlete moves through either a D1 or a D2 pattern, the sports therapist applies resistance at the appropriate scapular border.

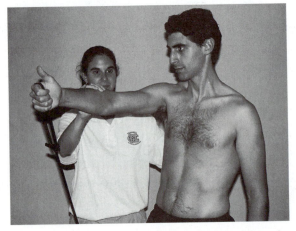

Figure 19-47 PNF using both manual resistance and surgical tubing. Rhythmic stabilization can be performed as the athlete isometrically holds a specific position in the ROM with surgical tubing and force applied by the sports therapist.

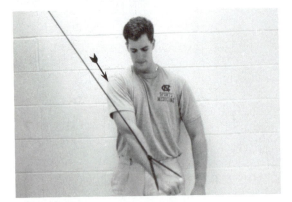

Figure 19-46 The athlete can use resistance from tubing through a PNF movement pattern.

Stretching Exercises

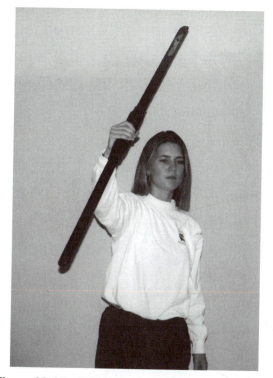

Figure 19-48 PNF using a Body Blade. In a standing position, the athlete moves an oscillating Body Blade through a D2 pattern.

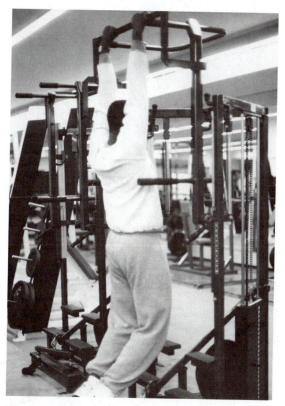

Figure 19-50 Static hanging. Hanging from a chinning bar is a good general stretch for the musculature in the shoulder complex.

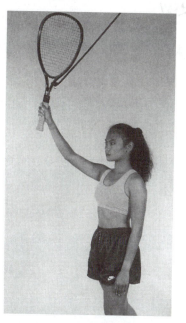

Figure 19-49 Surgical tubing may be attached to a tennis racket as the athlete practices an overhead serve technique. This is useful as a functional progression technique.

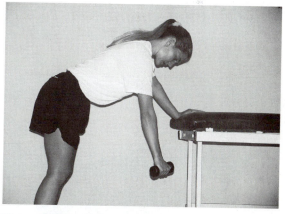

Figure 19-51 Codman's circumduction exercise. The athlete holds a dumbbell in the hand and moves it in a circular pattern, reversing direction periodically. This technique is useful as a general stretch in the early stages of rehabilitation when motion above 90 degrees is restricted.

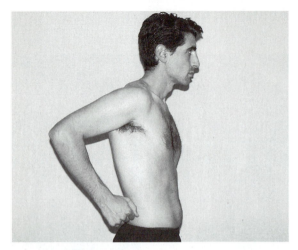

Figure 19-52 Sawing. The athlete moves the arm forward and backward as if performing a sawing motion. This technique is useful as a general stretch in the early stages of rehabilitation when motion above 90 degrees is restricted.

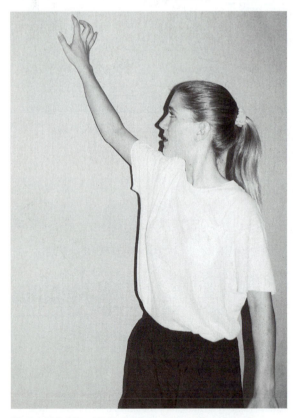

Figure 19-53 Wall climbing. The athlete uses the fingers to "walk" the hand up a wall. This technique is useful when attempting to regain full-range elevation. ROM should be restricted to a pain-free arc.

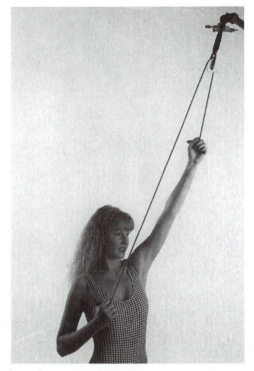

Figure 19-54 Rope and pulley exercise. This exercise may be used as an active-assistive exercise when trying to regain full overhead motion. ROM should be restricted to a pain-free arc.

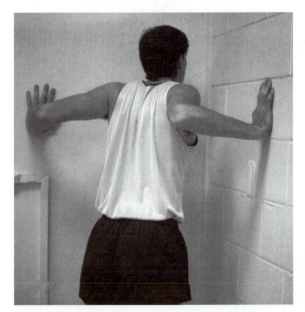

Figure 19-55 Wall/corner stretch. Used to stretch the pectoralis major and minor, anterior deltoid, and coracobrachialis, and the anterior joint capsule.

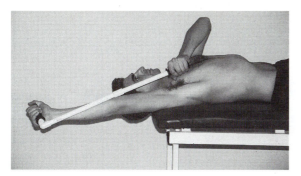

Figure 19-56   Shoulder extensor stretch using an L-bar. Used to stretch the latissimus dorsi, teres major and minor, posterior deltoid, and triceps muscles, and the inferior joint capsule.

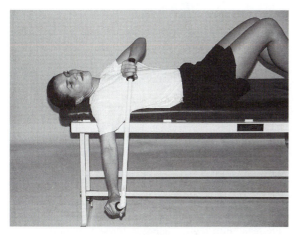

Figure 19-57   Shoulder flexors stretch using an L-bar. Used to stretch the anterior deltoid, coracobrachialis, pectoralis major, and biceps muscles and the anterior joint capsule.

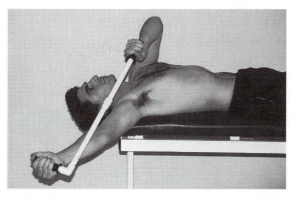

Figure 19-58   Shoulder adductors stretch using an L-bar. Used to stretch the latissimus dorsi, teres major and minor, pectoralis major and minor, posterior deltoid, and triceps muscles, and the inferior joint capsule.

A
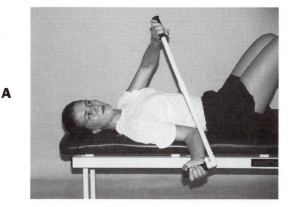

B
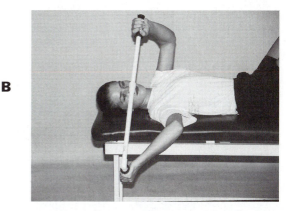

C
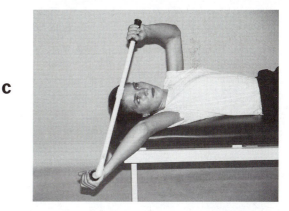

Figure 19-59   Shoulder medial rotators stretch using an L-bar. Used to stretch the subscapularis pectoralis major, latissimus dorsi, teres major, and anterior deltoid muscles, and the anterior joint capsule. This stretch should be done at **A,** 0 degrees, **B,** 90 degrees, and **C,** 135 degrees.

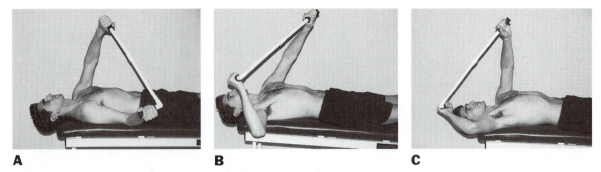

A   **B**   **C**

Figure 19-60   Shoulder lateral rotators using an L-bar. Used to stretch the infraspinatus, teres minor, and posterior deltoid muscles, and the posterior joint capsule. This stretch should be done at **A,** 0 degrees, **B,** 90 degrees, and **C,** 135 degrees.

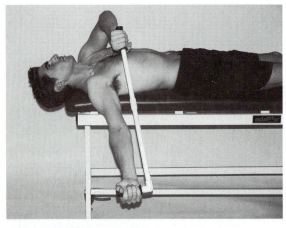

Figure 19-61   Horizontal adductors stretch using an L-bar. Used to stretch the pectoralis major, anterior deltoid, and long head of the biceps muscles, and the anterior joint capsule.

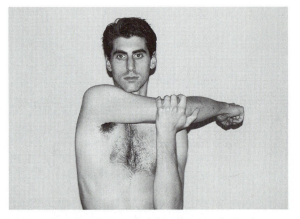

Figure 19-62   Horizonal abductors stretch. Used to stretch the posterior deltoid, infraspinatus, teres minor, rhomboids, and middle trapezius muscles, and the posterior capsule. This position might be uncomfortable for athletes with shoulder impingement syndrome.

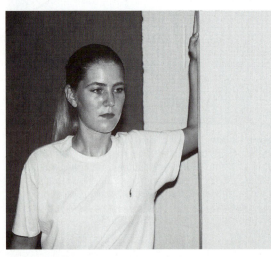

Figure 19-63   Anterior capsule stretch. Self-stretch using the wall.

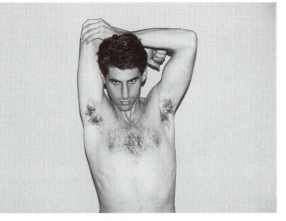

Figure 19-64   Inferior capsule stretch. Self-stretch done with the arm in the fully elevated overhead position. This position might be uncomfortable for athletes with shoulder impingement syndrome.

Joint Mobilization Techniques

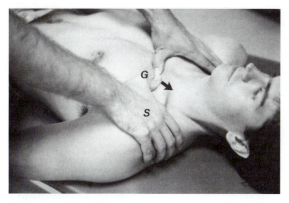

Figure 19-65   When posterior or superior clavicular glides are done at the sternoclavicular joint, use the thumbs to glide the clavicle. Posterior glides are used to increase clavicular retraction, and superior glides increase clavicular retraction and clavicular depression.

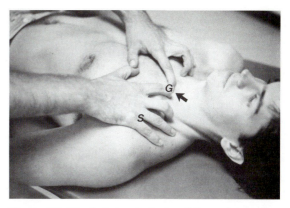

Figure 19-66   Inferior clavicular glides at the sternoclavicular joint use the index fingers to mobilize the clavicle, which increases clavicular elevation.

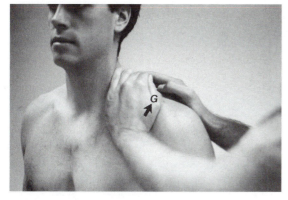

Figure 19-67   Posterior clavicular glides done at the acromioclavicular (AC) joint apply posterior pressure on the clavicle while stabilizing the scapula with the opposite hand. They increase mobility of the AC joint.

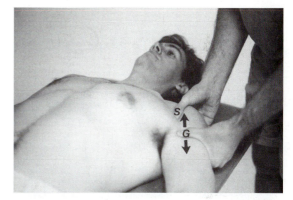

Figure 19-68   Anterior/posterior glenohumeral glides are done with one hand stabilizing the scapula and the other gliding the humeral head. They initiate motion in the painful shoulder.

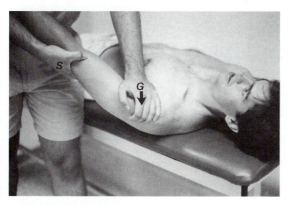

Figure 19-69   Posterior humeral glides use one hand to stabilize the humerus at the elbow and the other to glide the humeral head. They increase flexion and medial rotation.

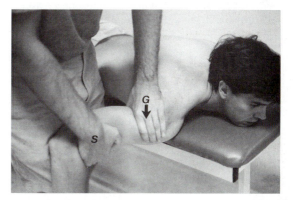

Figure 19-70   In anterior humeral glides, the patient is prone. One hand stabilizes the humerus at the elbow, and the other glides the humeral head. They increase extension and lateral rotation.

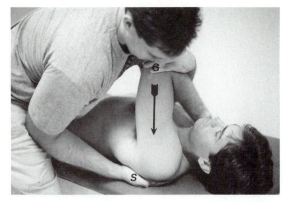

Figure 19-71 Posterior humeral glides may also be done with the shoulder at 90 degrees. With the patient in supine position, one hand stabilizes the scapula underneath while the patient's elbow is secured at the sports therapist's shoulder. Glides are directed downward through the humerus. They increase horizontal adduction.

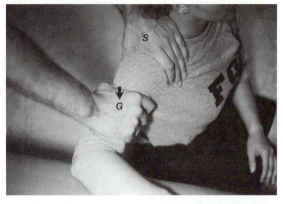

Figure 19-72 For inferior humeral glides, the patient is in the sitting position with the elbow resting on the treatment table. One hand stabilizes the scapula, and the other glides the humeral head inferiorly. These glides increase shoulder abduction.

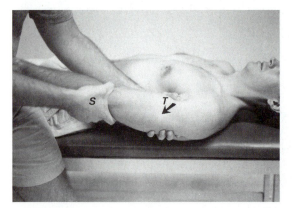

Figure 19-73 Lateral glenohumeral joint traction is used for initial testing of joint mobility and for decreasing pain. One hand stabilizes the elbow while the other applies lateral traction at the upper humerus.

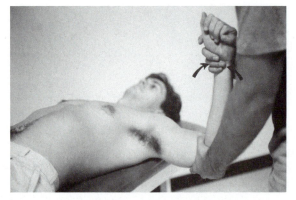

Figure 19-74 Medial and lateral rotation oscillations with the shoulder abducted at 90 degrees can increase medial and lateral rotation in a progressive manner according to patient tolerance.

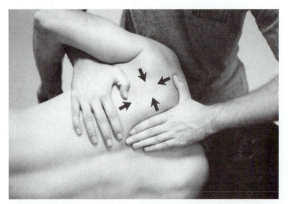

Figure 19-75 General scapular glides may be done in all directions, applying pressure at the medial, inferior, lateral, or superior border of the scapula. Scapular glides increase general scapulothoracic mobility.

Exercises to Reestablish Neuromuscular Control

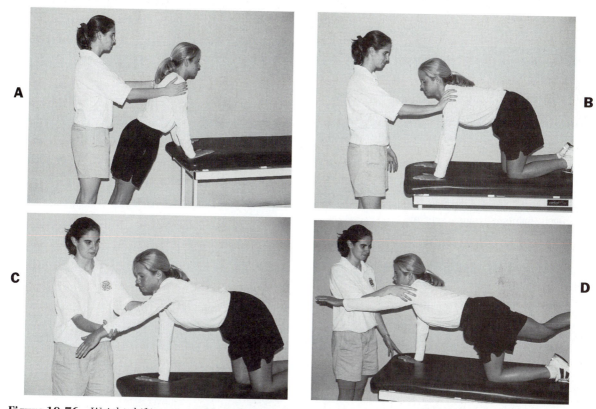

Figure 19-76 Weight shifting on a stable surface may be done **A,** standing with hands supporting weight on table, **B,** kneeling in a four-point position, **C,** kneeling in a three-point position, **D,** kneeling in a two-point position. The sports therapist can apply random directional pressure to which the athlete must respond to maintain a static position. In the two- and three-point positions, the arm that is supported in a closed-kinetic-chain is using shoulder force couples to maintain neuromuscular control.

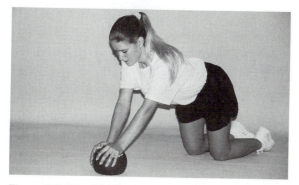

Figure 19-77 Weight shifting on a ball. In a push-up position with weight supported on a ball, the athlete shifts weight from side to side and/or forward and backward. Weight shifting on an unstable surface facilitates co-contraction of the muscles involved in the force couples that collectively maintain dynamic stability.

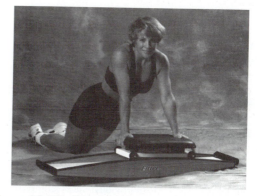

Figure 19-78 Weight shifting on a Fitter. In a kneeling position the athlete shifts weight from side to side using a Fitter. Weight shifting on an unstable surface facilitates co-contraction of the muscles involved in the force couples that collectively maintain dynamic stability.

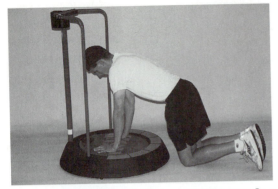

Figure 19-79 Weight shifting on a KAT system. In a kneeling position the athlete shifts weight from side to side and/or backward and forward using a KAT. Weight shifting on an unstable surface facilitates co-contraction of the muscles involved in the force couples that collectively maintain dynamic stability.

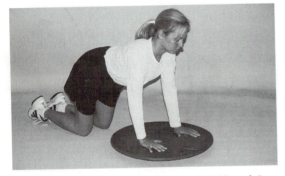

Figure 19-80 Weight shifting on a BAPS board. In a kneeling position the athlete shifts weight from side to side and/or backward and forward using a BAPS board. Weight shifting on an unstable surface facilitates co-contraction of the muscles involved in the force couples that collectively maintain dynamic stability.

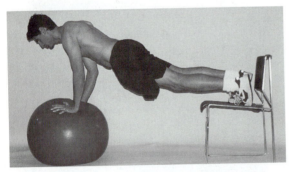

Figure 19-81 Weight shifting on a Swiss ball. With the feet supported on a chair, the athlete shifts weight from side to side and/or backward and forward using a Swiss ball. Weight shifting on an unstable surface facilitates co-contraction of the muscles involved in the force couples that collectively maintain dynamic stability.

A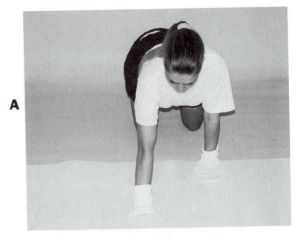

B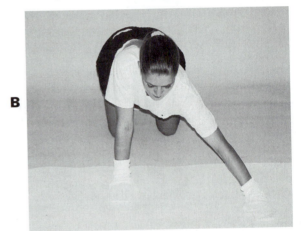

C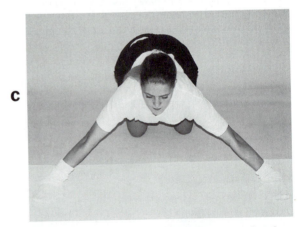

Figure 19-82 Slide board exercises. **A,** Forward and backward motion. **B,** Wax-on/wax-off motion. **C,** Hands lateral motion. The athlete shifts weight from side to side and/or backward and forward using a BAPS board. Weight shifting on an unstable surface facilitates co-contraction of the muscles involved in the force couples that collectively maintain dynamic stability.

REHABILITATION TECHNIQUES FOR SPECIFIC INJURIES

Sternoclavicular Joint Sprains

Pathomechanics. Sternoclavicular joint sprains are not commonly seen as athletic injuries. Although they are rare, the joint's complexity and integral interaction with the other joints of the shoulder complex warrant its discussion. The SC joint has multiple axis of rotation and articulates with the manubrium with an interposed fibrocartilaginous disc. Pathology of this joint can include injury to the fibrocartilage and sprains of the sternoclavicular ligaments and/or the costoclavicular ligaments.[27]

As stated earlier in this chapter, the sternoclavicular joint is extremely weak because of its bony arrangement. It is held in place by its strong ligaments, which tend to pull the sternal end of the clavicle downward and toward the sternum. A sprain of these ligaments often results in either a subluxing SC joint or a dislocated SC joint. This can be significant because the joint plays an integral role in scapular motion through the clavicle's articulation with the scapula. Combined movements at the acromioclavicular and sternoclavicular joints have been reported to account for up to 60 degrees of upward scapular rotation inherent in glenohumeral abduction.[3]

When this joint incurs an injury, a resultant inflammatory process occurs. The inflammatory process can cause an increase in the joint capsule pressure as well as a stiffening of the joint due to the collagen tissue being produced for the healing tissues. The pathogenesis of this inflammatory process can cause an altering of the joint mechanics as well as an increase in pain felt at the joint. This often results adversely on the shoulder complex.[59]

Injury Mechanism. After motor vehicle accidents, the most common source of injuries to the sternoclavicular joint is sports participation.[48] The SC joint can be injured by direct or indirect forces, resulting in sprains, dislocations, or physical injuries.[27] Direct force injuries are usually the result of a blow to the anteromedial aspect of the clavicle and produce a posterior dislocation.[27] Indirect force injuries can occur in many different sporting events, usually when the athlete falls and lands with an outstretched arm in either a flexed and adducted position or extended and adducted position of the upper extremity. The flexed position causes an anterior lateral compression force to the adducted arm, producing a posterior dislocation. The extended position causes a posterior lateral compression force to the adducted arm, leading to an anterior dislocation. Lesser forces can also lead to varying degrees of sprains to the SC joint. Additionally, there have been reports of repetitive microtrauma to this joint in sports such as golf, gymnastics, and rowing.[53,59]

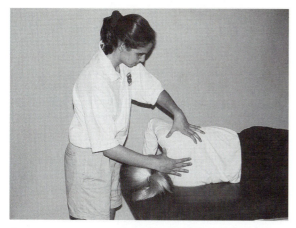

Figure 19-83 Scapular neuromuscular control exercises. The athlete's hand is placed on the table, creating a closed-kinetic chain, and the sports therapist applies pressure to the scapula in a random direction. The athlete moves the scapula isotonically into the direction of resistance.

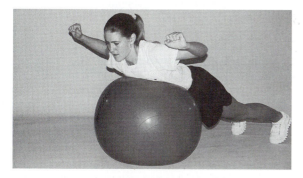

Figure 19-84 Swiss ball exercises. The athlete lies in a prone position on the Swiss ball and maintains a stable position.

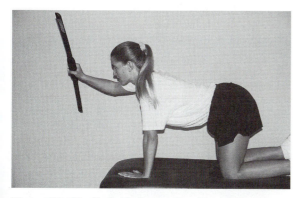

Figure 19-85 Body Blade exercises. The athlete is in a three-point kneeling position holding an oscillating Body Blade in one hand while working on neuromuscular control in the weight-bearing shoulder.

In golf, an example of mechanism of injury is during the backswing.[41] For a right-handed golfer, the sternoclavicular joint is subject to medially directed forces on the left at the top of the backswing and on the right at the end of the backswing. When the right arm is abducted and fully coiled at the end of the backswing and the beginning of the downswing, there is a posterior retraction of the shoulder complex, resulting in an anterior sternoclavicular joint stress. Due to the repetitive nature of golf, this can cause repetitive microtrauma leading to irritation of the joint. Over time the joint may become hypermobile relative to its normal stable condition, allowing for degeneration of the soft tissue and fibrocartilaginous disc. This often results in a painful syndrome affecting the mechanics of the joint and muscular control of the shoulder complex.[53] Similar examples are found in gymnastics and rowing.

Rehabilitation Concerns. In addressing the rehabilitation of an athlete with a sternoclavicular joint injury, it is important to address the function of the joint on shoulder complex movement. The sternoclavicular joint acts as the sole passive attachment of the shoulder complex to the axial skeleton. As noted earlier in the chapter, the clavicle must elevate approximately 40 degrees to allow upward scapular rotation.[51]

In most cases the primary problem reported by the injured athlete is discomfort associated with end-range movement of the shoulder complex. It is important to identify the cause of the pain (i.e., ligamentous instability, disc degeneration, or ligamentous trauma).

In cases where there is ligamentous instability as well as disc degeneration, the rehabilitation should focus on strengthening the muscles attached to the clavicle in a range that does not put further stress on the joint. Muscles such as the pectoralis minor, sternal fibers of the pectoralis major, and upper trapezius are strengthened to help control the motion of the clavicle during motion of the shoulder complex. Exercises include incline bench, shoulder shrugs, and the seated press-up, in a limited range of motion (see Figures 19-8, 19-21, 19-28). In addition to addressing the dynamic supports of the sternoclavicular joint, the sports therapist should employ the appropriate modalities necessary to control pain and the inflammatory process. It is also noteworthy, in cases where dislocation or subluxation has occurred, to consider the structures in close proximity to the sternoclavicular joint. In the case of a posterior dislocation, signs of circulatory vessel compromise nerve tissue impingement, and difficulty swallowing may be seen. It is important to avoid these symptoms and communicate with the athlete's physician regarding any lasting symptoms.[59]

When dealing with ligamentous trauma that lacks instability, the sports therapist should also address the associated pain with the appropriate modalities and utilize exercises that strengthen muscle with clavicular attachments. In all of the above scenarios, it is important to address the role of the SC joint on shoulder complex movement. A full evaluation of the shoulder complex should be performed to address issues related to scapular elevation. Exercises such as Superman, bent-over row, rhomboids, and push-ups with a plus should be included to help control upward rotation of the scapula (see Figures 19-22, 19-23, 19-24, 19-25). Appropriate progression should be followed while addressing the healing stages for the appropriate tissues.

Rehabilitation Progression. In the initial stages of rehabilitation, the primary goal is to minimize pain and inflammation associated with shoulder complex motion. The sports therapist should limit activities to midrange exercises and incorporate the use of therapeutic modalities along with the use of NSAID intervention from the physician. Ultrasound is often useful for increasing blood flow and facilitating the process of healing. Occasionally a shoulder sling or figure 8 strap can help minimize stress at the joint. During this phase of the rehabilitation progression, the sports therapist should identify the sport-specific needs of the athlete in order to tailor the later phases of rehabilitation to the athlete's demands. The athlete should also continue to work on exercises that maintain cardiorespiratory fitness.

When the pain and inflammation have been controlled, the athlete should gradually engage in a controlled increase of stress to the tissues of the joint. This is a good time to begin low-grade joint mobilizations resisted exercises for the muscles attaching to the clavicle. Exercises in this phase are best done in the midrange to minimize pain. As the athlete's tolerance increases, the resistance and range of motion can be increased. During this phase it is also important to address any limitations there might be in the athlete's range of motion. Emphasis should be placed on restoring the normal mechanics of the shoulder complex during shoulder movements.

As the athlete begins to enter the pain-free stages of the progression, the sports therapist should gradually incorporate sport-specific demands into the exercise program. Examples of this are PNF with rubber tubing, for the golfer (see Figures 19-46, 19-47); Stair Climber with feet on chair, for the gymnast (Figure 19-30); and rowing machine for the rower.

Criteria for Returning to Full Activity. The athlete may return to full activity when (1) the rehabilitation program has been progressed to the appropriate time and stress for the specific demands of the athlete's sport, (2) the athlete shows improved strength in the muscles used to protect the sternoclavicular joint when compared to the uninjured side, and (3) the athlete no longer has associated pain with movements of the shoul-

■ **TABLE 19-1** Acromioclavicular Sprain Classification

Type I

• Sprain of the acromioclavicular ligaments
• Acromioclavicular ligament intact
• Coracoclavicular ligament, deltoid and trapezius muscles intact

Type II

• Acromioclavicular joint disrupted with tearing of the acromioclavicular ligament
• Coracoclavicular ligament sprained
• Deltoid and trapezius muscles intact

Type III

• Acromioclavicular ligament disrupted
• Acromioclavicular joint displaced and the shoulder complex displaced inferiorly
• Coracoclavicular ligament disrupted with a coracoclavicular interspace 25 to 100 percent greater than the normal shoulder
• Deltoid and trapezius muscles usually detached from distal end of the clavicle

Type IV

• Acromioclavicular ligaments disrupted with the acromioclavicular joint displaced and the clavicle anatomically displaced posteriorly through the trapezius muscle
• Coracoclavicular ligaments disrupted with wider interspace
• Deltoid and trapezius muscles detached

Type V

• Acromioclavicular and coracoclavicular ligaments disrupted
• Acromioclavicular joint dislocated and gross displacement between the clavicle and the scapula
• Deltoid and trapezius muscles detached from distal end of the clavicle

Type VI

• Acromioclavicular and coracoclavicular ligaments disrupted
• Distal clavicle inferior to the acromion or the coracoid process
• Deltoid and trapezius muscles detached from distal end of the clavicle

der complex that will inevitably occur with the demands of their sport.

Acromioclavicular Joint Sprains

Pathomechanics. The acromioclavicular joint is composed of a bony articulation between the clavicle and the scapula. The soft tissues included in the joint are the hyaline cartilage coating the ends of the bony articulations, a fibrocartilaginous disc between the two bones, the acromioclavicular ligaments, and the costoclavicular ligaments. There have been two conflicting papers regarding the motion available at the joint. Codman reported little movement at the joint, whereas Inman reported exactly the opposite.[12,26] Multiple authors have reported degenerative changes at the AC joint by age 40 in the average healthy adult.[16,57]

The acromioclavicular joint provides the bridge between the clavicle and the scapula. When an injury occurs to the joint, all soft tissue should be considered in the rehabilitation process. An elaborate grading system has been reported to categorize injuries based on the soft tissue that is involved in the injury[55] (Table 19-1). Through evaluation by X-ray, the athlete's injury should be categorized in order to provide the sports therapist with a guideline for rehabilitation.

Injury Mechanism. Type I or type II acromioclavicular joint sprains are most commonly seen in athletics due to a direct fall on the point of the shoulder with the arm at the side in an adducted position or falling on an outstretched arm. The injury mechanism for type III and type IV sprains usually involves a direct impact that forces the acromion process downward, backward, and inward while the clavicle is pushed down against the rib cage. The impact can produce a number of injuries: (1) fracture of the clavicle; (2) AC joint sprain; (3) AC and coracoclavicular joint sprain; or (4) a combination of the previous injury with concomitant muscle tearing of the deltoid and trapezius at their clavicular attachments.[3] Another possible mechanism for injury to the acromio-clavicular joint is repetitive compression of the joint often seen in weight lifting.[59]

Rehabilitation Concerns. Management of acromioclavicular injuries is dependent on the type of injury.[20] Age, level of play, and the demand on the athlete can also factor into the management of this injury. Most physicians prefer to handle type I and type II injuries conservatively, but some authors have suggested that type I and type II injuries can cause further problems to the athlete later in life.[5,13] These injuries might require surgical excision of the distal 2 cm of the clavicle. The sports therapist should consider when developing a treatment plan (1) the stability of the AC joint; (2) the amount of time the athlete was immobilized; (3) pain, as a guide for the type of exercises being used; and (4) the soft tissue that was involved in the injury. Rehabilitation of these injuries should focus on strengthening the deltoid and trapezius muscles. Additional strengthening of the clavicular fibers of the pectoralis major should also be done. Other muscles that help restore the proper mechanics to the shoulder complex should also be done.

Type I. Treatment for the type I injury consists of ice to relieve pain and a sling to support the extremity for several days. The amount of time in the sling usually depends on the patient's ability to tolerate pain and begin carrying their involved extremity with the appropriate posture. The sports therapist can have the athlete begin active assisted range of motion immediately and then incorporate isometric exercises to the muscles with clavicular attachments. This will help restore the appropriate carrying posture for the involved upper extremity. When the athlete is able to remove the sling, the sports therapist should increase the exercise program to incorporate PRE exercises for the muscles with clavicular attachments and add exercises to encourage appropriate scapular motion. This will help prevent related shoulder discomfort due to poor glenohumeral mechanics after return to activity.

Type II. The treatment for type II injuries is also nonsurgical. Because this type of injury to the AC joint involves complete disruption of the acromioclavicular ligaments, immobilization plays a greater role in the treatment of these athletes. There is no consensus as to the duration of immobilization. Some authors have recommended 7 to 14 days, others have suggested using a sling that not only supports the upper extremity but depresses the clavicle.[1,59] This debate is fueled by disagreements regarding the time it takes the body to produce collagen and bridge the gap left from the injury. It has been reported that tissue mobilized too early shows a greater amount of type III collagen than the stronger type I collagen.[31] The time needed to heal the soft tissues involved in this injury must be considered prior to beginning exercises that stress the injury. Heavy lifting and contact sports should be avoided for 8 to 12 weeks.

Type III. Many authors have recommended a nonoperative approach for this type of injury, most agreeing that a sling is adequate for allowing the athlete to rest comfortably.[3] Use of this nonoperative technique has been reported to have limited success. Cox reported improved results without support of the arm in 62 percent of his patients, whereas only 25 percent had relief after 3 to 6 weeks of immobilization and a sling.[13]

Operative management of this type of injury can be summarized with the following options:

1. Stabilization of clavicle to coracoid with a screw
2. Resection of distal clavicle
3. Transarticular acromioclavicular fixation with pins
4. Use of coracoclavicular ligament as a substitute acromioclavicular ligament

Taft et al. found superior results with coracoclavicular fixation. They found that patients with acromioclavicular fixation had a higher rate of post-traumatic arthritis than those managed with a coracoclavicular screw.[62]

Type IV, V, and VI. Types IV, V, and VI injuries require open reduction and internal fixation. Operative procedures are designed to attempt realignment of the clavicle to the scapula. The immobilization for this type of injury is longer and therefore the rehabilitation time is longer. After immobilization, the concerns are similar to those previously discussed.

Rehabilitation Progression. Early in the rehabilitation progression, the sports therapist should be concerned with application of cold therapy and pressure for the first 24 to 48 hours to control local hemorrhage. Fitting the athlete for a sling is also important to control the athlete's pain. Time in the sling depends on the severity of the injury. After the athlete has been seen by a physician for differential diagnosis, the rehabilitation progression should be tailored to the type of sprain according to the diagnosis.

Type I, II, and III sprains should be handled similarly at first, with the time of progression accelerated with less severe sprains. Exercises should begin with encouraging the athlete to use the involved extremity for ADL activities and gentle range-of-motion exercises. Return of normal range of motion in the athlete's shoulder is the first objective goal. The athlete can also begin isometric exercises to maintain or restore muscle function in the shoulder. These exercises can be started while the athlete is in the sling. Once the sling is removed, pendulum exercises can be started to encourage movement. In type III sprains the sports therapist should hold off doing passive ROM exercises in the end ranges of shoulder elevation for the first 7 days. The athlete should have full passive ROM by 2 to 3 weeks. Once the athlete has full active range of motion, a program of progressive resistive exercises should begin. Strengthening of the deltoid and upper trapezius muscles should be emphasized. The sports therapist should evaluate the athlete's shoulder mechanics to identify problems with neuromuscular control and address specific deficiencies as noted. As the athlete regains strength in the involved extremity, sport-specific exercises should be incorporated into the rehabilitation program. Gradual return to activity should be supervised by the athlete's coach and sports therapist.

In the case of type IV, V, and VI acromioclavicular sprains a postsurgical progression should be followed. The sports therapist should design a program that is broken down into 4 phases of rehabilitation with the goal of returning the athlete to his or her activity as quickly as possible.[3] Contact with the physician is important to determine the time frame in which each phase may begin. Common surgeries for this injury include open reduction with pin or screw fixation and/or acromioplasty.

The early stage of rehabilitation should be designed with the goal of reestablishing pain-free range of motion, preventing muscle atrophy, and decreasing pain and inflammation. Range-of-motion exercises may include Codman's exercises (Figure 19-51), rope and pulley exercises (Figure 19-54), L-bar exercises (Figures 19-56 to 19-61), and self capsular stretches (Figures 19-63, 19-64). Strengthening exercises in this phase may include isometrics in all of the cardinal planes and isometrics for medial and lateral rotation of the glenohumeral joint at 0 degrees of elevation (Figure 19-6).

As rehabilitation progresses, the sports therapist has the goal of regaining and improving muscle strength, normalizing arthrokinematics, and improving neuromuscular control of the shoulder complex. Prior to advancing to this phase, the athlete should have full ROM, minimal pain and tenderness, and a 4/5 manual muscle test for internal rotation, external rotation, and flexion. Initiation of isotonic PRE exercises should begin. Shoulder medial and lateral rotation (Figures 19-17, 19-18), shoulder flexion and abduction to 90 degrees (Figures 19-12, 19-14), scaption (Figure 19-19), bicep curls, and

tricep extensions should be included. Additionally, a program of scapular stabilizing exercises should begin. Exercises should include: Superman exercises (Figure 19-22), rhomboids exercises (Figure 19-24), shoulder shrugs (Figure 19-21), and seated push-ups (Figure 19-28). To help normalize arthrokinematics of the shoulder, complex joint mobilization techniques should be used for the glenohumeral, acromioclavicular, sternoclavicular, and scapulothoracic joints (Figures 19-65 to 19-75). To complete this phase the athlete should begin neuromuscular control exercises (Figures 19-76 to 19-85), trunk exercises, and a low-impact aerobic exercise program.

During the advanced strengthening phase of rehabilitation, the goals should be to improve strength, power, and endurance of muscles as well as to improve neuromuscular control of the shoulder complex, and preparing the athlete to return to sport-specific activities. Prior to advancing to this phase, the sports therapist should use the criteria of full pain-free range of motion, no pain or tenderness, and strength of 70 percent compared to the uninvolved shoulder. The emphasis in this phase is on high-speed strengthening, eccentric exercises, and multiplanar motions. The athlete should advance to surgical tubing exercises (Figure 19-31), plyometric-style exercises (Figures 19-32 to 19-37), PNF-style diagonal strengthening (Figures 19-39 to 19-45), and isokinetic strengthening exercises (Figure 19-38).

When the athlete is ready to return to activity, the sports therapist should progressively increase activities that prepare the athlete for a fully functional return. An interval program of sport-specific activities should be started. Exercises from stage III should be continued. The athlete should progressively increase the time of participation in sport-specific activities as tolerated. For contact and collision sport athletes, the AC joint should be protected.

Criteria for Returning to Full Activity. Prior to returning to full activity the athlete should have full range of motion and no pain or tenderness. Isokinetic strength testing should meet the demands of the athlete's sport, and the athlete should have successfully completed the final phase of the rehabilitation progression.

Clavicle Fractures

Pathomechanics. Clavicle fractures are one of the most common fractures in sports. The clavicle acts as a strut connecting the upper extremity to the trunk of the body.[17] Forces acting on the clavicle are most likely to cause a fracture of the bone medial to the attachment of the coracoclavicular ligaments.[4] Intact acromioclavicular and coracoclavicular ligaments help keep fractures nondisplaced and stabilized.

Injury Mechanism. In athletics, the mechanism for injury often depends on the sport played. The mechanism can be direct or indirect. Fractures can result from a fall on an outstretched arm, a fall or blow to the point of the shoulder, or less commonly a direct blow as in stick sports like lacrosse and hockey.[53]

Rehabilitation Concerns. Early identification of the fracture is an important factor in rehabilitation. If stabilization occurs early, with minimal damage and irritation to the surrounding structures, the likelihood of an uncomplicated return to sports is increased. Other factors influencing the likelihood of complications are injuries to the acromioclavicular, coracoclavicular, and sternoclavicular ligaments. Treatment for clavicle fractures includes approximation of the fracture and immobilization for 6 to 8 weeks. Most commonly a figure-8 wrap is used, with the involved arm in a sling.

When designing a rehabilitation program for an athlete who has sustained a clavicle fracture, the sports therapist should consider the function of the clavicle. The clavicle acts as a strut offering shoulder girdle stability and allowing the upper extremity to move more freely about the thorax by positioning the extremity away from the body axis.[22] Mobility of the clavicle is therefore very important to normal shoulder mechanics. Joint mobilization techniques are started immediately after the immobilization period in order to restore normal arthrokinematics. The clavicle also serves as an insertion point for the deltoid, upper trapezius, and pectoralis major muscles, providing stability and aiding in neuromuscular control of the shoulder complex. It is important to address these muscles with the appropriate exercises in order to restore normal shoulder mechanics.

Rehabilitation Progression. For the first 6 to 8 weeks, the athlete is immobilized in the figure 8 brace and sling. If good approximation and healing of the fracture is occurring at 6 weeks, the athlete may begin gentle isometric exercises for the upper extremity. Utilization of the involved extremity below 90 degrees of elevation should be encouraged to prevent muscle atrophy and excessive loss of glenohumeral ROM. After the immobilization period, the athlete should begin a program to regain full active and passive ROM. Joint mobilization techniques are used to restore normal arthrokinematics (Figures 19-65 to 19-67). The athlete may continue to wear the sling for the next 3 to 4 weeks while regaining the ability to carry the arm in an appropriate posture without the figure 8 brace. The athlete should begin a strengthening program utilizing progressive resistance as range of motion improves. Once full ROM is achieved, the athlete should begin resisted diagonal PNF exercises and continue to increase the strength of the shoulder complex muscle, including the periscapular muscles, to enable normal neuromuscular control of the shoulder.

Criteria for Return. The athlete may return to activity when the fracture is clinically united, full active and passive range of motion is achieved, and the athlete has the strength and neuromuscular control to meet the demands of their sport.

Glenohumeral Dislocations/Instabilities (Surgical vs. Nonsurgical Rehabilitation)

Pathomechanics. Dislocations of the glenohumeral joint involve the temporary displacement of the humeral head from its normal position in the glenoid labral fossa. From a biomechanical perspective, the resultant force vector is directed outside the arc of contact in the glenoid fossa, creating a dislocating moment of the humeral head by pivoting about the labral rim.[18]

Shoulder dislocations account for up to 50 percent of all dislocations. The inherent instability of the shoulder joint necessary for the extreme mobility of this joint makes the glenohumeral joint susceptible to dislocation. The most common kind of dislocation is that occurring anteriorly. Posterior dislocations account for only 1 to 4.3 percent of all shoulder dislocations. Inferior dislocations are extremely rare. Of dislocations caused by direct trauma, 85 to 90 percent are recurring.[58]

In an anterior glenohumeral dislocation, the head of the humerus is forced out of its anterior capsule in an anterior direction past the glenoid labrum and then downward to rest under the coracoid process. The pathology that ensues is extensive, with torn capsular and ligamentous tissue, possibly tendonous avulsion of the rotator cuff muscles, and profuse hemorrhage. A tear or detachment of the glenoid labrum might also be present. Healing is usually slow, and the detached labrum and capsule can produce a permanent anterior defect on the glenoid labrum called a Bankart lesion. Another defect that can occur with anterior dislocation can be found on the posterior lateral aspect of the humeral head called a Hill-Sachs lesion. This is caused by compressive forces between the humeral head and the glenoid rim while the humeral head rests in the dislocated position. Additional complications can arise if the head of the humerus comes into contact with and injures the brachial nerves and vessels. Rotator cuff tears can also arise as a result of the dislocation. The bicipital tendon might also sublux from its canal as the result of a rupture of the transverse ligament.[58]

Posterior dislocations can also result in significant soft-tissue damage. Tears of the posterior glenoid labrum are common in posterior dislocation. A fracture of the lesser tubercle can occur if the subscapularis tendon avulses its attachment.

Glenohumeral dislocation is usually very disabling. The athlete assumes an obvious disabled posture and the deformity itself is obvious. A positive sulcus sign is usually present at the time of the dislocation, and the deformity can be easily recognized on X-ray. As detailed above, the damage can be extensive to the soft tissue.

Injury Mechanism. When discussing the mechanism of injury for dislocations of the glenohumeral joint, it is necessary to categorize the injury as traumatic or atraumatic, and anterior or posterior. An anterior dislocation of the glenohumeral joint can result from direct impact to the posterior or posterolateral aspect of the shoulder. The most common mechanism is forced abduction, external rotation, and extension that forces the humeral head out of the glenoid cavity.[40] An arm tackle in football or rugby or abnormal forces created in executing a throw can produce a sequence of events resulting in dislocation. The injury mechanism for a posterior glenohumeral dislocation is usually forced adduction and internal rotation of the shoulder or a fall on an extended and internally rotated arm.

The two mechanisms described for anterior dislocation can be categorized as traumatic or atraumatic. The following acronyms have been described to summarize the two mechanisms.[33]

Traumatic	Atraumatic
Traumatic	**A**traumatic
Unidirectional	**M**ultidirectional
Bankart lesion	**B**ilateral involvement
Surgery required	**R**ehabilitation effective
	Inferior capsular shift recommended

The AMBRI group can be characterized by subluxation or dislocation episodes without trauma, resulting in a stretched capsuloligamentous complex that lacks end-range stabilizing ability. Several authors report a high rate of recurrence for dislocations, especially those in the TUBS category.[56]

Rehabilitation Concerns. Management of shoulder dislocation depends on a number of factors that need to be identified. Mechanism, chronology, and direction of instability all need to be considered in the development of a conservatively managed rehabilitation program. No single rehabilitation program is an absolute solution for success in the treatment of a shoulder dislocation. The sports therapist should thoroughly evaluate the injury and discuss those objective findings and the physician's findings. The initial concern in rehabilitation focuses on maintaining appropriate reduction of the glenohumeral joint. The athlete is immobilized in a reduced position for a period of time, depending on the type of management used in the reduction (surgical vs. nonsurgical). For the purpose of this section, the discussion will continue with conservative management in mind. The principles of rehabilitation, however, remain constant regardless of whether the physician's management is surgical or nonsurgical. Surgical rehabilitation should be based on the healing time of tissue affected

by the surgery. The limitations of motion in the early stages of rehabilitation should also be based on surgical fixation. It is extremely important, because of this, that the sports therapist and physician communicate prior to the start of rehabilitation. After the immobilization period, the rehabilitation program should be focused on restoring the appropriate axis of rotation for the glenohumeral joint, optimizing the stabilizing muscle's length-tension relationship, and restoring proper neuromuscular control to the shoulder complex. In the uninjured shoulder complex with intact capsuloligamentous structures, the glenohumeral joint maintains a tight axis of rotation within the glenoid fossa. This is accomplished dynamically with complex neuromuscular control of the periscapular muscles, rotator cuff muscles, and intact passive structures of the joint. Because the extent of damage in this type of injury is variable, the exercises employed to restore these normal mechanics should also vary.[55] As the sports therapist helps the athlete regain full range of motion, a safe zone of positioning should be followed. Starting in the plane of the scapula is safe, because the axis of rotation for forces acting on the joint fall in the center of this plane. The least provocative position is somewhere between 20 and 55 degrees of scapular plane abduction. Keeping the humerus below 55 degrees prevents subacromial impingement, while avoiding full adduction minimizes excessive tension across the supraspinatus/coracohumeral and/or capsuloligamentous complex. As range of motion improves, the sports therapist should progress the exercise program into positions outside the safe zone, accommodating the demands that the athlete will need to meet. Specific strengthening should be given to address the muscles of the shoulder complex responsible for maintaining the axis of rotation, such as the supraspinatus, and rotator cuff muscles. The periscapular muscles should also be addressed in order to provide the rotator cuff muscles with their optimal length-tension relationship for more efficient usage. In the later stages of rehabilitation, neuromuscular control exercises are incorporated with sport-specific exercises to prepare the athlete for return to activity.[33]

Rehabilitation Progression. The first essential to a successful rehabilitation program is the removal of the athlete from activities that risk reinjury to the glenohumeral joint. A reasonable time frame for return to activity is approximately 12 weeks, with unrestricted activity coming closer to 20 weeks. This is variable, depending on the extent of soft-tissue damage and the type of intervention chosen by the athlete and physician. Some exercises previously used by the athlete might produce undesired forces on noncontractile tissues and need to be modified to be performed safely. Push-ups, pull-downs, and the bench press are performed with the hands in close and avoiding the last 10 to 20 degrees of shoulder extension. Pull-downs and military press performed with

■ **TABLE 19-2** Exercise Modification per Direction of Instability

Direction of Instability	Position to Avoid	Exercises to Be Modified or Avoided
Anterior	Combined position of external rotation and abduction	Fly, pull-down, push-up, bench press, military press
Posterior	Combined position of internal rotation, horizontal adduction, and flexion	Fly, push-up bench press, weight-bearing exercises
Inferior	Full elevation, dependent arm	Shrugs, elbow curls, military press

wide bars and machines are kept in front rather than behind the head. Supine fly exercises are limited to −30 degrees in the coronal plane while maintaining glenohumeral internal rotation. See Table 19-2 for further modifications dependent on directional instability.[3]

During phase I the athlete is immobilized in a sling. This lasts for up to 3 weeks with first-time dislocations. The goal of this phase is to limit the inflammatory process, decrease pain, and retard muscle atrophy. Passive range-of-motion exercises can be initiated along with low-grade joint mobilization techniques to encourage relaxation of the shoulder musculature. Isometric exercises are also started. The athlete begins with submaximal contractions and increases to maximal contractions for as long as 8 seconds. The protective phase is a good time to initiate a scapulothoracic exercise program, avoiding elevated positions of the upper extremity that put stability at risk. Athletes should begin an aerobic training regime with the lower extremity, such as stationary biking.

Phase II begins after the athlete has been removed from the sling. This phase lasts from 3 to 8 weeks postinjury and focuses on full return of active range of motion. The program begins with the use of an L-bar performing active assistive ROM (Figures 19-56 to 19-61). Manual therapy techniques can also begin using PNF techniques to help reestablish neuromuscular control (Figures 19-39 to 19-45). Exercises with the hands on the ground can help begin strengthening the scapular stabilizers more aggressively. These exercises should begin on a stable surface like a table, progressing the amount of weight bearing by advancing from the table to the ground (Figure 19-76). Advancing to a less stable surface like a BAPS board (Figure 19-80) or Swiss ball (Figure 19-81) will also help reestablish neuromuscular control.

At 6 to 12 weeks the sports therapist should gradually enter phase III of the rehabilitation progression. The goal of this phase is to restore normal strength and neuromuscular control. Prophylactic stretching is done, as full range of motion should already be present. Scapular and rotator cuff exercises should focus on strength and endurance. Weight-bearing exercises should be made more challenging by adding motion to the demands of the stabilization. Scapular exercises should be performed in the weight room with guidance from the sports therapist in order to meet the challenge of the athlete's strength. Weight shifting on a Fitter (Figure 19-78) and closed-kinetic-chain strengthening on a stair climber (Figure 19-30) for endurance are started. Strengthening exercises progress from PRE to plyometric. Rotator cuff exercises using surgical tubing with emphasis on eccentrics are added.[2] Progression to multiangle exercises and sport-specific positioning is started. The Body Blade is a good rehabilitation tool for this phase (Figure 19-85), progressing from static to dynamic stabilization and single-position to multiangular dynamic exercises.

Phase IV is the functional progression. Athletes are gradually returned to their sport with interval training and progressive activity increasing the demands on endurance and stability. This can last as long as 20 weeks, depending on the athlete's shoulder strength, lack of pain, and ability to protect the involved shoulder. The physician should be consulted prior to full return to activity.

Criteria for Return to Activity. At 20 to 26 weeks, the athlete should be ready for return to activity. This decision should be based on (1) full pain-free range of motion, (2) normal shoulder strength, (3) pain-free sport-specific activities, and (4) ability to protect the athlete's shoulder from reinjury. Some sports therapist and physicians like the athlete to use a protective shoulder harness during participation.

Multidirectional Instabilities of the Glenohumeral Joint

Pathomechanics. Multidirectional instabilities are an inherent risk of the glenohumeral joint. The shoulder has the greatest range of motion of all the joints in the human body. The bony restraints are minimal, and the forces that can be generated in overhead motions of throwing and other athletic activities far exceed the strength of the static restraints of the joint. Attenuation of force is multifactorial, with time, distance, and speed determining forces applied to the joint. Thus stability of the joint must be evaluated based on the athlete's ability to dynamically control all of these factors in order to have a stable joint. In cases of multidirectional instability, there are two categories for pathology: atraumatic and traumatic. The atraumatic category includes athletes who have congenitally loose joints or who have increased the demands on their shoulder prior to having developed the muscular maturity to meet these demands. When forces are generated at the glenohumeral joint that the stabilizing muscles are unable to handle (this occurs most commonly during the deceleration phase of throwing), the humeral head tends to translate anteriorly and inferiorly into the capsuloligamentous structures. Over time, repetitive microtrauma causes these structures to stretch. Lephart et al. document the essential importance of tension in the anterior capsule of the glenohumeral joint as a protective mechanism against excessive strain in these capsuloligamentous structures.[36] They theorized that the loss of this protective reflex joint stabilization can increase the potential for continuing shoulder injury. Increased translation of the humeral head also increases the demand on the posterior structures of the glenohumeral joint, leading to repetitive microtrauma and breakdown of those soft tissues. In this type of instability there will usually be some inferior laxity, leading to a positive sulcus sign. Although the anterior glenoid labrum is usually intact during the early stages of this instability, splitting and partial detachment can develop.[3] The athlete usually has some pain and clicking when the arm is held by the side. Any symptoms and signs associated with anterior or posterior recurrent instability may be present.

Injury Mechanism. It is generally believed that the cause of multidirectional instability is excessive joint volume with laxity of the capsuloligamentous complex. In the athlete, this laxity might be an inherent condition that becomes more pronounced with the superimposed trauma of sport. This type of instability might also occur due to extensive capsulolabral trauma in patients who do not appear to have laxity of other joints.[53]

Rehabilitation Concerns. The rehabilitation concerns for multidirectional instability are similar to those already discussed in relation to shoulder instabilities. The complexity of this program is increased due to the addition of inferior instability. The success of the program is often determined by the patient's tissue status and compliance.[61] Additionally, this program emphasizes the anterior and posterior musculature. These muscles working together are referred to as force couples and are believed to be essential stabilizers of the joint. The rehabilitation program should also address the neuromuscular control of these muscles to promote dynamic stability.[23] Compliance is often an extremely important factor in maintaining good results with this type of instability. The athlete must continue to do the exercise program even after symptoms have subsided. If the patient does not, subluxation usually recurs. For cases where conservative treatment is not successful, Neer recommended an inferior capsular shift surgical procedure that

has proven successful in restoring joint stability when used in conjunction with a rehabilitation program.[45]

Rehabilitation Progression. The rehabilitation program should begin with reestablishing muscle tone and proper scapulathoracic posture. This helps provide a steady base with appropriate length-tension relationships for the anterior and posterior muscles of the shoulder complex acting as force couples. Strengthening of the rotator cuff muscles in the plane of the scapula should progress to higher resistance, starting at 0 degrees of shoulder elevation. As the athlete becomes asymptomatic, the sports therapist should incorporate an emphasis on neuromuscular control exercises like PNF, rhythmic stabilization, and weight-bearing activity to establish co-contraction at the glenohumeral joint. Sport-specific training can then be added, first in the rehabilitation setting and then in the competitive setting. For successful results, the athlete might have to continue a program of maintenance for neuromuscular control for as long as they wish to be asymptomatic.

Criteria for Returning to Full Activity. The criteria for this instability are the same as described for other shoulder instabilities. Burkhead and Rockwood reported an 80 percent success rate using a conservative approach with athletes who had atraumatic multidirectional instability.[10,55]

Shoulder Impingement

Pathomechanics. Shoulder impingement syndrome was first identified by Dr. Charles Neer, who observed that impingement involves a mechanical compression of the supraspinatus tendon, the subacromial bursa, and the long head of the biceps tendon, all of which are located under the coracoacromial arch. This syndrome has been described as a continuum during which repetitive compression eventually leads to irritation and inflammation that progresses to fibrosis and eventually to rupture of the rotator cuff. Neer has identified three stages of shoulder impingement:

STAGE I

- Seen in patients less than 25 years of age with report of repetitive overhead activity
- Localized hemorrhage and edema with tenderness at supraspinatus insertion and anterior acromion
- Painful arc between 60 and 119 degrees; increased with resistance at 90 degrees
- Muscle tests revealing weakness secondary to pain
- Positive Neer or Hawkins-Kennedy impingement signs (Figures 19-86, 19-87)
- Normal radiographs, typically
- Reversible; usually resolving with rest, activity modification, and rehabilitation program

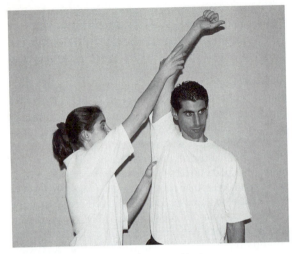

Figure 19-86 Neer impingement test.

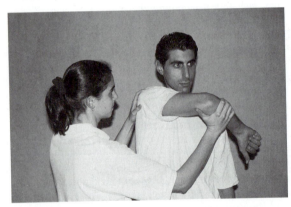

Figure 19-87 Hawkins-Kennedy impingement test.

STAGE II
- Seen in patients 25 to 40 years of age with report of repetitive overhead activity
- Many of the same clinical findings as in Stage I
- Severity of symptoms worse than Stage I, progressing to pain with activity and night pain
- More soft-tissue crepitus or catching at 100 degrees
- Restriction in passive ROM due to fibrosis
- Possibly radiographs showing osteophytes under acromion, degenerative AC joint changes
- No longer reversible with rest; possibly helped by a long-term rehabilitation program

STAGE III
- Seen in patients older than 40 years of age with history of chronic tendinitis and prolonged pain
- Many of the same clinical findings as Stage II
- Tear in rotator cuff usually less than 1 cm

- More limitation in active and passive ROM
- Possibly a prominent capsular laxity with multidirectional instability seen on radiograph
- Atrophy of infraspinatus and supraspinatus due to disuse
- Treatment typically surgical following a failed conservative approach

Neer's impingement theory was based primarily on the treatment of older, nonathletic patients. The older population will likely exhibit what has been referred to as "outside" or "outlet" impingement.[7,45] In outside impingement there is contact of the rotator cuff with the coracoacromial ligament or the acromion with fraying, abrasion, inflammation, fibrosis, and degeneration of the superior surface of the cuff within the subacromial space. There might also be evidence of degenerative processes, including spurring, decreased joint space due to fibrotic changes, and decreased vascularity.

"Inside" or "nonoutlet" impingement is more likely to occur in the younger overhead athlete. With inside impingement the subacromial space appears relatively normal. With forced humeral elevation and internal rotation, the rotator cuff can be impinged on the posterior superior glenoid labrum and the humeral head, potentially producing inflammation on the undersurface of the rotator cuff tendon, posterior superior tears in the glenoid labrum, and lesions in the posterior humeral head (Bankart lesion).

The mechanical impingement syndrome as originally proposed by Neer has been referred to as primary impingement. Jobe and Kvnite have proposed that an unstable shoulder permits excessive translation of the humeral head in an anterior and superior direction, resulting in what has been termed secondary impingement.[28] Based on the relationship of shoulder instability to shoulder impingement, Jobe and Kvnite have proposed an alternative system of classification:[28]

GROUP IA
- Found in recreational athletes more than 35 years of age with pure mechanical impingement and no instability
- Positive impingement signs
- Lesions on the superior surface of the rotator cuff, possibly with subacromial spurring
- Possibly some arthritic changes in the glenohumeral joint

GROUP IB
- Found in recreational athletes over 35 who demonstrate instability with impingement secondary to mechanical trauma
- Positive impingement signs

- Lesions found on the undersurface of the rotator cuff, superior glenoid, and humeral head

GROUP II
- Found in young overhead athletes (less than 35 years old) who demonstrate instability and impingement secondary to repetitive microtrauma
- Positive impingement signs with excessive anterior translation of humeral head
- Lesions on the posterior superior glenoid rim, posterior humeral head, or anterior inferior capsule
- Lesions on the undersurface of the rotator cuff

GROUP III
- Found in young overhead athletes (less than 35 years old)
- Positive impingement signs with atraumatic multidirectional, usually bilateral, humeral instabilities
- Demonstrated generalized laxity in all joints
- Humeral head lesions as in Group II but less severe

GROUP IV
- Found young overhead athletes (less than 35 years old) with anterior instability resulting from a traumatic event but without impingement
- Posterior defect in the humeral head
- Damage in the posterior glenoid labrum

It has also been proposed that wear of the rotator cuff is due to intrinsic tendon pathology, including tendinopathy and partial or small complete tears with age-related thinning, degeneration, and weakening. This permits superior migration of the humeral head, leading to secondary impingement, thus creating a cycle that can ultimately lead to full-thickness tears.[66]

A "critical zone" of vascular insufficiency has been proposed to exist in the tendon of the supraspinatus, which is found at about 1 cm proximal to its distal insertion on the humerus. It has been hypothesized that when the humerus is adducted and internally rotated, a "wringing out" of the blood supply occurs in this tendon. Should this occur repetitively, such as in the recovery phase on a swimming stroke, ultimately irritation and inflammation may lead to partial or complete rotator cuff tears.[54]

It is likely that some as yet unidentified combination of mechanical, traumatic, degenerative, and vascular processes collectively lead to pathology in the rotator cuff.

Injury Mechanism. Shoulder impingement syndrome occurs when there is compromise of the subacromial space under the coracoacromial arch. When the dynamic and static stabilizers of the shoulder complex fail for one reason or another to maintain this subacro-

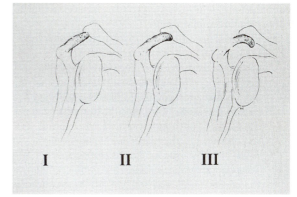

Figure 19-88   Acromion shapes. Type I, flat; type II, curved; and type III, hooked.

mial space, the soft-tissue structures are compressed, leading to irritation and inflammation. In athletes, impingement most often occurs in repetitive overhead activities such as throwing, swimming, serving a tennis ball, or spiking a volleyball, or during handstands in gymnastics. There is ongoing disagreement regarding the specific mechanisms that cause shoulder impingement syndrome. It has been proposed that mechanical impingement can result from either structural or functional causes. Structural causes can be attributed to existing congenital abnormalities or to degenerative changes under the coracoacromial arch and might include the following:

- An abnormally shaped acromion (Figure 19-88). Athletes with a type III or hook-shaped acromion are approximately 70 percent more likely to exhibit signs of impingement than those with a flat or slightly curved acromion.[6]
- Inherent capsular laxity compromises the ability of the glenohumeral joint capsule to act as both a static and a dynamic stabilizer.[28]
- Ongoing or recurring tendinitis or subacromial bursitis causes a loss of space under the coracoacromial arch, which can potentially lead to irritation of other, uninflamed structures, setting up a vicious degenerative cycle.[59]
- Laxity in the anterior capsule due to recurrent subluxation or dislocation can allow an anterior migration of the humeral head, which can cause impingement under the coracoid process.[69]
- Postural malalignments such as a forward head, round shoulders, and an increased kyphotic curve, which cause the scapular glenoid to be positioned such that the space under the coracoacromial arch is decreased, can also contribute to impingement.

Functional causes include adaptive changes that occur with repetitive overhead activities, altering the normal biomechanical function of the shoulder complex. These include the following:

- Failure of the rotator cuff to dynamically stabilize the humeral head relative to the glenoid, producing excessive translation and instability. The inferior rotator cuff muscles (infraspinatus, teres minor, subscapularis) should act collectively to both depress and compress the humeral head. In the overhead or throwing athlete, the internal rotators must be capable of producing humeral rotation on the order of 7,000 degrees per second.[64] The subcapularis tends to be stronger than the infraspinatus and teres minor, creating a strength imbalance in the existing force couple in the transverse plane. This imbalance produces excessive anterior translation of the humeral head. Furthermore, weakness in the inferior rotator cuff muscles creates an imbalance in the existing force couple with the deltoid in the coronal plane. The deltoid produces excessive superior translation of the humeral head, decreasing subacromial space. Weakness in the supraspinatus, which normally functions to compress the humeral head into the glenoid, allows for excessive superior translation of the humeral head.[67]

- Because the tendons of the rotator cuff blend into the joint capsule, we rely on tension created in the capsule by contraction of the rotator cuff to both statically and dynamically center the humeral head relative to the glenoid. Tightness in the posterior and inferior portions of the glenohumeral joint capsule causes an anterosuperior migration of the humeral head, again decreasing the subacromial space. In the overhead athlete, range of motion in internal rotation is usually limited by tightness of both the muscles that externally rotate and the posterior capsule. There tends to be excessive external rotation, primarily due to laxity in the anterior joint capsule.[9]

- The scapular muscles function to dynamically position the glenoid relative to the humeral head, maintaining a normal length-tension relationship with the rotator cuff. As the humerus moves into elevation, the scapula should also move so that the glenoid is able to adjust regardless of the position of the elevating humerus. Weakness in the serratus anterior, which elevates, upward rotates, and abducts the scapula, or weakness in the levator scapula or upper trapezius, which elevate the scapula, will compromise positioning of the glenoid during humeral elevation, interfering with normal scapulohumeral rhythm.

- It is critical for the scapula to maintain a stable base on which the highly mobile humerus can move. Weakness in the rhomboids and/or middle trapezius, which function eccentrically to decelerate the scapula in high-velocity throwing motions, can contribute to scapular hypermobility. Likewise, weakness in the inferior trapezius creates an imbalance in the force couple with the upper trapezius and levator scapula, contributing to scapular hypermobility.

- An injury that affects normal arthokinematic motion at either the sternoclavicular joint or the acromioclavicular joint can also contribute to shoulder impingement. Any limitation in posterior superior clavicular rotation and/or clavicular elevation will prevent normal upward rotation of the scapula during humeral elevation, compromising the subacromial space.

Rehabilitation Concerns. Management of shoulder impingement involves gradually restoring normal biomechanics to the shoulder joint in an effort to maintain space under the coracoacromial arch during overhead activities.[63] The sports therapist should address the pathomechanics and the adaptive changes that most often occur with overhead activities.

Overhead activities that involve humeral elevation (full abduction or forward flexion) or a position of humeral flexion, horizontal adduction, and internal rotation are likely to increase the pain.[38] The athlete complains of diffuse pain around the acromion or glenohumeral joint. Palpation of the subacromial space increases the pain.

Exercises should concentrate on strengthening the dynamic stabilizers, the rotator cuff muscles that act to both compress and depress the humeral head relative to the glenoid[32,44,63] (Figures 19-17, 19-18). The inferior rotator cuff muscles in particular should be strengthened to recreate a balance in the force couple with the deltoid in the coronal plane. The supraspinatus should be strengthened to assist in compression of the humeral head into the glenoid (Figures 19-19, 19-20). The external rotators, the infraspinatus and teres minor, are generally weaker concentrically but stronger eccentrically than the internal rotators and should be strengthened to recreate a balance in the force couple with the subscapularis in the transverse plane.

The external rotators and the posterior portion of the joint capsule are tight and tend to limit internal rotation and should be stretched (Figures 19-60, 19-62, 19-64). There is excessive external rotation due to laxity in the anterior portion of the joint capsule, and stretching should be avoided. There might be some tightness in both the inferior and the posterior portions of the joint capsule; this can be decreased by using posterior and inferior glenohumeral joint mobilizations (Figures 19-69, 19-71, 19-72, 19-73).

Strengthening of the muscles that abduct, elevate, and upward rotate the scapula (these include the serratus anterior, upper trapezius, and levator scapula) should also be incorporated (Figures 19-21, 19-25). The middle trapezius and rhomboids should be strengthened eccentrically to help decelerate the scapula during throwing activities (Figure 19-23, 19-24). The inferior trapezius should also be strengthened to recreate a balance in the force couple with the upper trapezius, facilitating scapular stability (Figure 19-22).

Anterior, posterior, inferior, and superior joint mobilizations at both the sternoclavicular and the acromioclavicular joint should be done to assure normal arthrokinematic motion at these joints (Figures 19-65, 19-66, 19-67).

Strengthening of the lower-extremity and trunk muscles to provide core stability is essential for reducing the stresses and strains placed on the shoulder and arm, and this is also important for the overhead athlete (Figure 19-32).

Rehabilitation Progression. In the early stages of a rehabilitation program, the primary goal of the sports therapist is to minimize the pain associated with the impingement syndrome. This can be accomplished by utilizing some combination of activity modification, therapeutic modalities, and appropriate use of NSAIDs.

Initially, the sports therapist should have a coach evaluate the athlete's technique in performing the overhead activity, to rule out faulty performance techniques. Once existing performance techniques have been corrected, the sports therapist must make some decision about limiting the activity that caused the problem in the first place. Activity limitation, however, does not mean immobilization. Instead, a baseline of tolerable activity should be established. The key is to initially control the frequency and the level of the load on the rotator cuff and then to gradually and systematically increase the level and the frequency of that activity. It might be necessary to initially restrict activity, avoiding any exercise that places the shoulder in the impingement position, to give the inflammation a chance to subside. During this period of restricted activity, the athlete should continue to engage in exercises to maintain cardiorespiratory fitness. Working on an upper-extremity erogometer will help to improve both cardiorespiratory fitness and muscular endurance in the shoulder complex.

Therapeutic modalities such as electrical stimulating currents and/or heat and cold therapy may be used to modulate pain. Ultrasound and the diathermies are most useful for elevating tissue temperatures, increasing blood flow, and facilitating the process of healing. NSAIDs prescribed by the team physician are useful not only as analgesics, but also for their long-lasting anti-inflammatory capabilities.

Once pain and inflammation have been controlled, exercises should concentrate on strengthening the dynamic stabilizers of the glenohumeral joint, stretching the inferior and posterior portions of the joint capsule, strengthening the scapular muscles that collectively produce normal scapulohumeral rhythm, and maintaining normal arthrokinematic motions of the acromioclavicular and sternoclavicular joints.

Strengthening exercises are done to establish neuromuscular control of the humerus and the scapula (Figures 19-76 through 19-82). Strengthening exercises should progress from isometric pain-free contractions to isotonic full-range pain-free contractions. Humeral control exercises should be used to strengthen the rotator cuff to restrict migration of the humeral head and to regain voluntary control of the humeral head positioning through rotator cuff stabilization.[70] Scapular control exercises should be used to maintain a normal relationship between the glenohumeral and scapulothorasic joints.[38]

Closed-kinetic-chain exercises for the shoulder should be primarily eccentric. They tend to compress the joint, providing stability, and are perhaps best used for establishing scapular stability and control.[39]

Gradually, the duration and intensity of the exercise may be progressed within individual patient tolerance limitations, using increased pain or stiffness as a guide for progression, eventually progressing to full-range overhead activities.

Criteria for Returning to Full Activity. The athlete may return to full activity when (1) the gradual program used to increase the duration and intensity of the workout has allowed him or her to complete a normal workout without pain; (2) the athlete exhibits improved strength in the appropriate rotator cuff and the scapular muscles; (3) there is no longer a positive impingement sign, drop arm test, or empty can test; and (4) the athlete can discontinue use of anti-inflammatory medications without a return of pain.

Rotator Cuff Tendinitis and Tears

Pathomechanics. Rotator cuff injury has often been described as a continuum starting with impingement of the tendon that, through repetitive compression, eventually leads to irritation and inflammation and eventually fibrosis of the rotator cuff tendon. This idea began with the work of Codman in 1934 when he identified a critical zone near the insertion of the supraspinatus tendon.[42] Since then many researchers in sports medicine have studied this area and have expanded the information base, leading to the identification of other causative factors.[29,49] Neer is also credited with developing a system of classification for rotator cuff disease. This system seemed to be appropriate until sports medicine professionals began dealing with overhead athletes as a separate entity due to the acceleration of repetitive stresses applied to the shoulder. Disease in the overhead athlete usually results from failure due to one or both of these chronic stresses: repetitive tension or compression of the tissue. We now regard rotator cuff injury in athletics as an accumulation of microtrauma to both the static and the dynamic stabilizers of the shoulder complex. In 1993, Meister and Andrews classified these causative traumas based on the pathophysiology of events leading to rotator cuff failure. Their five categories of classification for modes of failure are primary compressive, secondary compressive, primary tensile overload, secondary tensile overload, and macrotraumatic.[42]

Injury Mechanism. Rotator cuff tendonopathy is a gradation of tendon failure, so it is important to identify the causative factors. The following classification system helps group injury mechanisms to better aid the sports therapist in developing a rehabilitation plan.

Primary compressive disease results from direct compression of the cuff tissue. This occurs when something interferes with the gliding of the cuff tendon in the already tight subacromial space. A predisposing factor in this category is a type III hooked acromion process, a common factor seen in younger athletes with rotator cuff disease. Other factors in younger athletes include a congenitally thick coracoacromial ligament and the presence of an os acromiale. In younger athletes, a primary impingement without one of these associated factors is rare. In middle-aged athletes/patients, degenerative spurring on the undersurface of the acromion process can cause irritation of the tendon and eventually lead to complete tearing of the tendon. These individuals are often seen because they experience pain during such activities as tennis and golf.

Secondary compressive disease is a primary result of glenohumeral instability. The high forces generated by the overhead athlete can cause chronic repetitive trauma to the glenoid labrum and capsuloligamentous structures, leading to subtle instability. Athletes with inherent multidirectional instability, such as swimmers, are also at risk. The additional volume created in the glenohumeral capsule allows for extraneous movement of the humeral head, leading to compressive forces in the subacromial space.

Primary tensile overload can also cause tendon irritation and failure. The rotator cuff resists horizontal adduction, internal rotation, anterior translation of the humeral head, and distraction forces in the deceleration phase of throwing and overhead sports. The repetitive high forces generated by eccentric activity in the rotator cuff while attempting to maintain a central axis of rotation can cause microtrauma to the tendon and eventually lead to tendon failure. This type of mechanism is not associated with previous instability of the joint. Causes for this mechanism often are found when evaluating the athlete's mechanics and taking a complete history during the evaluation. The sports therapist might find that the throwing athlete had a history of injury to another area of the body where the muscles are used in the deceleration phase of overhead motion (for example, the right-handed pitcher who sprained his left ankle).

Secondary tensile disease is often a result of primary tensile overload. In this case the repetitive irritation and weakening of the rotator cuff allows for subtle instability. In contrast to secondary compressive disease of the tendon, the rotator cuff tendon experiences greater distractive and tensile forces because the humeral head is allowed to translate anteriorly. Over time, the increased tensile force causes failure of the tendon.

Macrotraumatic failure occurs as a direct result of one distinct traumatic event. The mechanism for this is often a fall on an outstretched arm. This is rarely seen in athletes with normal, healthy rotator cuff tendons. For this to occur, forces generated by the fall must be greater than the tensile strength of the tendon. Because the tensile strength of bone is less than that of young healthy tendon, it is rare to see this in an athlete. It is more common to see a longitudinal tear in the tendon with an avulsion of the greater tubercle.

Rehabilitation Concerns. When designing a rehabilitation program for rotator cuff tendonopathy, the basic concerns remain the same regardless of the extent to which the tendon is damaged. Instead, rehabilitation should be based on why and how the tendon has been damaged. Once the cause of the tendonopathy is identified and secondary factors are known, a comprehensive program can be designed. If a comprehensive rehabilitation program does not relieve the painful shoulder, surgical repair of the tendon and alteration of the glenohumeral joint are performed. Surgical rehabilitation is similar to the nonsurgical plan, with the time of progression altered based on tissue healing and tendon histology.

Conservative management. Stage I of the rehabilitation process is focused on reducing inflammation and removing the athlete from the activity that caused pain. Pain should not be a part of the rehabilitation process. The sports therapist may employ therapeutic modalities to aid in athlete comfort. A course of NSAIDs is usually followed during this stage of rehabilitation. Range-of-motion exercises begin, avoiding further irritation of the tendon. Attention is paid to restoring appropriate arthrokinematics to the shoulder complex. If the injury is a result of a compressive disease to the tendon, capsular stretching may be done (Figures 19-65 to 19-75). Active strengthening of the glenohumeral joint should begin, concentrating on the force couples acting around the joint. Beginning with isometric exercises for the medial and lateral rotators of the joint (Figure 19-6*A*, *B*), and progressing to isotonic exercises if the athlete does not experience pain (Figures 19-17 and 19-18). A towel roll under the athlete's arm can help initiate co-contraction of the shoulder muscles, increasing joint stability. Exercises might need to be altered to limit translational forces of the humeral head. Strengthening of the supraspinatus may begin if 90 degrees of elevation in the scapular plane is available (Figures 19-19, 19-20). Aggressive pain-free strengthening of the periscapular muscle should also start, as the restoration of normal scapular control will be essential to removal of abnormal stresses of the rotator cuff tendon in later stages. The sports therapist might want to begin with manual resistance (Figure 19-26), progressing to free-weight exercises (Figures 19-21 to 19-25).

In stage II, the healing process progresses and range of motion will need to be restored. The sports therapist might need to be more aggressive in stretching techniques, addressing capsular tightness as it develops. The prone-on-elbows position is a good technique for self-mobilization (Figure 19-63*B*). This position should be avoided if compressive disease was part of the irritation. If pain continues to be absent, strengthening gets increasingly aggressive. Isokinetic exercises at speeds greater than 200 degrees per second for shoulder medial and lateral rotation may begin (Figure 19-38).

Aggressive neuromuscular control exercises are started in this stage: quick reversals during PNF diagonal patterns, starting with manual resistance from the sports therapist and advancing to resistance applied by surgical tubing (Figures 19-46 and 19-47). A Body Blade may also be used for rhythmic stabilization (Figure 19-48).

The exercise program should now progress to free weights, and eccentric exercises of the rotator cuff should be emphasized to meet the demands of the shoulder in overhead activities. Strengthening of the deltoid and upper trapezius muscles can begin above 90 degrees of elevation. Exercises include the military press (Figure 19-10), shoulder flexion (Figure 19-12), and reverse flys (Figure 19-16). Push-ups can also be added. It might be necessary to restrict range of motion so the body does not go below the elbow, to prevent excessive translation of

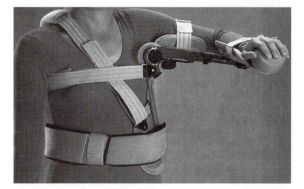

Figure 19-89 Airplane splint.

the glenohumeral joint. This author prefers combining this exercise with serratus anterior strengthening in a modified push-up with a plus (Figure 19-25).

In the later part of this stage, exercises should progress to plyometric strengthening. Surgical tubing is used to allow the athlete to exercise in 90 degrees of elevation with the elbow bent to 90 degrees (Figure 19-31). Plyoball exercises are initiated (Figures 19-32, 19-33). The weight and distance of the exercises can be altered to increase demands. The Shuttle 2000-1 is an excellent exercise to increase eccentric strength in a plyometric fashion (Figure 19-36).

Stage III of the rehabilitation focuses on sport-specific activities. With throwing and overhead athletes, an interval overhead program begins. Total body conditioning, return of strength, and increased endurance are the emphasis. The athlete should remain pain-free as sport-specific activities are advanced and a gradual return to sport is achieved.

Postsurgical management. If conservative management is insufficient, surgical repair is often indicated. The type of repair done depends on the classification of the injury. Subacromial decompression has been described by Neer as a method to stimulate tissue healing and increase the subacromial space.[45] Additional procedures may be done as open repairs of the tendon along with a capsular tightening procedure. One example is a modified Bankart procedure and capsulolabral reconstruction.[27]

Stage I is often begun with some form of immobilization. This does not mean complete lack of movement. Instead it refers to restricting positions based on the surgical repair. In open repairs, flexion and abduction might be restricted for as long as 4 weeks. When the repair addresses the capsulolabral complex, the athlete might spend up to 2 weeks in an airplane splint (Figure 19-89).

Pain control and prevention of muscle atrophy are addressed in this stage. Shoulder shrugs, isometrics, and joint mobilization for pain control can be done. Later in this stage, active assistive exercises with the L-bar and multiangle isometrics are done in the pain-free range of motion.

Stage II collagen and elastin components have begun to stabilize. Healing tissue should have a decreased level of elastin and an increased level of collagen by now.[59] Regaining full range of motion and increasing the stress to healing tissue for better collagen alignment is important in this stage. Having the athlete hang from an overhead bar (Figure 19-50) or using a rope and pulley system (Figure 19-54) can help achieve desired ROM.

Active range-of-motion exercises are added, progressing from no resistance to resistance with surgical tubing. If a primary repair has been done to the tendon, resisted supraspinatus exercises should be avoided until 10 weeks.

The restoration of normal arthrokinematics and scapulothoracic rhythm is addressed with exercises emphasizing neuromuscular control. The athlete can use a mirror to judge progress.

Stage III remains similar to conservative management. However, the time frame might lag getting to this stage.

Rehabilitation Progression.   The rehabilitation progression for conservatively managed rotator cuff injury should follow along with the progression outlined in the section on impingement syndrome. The following progression is the author's preference for postsurgical progression. The principles followed for rehabilitation progression are based on the dynamics of healing tissue. Depending on the surgical procedure, the time frame for this progression may be altered. A simple way to stage the rehabilitation of the postsurgical athlete is by following the rule of six. During the first 6 weeks after the surgery, the goal is to decrease pain, address inflammation, and prevent muscle atrophy. Therapeutic modalities and gentle ROM are initiated.

The second 6-week period (6 to 12 weeks) begins the stage of rehabilitation where full active and passive range of motion need to be achieved prior to maturation of the healing tissue. Other emphasis is placed on regaining normal static and dynamic joint mechanics. Proprioceptive and neuromuscular exercises are used to achieve this goal.

In the last 6 weeks (12 to 18 weeks), the repair should be mature enough to tolerate progression to activities that prepare the athlete for return to activity. Speed and control of resisted exercises are increased. Plyometric training and interval progression to sport-specific activities are used. This stage ends with the athlete's return to activity.

Criteria for Return to Activity.   Return to full activity should be based on these criteria: (1) The athlete has full active range of motion. (2) Normal mechanics have been restored in the shoulder complex. (3) The athlete has at least 90 percent strength in the involved shoulder as compared to the uninvolved side. (4) There is no pain present during overhead activity.

Adhesive Capsulitis (Frozen Shoulder)

Pathomechanics.   Adhesive capsulitis is characterized by the loss of motion at the glenohumeral joint. The cause of this arthrofibrosis is not well defined. One set of criteria used for diagnosis of a frozen shoulder was described by Jobe et al. in 1996, included: (1) decreased glenohumeral motion and loss of synchronous shoulder girdle motion; (2) restricted elevation (less than 135 degrees or 90 degrees, depending on the author); (3) external rotation 50 to 60 percent of normal; and (4) arthrogram findings of 5 to 10 cc volume with obliteration of the normal axillary fold.[30] Other authors have identified histological changes in different areas surrounding the glenohumeral joint.[59] Travell and Simons explained that a reflex autonomic reaction could be the underlying cause, due to the presence of subscapularis trigger points.[65] The result is a chronic inflammation with fibrosis and rotator cuff muscles that are tight and inelastic.

Injury Mechanism.   For the purposes of this chapter, we will separate this diagnosis into two categories: primary versus secondary frozen shoulder. Adhesive capsulitis may be considered primary when it develops spontaneously; it is considered secondary when a known underlying condition (e.g., a fractured humeral head) is present.

Primary frozen shoulder usually has a insidious onset. The patient often describes a sequence of painful restrictions in their shoulder, followed by a gradual stiffness with less pain. Factors that have been found to predispose a patient to idiopathic capsulitis include diabetes, hypothyroidism, and underlying cardiopulmonary involvement.[59] These factors were identified through epidemiological studies and might have more to do with characteristic personalities of these patients. It is rare to see this type of frozen shoulder in the athletic population.

Secondary frozen shoulder is more commonly seen in the athletic population. It has been associated with many different underlying diagnoses. Rockwood and Matsen listed eight categories of conditions that should be considered in the differential diagnosis of frozen shoulder: trauma, other soft-tissue disorders about the shoulder, joint disorders, bone disorders, cervical spine disorders, intrathoracic disorders, abdominal disorders, and psychogenic disorder[55] (Table 19-3).

■ **TABLE 19-3**   Differential Diagnosis
of Frozen Shoulder

Trauma

Fractures of the shoulder region
Fractures anywhere in the upper extremity
Misdiagnosed posterior shoulder dislocation
Hemarthrosis of shoulder secondary to trauma

Other Soft-Tissue Disorders About the Shoulder

Tendinitis of the rotator cuff
Tendinitis of the long head of biceps
Subacromial bursitis
Impingement
Suprascapular nerve impingement
Thoracic outlet syndrome

Joint Disorders

Degenerative arthritis of the AC joint
Degenerative arthritis of the glenohumeral joint
Septic arthritis
Other painful forms of arthritis

Bone Disorders

Avascular necrosis of the humeral head
Metastatic cancer
Paget's disease
Primary bone tumor
Hyperparathyroidism

Cervical Spine Disorders

Cervical spondylosis
Cervical disc herniation
Infection

Intrathoracic Disorder

Diaphragmatic irritation
Pancoast tumor
Myocardial infarction

Abdominal Disorder

Gastric ulcer
Cholecystitis
Subphrenic abscess

Psychogenic

From C. A. Rockwood and F. A. Matsen. 1990. The Shoulder.
Philadelphia: W. B. Saunders.

Rehabilitation Concerns.   The primary concern for rehabilitation is proper differential diagnosis. Attempting to progress the patient into the strength or functional activities portion of a rehabilitation program can lead to exacerbation of the motion restriction. The single best treatment for adhesive capsulitis is prevention.

Depending on the stage of pathology when intervention is started, the rehabilitation program time frame can be shortened. In all cases, the goals of rehabilitation are the same: first relieving the pain in the acute stages of the disorder, gradually restoring proper arthrokinematics, gradually restoring range of motion, and strengthening the muscles of the shoulder complex.

Rehabilitation Progression.   In the acute phase, Codman's exercises and low-grade joint mobilization techniques can be used to relieve pain. This may be accompanied by therapeutic modalities and passive stretching of the upper trapezius and levator scapulae muscles. The sports therapist may also want to suggest that the patient sleep with a pillow under the involved arm to prevent internal rotation during sleep.

In the subacute phase, range of motion is more aggressively addressed. Incorporating PNF techniques such as hold-relax can be helpful. Progressive demands should be placed on the patient with rhythmic stabilization techniques. Wall climbing (Figure 19-53) and wall/corner stretches (Figure 19-55) are also good additions to the rehabilitation program. As ROM returns, the program should start to address strengthening. Isometric exercises for the shoulder are often the best way to begin. Progressive strengthening will continue in the next phase.

The final phase of rehabilitation is a progressive strengthening of the shoulder complex. Exercises for maintenance of ROM continue, and a series of strengthening exercises should be added. The rehabilitation program should be tailored to meet the needs of the patient based on the differential diagnosis.

Criteria for Return to Activity.   The patient may return to their previous level of activity once the proper physiological and arthrokinematic motion has been restored to the glenohumeral joint. How long the patient went untreated and undiagnosed will affect how long it takes to reach this point.

Thoracic Outlet Syndrome

Pathomechanics.   Thoracic outlet syndrome is the compression of neurovascular structures within the thoracic outlet. The thoracic outlet is a cone-shaped passage, with the greater circumferential opening proximal to the spine and the narrow end passing into the distal extremity. On the proximal end, the cone is bordered anteriorly by the anterior scalene muscles, and posteriorly by the middle and posterior scalene muscles. Structures traveling through the thoracic outlet are the brachial plexus, subclavian artery and vein, and axillary vessels. The neurovascular structures pass distally under the clavicle and subclavius muscle. Beneath the neurovascular bundle is the first rib. At the narrow end of the cone, the bundle passes under the coracoid process of the scapula and into the upper extremity through the axilla. The distal end is bordered anteriorly by the pectoralis minor and posteriorly by the scapula.

Based on the anatomy of the thoracic outlet, there are several areas where neurovascular compression can occur. Therefore, pathology of the thoracic outlet syndrome is dependent on the structures being compressed.

Injury Mechanism. In 60 percent of the population affected by thoracic outlet syndrome, there is no report from the patient of an inciting episode.[35] Some of the theories presented by authors regarding the etiology of thoracic outlet syndrome include trauma, postural components, shortening of the pectoralis minor, shortening of the scalenes, and muscle hypertrophy.

There are four areas of vulnerability to compressive forces: the superior thoracic outlet, where the brachial plexus passes over the first rib; the scalene triangle, at the proximal end of the thoracic outlet, where there might be overlapping insertions of the anterior and middle scalenes onto the first rib; the costoclavicular interval, which is the space between the first rib and clavicle where the neurovascular bundle passes (the space can be narrowed by poor posture, inferior laxity of the glenohumeral joint, or an exostosis from a fracture of the clavicle); and under the coracoid process where the brachial plexus passes and is bordered anteriorly by the pectoralis minor.[59]

Rehabilitation Concerns. As described, thoracic outlet syndrome is an anatomy-based problem involving compressive forces applied to the neurovascular bundle. Conservative management of thoracic outlet syndrome is moderately successful, resulting in decreased symptoms 50 to 90 percent of the time. As the first course of treatment, rehabilitation should be based on encouraging the least provocative posture. Leffert advocated a detailed history and evaluation of the athlete's activities and lifestyle to help identify where and when postural deficiency is occurring.[35]

Through a detailed history and evaluation of an athlete's activity, the sports therapist can identify the cause of compression in the thoracic outlet. The rehabilitation program should be tailored to encourage good posture throughout the athlete's day. Therapeutic exercises should be used to strengthen postural muscles, such as

the rhomboids (Figure 19-24), middle trapezius (Figure 19-23), and upper trapezius (Figure 19-21). Flexibility exercises are also used to increase the space in the thoracic outlet. Scalene stretches and wall/corner stretches (Figure 19-55) are used to decrease the incidence of muscle impinging on the neurovascular bundle. Proper breathing technique should also be reviewed with the athlete. The scalene muscles act as accessory breathing muscles, and improper breathing technique can lead to tightening of these muscles.

Rehabilitation Progression. The rehabilitation process begins by detailed evaluation of the athlete's activities and symptoms. First, the athlete is removed from activities exacerbating the neurovascular symptoms until the athlete can maintain a symptom-free posture. During this time an erect posture is encouraged using stretching and strengthening exercises. Gradually encourage the athlete to return to their sport, for short periods of time, while maintaining a pain-free posture. The time of participation is increased at regular intervals if the athlete remains pain-free. This helps build endurance of the postural muscles. Exercising on an upper-body ergometer, by pedaling backward, can help build endurance. As the athlete returns to sports, it may be necessary to alter strength-training methods that place the athlete in a flexed posture.

Criteria for Return to Activity. If the athlete responds to the rehabilitation program and can maintain a pain-free posture during their sport-specific activity, participation can be resumed. The athlete should have no muscular weakness, neurovascular symptoms, or pain. If the athlete fails to respond to therapy, and functionally significant pain and weakness persist, surgical intervention might be indicated. Surgical procedure depends on the anatomical basis for the patient's symptoms.

Brachial Plexus Injuries (Stinger or Burner)

Pathomechanics. The brachial plexus begins at cervical roots c5 through c8 and thoracic root t1. The ventral rami of these roots are formed from a dorsal (sensory) and ventral (motor) root. The ventral rami join to form the brachial plexus. The ventral rami lie between the anterior and middle scalene muscles, where they run adjacent to the subclavian artery. The plexus continues distally passing over the first rib. It is deep to the sternocleidomastoid muscle in the neck.[46] Just caudal to the clavicle and subclavius muscle, the five ventral rami unite to form the three trunks of the plexus: superior, middle, inferior. The superior trunk is composed of the c5 and c6 ventral roots. The middle trunk is formed by the c7 root, and the inferior trunk is formed by c8 and t1 ventral roots. After passing under the clavicle, the three trunks divide into three divisions that eventually contribute to the three cords of the brachial plexus.

The typical picture of a brachial plexus injury in sports is that of a traction injury. This syndrome is commonly referred to as burner or stinger syndrome. These injuries usually involve the c5 to c6 nerve roots. The athlete will complain of a sharp, burning pain in the shoulder that radiates down the arm into the hand. Weakness in the muscles supplied by c5 and c6 (deltoid, biceps, supraspinatus, and infraspinatus) accompany the pain. Burning and pain are often transient, but weakness might last a few minutes or indefinitely.

Clancy et al. have classified brachial plexus injuries into three categories.[11] A grade I injury results in a transient loss of motor and sensory function, which usually resolves completely within minutes. A grade II injury results in significant motor weakness and sensory loss that might last from 6 weeks to 4 months. EMG evaluation after 2 weeks will demonstrate abnormalities. Grade III lesions are characterized by motor and sensory loss for at least 1 year in duration.

Injury Mechanism. The structure of the brachial plexus is such that it winds its way through the musculoskeletal anatomy of the upper extremity as described above. Clancy et al. identified neck rotation, neck lateral flexion, shoulder abduction, shoulder external rotation, and simultaneous scapular and clavicular depression as potential mechanisms of injury.[11]

During neck rotation and lateral flexion to one side, the brachial plexus and the subclavius muscle on the opposite side are put on stretch and the clavicle is slightly elevated about its A-P axis. If the arm is not elevated, the superior trunk of the plexus will assume the greatest amount of tension. If the shoulder is abducted and externally rotated, the brachial plexus migrates superiorly toward the coracoid process and the scapula retracts, putting the pectoralis minor on stretch. As the shoulder is moved into full abduction, a condition similar to a movable pully is formed, where the coracoid process of the scapula acts as the pulley. In full abduction, most stress falls on the lower cords of the brachial plexus.[60] The addition of clavicular and scapula depression to the above scenarios would produce a downward force on the pulley system, bringing the brachial plexus into contact with the clavicle and the coracoid process. The portion of the plexus that receives the greatest amount of tensile stress depends on the position of the upper extremity during a collision.

Rehabilitation Concerns. Management of brachial plexus injuries begins with the gradual restoration of the athlete's cervical range of motion. Muscle tightness caused by the direct trauma, and by reflexive guarding that occurs because of pain, needs to be addressed. Gentle passive range-of-motion exercises and stretching for the upper trapezius, levator scapulae, and scalene muscles should be done. The sports therapist should be careful not to cause sensory symptoms.

Strengthening of the involved muscles is also addressed in the rehabilitation program. Supraspinatus strengthening exercises like scaption (Figure 19-19) and alternative supraspinatus exercises (Figure 19-20) should be done. Other exercises for involved musculature are shoulder lateral rotation (Figure 19-18) for the infraspinatus, forward flexion and abduction to 90 degrees (Figures 19-12 and 19-14) to strengthen the deltoid, and bicep curls for elbow flexion.

The sports therapist should also work closely with the athlete's coach to evaluate the athlete's technique and correct any alteration in form that might be putting the athlete at risk for burners. Prior to return to activity, the athlete's equipment should be inspected for proper fitting, and a cervical neck roll should be used to decrease the amount of lateral flexion that occurs during impact, as in tackling.

Rehabilitation Progression. The athlete is removed from activity immediately after the injury. The rehabilitation progression should begin with the restoration of both active and passive range of motion at the neck and shoulder. As the athlete gets return of ROM, strengthening of the neck and shoulder are incorporated into the rehabilitation program. Strengthening should progress from PRE-type strengthening with free weights to exercises that emphasize power and endurance. Functional progression begins with teaching proper technique for sport-specific demands that mimic the position of injury. The progressive return and proper technique are important to the rehabilitation program, as they address the psychological component of preparing the athlete for return to sport.

Criteria for Return to Activity. Athletes are allowed to return to play when they have full, pain-free range of motion, full strength, and no prior episodes in that contest.[68] Additionally, football players should use a cervical neck roll. The athlete's psychological readiness should also be considered prior to return to sport. Athletes who are too protective of their neck and shoulder can expose themselves to further injury.

Myofascial Trigger Points

Pathology. Clinically, a trigger point (TP) is defined as a hyperirritable foci in muscle or fascia that is tender to palpation and may, upon compression, result in referred pain or tenderness in a characteristic "zone." This zone is distinct from myotomes, dermatomes, schlerotomes, or peripheral nerve distribution. TPs are identified via palpation of taut bands of muscle or discrete nodules or adhesions. Snapping of a taut band will usually initiate a local twitch response.[59]

Physiologically, the definition of a trigger point is not as clear. Muscles with myofascial trigger points reveal no diagnostic abnormalities upon EMG examination. Routine laboratory tests show no abnormalities or significant changes attributable to TPs. Normal serum enzyme concentrations have been reported with a shift in the distribution of LDH- isoenzymes. Skin temperature over active TPs might be higher in a 5 to 10 cm diameter.[65]

Travell and Simons classify TPs as follows:[65]

1. *Active Tps.* Symptomatic at rest with referral pain and tenderness upon direct compression. Associated weakness and contracture are often present.
2. *Latent Tps.* Pain is not present unless direct compression is applied. These might show up on clinical exam as stiffness and/or weakness in the region of tenderness.
3. *Primary Tps.* Located in specific muscles.
4. *Associated Tps.* Located within the referral zone of a primary TP's muscle or in a muscle that is functionally overloaded in compensation for a primary TP.

Pathology of a myofascial trigger point is identified with (1) a history of sudden onset during or shortly after an acute overload stress or chronic overload of the affected muscle; (2) characteristic patterns of pain in a muscle's referral zone; (3) weakness and restriction in the end range of motion of the affected muscle; (4) a taut, palpable band in the affected muscle; (5) focal tenderness to direct compression, in the band of taut muscle fibers; (6) a local twitch response elicited by snapping of the tender spot; and (7) reproduction of the patient's pain through pressure on the tender spot.

Injury Mechanism. The most common mechanism for myofascial trigger points in the shoulder region is acute muscle strain (Table 19-4). The damaged muscle tissue causes tearing of the sarcoplasmic reticulum and release of its stored calcium, with loss of the ability of that portion of the muscle to remove calcium ions. The chronic stress of sustained muscle contraction can cause continued muscle damage, repeating the above cycle of damage. The combined presence of the normal muscle ATP supplies and excessive calcium initiate and maintain a sustained muscle band contracture. This produces a region of the muscle with an uncontrolled metabolism, to which the body responds with local vasoconstriction.

■ **TABLE 19-4** Trigger Points of the Shoulder

Posterior shoulder pain

Deltoid
Levator scapulae
Supraspinatus
Subscapularis
Teres minor
Teres major
Serratus posterior superior
Triceps
Trapezius

Anterior shoulder pain

Infraspinatus
Deltoid
Scalene
Supraspinatus
Pectoralis major
Pectoralis minor
Biceps
Coracobrachialis

Adapted from Travell and Simons.[65]

This region of increased metabolism and decreased local circulation, with muscle fibers passing through that area, causes muscle shortening independent of local motor unit action potentials. This taut band can be palpated in the muscle.

Rehabilitation Concerns. The principal mechanism of myofascial trigger points is related to muscular overload and fatigue, so the primary concern is identification of the incriminating activity. The sports therapist should take a detailed history of the athlete's daily activity demands, as well as the changing demands of their sport activities.

The cyclic nature of TPs requires interruption of the cycle for successful treatment. Interrupting the shortening of the muscle fibers and prevention of further breakdown of the muscle tissue components should be attempted using modified hold-relax techniques and post-isometric stretching. Travell and Simons advocate a spray-and-stretch method, where vapocoolant spray is applied and passive stretching follows. Theoretically, when the muscle is placed in a stretched position and the skin receptors are cooled, a reflexive inhibition of the contracted muscle is facilitated, allowing for increased passive stretching.[65]

After a treatment session where passive range of motion has been achieved, the muscle must be activated to stimulate normal actin and myosin crossbridging. Gentle active range-of-motion exercises or active assistive exercises with the L-bar might be a good activity to use as post-treatment activity. Normal muscle activity and endurance must be encouraged after range of motion is restored. A gradual progression of shoulder exercises with an endurance emphasis should be used.

Rehabilitation Progression. Treatment progression for TPs should begin with temporary removal from activities that overload the contracted tissue. The athlete is then treated with myofascial stretching techniques to increase the length of the contracted tissue. Immediate use of the extended range of motion should be emphasized. Strengthening exercises are added once the athlete can maintain the normal muscle length without initiating the return of the contracted myofascial band. As strength and function of the involved muscles return, the athlete may gradually return to their sport.

Criteria for Return to Activity. The athlete may return to activity in a relatively short period of time if they can demonstrate the ability to function without reinitiating the myofascial trigger points and associated taut bands. Early return without meeting this criterion can lead to greater regionalization of the symptoms.

Summary

1. The high degree of mobility in the shoulder complex requires some compromise in stability, which in turn increases the vulnerability of the shoulder joint to injury, particularly in dynamic overhead athletic activities.

2. In rehabilitation of the sternoclavicular joint, effort should be directed toward regaining normal clavicular motion that will allow the scapula to abduct and upward rotate throughout 180 degrees of humeral abduction. The clavicle must elevate approximately 40 degrees to allow upward scapular rotation.

3. Acromioclavicular joint sprains are most commonly seen in athletes due to a direct fall on the point of the shoulder with the arm at the side in an adducted position or falling on an outstretched arm.

4. Management of acromioclavicular injuries depends on the type of injury. Types I and II injuries are usually handled conservatively, focusing on strengthening of the deltoid, trapezius, and the clavicular fibers of the pectoralis major. Occasionally AC injuries require surgical excision of the distal portion of the clavicle.

5. Treatment for clavicle fractures includes approximation of the fracture and immobilization for 6 to 8 weeks, using a figure 8 wrap with the involved arm in a sling. Because mobility of the clavicle is important for normal shoulder mechanics, rehabilitation should focus on joint mobilization and strengthening of the deltoid, upper trapezius, and pectoralis major muscles.

6. Following a short immobilization period, rehabilitation for a dislocated shoulder should focus on restoring the appropriate axis of rotation for the glenohumeral joint, optimizing the stabilizing muscle's length-tension relationship, and restoring proper neuromuscular control of the shoulder complex. Similar rehabilitation strategies are applied in cases of multidirectional instabilities, which can occur as a result of recurrent dislocation.

7. Management of shoulder impingement involves gradually restoring normal biomechanics to the shoulder joint in an effort to maintain space under the coracoacromial arch during overhead activities. Techniques include strengthening of the rotator cuff muscles, strengthening of the muscles that abduct, elevate, and upward rotate the scapula, and stretching both the inferior and the posterior portions of the joint capsule.

8. The basic concerns of a rehabilitation program for rotator cuff tendonopathy are based on why and how the tendon has been damaged. If a comprehensive rehabilitation program does not relieve the painful shoulder, surgical repair of the tendon and alteration of the glenohumeral joint are performed. Surgical rehabilitation is similar to the nonsurgical plan, with the time of progression altered, based on tissue healing and tendon histology.

9. In cases of adhesive capsulitis, the goals of rehabilitation are relieving the pain in the acute stages of the disorder, gradually restoring proper arthrokinematics, gradual restoration of range of motion, and strengthening the muscles of the shoulder complex.

10. Rehabilitation for thoracic outlet syndrome should be directed toward encouraging the least provocative posture combined with exercises to strengthen postural muscles (rhomboids, middle trapezius, upper trapezius) and stretching exercises for the scalenes to increase the space in the thoracic outlet in order to reduce muscle impingement on the neurovascular bundle.

11. Management of brachial plexus injuries includes the gradual restoration of cervical range of motion, and stretching for the upper trapezius, levator scapulae, and scalene muscles.
12. After identifying the cause of myofascial trigger points, rehabilitation may include a spray-and-stretch method with passive stretching, gentle active range-of-motion exercises or active assistive exercises, encouraging normal muscle activity and endurance, and gradual improvement of muscle endurance.

References

1. Allman, F. L. 1967. Fractures and ligamentous injuries of the clavicle and its articulations. *Journal of Bone and Joint Surgery* 49A:774.
2. Anderson, L., R. Rush, and L. Shearer. 1992. The effects of a TheraBand exercise program on shoulder internal rotation strength. Phys Ther (Suppl) 72(6): 540.
3. Andrews, J. R., and K. E. Wilk. eds. 1994. *The athlete's shoulder.* New York: Churchill Livingstone.
4. Bateman, J. E. 1971. *The shoulder and neck.* Philadelphia: W. B. Saunders.
5. Bergfeld, J. A., J. T. Andrish, and W. G. Clancy. 1978. Evaluation of the acromioclavicular joint following first and second degree sprains. *American Journal of Sports Medicine* 6:153.
6. Bigliani, L., J. Kimmel, and P. McCann. 1992. Repair of rotator cuff tears in tennis players. *American Journal of Sports Medicine* 20(2): 112–17.
7. Bigliani, L., D. Morrison, and E. April. 1986. The morphology of the acromion and its relation to rotator cuff tears. *Ortho Trans* 10:216.
8. Blackburn, T., W. McCloud, and B. White. 1990. EMG analysis of posterior rotator cuff exercises. *Ath Train* 25(1): 40–45.
9. Brewster, C., and D. Moynes. 1993. Rehabilitation of the shoulder following rotator cuff injury or surgery. *Journal of Orthopaedic and Sports Physical Therapy* 18(2): 422–26.
10. Burkhead, W., and C. Rockwood. 1992. Treatment of instability of rotator cuff injuries in the overhead athlete. *Journal of Bone and Joint Surgery* 74A:890.
11. Clancy, W. G., R. I. Brand, and J. A. Bergfeld. 1977. Upper trunk brachial plexus injuries in contact sports. *American Journal of Sports Medicine* 5:209.
12. Codman, E. A. 1934. Ruptures of the supraspinatus tendon and other lesions in or about the subacromial bursa. In *The shoulder,* edited by E. A. Codman. Boston: Thomas Todd.
13. Cox, J. S. 1981. The fate of the acromioclavicular joint in athletic injuries. *American Journal of Sports Medicine* 9:50.
14. Culham, E., and P. Malcolm. 1993. Functional anatomy of the shoulder complex. *Journal of Orthopaedic and Sports Physical Therapy* 18(1): 342–50.
15. Davies, G., and S. Dickoff-Hoffman. 1993. Neuromuscular testing and rehabilitation of the shoulder complex. *Journal of Orthopaedic and Sports Physical Therapy* 18(2): 449–58.
16. Depalma, A. F. 1973. *Surgery of the shoulder.* 2d ed. Philadelphia: Lippincott.
17. Dvir, Z., and N. Berme. 1978. The shoulder complex in elevation of the arm: A mechanism approach. *Journal of Biomechanics* 11:219–25.
18. Duncan, A. 1977. Personal communication to the author. August.
19. Greenfield, B. 1993. Special considerations in shoulder exercises: Plane of the scapula. In *The athlete's shoulder,* edited by J. Andrews and K. Wilk. New York: Churchill Livingstone.
20. Gryzlo, S. M. 1996. Bony disorders: Clinical assessment and treatment. In *Operative techniques in upper extremity sports injuries,* edited by F. W. Jobe. St. Louis: Mosby.
21. Hageman, P., D. Mason, and K. Rydlund. 1989. Effects of position and speed on concentric isokinetic testing of the shoulder rotators. *Journal of Orthopaedic and Sports Physical Therapy* 11:64–69.
22. Hart, D. L., and S. W. Carmichael. 1985. Biomechanics of the shoulder. *Journal of Orthopaedic and Sports Physical Therapy* 6(4): 229–34.
23. Hawkins, R., and R. Bell. 1990. Dynamic EMG analysis of the shoulder muscles during rotational and scapular strengthening exercises. In *Surgery of the shoulder,* edited by M. Post, B. Morey, and R. Hawkins. St. Louis: Mosby.
24. Hawkins, R., and J. Kennedy. 1980. Impingement syndrome in athletes. *American Journal of Sports Medicine* 8:151.
25. Howell, S., and T. Kraft. 1991. The role of the supraspinatus and infraspinatus muscles in glenohumeral kinematics of anterior shoulder instability. *Clin Ortho* 263:128–34.
26. Inman, V. T., J. B. Saunders, and L. C. Abbott. 1944. Observations on the function of the shoulder joint. *Journal of Bone and Joint Surgery* 26:1.
27. Jobe, F. W., ed. 1996. *Operative techniques in upper extremity sports injuries.* St. Louis: Mosby.
28. Jobe, F., and R. Kvnite. 1989. Shoulder pain in the overhand and throwing athlete: The relationship of anterior instability and rotator cuff impingement. *Ortho Rev* 18:963.
29. Jobe, F., and D. Moynes. 1982. Delineation of diagnostic criteria and a rehabilitation program for rotator cuff injuries. *American Journal of Sports Medicine* 10(6): 336–39.
30. Jobe, F. W., Schwab, K. E. Wilk, and J. E. Andrews. 1996. Rehabilitation of the shoulder. In *Clinical orthopedics rehabilitation,* edited by S. B. Brotzman. St. Louis: Mosby.
31. Kannus, P., L. Josza, P. Renstrom, M. Jarvinen, M. Kvist, M. Lehto, P. Oja, and L. Vuori. 1992. The effects of training, immobilization and remobilization on musculoskeletal tissue: 2. Remobilization and prevention of immobilization atrophy. *Scand J Med Sci Sports* 2:164–76.

32. Keirns, M. 1993. Conservative management of shoulder impingement. In *The athlete's shoulder,* edited by J. Andrews and K. Wilk. New York: Churchill Livingstone.

33. Kelley, M. J. 1995. Anatomic and biomechanical rationale for rehabilitation of the athlete's shoulder. *Journal of Sport Rehabilitation* 4:122–54.

34. Kibbler, B. 1991. Role of the scapula in the overhead throwing motion. *Contemp Ortho* 22:525–32.

35. Leffert, R. D. 1990. Neurological problems. In *The shoulder,* edited by C. A. Rockwood and F. A. Matsen. Philadelphia: W. B. Saunders.

36. Lephart, S. M., J. P. Warner, P. A. Borsa, and F. H. Fu. 1994. Proprioception of the shoulder joint in healthy, unstable, and surgically repaired shoulders. *Journal of Shoulder and Elbow Surgery* 3(6): 371–80.

37. Lew, W., J. Lewis, and E. Craig. 1993. Stabilization by capsule ligaments and labrum: Stability at the extremes of motion. In *The shoulder: A balance of mobility and stability,* edited by F. Masten, F. Fu, and R. Hawkins. Rosemont, IL: Am Acad Ortho Surg.

38. Litchfield, R., R. Hawkins, and C. Dillman. 1993. Rehabilitation for the overhead athlete. *Journal of Orthopaedic and Sports Physical Therapy* 18(2): 433–41.

39. Magee, D., and D. Reid. 1995. Shoulder injuries. In *Athletic injuries and rehabilitation,* edited by J. Zachazewski, D. Magee, and W. Quillen. Philadelphia: W. B. Saunders.

40. Matsen, F. A., S. C. Thomas, and C. A. Rockwood. 1990. Glenohumeral instability. In *The shoulder,* edited by C. A. Rockwood and F. A. Matsen. Philadelphia: W. B. Saunders.

41. McCarroll, J. 1995. Golf. In *Athletic injuries of the shoulder,* edited by F. A. Pettrone. New York: McGraw-Hill.

42. Meister, K., and J. R. Andrews. 1993. Classification and treatment of rotator cuff injuries in the overhead athlete. *Journal of Orthopaedic and Sports Physical Therapy* 18(2): 413–21.

43. Moseley, J, F. Jobe, and M. Pink. 1992. EMG analysis of the scapular muscles during a shoulder rehabilitation program. *American Journal of Sports Medicine* 20:128–34.

44. Mulligan, E. 1988. Conservative management of shoulder impingement syndrome. *Ath Train* 23(4): 348–53.

45. Neer, C. 1972. Anterior acromioplasty for the chronic impingement syndrome in the shoulder: A preliminary report. *Journal of Bone Joint Surgery* 54A:41.

46. Nicholas, J. A., and E. B. Hershmann, eds. 1990. *The upper extremity in sports medicine.* St. Louis: Mosby.

47. O'Brien, S., M. Neeves, and A. Arnoczky. 1990. The anatomy and histology of the inferior glenohumeral ligament complex of the shoulder. *American Journal of Sports Education* 18:451.

48. Omer, G. E. 1967. Osteotomy of the clavicle in surgical reduction of anterior sternoclavicular dislocations. *J Trauma* 7(4): 584–90.

49. Ozaki, J., S. Fujimoto, and Y. Nakagawa. 1988. Tears of the rotator cuff of the shoulder associated with pathological changes in the acromion: A study of cadavers. *Journal of Bone Joint Surgery* 70A:1224.

50. Paine, R., and M. Voight. 1993. The role of the scapula. *Journal of Orthopaedic and Sports Physical Therapy* 18(1): 386–91.

51. Peat, M., and E. Culham. 1993. Functional anatomy of the shoulder complex. In *The athlete's shoulder,* edited by J. Andrews and K. Wilk. New York: Churchill Livingstone.

52. Petersson, C., and I. Redlund-Johnell. 1984. The subacromial space in normal shoulder radiographs. *Acta Ortho Scanda* 55:57.

53. Pettrone, F. A., ed. 1995. *Athletic injuries of the shoulder.* New York: McGraw-Hill.

54. Rathburn, J., and I. McNab. 1970. The microvascular pattern of the rotator cuff. *Journal of Bone Joint Surgery* 52B:540.

55. Rockwood, C., and F. Masten. 1990. *The shoulder.* Vols. 1 and 2. Philadelphia: W. B. Saunders.

56. Rowe, C. R. 1956. Prognosis in dislocation of the shoulder. *Journal of Bone Joint Surgery* 38A:957.

57. Salter, E. G., B. S. Shelley, and R. Nasca. 1985. A morphological study of the acromioclavicular joint in humans [Abstract] *Anat Rec* 211:353.

58. Skyhar, M., R. Warren, and D. Altcheck. 1990. Instability of the shoulder. In *The upper extremity in sports medicine,* edited by A. Nicholas and E. B. Hershmann. St. Louis: Mosby.

59. Souza, T. A. 1994. *Sports injuries of the shoulder: Conservative management.* New York: Churchill Livingstone.

60. Stevens, J. H. 1934. The classic brachial plexus paralysis. In *The Shoulder,* edited by E. A. Codman, pp. 344–50. Boston: n.p.

61. Sutter, J. S. 1994. Conservative treatment of shoulder instability. In *The athlete's shoulder,* edited by J. Andrews and K. E. Wilk. New York: Churchill Livingstone.

62. Taft, T. N., F. C. Wilson, and J. W. Ogelsby. 1987. Dislocation of the AC joint, an end result study. *Journal of Bone and Joint Surgery* 69A:1045.

63. Thein, L. 1989. Impingement syndrome and its conservative management. *Journal of Orthopaedic and Sports Physical Therapy* 11(5): 183–91.

64. Townsend, H., F. Jobe, and M. Pink. 1991. EMG analysis of the glenohumeral muscles during a baseball rehabilitation program. *American Journal of Sports Medicine* 19(3): 264–72.

65. Travell, J. G., and D. G. Simons. 1983. *Myofascial pain and dysfunction. The trigger point manual.* Baltimore: Williams & Wilkins.

66. Uthoff, H., J. Loeher, and K. Sarkar. 1987. The pathogenesis of rotator cuff tears. In *The shoulder,* edited by N. Takagishi. Philadelphia: Professional Post Graduate Services.

67. Warner, J., L. Michili, and L. Arslanin. 1990. Patterns of flexibility, laxity, and strength in normal shoulders and shoulders with instability and impingement. *American Journal of Sports Medicine* 18(4): 366–75.

68. Warren, R. F. 1989. Neurological injuries in football. In *Sports Neurology,* edited by B. D. Jordan, P. Tsiaris, and R. F. Warren. Rockville, MD: Aspen.

69. Wilk, K., and J. Andrews. 1993. Rehabilitation following subacromial decompression. *Orthopaedics* 16(3): 349–58.

70. Wilk, K., and C. Arrigo. 1992. An integrated approach to upper extremity exercises. *Ortho Phys Ther Clinics of North Am* 9(2): 337–60.

71. Wilk, K., and C. Arrigo. 1993. Current concepts in the rehabilitation of the athletic shoulder. *Journal of Orthopaedic and Sports Physical Therapy* 18(1): 365–78.

72. Wilk, K., and C. Arrigo. 1993. Current concepts in rehabilitation of the shoulder. In *The athlete's shoulder,* edited by J. Andrews and K. Wilk. New York: Churchill Livingstone.

73. Wilk, K., M. Voight, and M. Kearns. 1993. Stretch shortening drills for the upper extremity: Theory and application. *Journal of Orthopaedic and Sports Physical Therapy* 17(5): 225–39.

CHAPTER 20

Rehabilitation of Elbow Injuries

Pete Zulia
William E. Prentice

After completion of this chapter, the student should be able to do the following:

- Discuss the functional anatomy and biomechanics associated with normal function of the elbow.

- Discuss the various rehabilitative strengthening techniques for the elbow, including both open- and closed-kinetic-chain isometric, isotonic, plyometric, isokinetic, and PNF exercises.

- Identify the various techniques for regaining range of motion, including stretching exercises and joint mobilizations.

- Discuss exercises that may be used to reestablish neuromuscular control.

- Discuss criteria for progression of the rehabilitation program for different elbow injuries.

FUNCTIONAL ANATOMY AND BIOMECHANICS

Anatomically, the elbow joint is three joints in one. The humeroulnar joint, the humeroradial joint, and the proximal radioulnar joint are the articulations that make up the elbow complex (Figure 20-1). The elbow allows for flexion, extension, pronation, and supination movement patterns about the joint complex. The bony limitations, ligamentous support, and muscular stability will help to protect it from vulnerability of overuse and resultant injury. In the athletic environment, the elbow complex can be subjected to forces that can result in various injuries ranging from overhead throwing injuries to blunt trauma.

The elbow complex is composed of three bones: the distal humerus, proximal ulna, and proximal radius. The articulations between these three bones dictate elbow movement patterns.[32] It is also important to mention that the appropriate strength and function of the upper quarter (cervical spine to the hand) needs to be addressed when evaluating the elbow specifically. The elbow complex has an intricate articulation mechanically between the three separate joints of the upper quarter to allow for function to occur.

In the elbow, the joint capsule plays an important role. The capsule is continuous (Figure 20-2A) between the three articulations[19,20] and highly innervated. This is important for not only support of the complex, but also for proprioception of the joint. The capsule of the elbow functions as a neurological link between the shoulder and the hand. This has an affect on upper-quarter activity and is an obvious aspect of the rehabilitation process if injury does occur.

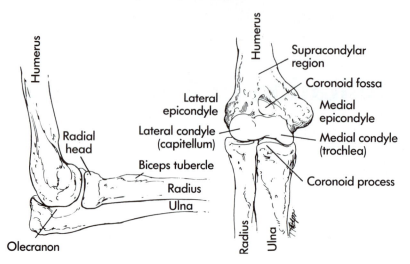

Figure 20-1 Bony anatomy of the elbow (anterior).-

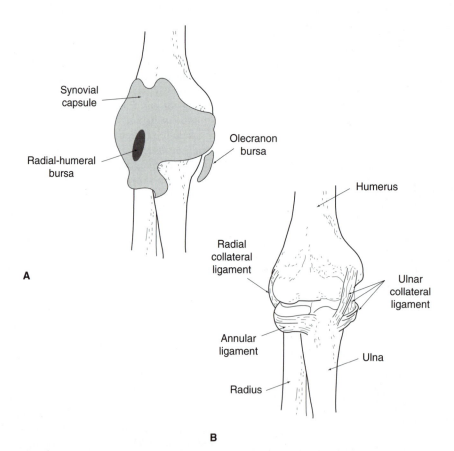

Figure 20-2 **A,** Joint capsule at the elbow joint. **B,** Major supporting ligaments of the elbow.

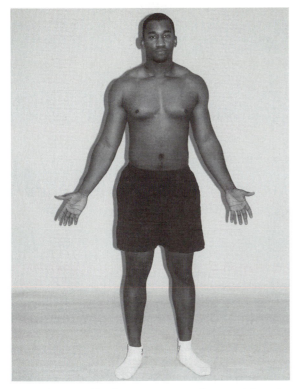

Figure 20-3 The elbow carrying angle is an abducted position of the elbow in the anatomical position. The normal carrying angle in females is 10 to 15 degrees and in males 5 degrees.

Humeroulnar Joint

The humeroulnar joint is the articulation between the distal humerus medially and the proximal ulna. The humerus has distinct features distally. The medial aspect has the medial epicondyle and an hourglass-shaped trochlea[1,15] located anteromedially on the distal humerus. The trochlea extends more distally than the lateral aspect of the humerus. The trochlea articulates with the trochlear notch of the proximal ulna.

Because of the more distal projection of the humerus medially, the elbow complex demonstrates a carrying angle that is an abducted position of the elbow in the anatomical position. The normal carrying angle (Figure 20-3) in females is 10 to 15 degrees and in males 5 degrees.[3] When the elbow is in flexion, the ulna slides forward until the coronoid process of the ulna stops in the floor of the coronoid fossa of the humerus. In extension, the ulna will slide backward until the olecranon process of the ulna makes contact with the olecranon fossa of the humerus posteriorly.

Humeroradial Joint

The humeroradial joint is the articulation of the laterally distal humerus and the proximal radius. The lateral aspect of the humerus has the lateral epicondyle and the capitellum, which is located anteriolaterally on the distal humerus. With flexion, the radius is in contact with the radial fossa of the distal humerus, whereas in extension the radius and the humerus are not in contact.

Proximal Radioulnar Joint

The proximal radioulnar joint is the articulation between the radial notch of the proximal lateral aspect of the ulna, the radial head, and the capitellum of the distal humerus. The proximal and distal radioulnar joints are important for supination and pronation. When evaluating this motion, it is important to look at them as one, functionally. The proximal and distal aspects of this joint cannot function one without the other. Proximally, the radius articulates with the ulna by the support of the annular ligament, which attaches to the ulnar notch anteriorly and posteriorly. The ligament circles the radial head for support. The interosseous membrane is the connective tissue that functions to complete the interval between the two bones. When there is a fall on the outstretched arm, the interosseous membrane can transmit some forces off the radius, the main weight-bearing bone to the ulna. This can help prevent the radial head from having forceful contact with the capitellum. Distally, the concave radius will articulate with the convex ulna. With supination and pronation, the radius will move on the ulna.

Ligamentous Support

The stability of the elbow first starts with the joint capsule that is continuous between all three articulations. The capsule is loose anteriorly and posteriorly to allow for movement in flexion and extension.[38,39] It is taut medially and laterally due to the added support of the collateral ligaments. The capsule is highly innervated for proprioception, as stated earlier.

The medial (ulnar) collateral ligament (MCL) is fan-shaped and has three aspects (Figure 20-2B). The anterior aspect of the MCL is the primary stabilizer in the MCL from approximately 20 degrees to 120 degrees of motion.[34] The posterior and the oblique aspect of the MCL add support and assist in stability to the MCL.

The lateral elbow complex consists of four structures. The radial collateral ligament attachments are from the lateral epicondyle to the annular ligament. The lateral ulnar collateral ligament is the primary lateral stabilizer

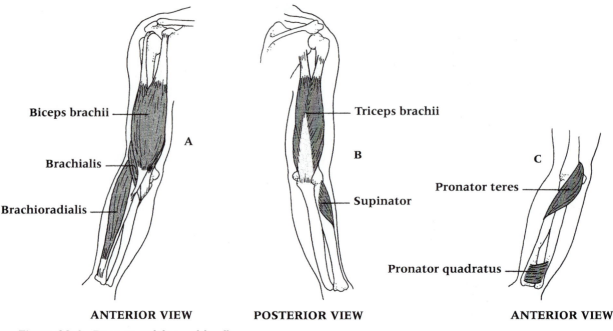

Biceps brachii

Brachialis

Brachioradialis

A

Triceps brachii

B

Supinator

C

Pronator teres

Pronator quadratus

ANTERIOR VIEW   **POSTERIOR VIEW**   **ANTERIOR VIEW**

Figure 20-4   Dynamic stabilizers of the elbow.

and passes over the annular ligament into the supinator tubercle. It reinforces the elbow laterally, and reinforces the humeroradial joint.[24,34] The assessory lateral collateral ligament passes from the tubercle of the supinator into the annular ligament. The annular ligament, as previously stated, is the main support of the radial head in the radial notch of the ulna. The interosseous membrane is a syndesmotic condition that connects the ulna and the radius in the forearm. This structure prevents the proximal displacement of the radius on the ulna.

The Dynamic Stabilizers of the Elbow Complex

The elbow flexors are the biceps brachii, brachialis, and brachioradialis muscles (Figure 20-4). The biceps brachii originate via two heads proximally at the shoulder: the long head from the supraglenoid tuberosity of the scapula and the short head from the coracoid process of the scapula. The insertion is from a common tendon at the radial tuberosity and lacertus fibrosis to origins of the forearm flexors. The biceps brachii function is flexion of the elbow and supination the forearm.[35] The brachialis originates from the lower two-thirds of the anterior humerus to the cornoid process and tuberosity of the ulna. It functions to flex the elbow. The brachioradialis, which originates from the lower two-thirds of the lateral

humerus and attaches to the lateral styloid process of the distal radius, functions as an elbow flexor, semipronator, and semisupinator.

The elbow extensors are the triceps brachii and the anconeus muscles. The triceps brachii has a long, medial and lateral head origination. The long head originates at the infraglenoid tuberosity of the scapula, the lateral and medial heads to the posterior aspect of the humerus. The insertion is via the common tendon posteriorly at the olecranon. Through this insertion along with the anconeus muscle that assists the triceps, extension of the elbow complex is accomplished.

The Elbow in the Upper Quarter

The elbow plays an important part in functional activity in the upper quarter. Anatomical position places the elbow in full extension and full supination. The elbow functions in flexion, extension, supination, and pronation movement patterns. The elbow allows for approximately 145 degrees of flexion and 90 degrees of both supination and pronation, although normals for range of motion are individual for the involved and for the noninvolved joint.[23] The capsule, as previously stated, is a proprioceptive link of the upper quarter to the hand. Functionally, the relationship between the hand and the shoulder needs the elbow for normal movement to occur. The connection between multijoint muscles that affect the elbow will work proximally and distally in the upper quarter as a whole.

The hand and wrist muscles add to the support of the capsule for stability. Function of the cervical spine and shoulder can also affect the elbow. Limitations in motion in either area can cause accommodations in the elbow complex. For example, for an athlete who has a decrease in supination due to injury, an accommodation of the injury is an increase in adduction and external rotation at the shoulder and an increased valgus stress to the elbow to allow function to continue. This is why proper knowledge of biomechanics in the elbow complex and associated joints is essential for proper assessment of injury and rehabilitation.

REHABILITATION TECHNIQUES FOR THE ELBOW COMPLEX

Isotonic Open-Kinetic-Chain Strengthening Exercises

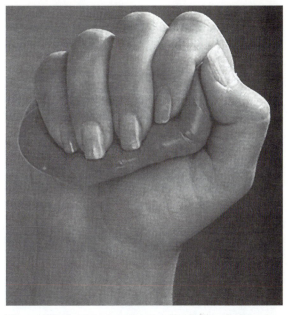

Figure 20-5 Gripping exercise. Used to strengthen the wrist flexors and the intrinsic muscles of the hand.

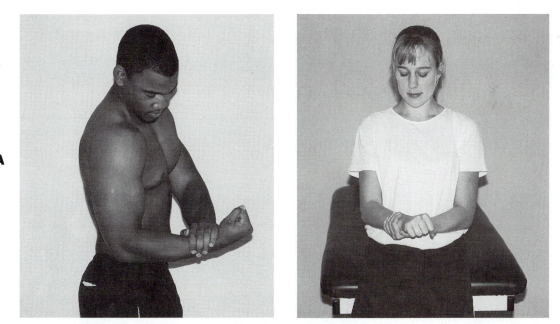

A   B

Figure 20-6 **A,** Isometric elbow flexion; resist elbow flexion with the opposite hand. **B,** Isometric elbow extension; resist elbow extension with the opposite hand. The reeducation that the isometric contractions provide is a safe technique for the early stages of rehabilitation. Contractions can be performed in various angles prior to isotonic exercise.

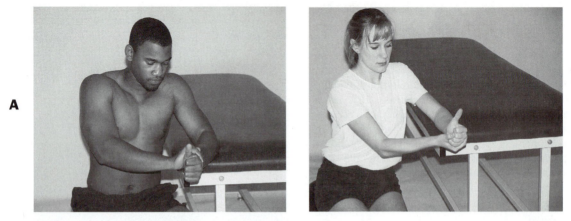

Figure 20-7 **A,** Isometric wrist supination; resist supination with the opposite hand. **B,** Isometric wrist pronation; resist pronation with the opposite hand. This exercise is performed with the same benefits for safe muscle reeducation in the early rehabilitation stages. Resistance can be performed in various angles prior to isotonic exercise.

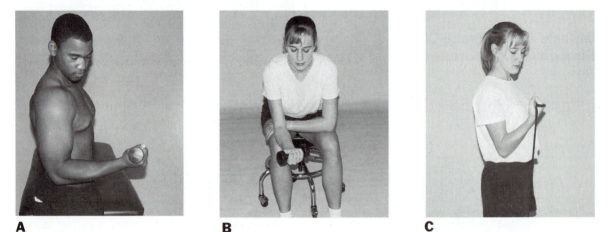

Figure 20-8 Isotonic elbow flexion. The biceps brachii, the brachialis, and the brachioradialis muscles are used when moving the elbow from full extension into full flexion. **A,** Used in the standing position; **B,** in the seated position and the distal humerus resting on the opposite forearm; **C,** with the use of tension band.

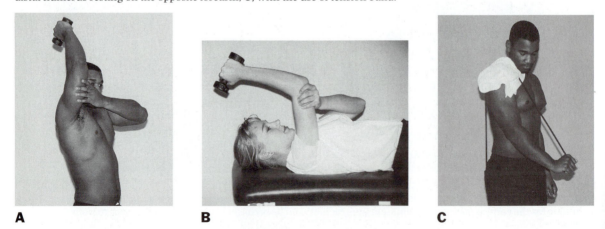

Figure 20-9 Isotonic elbow extension. The triceps brachii muscle moves the arm from full flexion to full extension. **A,** Standing position; **B,** in the supine position; **C,** with the use of tension band.

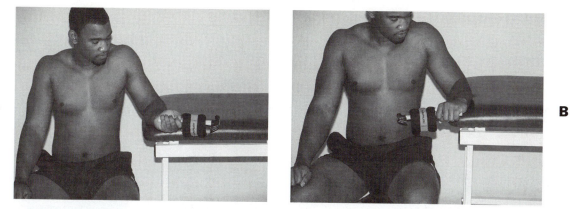

Figure 20-10 Isotonic wrist supination/pronation. The forearm is in a stable position on the table, and the elbow is in a 90-degree position. **A,** Supinate the forearm while holding onto a hammer. **B,** Pronate the forearm while holding a hammer.

Figure 20-11 Concentric/eccentric flexion with the use of tension band for the benefits of maximum load on the muscle. **A,** Concentric: This is done slowly, at first, then the speed is increased to mimic functional activity. **B,** Eccentric: This is done by pulling the muscle into a shortened position, then allowing a lengthening contraction to take place by lowering the hand in control. Increased speed is introduced when proficiency is obtained.

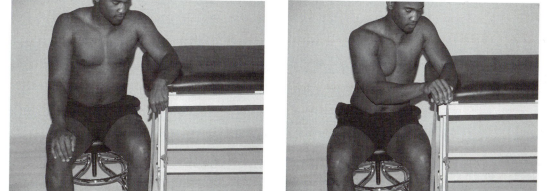

Figure 20-12 Concentric/eccentric extension with the use of tension band for the benefits of maximum load on the muscle. **A,** Concentric: This is done slowly at first, then the speed is increased to mimic functional activity. **B,** Eccentric: This is done by pulling the muscle into a shortened position, then allowing a lengthening contraction to take place by lowering the hand in control. Increased speed is introduced when proficiency is obtained.

Closed-Kinetic-Chain Exercises

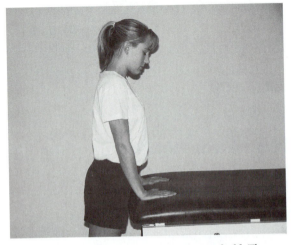

Figure 20-13   Closed-kinetic-chain static hold. The body weight is over the elbow in varying degrees for the purpose of bearing weight and initiating kinesthetic awareness in the elbow joint.

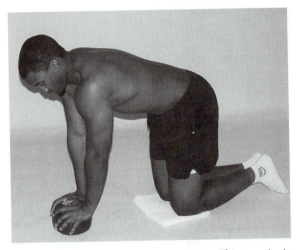

Figure 20-14   Gymnastic ball exercises. This exercise is used for sport-specific rehabilitation in sports that require closed-kinetic-chain activity. There is stimulation of the joint receptors.

A

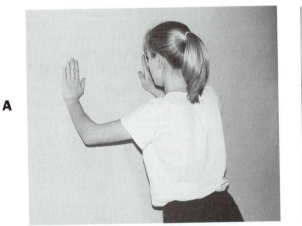

B

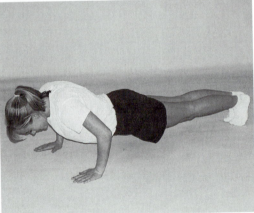

Figure 20-15   Push-ups. **A,** Standing, **B,** prone.

Plyometric Exercises

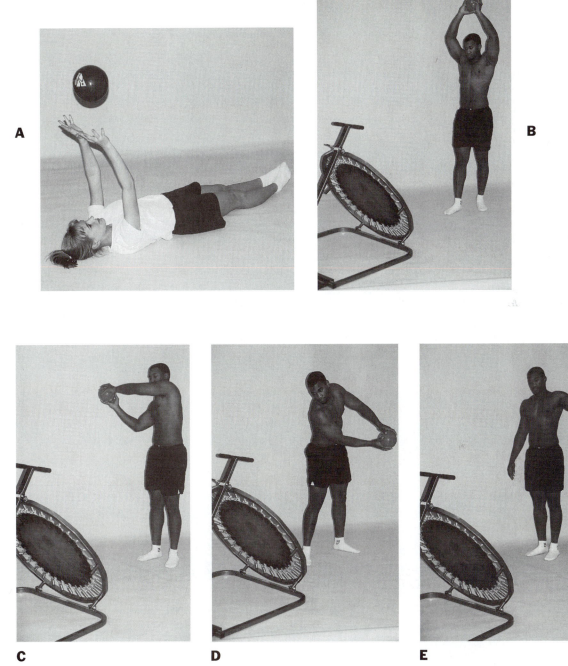

Figure 20-16 Plyometric exercise drills. Plyometric exercise working on a Plyoback has three phases: a quick eccentric load (stretch), a brief amortization phase, and a concentric contraction. **A,** Elbow extensors. **B,** Two-hand overhead toss. **C,** Two-hand side throws. **D,** Side-to-side throws. **E,** One-arm overhead throw.

Isokinetic Exercises

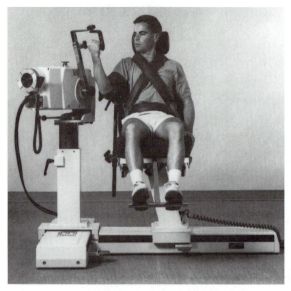

Figure 20-17 Isokinetic elbow flexion (hand positioned in supination).

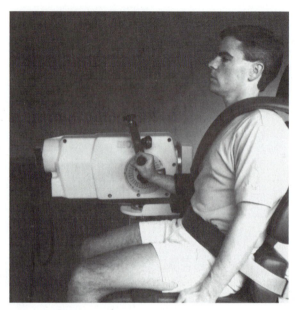

Figure 20-18 Isokinetic wrist flexion/extension.

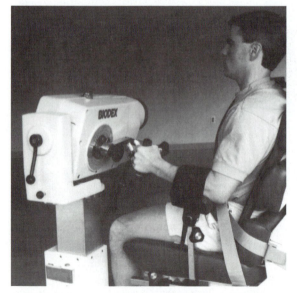

Figure 20-19 Isokinetic wrist supination/pronation.

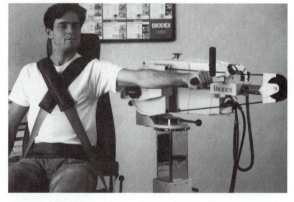

Figure 20-20 Isokinetic elbow flexion/extension with scapular retraction/protraction.

PNF Strengthening Exercises

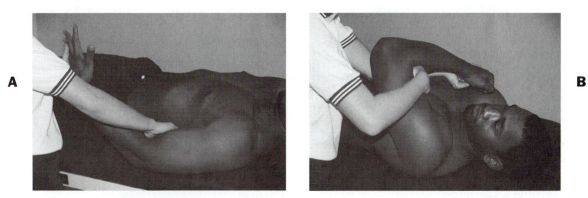

Figure 20-21   D1 pattern moving into flexion **A,** Starting position, **B,** Terminal position.

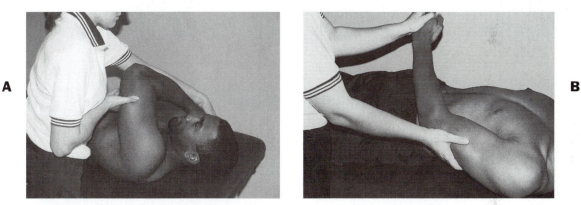

Figure 20-22   D1 Pattern moving into extension. **A,** Starting position. **B,** Terminal position.

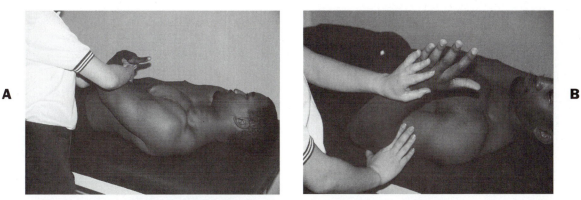

Figure 20-23   D2 pattern moving into flexion. **A,** Starting position. **B,** Terminal position.

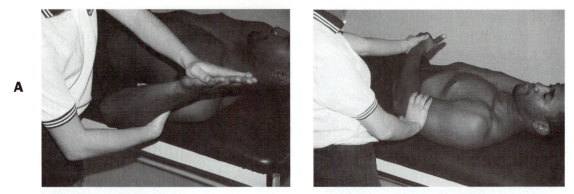

Figure 20-24 D2 pattern moving into extension. **A,** Starting position. **B,** Terminal position.

Stretching Exercises

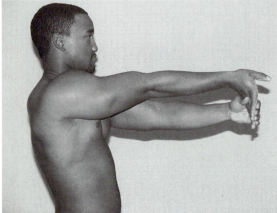

Figure 20-25 Stretching of the elbow and wrist flexors. The elbow is extended with the wrist in extension, the force is applied to stretch the brachialis and brachioradialis.

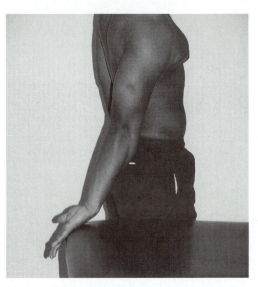

Figure 20-26 Stretching of the biceps brachii. Extend the elbow and pronate the wrist, bring the arm into extension.

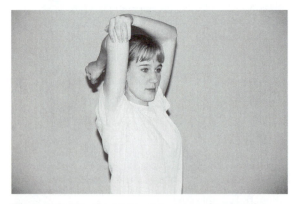

Figure 20-27 Stretching of the triceps brachii. Flex arm with the elbow in flexion, passive force is applied by pulling the arm into flexion.

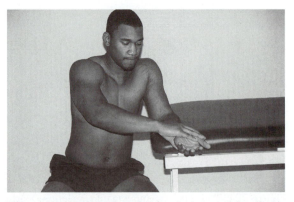

Figure 20-28 Stretching of the pronators of the elbow. Place the forearm on a table. With the opposite hand, pull the wrist into supination.

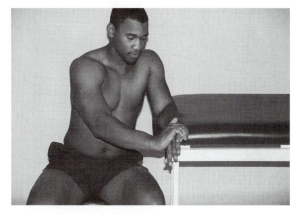

Figure 20-29   Stretching of the supinators of the elbow. Place the forearm on a table. To stretch the supinators, pull the wrist into pronation.

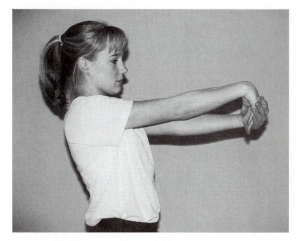

Figure 20-30   Stretching of the wrist extensors.

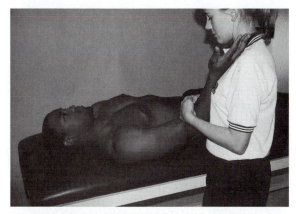

Figure 20-31   Passive distraction. The elbow is at 90 degrees while the athlete is supine, and the arm is in the plane of the body, hands are clasped while a pull on the proximal radius and ulna is performed. Used to increase elasticity of the adhesed joint capsule to enhance range of motion in all planes of motion.

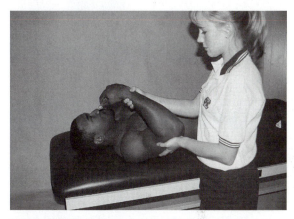

Figure 20-32   Passive flexion. While the athlete is supine and the arm is in the plane of the body, a push of the forearm toward the shoulder is performed to increase the angle of the elbow toward a straight position. Used to increase elasticity of the adhesed joint capsule to enhance range of motion in all planes of motion.

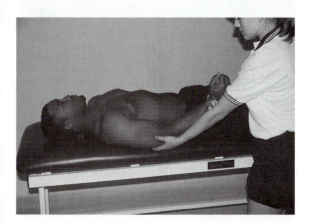

Figure 20-33   Passive extension. While the athlete is supine and the arm is in the plane of the body, a push of the forearm away from the shoulder is performed to decrease the angle of the elbow toward a straight position. Used to increase the elasticity of the adhesed joint capsule to enhance range of motion in all planes of motion.

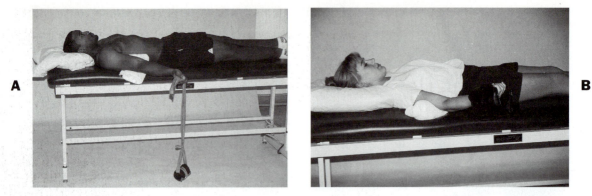

Figure 20-34 Long-duration, low-intensity passive range of motion. **A,** With the use of tension band. **B,** Cuff weight at the wrist. This will increase range of motion by stretching the joint capsule while the athlete is supine and the arm is in anatomic position at the shoulder and the wrist.

Joint Mobilization Techniques

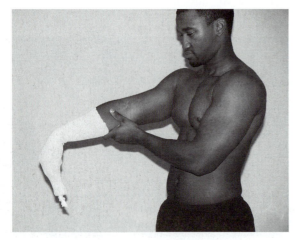

Figure 20-35 Long-duration, low-intensity stretching to increase flexibility to the wrist extensors (can be used for wrist flexors by supinating wrist).

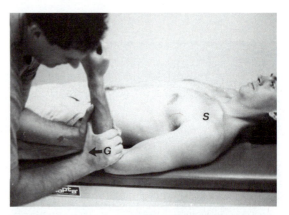

Figure 20-36 Inferior humeroulnar glides increase elbow flexion and extension. They are performed using the body weight to stabilize proximally with the hand grasping the ulna and gliding inferiorly.

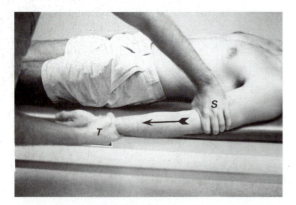

Figure 20-37 Humeroradial inferior glides increase the joint space and improve flexion and extension. One hand stabilizes the humerus above the elbow; the other grasps the distal forearm and glides the radius inferiorly.

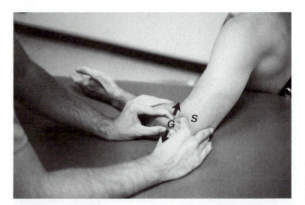

Figure 20-38 Proximal anterior/posterior radial glides use the thumbs and index fingers to glide the radial head. Anterior glides increase flexion, while posterior glides increase extension.

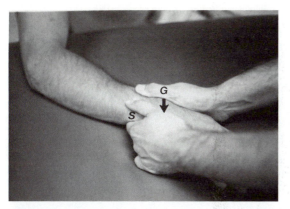

Figure 20-39 Distal anterior/posterior radial glides are done with one hand stabilizing the ulna and the other gliding the radius. These glides increase pronation.

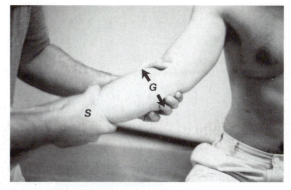

Figure 20-40 Medial and lateral ulnar oscillations increase flexion and extension. Valgus and varus forces are used with a short lever arm.

Exercises to Reestablish Neuromuscular Control

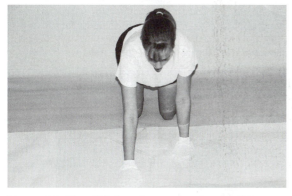

Figure 20-41 Slide board exercises. The closed-kinetic-chain patterns as shown incorporate joint awareness and movement for proprioceptive benefits. Stress to the athlete the importance of developing the weight over the upper quarter while movement patterns are worked.

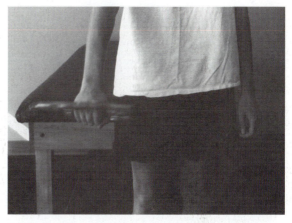

Figure 20-42 Proprioceptive oscillation. This is for kinesthetic/proprioceptive exercises for the elbow and the entire upper quarter. An upper-quarter exercise tool, there are three metal balls in the ring that moves when the upper extremity generates the movement. This can be performed in various positions to mimic arm positioning in sport.

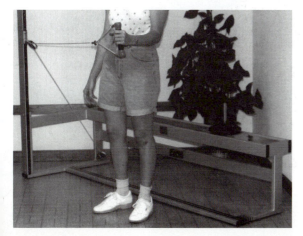

Figure 20-43 Kinesthetic training for timing. This device is used for the purpose of improving proprioception and timing with functional activity. The pulling of the handle causes the weight to move, and with the benefit of inertia, proprioceptive and kinesthetic awareness can improve.

Bracing and Taping.

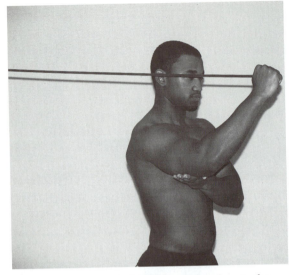

Figure 20-44 Surgical tubing exercises done in the scapular plane to mimic the throwing motion using internal and external rotation.

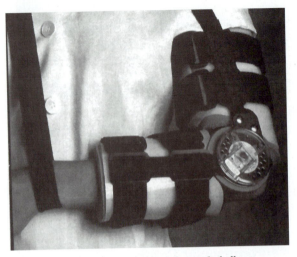

Figure 20-45 Brace to protect the medial elbow structures. This brace is used when injury stress has occurred to the medial aspect of the elbow. The hinge design is developed for valgus and also varus stress, and can have limits on range of motion as well.

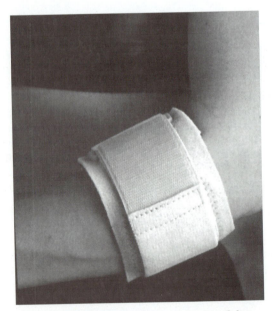

Figure 20-46 Elbow brace for lateral epicondylitis. This brace is used to decrease the tension of the extensor muscles at the elbow. The brace is applied over the extensor muscles just distal to the elbow joint.

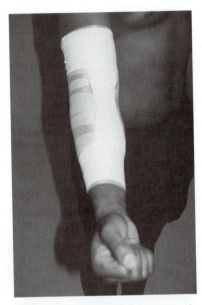

Figure 20-47 Elbow taping for hyperextension of the elbow uses a checkrein to limit extension in the joint.

Functional Exercises.

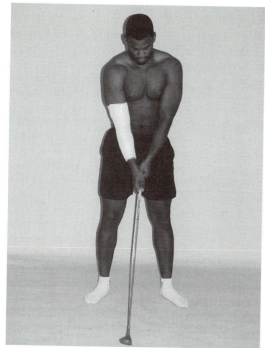

Figure 20-48   Functional exercise. **A,** Baseball/golf swing. **B,** Volleyball drills on a slide board.

REHABILITATION TECHNIQUES FOR SPECIFIC INJURIES

Fractures of the Elbow

Pathomechanics.   Fractures to the elbow proper will be specific to one or more bones in the elbow, with effects to the joint as a whole. The fractures seen in the humeral shaft and distal humerus, the radial head, and the proximal ulna will affect the function of the entire elbow complex as well as the individual bones themselves. Dislocations might accompany an elbow fracture, depending on the specific mechanism of injury. With elbow fractures, properly evaluating the neurovascular system is critical. The ulnar, radial, median, and musculocutaneous nerves pass the elbow in various positions anatomically. The brachial artery has various branches that provide the blood supply from the proximal elbow to the digits.

The radial, ulnar, and common interosseous arteries (and the collateral and recurrent arteries), specifically, provide the circulation off the brachial artery to the structures at and distal to the elbow.

Mechanism of Injury.   The fracture of an elbow bone can have various injury mechanisms. The shaft of the humerus can fracture as a result of a direct force, as well as from a rotational component with the hand in a fixed position. There is also evidence that a direct blow can fracture the bones of the elbow, via a stick, helmet, or bat.[28] A rotational or twisting mechanism can also occur when pushing off on a fixed hand (e.g., a gymnast on a vault)[26] and can cause the onset of immediate pain and loss of function. The increased load on the joint structures from a direct blow can increase the possibility of supracondylar fractures. Olecranon process fractures will occur with a fall directly on the tip of the elbow (e.g., when a volleyball player falls on an elbow). A forearm fracture will often occur in the shafts of both the radius and ulna. A fracture of one of the forearm bones can result in a dislocation of the other bone.[8,30] Radial head fractures make up a third of all elbow fractures and a fourth of all elbow trauma. They are more common in females than in males by a 2:1 ratio.[30] The mechanism of injury is an axial load being placed on a pronated arm. This can occur in skating falls and biking accidents when the posterolateral aspect of the radius is in contact with the capitellum.

This type of stress makes the medial collateral ligament susceptible to injury. A valgus stress can also injure the epiphyseal plate of an adolescent athlete with an avulsion fracture as a possible result.

Rehabilitation Concerns. Undisplaced or minimally displaced fractures in adults and children are treated conservatively and require little or no immobilization. Cases managed using open reduction and internal fixation (ORIF) surgical procedures require only slightly longer periods of immobilization. The joint may be aspirated if the swelling is extremely painful. With the elbow flexed 90 degrees, a posterior plaster splint and sling are applied. Early motion is encouraged, and the splint is removed in 1 to 2 weeks, while a sling is continued for another 1 to 2 weeks as tolerated.

Displaced or comminuted radial head fractures in adults are usually treated by early surgery (within 24 to 48 hours), to minimize the likelihood of permanent restriction of joint motion, traumatic arthritis, soft-tissue calcification in the anterior elbow region, and myositis ossificans.

Fractures in children with less than 15 to 30 degrees of angulation are treated as undisplaced fractures. Displaced fractures, or fractures angulated greater than 15 to 30 degrees, are treated by closed or open reduction.

Fractures of the olecranon can be either displaced or undisplaced. The extensor mechanism is intact in undisplaced fractures, and further displacement is unlikely. The undisplaced fracture is treated with a posterior plaster splint for 2 weeks, followed by a sling and progressive range-of-motion exercises. Displaced fractures usually require open reduction and internal fixation to restore the bony alignment and repair the triceps insertion.

Regardless of the method of treatment, some loss of extension at the elbow is very likely however, little functional impairment usually results.

Rehabilitation Progression. Immediately following the injury or with ORIF surgical procedures, the goal is to minimize pain and swelling by using cold, compression, and electrical stimulation. Active and passive ROM exercises (Figures 20-25 through 20-35) should begin immediately after injury.The goal should be to achieve 15 to 105 degrees of motion by the end of week 2. Within the first week isometric elbow flexion and extension exercises (Figure 20-6) and gentle isometric pronation/supination exercises (Figure 20-7) should begin. Isotonic shoulder and wrist exercises should also be used and should continue to progress throughout the rehabilitation program. Joint mobilizations should begin during the second week in an attempt to minimize loss of extension (Figures 20-37 through 20-40).

Progressive lightweight (1–2 lb) isotonic elbow flexion exercises (Figure 20-8) and elbow extension exercises (Figure 20-9) can be incorporated during the third week and should continue for as long as 12 weeks. Active-assisted passive pronation/supination exercises (Figure 20-10) should begin at week 6, progressing as tolerated.

Beginning at week 7, eccentric elbow flexion and extension exercises (Figures 20-11 and 20-12) along with plyometric exercises can be used. Exercises designed to establish neuromuscular control, including closed-kinetic-chain activities, should also be used to help regain dynamic stability about the elbow joint (Figures 20-13 through 20-15, 20-41 through 20-44). Functional training activities will also begin about this time and should progressively incorporate the stresses, strains, and forces that occur during normal activities. Each of these exercises should continue in a progressive manner throughout the rehabilitative period.

Criteria for Return. Full return to activity is expected at about 12 weeks. The athlete may return to full activity when specific criteria have been successfully completed. There should be clinical healing of the fracture site. Range of motion in flexion, extension, supination, and pronation should be within normal limits. Strength should be at least equal to the uninvolved elbow, and the athlete should have no complaint of pain in the elbow while performing a progression of activities in normal conditions. The return to sport is progressed with the use of restrictions (e.g., pitch counts in baseball), which can be helpful in objectively measuring activity and progression. The throwing progression for the elbow shows a gradual increase in activity in terms of time, repetitions, duration, and intensity (see Table 20-1).

Osteochondritis Dissecans/ "Panner's Disease"

Pathomechanics. Osteochondritis dissecans and "Panner's disease" are injuries that affect the lateral aspect of the elbow. Osteochondritis dissecans is a condition that affects the central and/or lateral aspect of the capitellum or radial head in which an underlying osteochondral bone fragment becomes detached from the articular surface, forming a loose body in the joint. It can also be found in the knee and ankle joints.

Osteochondritis dissecans is considered to be different from osteochondrosis but might represent different stages of the same disease.[29,30] With osteochondritis there is no inflammation. It is the most common cause of loose bodies in adolescents, and although it is most often seen in pitchers, it can also be seen in gymnasts or basketball players between the ages of 12 and 15.[7,22] The primary cause is thought to be trauma due to a repetitive compressive force between the radial head and the capitellum at the radiocapitular joint with valgus forces that load the joint during throwing.[6]

Some confusion exists as to whether there is any difference between osteochondritis dissecans and Panner's disease. Although Panner's disease might just be a part of the spectrum of osteochondritis dissecans, it is probably better to limit the diagnosis of Panner's disease to children age 10 or younger at the time of onset.[31] Panner's disease is an osteochondrosis of the capitellum in which there is a localized avascular necrosis leading to loss of the subchondral bone of the capitellum that can cause softening and fissuring of articular surfaces of the radiocapitellar joint. If loose bodies develop, Panner's disease will produce osteochondritis dissecans.[4]

Mechanism of Injury. Osteochondritis dissecans occurs due to compressive forces at the lateral aspect of the elbow. When the elbow is in the late cocking and acceleration phases of throwing motion, there is a valgus condition that causes a compressive force to the articular surface between the radial head and the capitellum. The repetitive throwing motion causes vascular defects in the area. Panner's disease is an idiopathic condition that encompasses the entire capitellum.[15,18]

Rehabilitation Concerns. Impaired motion and pain to the lateral aspect of the elbow are among the most common complaints. The caution is to avoid excessive and repetitive compression of the joint surfaces, which can lead to degenerative changes and the formation of loose bodies within the joint.[12,18]

Treatment of osteochondritis dissecans is variable. In some cases lesions in the skeletally immature elbow will heal if properly managed. Treatment includes totally avoiding any throwing or impact loading activities as seen in gymnastics. Pain, tenderness, contracture, and radiographic changes provide objective parameters to determine the activity of the disease. If there is formation of loose bodies or if healing has been incomplete (as is usually the case) and symptoms persist, surgical intervention is necessary. Arthroscopic joint debridement and loose body removal has been advocated.

Rehabilitation Progression. The functional progression after the injury has been diagnosed should be first and foremost pain-free. The injury is articular in nature, and a cautious rehabilitation program should be followed. Range-of-motion exercises should be full and pain-free (Figures 20-25 through 20-33). Strengthening exercises (Figures 20-8 through 20-10) will progress at the pain-free level and with restriction from increased pressure between the radius and the capitellum. The athlete might have to decrease or modify the activity level to avoid the compressive nature in the joint. A slow, progressive program that gradually increases the load on the injured structure is essential.

Following arthroscopic debridement and removal of loose bodies, the goal is to minimize pain and swelling by using cold, electrical stimulation, and compression using a bulky dressing initially followed by an elastic wrap. Active and passive ROM exercises (Figures 20-25 through 20-35) should begin immediately after surgery, as tolerated. The goal should be to achieve full ROM within 7 to 14 days after surgery, although the athlete must continue to work on ROM throughout the rehabilitation period. Within the first 2 days, isometric elbow flexion and extension exercises (Figure 20-6), and isometric pronation/supination exercises (Figure 20-7) should begin. Isometric shoulder and wrist exercises (Figure 20-5) should also be used and should continue to progress throughout the rehabilitation program.

Progressive lightweight (1–2 lb) isotonic elbow flexion exercises (Figure 20-8), elbow extension exercises (Figure 20-9), and pronation/supination exercises can be incorporated between days 3 and 7. Isotonic shoulder and wrist exercises should begin during this period and continue to progress throughout the rehabilitation program.

At 3 weeks, eccentric elbow flexion and extension exercises (Figures 20-11 and 20-12) can be used. Joint mobilizations should begin in an attempt to normalize joint arthrokinematics. (Figures 20-37 through 20-40).

Beginning at week 5, in addition to continuing strengthening and ROM exercises, activities that progressively incorporate the stresses, strains, and forces that prepare the athlete for gradual return to functional activities should begin. For throwing athletes, the interval throwing program can be initiated. Exercises designed to establish neuromuscular control, including closed-kinetic-chain activities, should also be used to help regain dynamic stability about the elbow joint (Figures 20-13 through 20-15, 20-41 through 20-44).

Criteria for Return. The athlete may return to full competitive activity when (1) full range of motion in flexion, extension, supination, and pronation has been regained, (2) strength is at least equal to that in the uninvolved elbow, (3) there is no complaint of pain in the elbow while performing throwing or loading activities, and (4) the interval throwing program has been completed.

Realistically, the prognosis for full return to throwing or to loading activities, as in gymnastics and wrestling, especially at a competitive level, should be cautious. The sports therapist should educate parents, coaches, and children about this problem so that early recognition and subsequent intervention and referral to medical personnel can reduce the likelihood of need for surgical intervention. Following an arthoscopic procedure, the athlete might be able to return to full throwing activities in 7 to 8 weeks.

Ulnar Collateral Ligament Injuries

Pathomechanics. The medial complex of the elbow is susceptible to various injuries in the athletic population.[5] The repetitive stresses that are placed on the medial elbow increase the possibilities of injury. The ulnar collateral ligament, the medial aspect of the joint capsule, and the ulnar nerve can individually or collectively be stressed when valgus forces are applied to the elbow. The ulnar collateral ligament is composed of three bands: the anterior oblique ligament, which remains tight throughout full ROM; the posterior oblique ligament, which is tight during flexion and loose during extension; and the transverse oblique ligament, which remains tight throughout the range but provides little medial stability.[36] The anterior band of the ulnar collateral ligament has been demonstrated to be the primary structure resisting valgus stress at the elbow and is tight from 20 to 120 degrees of flexion. The osseous articulation of the elbow contributes little to medial stability with the arm in this position.[14]

The ulnar collateral ligament provides the primary resistance to valgus stresses that occur during the late cocking and early acceleration phases of throwing.[21] On examination the athlete typically complains of pain along the medial aspect of the elbow. There is tenderness over the medial collateral ligament, usually at the distal insertion and occasionally in a more diffuse distribution. In some cases the athlete might describe associated paresthesias in the distribution of the ulnar nerve with a positive Tinel's sign. When valgus stress is applied to the elbow at 20 to 30 degrees of flexion, local pain, tenderness, and end-point laxity are assessed. On standard X-ray, hypertrophy of the humeral condyle and posteromedial aspect of the olecranon, marginal osteophytes of the ulnohumeral or radiocapitellar joints, calcification within the medial collateral ligament, and/or loose bodies in the posterior compartment might be present.[11]

The adolescent elbow has an increased injury potential due to ligament laxity, which can produce stress on the epiphyseal growth plate and an avulsion fracture of the medial epicondyle from the pull of the medial collateral ligament. This can occur in athletes at or around the age of 13.[16]

Mechanism of Injury. In athletes, the ulnar collateral ligament is most often injured as a result of a valgus force from the repetitive trauma of overhead throwing. It can also be injured during a forehand stroke in tennis, or in the trail arm during an improper golf swing. In the general population acute injury to the ulnar collateral ligament rarely results in recurrent instability of the elbow. Stress of the medial complex can also result in ulnar nerve inflammation or impairment, or wrist flexor tendinitis.

During the late cocking phase through the early acceleration phase of throwing, tremendously high, repetitive stresses are applied to the medial elbow joint, frequently resulting in ligament failure, tendinitis, or osseous changes. Injuries can vary in degree from an overuse flexor/pronator muscular strain to ligamentous sprains of the ulnar collateral ligament. These injuries can result in elbow flexion contractures or potentially increase the instability of the elbow in adolescents.

Rehabilitation Concerns. Conservative treatment of athletes with chronic ulnar collateral ligament injury should begin with rest and nonsteroidal anti-inflammatory medication. With resolution of symptoms, rehabilitation should be instituted with emphasis on strengthening. The sports therapist along with the coach should analyze the athlete's throwing mechanics, which might include video assessment, to correct any existing faulty mechanics. If periods of rest and rehabilitation fail to result in a resolution of symptoms, surgical intervention might be necessary.

Operative management consists of repair or reconstruction. In the case of an acute rupture, surgical repair can be considered; however, the indications are extremely limited. The avulsed ligament should be without evidence of calcification, and if there is any question as to the quality of the tissue, reconstruction should be performed.

The ulnar collateral ligament is the primary stabilizer to valgus stress at the elbow, so reconstruction is vital to competitive throwing athletes who wish to return to their previous levels of performance. An autograft, using either the palmaris longus or extensor hallucis, is used to reconstruct the ulnar collateral ligament. The graft then simulates function of the ulnar collateral ligament, particularly the anterior oblique portion, providing the primary restraint to valgus stress during throwing. During this surgical procedure, the ulnar nerve is transposed medially and is held in place with fascial slings. Immediate postoperative precautions must be observed, especially in relation to the soft tissue of the fascial slings that stabilize the ulnar nerve.

Rehabilitation Progression. Following a requisite period of rest and rehabilitation techniques designed to reduce inflammation, the rehabilitation progression for ulnar collateral ligament injuries should concentrate primarily on strengthening of the flexor muscles, particularly the flexor carpi ulnaris and flexor digitorum superficialis, which can help prevent medial injury by providing additional support to medial elbow structures.[32] Strengthening exercises (Figures 20-5 through 20-12) should be done initially in the pain-free midrange of motion with a gradual increase of forces at the end ranges of motion. Exercises to increase both static and dynamic flexibility of the elbow without producing valgus stress should be incorporated (Figures 20-13 through 20-15). Support taping can also assist in the protection for return to activity (Figure 20-47).

Following a reconstruction of the ulnar collateral ligament, the initial goal is to decrease pain and swelling (using a compression dressing for 2 to 3 days) and to protect the healing reconstruction. The athlete is placed in a 90-degree posterior splint for 1 week, during which time submaximal isometrics for the wrist musculature (Figure 20-5) and the elbow flexors and extensors (Figures 20-6, 20-7) are performed at multiple angles as long as all valgus stress is eliminated. Isometric shoulder exercises, except for external rotation, along with isometric biceps exercises should be used.

In the second week the athlete is placed into a ROM brace set at 30 to 100 degrees (Figure 20-45). Range of motion should be increased by 5 degrees of extension and 10 degrees of flexion each week, with full range of motion at 6 to 7 weeks. In addition to the exercises used during the first week, wrist isometrics and elbow flexion and extension isometrics (Figure 20-6) should begin.

At 4 weeks, progressive lightweight (1–2 lb) isotonic elbow flexion exercises (Figure 20-8), elbow extension exercises (Figure 20-9), and pronation/supination exercises (Figure 20-10) can be incorporated. Isotonic shoulder exercises (avoiding external rotation for 6 weeks) should begin during this period and continue to progress throughout the rehabilitation program. Passive elbow flexion and extension ROM exercises (Figures 20-32, 20-33) may begin during this period.

At 6 weeks, isotonic strengthening exercises for the shoulder (now including external rotation), elbow, and wrist should continue to progress.

At 9 weeks, as strength continues to increase, more functional activities can be incorporated, including eccentric elbow flexion and extension exercises (Figures 20-11 and 20-12), PNF diagonal strengthening patterns (Figures 20-21 through 20-24), and plyometric exercises. (Figure 20-16). Exercises designed to establish neuromuscular control, including closed-kinetic-chain activities, should also be used to help regain dynamic stability about the elbow joint (Figures 20-13 through 20-15, 20-41 through 20-44).

Beginning at week 11, in addition to continuing strengthening and ROM exercises, activities that progressively incorporate the stresses, strains, and forces that prepare the athlete for gradual return to throwing activities should begin. For throwing athletes, the interval throwing program can be initiated at week 14 (see Table 20-1).

Criteria for Full Return. Generally the throwing athlete can return to competitive levels at about 22 to 26 weeks postsurgery. The athlete may return to full competitive activity when (1) full range of motion in flexion, extension, supination, and pronation has been regained, (2) strength is at least equal to that of the uninvolved elbow, (3) there is no complaint of pain in the elbow while performing throwing or loading activities, and (4) the interval throwing program has been completed.

Nerve Entrapments

Pathomechanics and Injury Mechanism. The ulnar, median, and radial nerves are susceptible to injury and entrapment in the elbow. The ulnar nerve, which passes through the medial epicondylar groove, can be injured with medial stress to the elbow as previously described. The median nerve passing between the supracondylar process, and the medial epicondyle can become compressed. The radial nerve passes under the lateral head of the triceps and, if compressed, can cause weakness in the forearm extensors. Whenever nerve compression conditions at the elbow are considered, the sports therapist should also consider the possibility of compression lesions at other levels such as the cervical spine, brachial plexus, and wrist.

Ulnar nerve entrapment. Ulnar nerve compression can occur from a number of causes, including (1) direct trauma, (2) traction due to an increase of laxity in the medial complex, which causes a compressive force to be placed on the nerve resulting in a tension neuropathy, (3) compression due to a thickened retinaculum or a hypertrophied flexor carpi ulnaris muscle, (4) recurrent subluxation or dislocation, and (5) osseous degenerative changes.[10] In throwing athletes, ulnar nerve irritation is most likely to develop secondary to mechanical factors that occur during the late cocking and early acceleration phases of the throwing motion. In these athletes, ulnar neuritis often occurs along with medial instability and medial epicondylitis.[10]

The term **cubital tunnel syndrome** is used to identify a specific anatomic site for entrapment of the ulnar nerve. The ulnar nerve can be compromised by any swelling that occurs within the canal or with inflammatory changes that result in thickening of the fascial sheath.

The athlete generally complains of medial elbow pain associated with numbness and tingling in the ulnar nerve distribution. Paresthesias may be present that radiate from the medial epicondyle distally along the ulnar aspect of the forearm into the fourth and fifth fingers. These sensory symptoms usually precede the development of motor deficits. There is tenderness at the cubital tunnel, which may include the medial epicondyle. Tinel's sign is generally present at the cubital tunnel. Subluxation of the ulnar nerve occurs in as many as 16 percent of athletes with symptoms, particularly in those with a shallow medial epicondylar groove. Radiographs might show osteophytes on the humerus and olecranon, calcifications of the medial collateral ligament, and loose bodies.[10]

Median nerve entrapment.   The median nerve can be compressed under the ligament of Struthers, within the pronator teres muscle, and under the superficial head of the flexor digitorum superficialis. The compression can occur as a result of hypertrophy of the proximal forearm muscles, particularly the pronator teres muscle, that occurs with repetitive grip-related activity or pronation and extension of the forearm, as occurs in the racket sports and other grip/hold activities. The athlete will usually describe aching pain and fatigue or weakness of the forearm muscles along with paresthesia in the distribution of the median nerve. Symptoms seem to worsen with repetitive pronation, as in practicing tennis serves. There is usually tenderness of the proximal pronator teres with a positive Tinel's sign. The athlete might also complain of increased pain while sleeping.

Radial nerve entrapment.   Entrapment of the radial nerve, specifically the posterior interosseous nerve, occurs within the radial tunnel and has been referred to as either **radial tunnel syndrome** in which there is pain with no motor weakness, or **posterior interosseous nerve compression** where there is motor weakness in the absence of pain.[10] The radial nerve innervates the brachioradialis as well as the extensor muscles of the proximal forearm. Radial nerve compression occurs in throwing mechanisms and overhead activities such as swimming and playing tennis. The athlete typically complains of lateral elbow pain that is sometimes confused with lateral epicondylitis. There is tenderness distal to the lateral epicondyle over the supinator muscle. The pain is described as an ache that spreads into the extensor muscles and occasionally radiates distally to the wrist. Nocturnal pain might be present.

Rehabilitation Concerns.   If rehabilitation begins early after onset of symptoms, treatment should include rest, avoiding activities that seem to exacerbate pain, use of anti-inflammatory medications, protective padding, and occasionally use of extension night splints. This should be followed by a rehabilitation program that concentrates on range-of-motion exercises before return to sport. A concern that will arise and needs to be addressed with regard to nerve entrapments is that of decreased muscle function, which can lead to accommodative activity and possible muscle imbalance. If the athlete remains symptomatic despite a conservative program, surgery is generally recommended. It should be noted that, although physical findings other than local tenderness might be minimal and electrodiagnostic tests are rarely positive, good to excellent results can be obtained by surgery. The surgical treatment options include decompression alone and subcutaneous, intramuscular, or submuscular transposition.

Rehabilitation Progression.   Following a course of conservative care involving rest and anti-inflammatory medication, the rehabilitation program should concentrate on strengthening of the involved muscles to maintain a balance between agonist and antagonist muscles (Figures 20-5 through 20-12). In addition, maintaining range of motion through aggressive stretching exercises will help to free up entrapped nerves (Figures 20-25 through 20-35). Massage techniques that can be utilized in the affected area can prevent the development of adhesions that would restrict injured nerves. Mobility of the nerve is critical in reducing nerve entrapment.

Following surgical decompression or transposition of an entrapped nerve, the initial goal is to decrease pain and swelling (using a compression dressing for 2 to 3 days). The athlete is placed in a 90-degree posterior splint for 1 week, during which time gripping exercises (Figure 20-5), isometric shoulder exercises, and wrist ROM exercises are used. During weeks 2 and 3, the posterior splint ROM is limited to 30 to 90 degrees initially, progressing to 15 to 120 degrees. The splint may be removed for exercise. Isometric flexion and extension exercises (Figures 20-6, 20-7) are begun, and shoulder isometrics continue.

At 3 weeks, the splint can be discontinued. Progressive isotonic elbow flexion exercises (Figure 20-8), elbow extension exercises (Figure 20-9), and pronation/supination exercises (Figure 20-10) can be incorporated. Isotonic shoulder exercises should begin during this period and continue to progress throughout the rehabilitation program. Passive elbow flexion and extension ROM exercises (Figures 20-32, 20-33) continue during this period with particular emphasis placed on regaining extension.

At 7 weeks, as strength continues to increase, more functional activities can be incorporated, including eccentric elbow flexion and extension exercises (Figures 20-11 and 20-12), PNF diagonal strengthening patterns (Figures 20-21 through 20-24), and plyometric exercises (Figure 20-16). Exercises designed to establish neuromuscular control, including closed-kinetic-chain activities, should also be used to help regain dynamic stability about the elbow joint (Figures 20-13 through 20-15, 20-41 through 20-44). For throwing athletes, the interval throwing program can be initiated (Table 20-1).

Criteria for Return. The throwing athlete can return to competitive activity at about 12 weeks. The athlete must be able to demonstrate full function of the elbow after nerve injury. Range of motion, strength, neuromuscular control, and functional activities must be comparable to preinjury levels. The athlete must also appropriately demonstrate activities related to his or her sport, and perform these tasks without compensation or substitution of other structures. For example, a swimmer must demonstrate the proper mechanics in the elbow while performing the stroke with the involved extremity comparably to the uninvolved extremity. If it is not performed in a satisfactory manner, the rehabilitation will be continued until the stroke can be performed appropriately.

Elbow Dislocations

Pathomechanics. Generally elbow dislocations are classified as either anterior or posterior dislocations. Anterior dislocations and radial head dislocations are not common, occurring in only 1 to 2 percent of cases. There are several different types of posterior dislocations, which are defined by the position of the olecranon relative to the humerus: (1) posterior, (2) posterolateral (most common), (3) posteromedial (least common), or (4) lateral. Dislocations can be complete or *perched.* As compared with complete dislocations, perched dislocations have less ligament tearing, and thus they have a more rapid recovery and rehabilitation period.[2,36] In a complete dislocation there is rupture of the ulnar collateral ligament, a possibility that the anterior capsule will rupture, along with possible ruptures of the lateral collateral ligament, brachialis muscle, or wrist flexor/extensor tendons.[33] Fractures occur in 25 to 50 percent of patients with elbow dislocations, with a fracture of the radial head being most common.

With rupture of the anterior oblique band of the ulnar collateral ligament, repair is sometimes necessary in athletes if the injury occurs in the dominant arm.

Injury Mechanism. Elbow dislocations most frequently occur as a result of elbow hyperextension from a fall on the outstretched or extended arm, although dislocation can occur in flexion. The radius and ulna are most likely to dislocate posterior or posterolateral to the humerus. The olecranon process is forced into the olecranon fossa with such impact that the trochlea is levered over the coronoid process. Flexion dislocation is often associated with radial head fractures.

If the dislocation is simple without associated fractures, reduction can result in a stable elbow if the forearm flexors, extensors, and annular ligament have maintained their continuity. In these cases early motion is resumed and the ultimate prognosis is good. The injury will present with rapid swelling, severe pain at the elbow, and a deformity with the olecranon in posterior position, giving the appearance of a shortened forearm.

Elbow dislocations that involve fractures of the bony stabilizing forces about the elbow, such as a radial head or capitular fracture/dislocation, creates a significant instability pattern that cannot completely be corrected on either the medial or the lateral side of the elbow alone for maximum functional return. These injuries must be treated surgically.

Rehabilitation Concerns. Following reduction of an elbow dislocation, the degree of stability present will determine the course of rehabilitation. If the elbow is stable, best results are obtained with a brief period of immobilization followed by rehabilitation that is focused on restoring early range of motion within the limits of elbow stability. Prolonged immobilization after dislocation has been closely associated with flexion contractures and more increased pain, with no decrease in instability. An unstable dislocation requires surgical repair of the ulnar collateral ligament and thus a longer period of immobilization.

Recurrent elbow dislocation is uncommon, occurring after only 1 to 2 percent of simple dislocations. Recurrent instability is more likely if the initial dislocation involved a fracture or if the first incident took place during childhood.

An overly aggressive rehabilitation program is more likely to result in chronic instability, while being overly conservative can lead to a flexion contracture. Typically, flexion contracture is much more likely. It is not uncommon to have a flexion contracture of 30 degrees at 10 weeks. After 2 years a 10-degree flexion contracture is often still present.[2] Unfortunately this flexion contracture does not improve with time. For the athlete it is most desirable to regain full elbow extension. For nonathletes, it is more important to ensure that the joint structure and ligaments are given sufficient time to heal, to decrease the risk of recurrent subluxation or dislocation.

Loss of motion, joint stiffness, and heterotopic ossification are more likely complications following dislocation.

Rehabilitation Progression. The rehabilitation progression is determined by whether the elbow is stable or unstable following reduction. If the elbow is stable, it should be immobilized in posterior splint at 90 degrees of flexion for 3 to 4 days. During that period, gripping exercises (Figure 20-5) and isometric shoulder exercises are used. All exercises that place valgus stress on the elbow should be avoided. Therapeutic modalities should also be used to modulate pain and control swelling. On day 4 or 5, gentle active ROM elbow exercises (Figures 20-8 through 20-10) and gentle isometric elbow flexion and extension exercises (Figures 20-6, 20-7) can be done out of the splint. Passive stretching is absolutely avoided because of the tendency toward scarring of the traumatized soft tissue and the possibility of recurrent posterior dislocation. Shoulder and wrist isotonic exercises may be done in the splint. Gentle joint mobilizations can be used to regain normal joint arthokinematics (Figures 20-36 through 20-40).

At 10 days the splint can be discontinued. Passive ROM exercises (Figures 20-32 through 20-35) can begin, progressing to stretching exercises (Figure 20-25 through 20-29). Progressive isotonic elbow flexion exercises (Figure 20-8), elbow extension exercises (Figure 20-9), and pronation/supination exercises (Figure 20-10) should continue and progress as tolerated. Isotonic shoulder exercises should continue to progress throughout the rehabilitation program. Eccentric elbow flexion and extension exercises (Figures 20-11 and 20-12) , PNF diagonal strengthening patterns (Figures 20-21 through 20-24), and plyometric exercises (Figure 20-16) may be incorporated as tolerated. Exercises designed to establish neuromuscular control, including closed-kinetic-chain activities, should also be used to help regain dynamic stability about the elbow joint (Figures 20-13 through 20-15, 20-41 through 20-44). The athlete should continue to wear the brace or use taping (Figure 20-47) to prevent elbow hyperextension and valgus stress during return to activities.

For an unstable elbow, the goal during the first 3 to 4 weeks is to protect the healing soft tissue while decreasing pain and swelling. During this period the protective brace should be set initially at 10 degrees less that the active ROM extension limit. Starting at week 1, a ROM brace preset at 30 to 90 degrees is implemented. Each week, motion in this brace is increased by 5 degrees of extension and 10 degrees of flexion. The brace can be discontinued when full ROM is achieved. During this period, gripping exercises (Figure 20-5) and wrist ROM exercises are used. All exercises that place valgus stress on the elbow should be avoided. Shoulder isometric exercises avoiding internal or external rotation may be used.

At 4 weeks, progressive lightweight (1–2 lb) isotonic elbow flexion exercises (Figure 20-8), elbow extension exercises (Figure 20-9), and pronation/supination exercises (Figure 20-10) may be incorporated. Isotonic shoulder exercises (avoiding internal and external rotation for 6 weeks) should begin during this period and continue to progress throughout the rehabilitation program. Passive elbow flexion and extension ROM exercises (Figures 20-32, 20-33) may begin during this period.

At 6 weeks, isotonic strengthening exercises for the shoulder external and internal rotation should begin and continue to progress.

At 9 weeks, as strength continues to increase, more functional activities can be incorporated, including eccentric elbow flexion and extension exercises (Figures 20-11 and 20-12) , PNF diagonal strengthening patterns (Figures 20-21 through 20-24), and plyometric exercises (Figure 20-16). Exercises designed to establish neuromuscular control, including closed-kinetic-chain activities, should also be used to help regain dynamic stability about the elbow joint (Figures 20-13 through 20-15, 20-41 through 20-44).

At 11 weeks, the athlete can begin some sport activities as tolerated while continuing to progress the strengthening program. The protective brace should be worn whenever the athlete is engaging in any type of sport activity.

Criteria for Full Return. The criteria for a return to full activity after an elbow dislocation are the same as for any return to full activity. The elbow must demonstrate full range of motion, and the athlete must demonstrate strength, endurance, and neuromuscular control skills appropriate to their own sport without limiting performance. A functional progression must be demonstrated, and success in terms of the criteria of the rehabilitation protocol must be reached.

Medial and Lateral Epicondylitis

Pathomechanics and Injury Mechanism. The medial and the lateral epicondyles of the distal humerus are the tendon attachments of the wrist flexors and extensors.[27] The medial epicondyle serves as the attachment for the wrist flexors, and the wrist extensors attach to the lateral epicondyle.

Medial epicondylitis. Medial epicondylitis (*golfer's elbow, racquetball elbow,* or *swimmer's elbow* in adults and *Little League elbow* in adolescents) generally occurs as a result of repetitive microtrauma to the pronator teres and the flexor carpi radialis muscles during pronation and flexion of the wrist. The athlete usually complains of pain on the medial aspect of the elbow, which is exacerbated when throwing a baseball, serving or hitting a forehand shot in racquetball, pulling during a swimming backstroke, or hitting a golf ball, in which case the trail arm is affected. There is tenderness at the medial epicondyle, and pain is exacerbated with resisted pronation, resisted volar flexion of the wrist, or passive extension of the wrist with the elbow extended. Associated ulnar neuropathy at the elbow has been reported in 25 to 60 percent of patients with medial epicondylitis.[10]

Lateral epicondylitis. Lateral epicondylitis (*tennis elbow*) occurs with repetitive microtrauma that results in either concentric or eccentric overload of the wrist extensors and supinators, most commonly the extensor carpi radialis brevis.[27] There is pain along the lateral aspect of the elbow, particularly at the origin of the extensor carpi radialis brevis. Pain increases with passive flexion of the wrist with the elbow extended, as it does with resisted wrist dorsiflexion. Pain with resisted wrist extension and full elbow extension indicates involvement of the extensor carpi radialis longus. Lateral epicondylitis usually results from repeated forceful wrist hyperextension, as often occurs in hitting a backhand stroke in tennis. For beginning tennis players, the backhand stroke is somewhat unnatural, and to get enough power to hit the ball over the net there is a tendency to use forced wrist hyperextension. In more advanced players lateral epicondylitis can develop in a number of ways, including hitting a topspin backhand stroke using a "flick" of the wrist instead of a long follow-through; hitting a serve with the wrist in pronation and "snapping" the wrist to impart spin; using a racquet that is strung with too much tension (55 to 60 lb is recommended); using a grip size that is too small; and hitting a heavy, wet ball.[30] It must be emphasized that any activity that involves repeated forceful wrist extension can result in lateral epicondylitis.

Rehabilitation Concerns. Medial and lateral epicondylitis, but particularly lateral epicondylitis, can be lingering, limiting, frustrating, painful pathological conditions for both the athlete and the sports therapist. Perhaps the first step in treating these conditions is altering faulty performance mechanics to minimize the repetitive stress created by these activities. The stressful components of high-level activities can also be alleviated by altering the frequency, intensity, or duration of play.[25]

Two rehabilitation approaches may be taken in treating medial and lateral epicondylitis. The first approach involves using all of the normal measures to reduce inflammation and pain. Treatment may include several weeks of rest or at least restricted activity during which painful movements, like gripping activities that aggravate the condition, are avoided; using therapeutic modalities such as cryotherapy, electrical stimulating currents, ultrasound phonophoresis with hyrocortisone, or iontophoresis using dexamethasone; and using nonsteroidal anti-inflammatory drugs. If pain persists, some physicians might recommend a steroid injection if they feel that the patient is incapable of progressing in the rehabilitation program. However, more than two or three steroid injections per year is inappropriate and probably harmful, because it can result in weakening of the surrounding normal tissues.

A second approach would be to realize that the athlete has a chronic inflammation. For one reason or another the inflammatory phase of the healing process has not accomplished what it is supposed to and thus the inflammatory process is in effect "stuck." The goal in this approach is to "jump start" the inflammatory process, using techniques that are likely to increase the inflammatory response, with the idea that increasing inflammation might allow healing to progress as normal to the fibroblastic and remodeling phases. To increase the inflammatory response, transverse friction massage can be used. This technique involves firm pressure massage over the point of maximum tenderness at the epicondyle in a direction perpendicular to the muscle fibers. This massage will be painful for the athlete, so it is recommended that a 5-minute ice treatment be used prior to the massage to minimize pain. Transverse friction massage should be done for 5 to 7 minutes, every other day, using a maximum of five treatments. It is our experience that if the symptoms do not begin to resolve in a week to 10 days, it is unlikely that this approach will eliminate the problem.

It must also be emphasized that during this treatment period, all measures previously described to reduce inflammation should be avoided. Remember that the idea is to increase the inflammatory response. In those individuals who have persistent pain that does not resolve after 1 year of conservative treatment, surgery should be considered.

Rehabilitation Progression. Rehabilitation time frames will differ somewhat, depending on which of the two approaches is utilized in the early treatment of medial and lateral epicondylitis. Regardless of which of the two techniques is used, some submaximal exercise can begin during this period as long as it does not cause pain. If rest and anti-inflammatory measures are used, 2 or 3 weeks of restricted activity with very limited or no submaximal exercise might be necessary to control pain and inflammation. If the more aggressive approach, using transverse friction massage, is chosen, submaximal exercises can begin immediately within pain-free limits.

Exercise intensity should be based on patient tolerance but should adhere to an exercise progression. Throughout the rehabilitation process pain should always be a guide for progression. Each of the following exercises should continue in a progressive manner throughout the rehabilitative period: gentle active and passive ROM exercises for both the elbow and wrist (Figures 20-25 through 20-35), gentle isometric elbow flexion and extension exercises (Figure 20-6), gentle isometric pronation/supination exercises (Figure 20-7), progressive isotonic elbow flexion exercises (Figure 20-8), elbow extension exercises (Figure 20-9), ronation/supination exercises (Figure 20-10) beginning with lightweight (1–2 lb). Lateral counterforce bracing should be used as a supplement to muscular strengthening exercises (Figure 20-46), with the athlete gradually weaning from use as appropriate. Eccentric elbow flexion and extension exercises (Figures 20-11 and 20-12), along with plyometric exercises (Figure 20-16) and functional training activities should progressively incorporate the stresses, strains, and forces that occur during normal sport activities, gradually increasing the frequency, intensity, and duration of play.

Criteria for Full Return. Perhaps the biggest mistake made with epicondylitis is trying to progress too quickly in the exercise program and rushing full return to play. The sports therapist should counsel the athlete about doing too much too soon, cautioning that rapid increases in activity levels often exacerbate the condition. The involved muscles must regain appropriate strength, flexibility, and endurance with reduced inflammation and pain. Functional activity needs to progress slowly to prepare the athlete for the return without restrictions.

THROWING PROGRAM FOR RETURN TO SPORT

The athlete progresses through a series of steps for return to his or her sport. For the throwing athlete, the progression described in Table 20-1 is one of the final criteria for full return.[37,38] During this throwing progression the athlete is doing upper-quarter exercises that work on the cervical spine, the shoulder rotator cuff, and muscles that affect the glenohumeral joint, as well as exercises that work on the elbow, hand, and wrist. The proprioceptive and neuromuscular control effects stressed by this throwing program are critical in returning the athlete back to full activity. The throwing program is progressive in distance, repetition, duration, and intensity. It is imperative that the athlete successfully complete the criteria at one level before progressing to the next.

TABLE 20-1 Interval Throwing Program

45-Foot Phase		60-Foot Phase		90-Foot Phase	
Step 1:	A. Warm-up throwing B. 45 feet (25 throws) C. *Rest 15 minutes* D. Warm-up throwing E. 45 feet (25 throws)	**Step 3:**	A. Warm-up throwing B. 60 feet (25 throws) C. *Rest 15 minutes* D. Warm-up throwing E. 60 feet (25 throws)	**Step 5:**	A. Warm-up throwing B. 90 feet (25 throws) C. *Rest 15 minutes* D. Warm-up throwing E. 90 feet (25 throws)
Step 2:	A. Warm-up throwing B. 45 feet (25 throws) C. *Rest 10 minutes* D. Warm-up throwing E. 45 feet (25 throws) F. *Rest 10 minutes* G. Warm-up throwing H. 45 feet (25 throws)	**Step 4:**	A. Warm-up throwing B. 60 feet (25 throws) C. *Rest 10 minutes* D. Warm-up throwing E. 60 feet (25 throws) F. *Rest 10 minutes* G. Warm-up throwing H. 60 feet (25 throws)	**Step 6:**	A. Warm-up throwing B. 90 feet (25 throws) C. *Rest 10 minutes* D. Warm-up throwing E. 90 feet (25 throws) F. *Rest 10 minutes* G. Warm-up throwing H. 90 feet (25 throws)
120-Foot Phase		**150-Foot Phase**		**180-Foot Phase**	
Step 7:	A. Warm-up throwing B. 120 feet (25 throws) C. *Rest 15 minutes* D. Warm-up throwing E. 120 feet (25 throws)	**Step 9:**	A. Warm-up throwing B. 150 feet (25 throws) C. *Rest 15 minutes* D. Warm-up throwing E. 150 feet (25 throws)	**Step 11:**	A. Warm-up throwing B. 180 feet (25 throws) C. *Rest 15 minutes* D. Warm-up throwing E. 180 feet (25 throws)
Step 8:	A. Warm-up throwing B. 120 feet (25 throws) C. *Rest 10 minutes* D. Warm-up throwing E. 120 feet (25 throws) F. *Rest 10 minutes* G. Warm-up throwing H. 120 feet (25 throws)	**Step 10:**	A. Warm-up throwing B. 150 feet (25 throws) C. *Rest 10 minutes* D. Warm-up throwing E. 150 feet (25 throws) F. *Rest 10 minutes* G. Warm-up throwing H. 150 feet (25 throws)	**Step 12:**	A. Warm-up throwing B. 180 feet (25 throws) C. *Rest 10 minutes* D. Warm-up throwing E. 180 feet (25 throws) F. *Rest 10 minutes* G. Warm-up throwing H. 180 feet (25 throws)

■ **TABLE 20-1** Interval Throwing Program—*Cont'd*

45-Foot Phase	60-Foot Phase	90-Foot Phase
		Step 13: A. Warm-up throwing
		B. 180 feet (25 throws)
		C. *Rest 15 minutes*
		D. Warm-up throwing
		E. 180 feet (25 throws)
		F. *Rest 15 minutes*
		G. Warm-up throwing
		H. 180 feet (25 throws)
		Step 14: Begin throwing off the mound or return to respective position

Interval Throwing Program—Phase 2

Stage 1: Fastball only

Step 1: Internal throwing
15 throws off mound 50%

Step 2: Interval throwing
30 throws off mound 50%

Step 3: Interval throwing
45 throws off mound 50%

Step 4: Interval throwing
60 throws off mound 50%

Step 5: Interval throwing
30 throws off mound 50%

Step 6: 30 throws off mound 75%
45 throws off mound 50%

Step 7: 45 throws off mound 75%
15 throws off mound 50%

Step 8: 60 throws off mound 50%
15 throws off mound 50%

Stage 2: Fastball Only

Step 9: 45 throws off mound 75%
15 throws in batting practice

Step 10: 45 throws off mound 75%
30 throws in batting practice

Step 11: 45 throws off mound 75%
45 throws in batting practice

Stage 3

Step 12: 30 throws off mound 75%
warm-up
15 throws off mound 50%
breaking balls
45–60 throws in batting practice (fastball only)

Step 13: 30 throws off mound 75%
30 breaking balls 75%
30 throws in batting practice

Step 14: 30 throws off mound 75 %
60 to 90 throws in batting practice
25% breaking balls

Step 15: Simulated game: progressing by 15 throws per workout

Note: *Use interval throwing to 120-foot phase as a warm-up. All throwing off the mound should be done in the presence of the pitching coach to stress proper throwing mechanics. Use a speed gun to aid in effort control.

Summary

1. The elbow joint is composed of the humeroulnar joint, humeroradial joint, and the proximal radioulnar joint. Motions in the elbow complex include flexion, extension, pronation, and supination.

2. Fractures in the elbow can occur from a direct blow or from falling on an outstretched hand. They may be treated by casting or in some cases by surgical reduction and fixation. Following surgical fixation the athlete might require 12 weeks for return.

3. Osteochondritis dissecans and Panner's disease are injuries that affect the lateral aspect of the elbow. Osteochondritis dissecans is associated with a loose body in the joint, whereas Panner's disease is an osteochondrosis of the capitellum. The prognosis for full return to throwing or loading activities should be cautious.

4. In athletes, injuries to the ulnar collateral ligament result from a valgus force from the repetitive trauma of overhead throwing, which occurs during the late cocking phase through the early acceleration phase of throwing. Reconstruction is vital to competitive throwing athletes, and rehabilitation can require as long as 22 to 26 weeks for full return.

5. In the case of entrapment of the ulnar, median, and radial nerves, mobility of the nerve is critical in reducing nerve entrapment. Rehabilitation should concentrate primarily on stretching to free up the nerve. If conservative treatment fails, surgical release might be indicated.

6. Elbow dislocations result from elbow hyperextension from a fall on an extended arm, with the radius and ulna dislocating posteriorly. The degree of stability present will determine the course of rehabilitation. If the elbow is stable, a brief period of immobilization is followed by rehabilitation. An unstable dislocation requires surgical repair and thus a longer period of immobilization.

7. Medial epicondylitis (*golfer's elbow, racquetball elbow, swimmer's elbow, Little League elbow*) results from repetitive microtrauma to flexor carpi radialis muscles during pronation and flexion of the wrist. Lateral epicondylitis (*tennis elbow*) occurs with concentric or eccentric overload of the wrist extensors and supinators, most commonly the extensor carpi radialis brevis.

References

1. An, K. N., and B. F. Morrey. 1993. Biomechanics of the elbow. In *The elbow and its disorders,* edited by B. F. Morrey. Philadelphia: W. B. Saunders.

2. Andrews, J. R., K. E. Wilk, and D. Groh. 1996. Elbow rehabilitation. In *Clinical orthopaedic rehabilitation,* edited by B. Brotzman. St. Louis: Mosby.

3. Andrews, J. R., K. E. Wilk, Y. E. Satterwhite, and J. L. Tedder. 1993. Physical examination of the throwers elbow. *Journal of Orthopaedic and Sports Physical Therapy* 17:296–304.

4. Andrich, J. 1995. Upper extremity injuries in the skeletally immature athlete. In *The upper extremity in sports medicine,* edited by J. Nicholas and E. Hershman. St. Louis: Mosby.

5. Azar, F. M., and K. E. Wilk. 1996. Nonoperative treatment of the elbow in throwers. *Operative Techniques in Sports Medicine* 4:91–99: W. B. Saunders.

6. Bauer, M., K. Jonsson, P. O. Josefsson, and B. Linden. Osteochondritis dissecans of the elbow: A long-term follow-up study. *Clinical Orthopaedics and Related Research* 284:156–60.

7. Brown, R., M. E. Blazina, and K. Kerlan. 1974. Osteochondritis of the capitellum. *Journal of Sports Medicine* 2(1): 27–46.

8. Bruckner, J. D., A. H. Alexander, and D. M. Lichtman. 1996. Acute dislocations of the distal radioulnar joint. *Instructional Course Lectures* 45:27–36.

9. Byron, P. 1997. Restoring function. *Journal of Hand Therapy* 10(1): 334–37.

10. Cordasco, F., and J. Parkes. 1995. Overuse injuries of the elbow. In *The upper extremity in sports medicine,* edited by J. Nicholas and E. Hershman. St. Louis: Mosby.

11. Davidson, P. A., M. Pink, J. Perry, and F. W. Jobe. 1995. Functional anatomy of the flexor pronator muscle group in relation to the medial collateral ligament of the elbow. *American Journal of Sports Medicine* 23(2): 245–50.

12. Ferlic, D. C., and B. F. Morrey. 1993. Evaluation of the painful elbow: The problem elbow. In *The elbow and its disorders,* 2d ed., edited by B. F. Morrey. Philadelphia: W. B. Saunders.

13. Fyfe, I., and W. D. Stanish. 1992. The use of eccentric training and stretching in the treatment and prevention of tendon injuries. *Clinics in Sports Medicine* 3:601–24.

14. Gore, R. M., L. F. Rogers, J. Bowerman, et al. 1980. Osseous manifestations of elbow stress associated with sports. *AJR* 134:971–77.

15. Guerra, J. J., and L. A. Timmerman. 1996. Clinical anatomy, histology, and pathomechanics of the elbow in sports. *Operative Techniques in Sports Medicine* 4:69–76.

16. Harrelson, G. L. 1991. Elbow rehabilitation. In *Physical rehabilitation of the injured athlete,* edited by J. Andrews and G. L. Harrelson. Philadelphia: W. B. Saunders.

17. Kao, J. T., M. Pink, F. W. Jobe, and J. Perry. 1995. Electromyographic analysis of the scapular muscles during a golfswing. *American Journal of Sports Medicine* 23(1): 19–23.

18. Lindholm, T. S., K. Osterman, and E. Vankka. 1980. Osteochondritis dissecans of the elbow, ankle, and hip: A comprehensive survey. *Clin Orthop* 148:245–53.

19. Magee, D. J. 1997. *Elbow. Orthopedic physical assessment.* Philadelphia: W. B. Saunders.

20. Morrey, B. F. 1993. Anatomy of the elbow joint. In *The elbow and its disorders,* 2d ed., edited by B. F. Morrey. Philadelphia: W. B. Saunders.

21. Morrey, B. F., and K. N. An. 1983. Articular and ligamentous contributions to the stability of the elbow joint. *American Journal of Sports Medicine* 11:315–18.

22. Morrey, B. F., K. N. An, and T. J. Stormont. 1988. Force transmissions through the radial head. *Journal of Bone and Joint Surgery* 70A:250–56.

23. Norkin, C. C., and P. K. Levangie. 1992. Function: Humeroulnar and humeroradial joints. *In joint structure and function,* 2d ed. Philadelphia: F. A. Davis.

24. Olsen, B. S., J. O. Sojbjerg, M. Dalstra, and O. Sneppen. 1996. Kinematics of the lateral ligamentous constraints of the elbow joint. *Journal of Shoulder and Elbow Surgery* 5(5): 333–41.

25. Plancher, K. D., J. Halbrecht, and G. M. Lourie. 1996. Medial and lateral epicondylitis in the athlete. *Clinics in Sports Medicine* 15(2): 283–305.

26. Priest, J. D. 1985. Elbow injuries in gymnastics. *Clinics in Sports Medicine* 4(1): 73–84.

27. Roetert, E. P., H. Brody, C. J. Dillman, J. L. Groppel, and J. M. Schultheis. 1995. The biomechanics of tennis elbow: An integrated approach. *Clinics in Sports Medicine* 14(1): 47–57.

28. Saliba, E. 1991. The upper arm, elbow, and forearm. In *AAOS athletic training and sports medicine,* 2d ed., edited by L. Y. Hunter. Park Ridge, IL: AAOS.

29. Singer, K. M., and S. P. Roy. 1984. Osteochondrosis of the humeral capitellum. *American Journal of Sports Medicine* 12(5): 351–60.

30. Sobel, J., and R. P. Nirschl. 1996. Elbow injuries. In *Athletic injuries and rehabilitation,* edited by J. Zachewski, D. Magee, and W. Quillen. Philadelphia: W. B. Saunders.

31. Stoane, J. M., M. R. Poplausky, J. O. Haller, and W. E. Berdon. 1995. Panner's disease: X-ray, MR imaging findings and review of the literature. *Computerized Medical Imaging and Graphics* 19(6): 473–76.

32. Stroyan, M., and K. E. Wilk. 1993. The functional anatomy of the elbow complex. *Journal of Orthopaedic and Sports Physical Therapy* 17(6): 279–88.

33. Thomas, P. J., and R. C. Noellert. 1995. Brachial artery disruption after closed posterior dislocation of the elbow. *American Journal of Orthopedics* 24(7): 558–60.

34. Tullos, H. S., and W. J. Ryan. 1985. Functional anatomy of the elbow. In *Injuries to the throwing arm,* edited by B. Zarins, J. R. Andres, and W. D. Carson. Philadelphia: W. B. Saunders.

35. Warfel, J. H. 1993. Muscles of the arm. In *The extremities, muscles and motor points.* Philadelphia: Lea & Febiger.

36. Wilk, K. E., C. Arrigo, and J. R. Andrews. 1993. Rehabilitation of the elbow in the throwing athlete. *Journal of Orthopaedic and Sports Physical Therapy* 17(6): 305–17.

37. Wilk, K. E. 1997. Personal communication with the author.

38. Williams, P. L., R. Warwick, M. Dyson, and L. Bannister. 1989. *Gray's anatomy,* 37th ed. London: Churchill Livingstone.

CHAPTER 21

Rehabilitation of Wrist, Hand, and Finger Injuries

Anne Marie Schneider

FUNCTIONAL ANATOMY AND BIOMECHANICS

The hand is an intricate balance of muscles, tendons, and joints working in unison. Hands are almost always exposed and for that reason can be especially prone to injuries, especially during sport contact. Changing the mechanics can greatly alter the function and appearance of the hand.

The Wrist

The wrist is the connecting link between the hand and the forearm.[52] The wrist joint is composed of eight carpal bones and their articulations with the radius and ulna proximally, and the metacarpals distally.

There is an intricate relationship between the carpal bones. They are connected by ligaments to each other, and to the radius and ulna. The palmar ligaments from the proximal carpal row to the radius are strongest, followed by the dorsal ligaments (scaphoid-triquetrum, and distal radius to lunate and triquetrum), with intrinsic ligaments (scapholunate and lunotriquetral) being the weakest.[7] The carpal bones are arranged in two rows, proximal and distal, with the scaphoid acting as the functional link between the two.[52] The distal carpal row determines the position of the scaphoid and thus the lunate. With radial deviation the distal row is displaced radially while the proximal row moves ulnarly. The distal portion of the scaphoid must shift to avoid the radial styloid. The scaphoid palmar flexes. This is reversed in ulnar deviation.[46] The total arc of motion for radial and ulnar deviation averages approximately 50 degrees, 15 degrees radially and 35 degrees ulnarly.[46] The uneven division is due to the buttressing effect of the radial styloid.[46]

Flexion and extension occur through synchronous movement of proximal and distal rows. The total excursion is equally distributed between the midcarpal and radiocarpal joints.[7] The arc of motion for flexion and extension is 121 degrees.[38]

There are no collateral ligaments in the wrist. Their presence would impede radial and ulnar deviation, allowing only flexion and extension. Cross sections through the wrist reveal that tendons of the extensor carpi ulnaris (ECU) at the ulnar aspect of the wrist, and the extensor pollicus brevis (EPB) and abductor pollicus longus (APL) on the radial side are in "collateral" position.[23] EMG studies show that ECU, EPB, and APL are active in wrist flexion and extension.[23] These muscles show only small displacement with flexion and extension so they are in an isometric position.[23] Their function can be described as an adjustable collateral system. The ECU shows activity in ulnar deviation and the APL and EPB in radial deviation.[23]

Stability of the ulnar side of the wrist is provided by the triangular fibrocartilage complex (TFCC).[52] This ligament arises from the radius and inserts into the base of the ulnar styloid, the ulnar carpus, and the base of the fifth metacarpal.[52] This ligament complex is the major stabilizer of the distal radioulnar joint (DRUJ) and is a load-bearing column between the distal ulna and ulnar carpus.[52]

There are no muscular or tendinous insertions on any carpal bones except the flexor carpi ulnaris (FCU) into the pisiform.[52] Muscles that move the wrist and fingers cross the wrist and insert on the appropriate bones. There is a dorsal retinaculum (fascia) with six vertical septa that attach to the distal radius and partition the first five dorsal compartments.[37] These define fibroosseous tunnels that position and maintain extensor tendons and their synovial sheaths relative to the axis of wrist motion.[37] The sixth compartment that houses the ECU is a separate tunnel formed from infratendinous retinaculum. This allows unrestricted ulnar rotation during pronation and supination.[37] The retinaculum prevents bowstringing of the tendons during wrist extension.

Volarly, the long finger flexors, long thumb flexor, median nerve, and radial artery pass through the carpal tunnel. Bowstringing is prevented by the thick transverse carpal ligament.

The Hand

The metacarpal phalangeal (MCP) joints allow for multiplanar motion; however, the primary function is flexion and extension.[52] The metacarpal head has a convex shape that fits with a shallow concave proximal phalanx. The stability of the MCP joint is provided by its capsule, collateral ligaments, accessory collateral ligaments, volar plate, and musculotendinous units.[52] The collateral liga-

ments are laterally positioned and are dorsal to the axis of rotation. In extension the collateral ligament is lax, in flexion it is taut.[22] This is important to remember if immobilizing the MCP joint. If the joint is casted or splinted in extension, the lax collateral ligament will tighten, which will then prevent flexion once mobilization has begun. The accessory collateral ligament is volar to the axis of rotation and is taut in extension and lax in flexion.

The volar plate helps prevent hyperextension of the MCP joint. It forms the dorsal wall of the flexor tendon sheath and the A1 pulley.[52]

Several muscles cross the MCP joints. On the flexor surface the flexor digitorum superficialis (FDS) and flexor digitorum profundus (FDP) are held close to the bones by pulleys. These pulleys prevent bowstringing during finger flexion. The FDS flexes the proximal interphalangeal (PIP) joint, and the FDP flexes the distal interphalangeal (DIP) joint. The interosseous muscles are lateral to the MCP joints and are responsible for abduction and adduction of the MCP joints. The lumbrical muscles are volar to the axis of rotation of the MCP joint, but then insert into the lateral bands and are dorsal to the PIP and DIP joints. Their function is MCP joint flexion and IP joint extension. (This is also the reason there can be IP extension with a radial nerve palsy.) Dorsally the extensor mechanism crosses the MCP joint. The tendon is held centrally by the sagittal bands.

The Fingers

The IP joints are bicondylar hinge joints allowing flexion and extension. Collateral and accessory collateral ligaments stabilize the joints on the lateral aspect. The collateral ligament is taut in extension and lax in flexion. This is important when splinting the PIP joint. If it is not a contraindication to the injury (i.e., PIP fracture dislocation), the joint should be splinted in full extension to help prevent flexion contractures.

On the flexor surface the FDS bifurcates proximal to the PIP joint, allowing the FDP to become more superficial as it continues to insert on the distal phalanx, allowing DIP flexion. The FDS inserts on the middle phalanx for PIP flexion. Five annular pulleys and three cruciate pulleys between the MCP and DIP joints prevent bowstringing of the tendons and help provide nutrition to the tendons.

On the extensor surface the common extensor tendon crosses the MCP joint then divides into three slips. The central slip inserts on the dorsal middle phalanx, allowing for PIP extension. The two lateral slips, called the lateral bands, get attachments from the lumbricals, travel dorsal and lateral to the PIP joint, rejoin after the PIP joint, and insert as the terminal extensor into the DIP joint. This is a delicately balanced system to extend the IP joints. Disruption of this system greatly alters the balance, and thus the dynamic function, of the hand.

REHABILITATION TECHNIQUES

Strengthening Techniques

Open-Kinetic-Chain Strengthening Exercises.

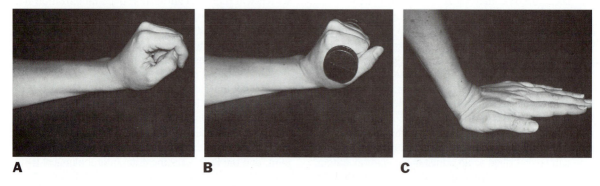

A   **B**   **C**

Figure 21-1   **A,** Wrist extension should be done in pronation to work against gravity. This exercise encourages strength and motion of the common wrist extensor tendons (ECRL, ECRB, ECU). MCP flexion should be maintained to eliminate EDC contribution and isolate wrist musculature. **B,** This position can be graded by adding weights. **C,** Passive wrist extension helps regain motion in the wrist, which then needs to be maintained actively.

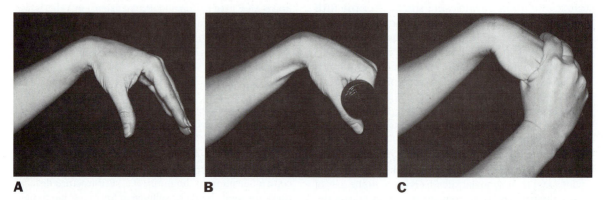

A   **B**   **C**

Figure 21-2   **A,** Wrist flexion actively works on FCR and FCU. It may be done in pronation as gravity assists or in supination with gravity. **B,** Position may be graded by adding weights. **C,** Passive wrist flexion should be done first by pulling out or distracting the wrist, then flexing.

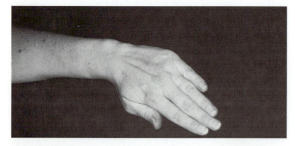

Figure 21-3   Wrist radial deviation with neutral flexion and extension will exercise the FCR and ECRL. It may be performed with palm flat on a table, or with arm in neutral over the edge of a table. It may be graded to include weights.

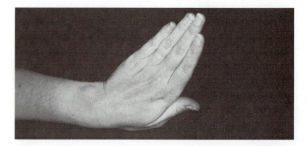

Figure 21-4   Wrist ulnar deviation with neutral flexion and extension will exercise the ECU and FCU. It may be performed in neutral rotation with gravity assisted, or with palm on the table. It is difficult to position for against gravity. It can be graded to include weights.

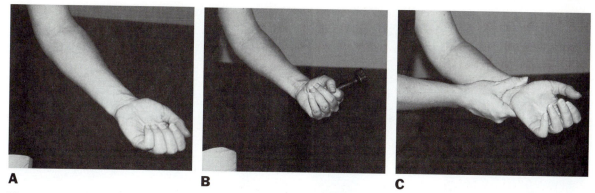

A   **B**   **C**

Figure 21-5   A, Active supination exercises the supinator and the biceps. It should be done with elbow at 90 degrees of flexion with the humerus by the side. This eliminates shoulder rotation. **B,** This can be graded using a hammer or weights for strengthening. The hammer with lever action being heavier on one end will also assist with passive motion. **C,** Passive stretching should be done in the same position, with force applied proximal to the wrist applying pressure over the radius rather than torquing the wrist.

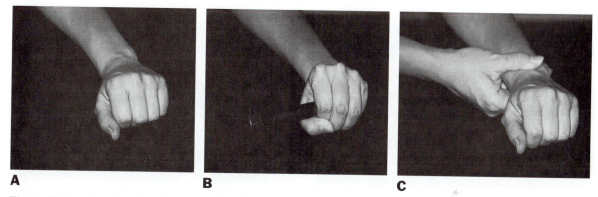

A   **B**   **C**

Figure 21-6   A, Active pronation exercises the pronator. It should be done with elbow flexed to 90 degrees with the humerus by the side. This eliminates shoulder rotation. **B,** This can be done with a hammer or weights for strengthening. **C,** Passive stretching should be done in the same position with the pressure applied proximal to the wrist.

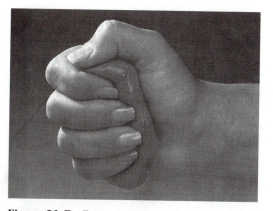

Figure 21-7   Putty exercises are for grip strengthening and wrist stabilization. Putty tends to be more effective than a ball because it gives resistance throughout the entire range of motion. Putty can be used for gross grasp, pinch, or extension.

Closed-Kinetic-Chain Strengthening Exercises.

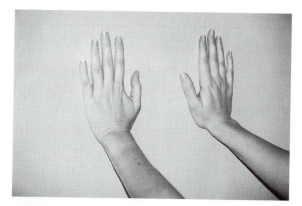

Figure 21-8   Wall push-ups encourage wrist motion and general upper-body strengthening. They also encourage weight bearing and closed-chain activities.

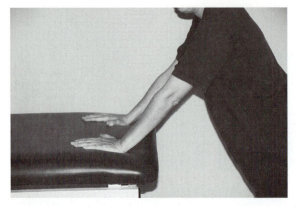

Figure 21-9 Push-ups can be progressed from the wall to a table or countertop. This encourages increased weight but not the full weight of floor push-ups.

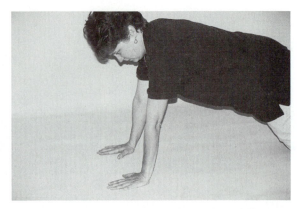

Figure 21-10 Push-ups on the floor require full, or close to full, wrist motion and encourage full upper-body weight bearing on the wrist.

Stretching and Range-of-Motion Exercises.

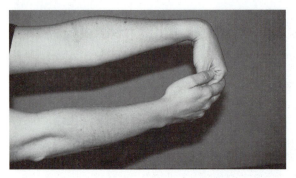

Figure 21-11 Stretching wrist extensor musculature is appropriate when tendinitis is present. The greatest stretch will occur with the elbow at full extension and the arm at shoulder height. If this stretch is too great, increase elbow flexion to a comfortable stretch point. Do not bounce at the end of a stretch.

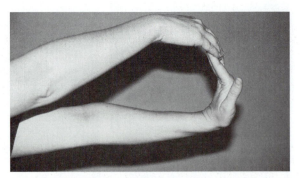

Figure 21-12 Stretching wrist flexor musculature is appropriate with flexor tendinitis. Again the largest stretch will occur with full elbow extension. Modify elbow flexion as necessary. Stretching should not be painful.

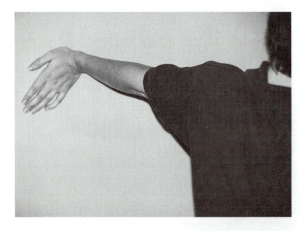

Figure 21-13 Butler describes median nerve gliding exercises to be done in the clinic. It is also important to teach athletes to stretch on their own. This is a median nerve glide that athletes can perform on their own against a wall. Start with arm at shoulder height, elbow extended, and wrist extension with palm against the wall. Rotate shoulder externally. Turn away from the wall so as to be perpendicular. The last step is to add lateral neck flexion. Stop at any point along this progression where numbness or burning is felt along the arm.

Tendon Mobilization Exercises.

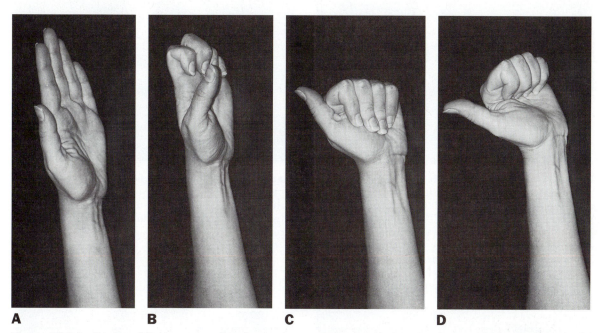

A   **B**   **C**   **D**

Figure 21-14 Tendon gliding exercises allow for maximum gliding of the FDS and FDP independent of each other. Start with full composite finger extension **A,** move to hook fisting which gives the maximum glide of the FDP **B,** return to extension, move to long fisting with MCP and PIP flexion and DIP extension for maximum FDS glide **C,** return to extension, then to composite flexion with full fisting **D.**

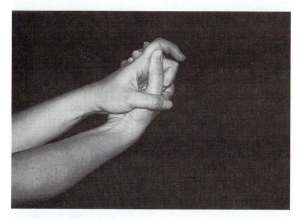

Figure 21-15 Blocked PIP exercises encourage FDS pull-through. Stabilizing the proximal phalanx then allows the flexion force to act at the PIP joint. It is most often used with tendon injuries, or finger fractures.

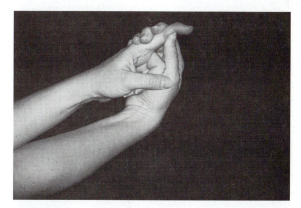

Figure 21-16 Blocked DIP exercises encourage FDP pull-through. Stabilizing the middle phalanx allows the flexion force to concentrate at the DIP joint. These are most often done with flexor tendon injuries, extensor tendon injuries, or finger fractures.

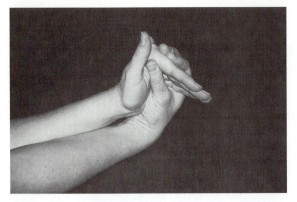

Figure 21-17 MCP flexion with IP extension exercises the intrinsic muscles of the hand. It may help with edema control and muscle pumping. This is most often done with distal radius fractures or MCP joint injuries. Performing IP extension with the MCP joints blocked in flexion concentrates the extension force at the IP joints. This is beneficial for IP joint injuries or tendon injuries.

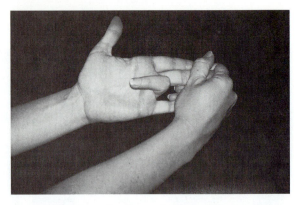

Figure 21-18 Isolated superficialis exercises are done for tendon gliding of the FDS. Noninvolved fingers should be held in full extension, allowing only the involved finger to flex. This is most helpful during flexor tendon lacerations.

Joint Mobilization Exercises.

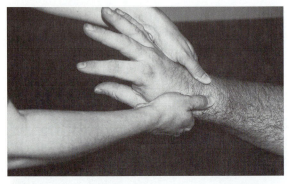

Figure 21-19 Distal anterior/posterior radial glides are done with one hand stabilizing the ulna and the other gliding the radius. These glides increase pronation.

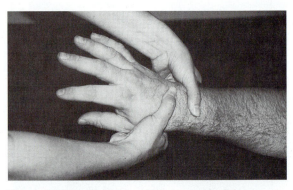

Figure 21-20 Radiocarpal joint anterior glides increase wrist extension.

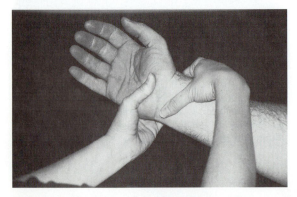

Figure 21-21 Radiocarpal joint posterior glides increase wrist flexion.

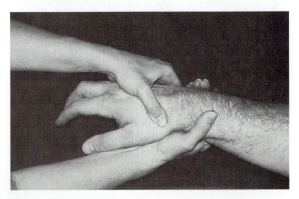

Figure 21-22 Radiocarpal joint ulnar glides increase radial deviation.

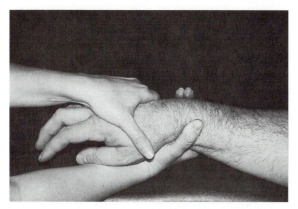

Figure 21-23 Radiocarpal joint radial glides increase ulnar deviation.

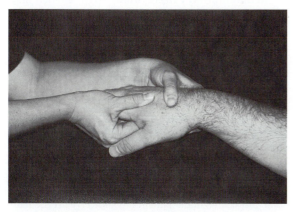

Figure 21-24 Carpometacarpal joint anterior/posterior glides increase mobility of the hand.

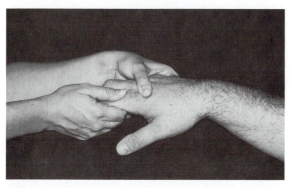

Figure 21-25 Metacarpophalangeal joint anterior/posterior glides. In metacarpophalangeal joint anterior or posterior glides, the proximal segment, in this case the metacarpal, is stabilized and the distal segment is mobilized. Anterior glides increase flexion of the MP joint. Posterior glides increase extension.

Exercises for Reestablishing Neuromuscular Control

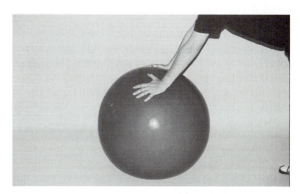

Figure 21-26 Push-ups on the ball allow for an unstable surface, to encourage strengthening and upper extremity control. Overhead plyometric activities encourage endurance and strength of entire upper extremity.

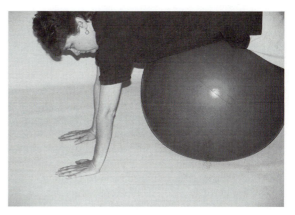

Figure 21-27 Exercising prone over a large gym ball allows for weight bearing throughout the upper extremity, weight shifting, and balance activities.

REHABILITATION TECHNIQUES FOR SPECIFIC INJURIES

Distal Radius Fractures

Pathomechanics. Fractures of the distal radius can be described in many different ways, by several classification systems. For treatment it is important to be able to describe the fracture and X ray. Is the fracture intra-articular or extra-articular? displaced or nondisplaced? simple or comminuted? open or closed? Is the radius shortened? Is the ulna also fractured? Answers to these questions help guide treatment and expected outcomes.

Simple, extra-articular, nondisplaced fractures tend to heal without incident with immobilization, with full or nearly full motion expected following treatment. As the fractures become more involved (intra-articular or comminuted), chances of full return of motion are decreased.

The normal anatomic radius is tilted volarly. If in a fracture the volar tilt becomes dorsal, motion will be affected. It can also lead to midcarpal instability, decreased strength, increased ulnar loading, and a dysfunctional DRUJ.[17]

The normal anatomic radius is longer than the ulna. If in a comminuted fracture the radius is shortened, this is the most disabling.[17,18] Radial shortening can lead to DRUJ problems, decreased mobility, and decreased power (strength). Articular displacement correction is critical. Radial shortening must be corrected via external fixation.

The external fixator will attach to the mid radius and to the second metacarpal shaft. Length may be restored and held with the traction bars of the external fixator. If the fixator was not in place and the fracture was not reduced, the weight and anatomy of the carpal bones and the force of the muscles would cause loss of reduction and shortening of the radius. The type of fracture, size of the fragments, and displacement determine initial treatment (cast vs. fixator). Once reduced, the fractures must be closely monitored to be sure reduction is being maintained.

Rehabilitation following a distal radius fracture is similar, regardless of method of fixation (cast, ORIF, or ex fix). Range of motion and edema control of noninvolved joints are essential, so that when immobilization is discontinued rehabilitation can be concentrated on the wrist and forearm rather than also on the fingers, elbow, and shoulder.

Injury Mechanism. As is true of most wrist injuries, distal radius fractures occur from a fall on an outstretched hand. It might be a high-impact event, but does not always have to be.

Rehabilitation Concerns. Early and proper reduction and immobilization are of utmost importance. The fracture must be closely watched initially to be sure reduction is being maintained. Early ROM to noninvolved joints is imperative. This helps prevent muscle atrophy, aids in muscle pumping to decrease edema, and most importantly maintains motion so treatment can focus on the wrist once the fracture is healed and fixation is removed.

Other concerns include complications of carpal tunnel or reflex sympathetic dystrophy (RSD).[26] If present and first noted in the therapy clinic or training room, referral should be made back to the physician as soon as possible. One other complication, which usually occurs late in a seemingly inconsequential nondisplaced distal radius fracture, is an extensor pollicus longus (EPL) rupture.[26] It is thought that this occurs from the EPL rubbing around the fracture site near Lister's tubercle. The athlete would be unable to extend the thumb IP joint. This would need to be surgically repaired.

Rehabilitation Progression. Rehabilitation may be initiated while the wrist is immobilized. This should include shoulder ROM in all planes, elbow flexion and extension, and finger flexion and extension. Finger exercises should include isolated MCP flexion, composite flexion (full fist), and intrinsic minus fisting (MCP extension with IP flexion) (Figure 21-14). Coban or an Isotoner glove may be used for edema control if necessary.

If a fixator or pins are present, pin site care may be performed, depending on physician preference. Most physicians this author works with prefer hydrogen peroxide with a cotton applicator to remove the crusted areas from around the pins. A different applicator should be used on each pin, to prevent possible spread of infection. Some physicians allow patients to shower with the fixator in place (not soaking while bathing); other physicians prefer to cover the pin sites with a plastic bag to keep them dry.

Once immobilization is discontinued (at approximately 6 weeks for casting, 8 weeks with an external fixator, 2 weeks for ORIF with plate and screws), ROM to the wrist is begun. Active motion is begun immediately. Wrist flexion, extension, and radial and ulnar deviation are evaluated, then instructed. Wrist extension should be taught with finger (especially MCP) flexion (Figure 21-1). This isolates the wrist extensors and prevents "cheating" with the extensor digitorum communis (EDC). The importance of wrist extensor isolation is for hand function. If the EDC is used to extend the wrist, then flexing the fingers to grasp something will cause the wrist to also flex, tenodesis will extend the fingers, and the object will be dropped. Isolating wrist extension should be the emphasis of treatment on the first visit.

Passive ROM (PROM) may depend on physician preference. Many let PROM begin immediately, others prefer waiting 1 to 2 weeks (Figures 21-1 and 21-2) for passive stretching exercises. Forearm rotation (supination and

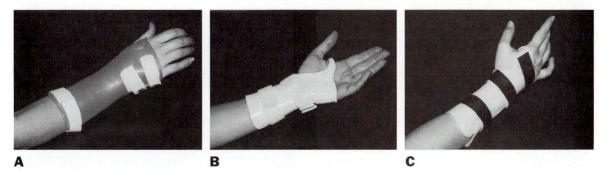

Figure 21-28 A wrist splint may be made dorsally, volarly, or circumferentially, depending on support needs and type of injury. These splints may be used for tendinitis, wrist fractures, wrist sprains, and carpal tunnel syndrome.

pronation) must not be ignored. Active ROM (AROM) and PROM are both important. When stretching rotation passively, pressure should be applied at the distal radius, proximal to the wrist, not at the hand. This will help apply pressure where the limitations are and not put unnecessary torque across the carpus (Figures 21-5, 21-26).

Active motion can be progressed to strengthening. Light weights, TheraBand, or tubing may be graded for all wrist and forearm motions. This can be in conjunction with weight-bearing wall push-ups in a countertop to mat to floor progression (Figures 21-8 through 21-10). Push-ups on a ball may be the next progression (Figure 21-26), along with lying prone over a large ball and "walking" out and back on extended wrists (Figure 21-27).

Using putty for grip strengthening can be started and upgraded to harder putty beginning about 1 week after immobilization. This also helps to strengthen the wrist musculature (Figure 21-7).

Plyometric exercises for the wrist and general upper-extremity strength are next. Activities are graded from a playground-type ball to a large gym ball to weighted balls. Activities can be done in supine, against a wall, or, if available, using a rebounder. Specific return-to-sport exercises and activities must also be done.

Criteria for Return. Return to play depends on the sport and the severity of the fracture. If the fracture is nondisplaced, the athlete usually may return to sport when it stops hurting (2 to 3 weeks, or sooner), with protection. There should be early signs of healing, no pain at rest, and no pain with a direct blow to the protection. If a nondisplaced fracture is treated by ORIF with plate and screw fixation, the athlete might be able to return to play at about 3 weeks without protection if the sport is noncontact. At approximately 6 weeks the athlete may play without protection. The sport must be taken into consideration. An athlete in a high-contact sport might need protection longer than an athlete in a noncontact sport.

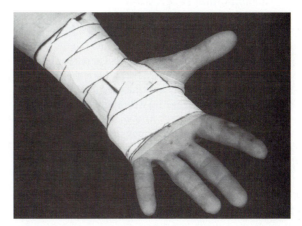

Figure 21-29 Wrist taping may be done when extra support is needed but hard plastic splinting is inappropriate.

If the fracture was displaced, the athlete is usually out of competition for about 6 weeks, then returns with protection for an additional 2 to 6 weeks (Figures 21-28 and 21-29).

As with all injuries, return to sport depends on the sport, position played, and physician. The athlete's strength must also be adequate for the position played, to prevent reinjury.

Wrist Sprain

Pathomechanics. The term *wrist sprain* is often seen when patients complain of pain and have a history of minor trauma. The diagnosis should be one of exclusion. Injuries that must be ruled out include scaphoid fracture, traumatic instability patterns, lunate fractures, dorsal chip fractures, other carpal fractures and injuries, and ligament tears.[17]

Injury Mechanism. The injury is usually a minor trauma, either a fall landing on an outstretched hand, a twisting motion, or some impact such as striking the ground with a club.

Rehabilitation Concerns. The primary concern is ruling out more serious injury. Once other diagnoses are ruled out, treatment is focused on edema control, pain control, maintaining (or increasing) active and passive ROM to the wrist and other, noninvolved joints. If necessary, splint immobilization (Figure 21-28) may also be tried for pain relief. If activities increase pain, those activities should be examined to determine whether modifications can be made to decrease pain and increase activity level for return to sports.

Rehabilitation Progression. Following decrease in pain and edema, and return of ROM, strengthening should be performed to all wrist motions and, if necessary, to grip strength and entire arm. Refer to the section on distal radius fracture for specific exercises (Figures 21-1 through 21-10, 21-26, 21-27). Joint mobilizations for the wrist can certainly help improve joint arthrokinematics and ROM (Figures 21-19 through 21-24).

Criteria for Return. Athletes may return to sport when they are comfortable. Taping the wrist (Figure 21-29) can help provide support and decrease pain. The athlete should not return to play until all other serious conditions are ruled out.

Scaphoid Fracture

Pathomechanics. Fractures of the scaphoid account for 60 percent of all carpal injuries.[3] The prognosis is related to the site of the fracture, obliquity, displacement, and promptness of diagnosis and treatment.[17] The blood supply of the scaphoid comes distal to proximal. Fracture through the waist of the proximal one-third of the scaphoid can result in delayed union or avascular necrosis secondary to poor blood supply. It can take 20 weeks for a proximal one-third fracture to heal, compared to 5 or 6 weeks at the scaphoid tuberosity.[17] Displacement of the fracture occurs at the time of injury and must be treated early using ORIF.

Ninety percent of scaphoid fractures heal without complications if treated early and properly.[27,28] If the fracture does go on to non-union, whether symptomatic or not, it should be treated. Not treating will lead to carpal instability and periscaphoid arthritis.[34,44]

Diagnosis is made by X ray. Patients will have wrist pain, especially in the anatomic snuffbox (Figure 21-30).

Injury Mechanism. Scaphoid fractures result from a fall on an outstretched hand. The radial styloid may impact against the scaphoid waist, causing a fracture.[7] The scaphoid fails in tension when the palmar surface experi-

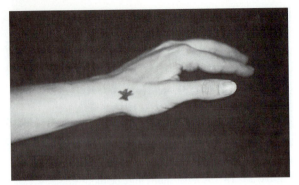

Figure 21-30 The * indicates the anatomic snuffbox, under which the scaphoid is positioned. This area will be painful to palpation with scaphoid fracture or scapholunate ligament injury.

ences an excessive bending movement.[45] Because the scaphoid blocks wrist extension, it is at risk for injury.[17]

Rehabilitation Concerns. Of primary concern is proper diagnosis. If the athlete has a history of falls on an outstretched hand and has pain in the anatomic snuffbox, but the initial X ray is negative, they should be treated conservatively in a thumb spica cast for 2 weeks, then be X rayed again.[9,29] If the X ray is negative after 2 weeks, the cast may be removed and ROM begun.

Another concern is non-unions, which can lead to carpal instability or periscaphoid arthritis. ROM of noninjured and noncasted joints must be maintained during prolonged periods of immobilization.

Rehabilitation Progressions. Treatment of the nondisplaced scaphoid is casting. Following casting, an additional 2 to 4 weeks of splinting (Figure 21-31) may be used, with the splint removed for the exercise program. AROM exercises of wrist flexion, wrist extension (with finger flexion to isolate wrist extensors), and radial and ulnar deviation are initiated following immobilization (Figures 21-1 through 21-4). Thumb flexion and extension, abduction and adduction, and opposition to each finger are also initiated. After approximately 2 weeks (sooner if cleared by the physician), PROM to the same motion is begun. Gentle strengthening with weights or putty may be started around the same time. Strengthening is progressed over the next several weeks to include weight-bearing activities, plyometrics, and general arm conditioning to return to sport-specific activity (Figures 21-8 through 21-10, 21-26, 21-27).

Surgical repair rehabilitation follows the same progression as for nonsurgical rehabilitation. The time frame of immobilization might be less because of the repair of the scaphoid with rigid fixation.

Criteria for Return. Return to play depends on the sport, location and type of fracture, and type of im-

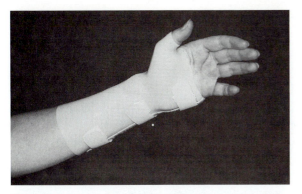

Figure 21-31 A thumb spica splint is circumferential and includes the thumb and wrist. It might or might not include the thumb IP joint. It is most commonly used for a scaphoid or thumb metacarpal fracture.

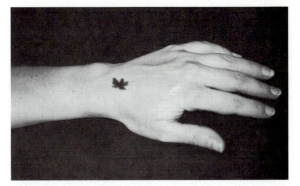

Figure 21-32 The * indicates the position of the lunate and the location of pain with lunate or scapholunate ligament injuries.

mobilization. If the fracture is nondisplaced and treated in a cast, return to play in a padded cast might be at 2 or 3 weeks or sooner—when the arm stops hurting, there are early signs of healing, and there is no pain with a blow to the cast. The athlete should continue to play with protection until the bone has healed and adequate strength has returned to help prevent reinjury, or new injury to a separate site. If the nondisplaced fracture has undergone ORIF or if the athlete is participating in a noncontact sport, the athlete may return, if cleared by the physician, in about 2 or 3 weeks without additional protection. An athlete in a contact sport should participate with protection. If the fracture is displaced and surgically repaired, time until return to play may be longer. The athlete must wear a padded protective cast upon return to play. In all cases, close communication is essential for return to competition.

Lunate Dislocations

Pathomechanics. Stability of the carpus is dependent upon the maintenance of bony architecture interlaced with ligaments.[17] Most carpal dislocations are of the dorsal perilunate type. Many people believe that a lunate dislocation is the end of a perilunate dislocation.[17] The lunate dislocates palmarly with the loss of ligamentous stability. It may be reduced, if seen early, by placing the wrist in extension and putting pressure on the lunate (Figure 21-32). The wrist is then brought into flexion and immobilized. It is very common for reduction to be lost over time with this injury, so percutaneous pinning or ORIF is recommended.[17]

Median nerve compression is frequently caused by this injury. The palmarly displaced lunate puts pressure on the nerve. Symptoms might continue for several weeks following reduction of the lunate secondary to swelling and contusion of the nerve.

Injury Mechanism. A violent hyperextension of the wrist is the injury mechanism.[7,17] A fall on the outstretched hand produces a translational compressive force when the lunate is caught between the capitate and the dorsal aspect of the distal radius articular surface.[17] If the lunate does not fracture, a periscaphoid or lunate dislocation can occur.

Rehabilitation Concerns. The primary concern is early surgical repair. Without surgical correction, complications include pain, weakness, wrist clicking, and bones slipping.[7] Carpal tunnel syndrome, if present, must be addressed at the time of surgery. ROM of noninvolved joints must be maintained during immobilization.

Rehabilitation Progressions. Progression is very similar to the rehabilitation of distal radius fractures and other wrist injuries. Following cast and pin removal (if applicable), AROM is begun. This is progressed to passive stretching and gentle strengthening. Strengthening becomes more aggressive with free weights and weight-bearing and plyometric activities. Motions that need to be addressed for ROM and strengthening are flexion, extension, radial deviation, ulnar deviation, supination, and pronation (Figures 21-1 through 21-10, 21-26, 21-27).

Criteria for Return. The severity of this injury, and the need for ORIF secondary to frequent loss of reduction if not repaired, will keep this athlete from competition for at least 8 weeks. Upon return at 8 weeks, the wrist may be taped for support and protection (Figure 21-29). The athlete should not be favoring or protecting the hand during periods of noncompetition. Athletes should have good ROM and strength prior to return to help prevent reinjury.

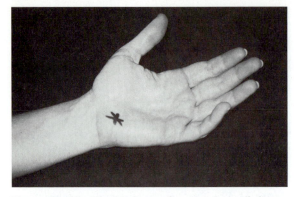

Figure 21-33 The * indicates the point that will elicit pain with palpation (especially deep) for a hamate hook fracture. Some pain might also be referred to the ulnar wrist.

Hamate Fractures

Pathomechanics. Fractures of the hook of the hamate are more common than hamate body fractures.[4] The hook is the attachment for the pisohamate ligament, short flexor and opponens to the small finger, and the transverse carpal ligament.[52] Because of these attachments, if there is a hamate hook fracture there are deforming forces on the fragment with intermittent tension. This makes it nearly impossible to align and immobilize the fracture, and as a result these often do not heal.[52] The hook can be palpated on the volar surface of the hand at the base of the hypothenar eminence deep and radial to the pisiform.

The hamate is in close proximity to the ulnar nerve and artery on the ulnar side, and flexor tendons to the ring and small finger in the carpal canal on the radial side (Figure 21-33). There is a possibility of an ulnar neuropathy, tendinitis, or tendon rupture with this injury.[10,40,41]

Injury Mechanism. The suspected injury mechanism is a shearing force transmitted from the handle of a club to the hamate. It often occurs when striking an unexpected object (as when a golfer strikes a rock or tree root). It most frequently occurs in golfers but can occur in any stick sport, such as baseball or field hockey. There is also a possibility of a stress fracture from tension from ligament and muscle attachments, but this is rare.[7]

Rehabilitation Concerns. The first concern is diagnosis. Athletes might have felt a snap or pop. They will have localized tenderness over the hamate hook, ulnar-side wrist pain, and weakness of grip that increases over time. A carpal tunnel view X ray will confirm the diagnosis. The trainer or therapist must also be concerned and watch for signs of ulnar neuritis or neuropathy, and flexor tendon rupture.

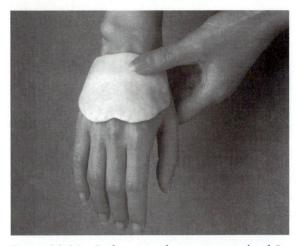

Figure 21-34 Otoform is used as a scar control pad. It comes in varying size containers. The needed amount of "putty" is taken from the jar, mixed with a catalyst, and applied directly to the scar area. Once it hardens, in 1 to 2 minutes, it can be rinsed and applied with Coban or a similar covering. It is usually worn 23 hours per day for scar control. It does need to be removed, as it does not breathe and skin can become macerated, or a rash can develop. It may also be worn during sport activity for additional protection to a sensitive area.

Rehabilitation Progressions. Treatment has been described as casting an acute hamate hook fracture[2,31] or bone grafting a non-union.[47] However, as described previously, these fractures do not usually heal secondary to forces applied to the fracture fragment. Treatment for symptomatic hamate fractures is fragment excision.[40,41]

Treatment following excision is edema control, scar massage (3 to 5 minutes, 5 times/day), and grip strengthening if necessary.

Criteria for Return. Acute injuries must be treated symptomatically. Tape or padding, if allowed, may be placed in the palm. Chronic fractures are also treated symptomatically, with pain being the limiting factor. It is not detrimental for the athlete to continue to play with a fracture and have the fragment removed at the end of the season, as long as they are able to play with their symptoms. Otherwise, the injury should be surgically addressed earlier.

Once the fragment has been excised, the athlete may return to sport as soon as they are comfortable. A small splint, padding, or scar control pad such as Topigel or Otoform (Figure 21-34) might be helpful initially for scar control and to decrease hypersensitivity around the incision area. Full return is expected.

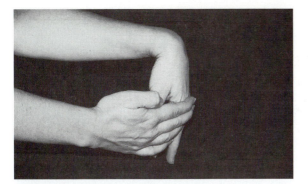

Fig 21-35   Phalen's test for carpal tunnel injury is extreme wrist flexion, which narrows the space in the carpal canal. The test is positive if there is numbness and tingling in the median nerve distribution within 60 seconds. Do not flex elbows or rest elbows on the table, as this can elicit ulnar nerve symptoms.

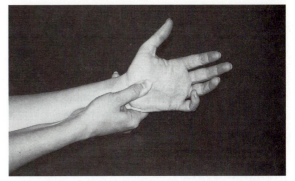

Figure 21-36   Firm pressure over the carpal tunnel can elicit numbness or tingling in the median nerve distribution. This alone is not indicative of carpal tunnel injury, but provides more information.

Carpal Tunnel Syndrome

Pathomechanics.   Carpal tunnel syndrome is compression of the median nerve at the level of the wrist. The carpal tunnel is made of the carpal bones dorsally and transverse carpal ligament volarly. Located in the carpal tunnel are the FDS and FDP to all digits, FPL, median nerve, and median artery.[19] If tendons become inflamed, the space within the carpal tunnel is decreased and the nerve becomes compressed. Excessive wrist flexion or extension will also increase pressure in the carpal tunnel. Symptoms of classic carpal tunnel are numbness and tingling in the thumb through the radial half of ring finger, pain or waking at night, and clumsiness or weakness in the hand. Symptoms might increase with static positioning (e.g., when driving or reading a newspaper).[19] Diagnosis is made by history, Phalen's test (Figure 21-35), Tinel's sign, nerve conduction studies, direct pressure over the carpal tunnel (Figure 21-36), and EMGs. Injection can help confirm diagnosis and may relieve symptoms.

Injury Mechanism.   The incidence of carpal tunnel is extremely low in most athletes,[33] but the injury is found in cyclists, throwers, and tennis players.[35] Pressure from resting on handlebars can cause symptoms. Sustained grip and the repetitive actions of throwers and racquet sports can also increase symptoms. Illnesses or injuries that have been associated with carpal tunnel include tenosynovitis from overuse or from rheumatoid arthritis, and external or internal pressure from conditions such as lipoma, diabetes, or pregnancy.[48] Acute carpal tunnel can occur following a fracture or other trauma, by either edema or a fracture fragment pressing on the median nerve.

Rehabilitation Concerns.   Conservative treatment is tried first and consists of night splinting with the wrist in neutral (Figure 21-28), anti-inflammatory medication, and relative rest from the aggravating source (if known). Occasionally physicians will recommend full-time wrist splinting. This author prefers that wrist splints not be worn during the day, as this leads to muscle weakness and arm pain from distribution of forces to new areas. Injections may be done by the physician for symptom relief—this is also diagnostic. If the symptoms disappear with injection, the diagnosis is correct. Symptoms can recur. Nerve-gliding exercises described by Butler[6] (Figure 21-13) and myofascial release might also help relieve symptoms. Activity analysis and biomechanical analysis of activities that increase symptoms should be done to see if changes in technique will decrease symptoms.

If conservative treatment fails, a carpal tunnel release may be performed. Rehabilitation following a release consists of wound care (if necessary), scar massage, and ROM exercises. Tendon-gliding exercises are done to improve ROM and isolation of tendons. These exercises start with full-finger extension, then a hooked fist to maximize FDP pull-through in relation to FDS, then a long fist to maximize FDS pull-through, then a composite fist. Full extension should be performed between each position (Figure 21-14). Wrist ROM should also be performed (Figures 21-1 and 21-2).

Rehabilitation Progressions.   Progression for carpal tunnel release includes grip strengthening. Exercises should begin slowly, to not increase the symptoms. Wrist strengthening may also be performed. Strengthening is generally begun 2 to 4 weeks postsurgery, after consultation with the physician. Upper-body conditioning should also be performed if necessary for return to sport.

Criteria for Return. Athletes may continue to play with carpal tunnel. Activity should be examined, though, to see whether it could be altered to decrease symptoms. Activity level is based on symptoms. If conservative treatment fails and a release is performed, athletes can typically return to sport once sutures are removed. Surgical release is rarely necessary in athletes.

Ganglion Cysts

Pathology. A ganglion cyst is the most common soft-tissue tumor in the hand.[5] It is a synovial cyst arising from the synovial lining of a tendon sheath or joint. The etiology is unclear. They are most common on the dorsal radial wrist, but can also be volar (Figure 21-37). They originate deep in the joint and can be symptomatic before they appear at the surface. The usual origin is from the area of the scapholunate ligament.[5] Ganglion cysts are translucent, which can help confirm the diagnosis.

Treatment is aspiration of the cyst. Results of recurrence are variable. In adults, multiple aspirations are suggested, with success rates of 51 to 85 percent.[25] If multiple aspirations are not successful and cysts recur, they may be surgically excised.

Injury Mechanism. In the athletic population, it appears that ganglions most often form with repeated forceful hyperextension of the wrist, as would occur in weight lifters, shot putters, wrestlers, and gymnasts. Pain is the indication for treatment.

Rehabilitation Concerns. These patients do not need to be seen for rehabilitation once diagnosed and aspirated. The aspiration usually decreases pain and allows for full ROM. Following ganglion cyst excision, patients may need to be seen for ROM, passive stretching, strengthening, and scar control. ROM emphasis should be on wrist flexion and extension and finger flexion and extension (Figures 21-1, 21-2, 21-14). Scar massage and desensitization may be done with lotion, rubbing on the scar, tapping on the scar, and performing vibration to the scar. Less noxious stimuli should be done first, with increasing difficulty being added to program. Scar control pads such as Otoform (see Figure 21-34) or Topigel sheeting may also be used, held in place with Coban.

Rehabilitation Progressions. Following excision and return of ROM, strengthening may be done as necessary for grip, wrist flexion and extension, and general upper-extremity return-to-play exercises.

Criteria for Return. Activity is limited by pain. Athletes may participate with a ganglion if it is not symp-

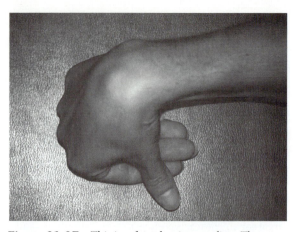

Figure 21-37 This is a dorsal wrist ganglion. These vary in size and shape and will transilluminate.

tomatic. If symptomatic, it may be aspirated with immediate return to activity. If it recurs, it may be aspirated again with no loss of playing time. If necessary, the ganglion may be excised at the end of the season. If excised, sport activity may begin once sutures are removed, at approximately 10 days. Full return is expected.

Boxer's Fracture

Pathomechanics. A boxer's fracture is a fracture of the fifth metacarpal neck. This is the most commonly fractured metacarpal.[21] It will frequently shorten and angulate on impact. There is a large amount of movement of the fifth metacarpal. For this reason, perfect anatomic reduction is not necessary. It should be noted, however, that excess angulation can lead to either an imbalance between the intrinsic and extrinsic muscles of the hand, leading to clawing, or to a mass in the palm.[32]

Injury Mechanism. This injury occurs most frequently from contact against an object with a closed fist. The impact is usually through the fifth metacarpal head.

Rehabilitation Concerns. Of concern is skin integrity. The injuries frequently occur as a result of a fight, and pieces of tooth might be in an open wound. If the injury is closed, concern is for proper immobilization, edema control, and ROM of noninvolved joints—especially the IP joints of the small finger. Occasionally ORIF is required. Edema control is critical. AROM may be initiated 72 hours after the ORIF.[32]

Treatment is immobilization in a plaster gutter splint, or in a thermoplastic splint fabricated by a hand therapist (Figure 21-38). The latter is often preferred as it allows for skin hygiene, wrist ROM, and IP joint ROM. The splint immobilizes only the ring and small finger MCP joints.

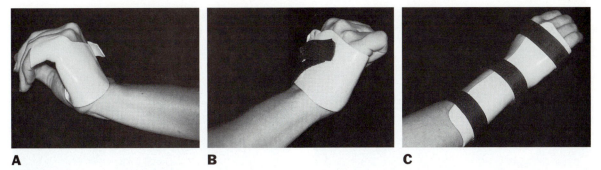

A   **B**   **C**

Figure 21-38 A boxer's fracture splint protects the ring and small finger proximal phalanxes and metacarpals, including the MCP joint. The splint may be modified for a different neck fracture (immobilizing the involved MCP joint), metacarpal shaft fracture (possibly only the metacarpal will need to be in the splint, leaving the wrist and MCP joints free), or metacarpal base fracture (this might need to include the wrist, usually leave the MCP joints free).

The splint is also easily remolded if necessary as edema decreases. Splinting is continued for approximately 4 weeks.

Rehabilitation Progression. During the time of immobilization, ROM to noninvolved joints is maintained by active and passive exercises. At approximately 4 weeks the splint is discontinued and ROM to MCP joints is begun. Buddy taping may be done to encourage ROM. Between 4 and 6 weeks gentle resistance may be performed, with vigorous activities at about 6 weeks.

Criteria for Return. An athlete may return when there is a sign that the fracture is healing, it feels stable, and there is no pain with the fracture or movement. This is generally at 3 to 4 weeks with protection. Generally by 6 weeks the athlete may play with only buddy taping protection. This, as always, depends on the sport, the athlete, and the physician.

DeQuervain's Tenosynovitis and Tendinitis

Pathomechanics. Tendinitis, most simply put, is inflammation of a tendon. It can occur on the dorsal wrist, volar wrist, or thumb. Symptoms are pain along the muscle, pain with resisted motions, or swelling. It is frequently caused by overuse. Injections can help relieve symptoms and confirm diagnosis.

DeQuervain's tenosynovitis is an inflammation in the first dorsal compartment; the abductor pollicus longus (APL) and extensor pollicus brevis (EPB) are affected.[1] The third dorsal compartment is usually not affected, and as such the IP joint of the thumb does not need to be included in any splint. The condition can be aggravated by excessive wrist radial and ulnar deviation, flexion and adduction of the thumb, or adduction of the thumb.[24]

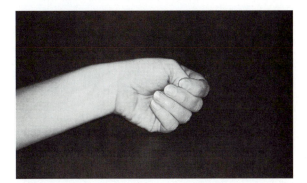

Figure 21-39 Finklestein's test will be positive for pain in DeQuervain's. Passive flexion of the thumb with wrist ulnar deviation is the provocative position. Always compare to the noninvolved side, as this test can be uncomfortable normally.

Finklestein's test,[15] passive thumb flexion into the palm with passive wrist ulnar deviation, will be positive for pain (Figure 21-39). Always compare to the noninjured side, as this test can be uncomfortable normally.

Injury Mechanism. Tendinitis is usually caused by overuse. It can also be caused by weakness, poor body mechanics, or abnormal postures. DeQuervain's can be caused by repeated wrist radial and ulnar deviation. Less frequent causes include a direct blow to the radial styloid, acute strain as in lifting, or a ganglion in the first dorsal compartment.[24]

Rehabilitation Concerns. Initial treatment is anti-inflammatory medication and rest from aggravating activities. Modalities for edema reduction and pain control, such as ultrasound, iontophoresis, or ice, can be effective. Analysis of activity should be done to see if poor mechanics are aggravating symptoms.

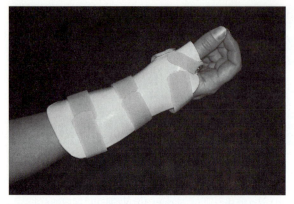

Figure 21-40 A DeQuervain's splint is a radial gutter thumb splint. It supports the wrist and thumb CMC and MCP joints. It is used to rest the thumb and wrist with DeQuervain's.

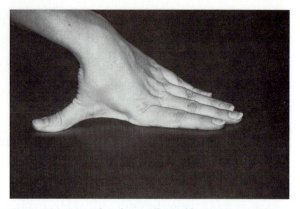

Figure 21-41 The ulnar collateral ligament provides support on the ulnar MCP joint. A fall on an abducted thumb can cause injury or rupture.

Splinting for wrist tendinitis includes the wrist only (Figure 21-28). Splinting for DeQuervain's includes the thumb MCP and CMC joints, and wrist, usually in a radial gutter fashion (Figure 21-40). Splinting is usually full-time except for hygiene for the first 2 to 3 weeks, then if symptoms are subsiding, wearing time is slowly decreased while activity is increased. If pain is persistent, splinting continues.

Rehabilitation Progressions. Stretching of the affected areas in a pain-free range (Figures 21-11, 21-12) three times per day should begin immediately with rest (splinting) and anti-inflammatory medication. Once pain has decreased, strengthening of grip and wrist musculature may begin. If strengthening is begun too early, symptoms will be re-exacerbated. If tendinitis is a result of muscle imbalance, the weak muscle groups must be strengthened. If symptoms do not subside, and injections are helpful but do not cure the symptoms, a release of the first dorsal compartment might need to be performed.

Criteria for Return. Pain and strength are limiting factors for return. Athletes should have pain-free ROM to the affected part. Strength should be significant to prevent reinjury. The athlete may participate prior to absence of pain if they are taped for support, use a splint for rest while they are not participating in sports, and pain does not impair performance.

If a release is performed, it may be done at the end of the season if symptoms permit play. If not, the athlete can return when comfortable, as early as 10 days post-surgery. Strength should be sufficient to prevent reinjury, aggravating forces should have been addressed, and support initially might be needed.

Ulnar Collateral Ligament Sprain (Gamekeeper's Thumb)

Pathomechanics. The ulnar collateral ligament (UCL) injury to the MCP joint of the thumb is the most common ligament injury.[36,39,50] The injury can be classified as grade I or grade II, in which the majority of the ligament remains intact. Grade III is a complete disruption of the UCL, and surgical repair is recommended. Rupture occurs most often at the distal attachment of the ligament[20,30] (Figure 21-41).

The athlete will complain of pain or tenderness on the ulnar side of the MCP joint. X rays should be taken to rule out fracture. Following X rays, MCP joint stability should be evaluated at full extension and at 30 degrees of flexion. These two positions will test the accessory collateral ligament and the proper collateral ligament, respectively. Angulation greater than 35 degrees or 15 degrees greater than the noninjured side indicates instability and surgery is recommended.[20]

If the ligament is completely torn, one must also worry about a Stener lesion. This is where the torn UCL protrudes beneath the adductor aponeurosis. This places the aponeurosis between the ligament and its insertion. If this occurs, reattachment will not occur and surgery is needed.[43]

A more appropriate term for this injury in an athlete would be *skier's thumb.* Initially, Campbell described gamekeeper's injury as being due to chronic repeated stress on the UCL.[8] It was not an acute injury, as it most commonly is in sports.

Injury Mechanism. UCL injuries occur when a torsional load is applied to the thumb.[7] It frequently oc-

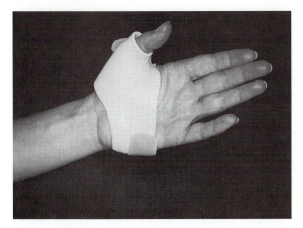

Figure 21-42 A gamekeeper's splint may also be called a hand-based thumb spica splint. It always includes the thumb MCP joint and may include the CMC or IP joint, depending on the injury or sport.

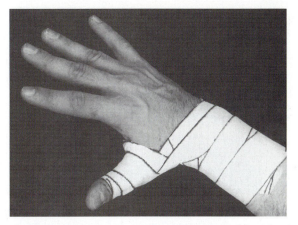

Figure 21-43 Thumb spica taping may be used when additional support is needed to the wrist and thumb. Tendinitis, gamekeeper's injuries, or healed fractures are some indications.

curs in pole or stick sports (e.g., skiing) where the thumb is abducted to hold the pole or stick and the athlete falls and tries to catch herself on an outstretched hand, landing on an abducted thumb.[30,36,50] Defensive backs in football might also sustain this injury while abducting the thumb before making a tackle.[30]

Rehabilitation Concerns. Early diagnosis and treatment is important. An unstable thumb or Stener lesion, if not treated, will become chronically and painfully unstable with weak pinch and arthritis as sequelae.[20]

Treatment for incomplete (grade I or II) tears is immobilization in a thumb spica cast (Figure 21-31) for 3 weeks, with additional protective splinting for 2 weeks (Figure 21-42). AROM to flexion and extension may be performed following the first 3 weeks.

Treatment for complete tears (grade III, unstable MCP joint) should be surgical repair. Late reconstruction is not as successful as early surgery, so early operative treatment is recommended.[30] Postoperatively, a thumb spica cast or splint is worn for 3 weeks, with an additional 2 weeks of splinting except for exercise sessions of active flexion and extension.

Concerns during the initial 5 or 6 weeks postinjury include protective immobilization, controlling edema, and maintaining motion in all noninvolved joints. An additional concern, is once movement is begun, is to not place radial stress on the thumb to stretch the UCL.

Rehabilitation Progression. After protective splinting is discontinued (at approximately 5 to 6 weeks), exercises are upgraded from AROM of flexion and exten-

sion to active assistive and passive exercises. Care should be taken not to apply abduction stress to the MCP joint during the first 2 to 6 weeks following immobilization. Putty exercises for strength may be performed at approximately 8 weeks postinjury. When measuring thumb ROM, always compare to the noninjured side. There is a large amount of variation in MCP and IP ROM from person to person.

Criteria for Return. Return-to-play decisions are made by the physician in conjunction with the sports medicine staff. Length of time to return to play is determined by the sport and position played, and whether the athlete needs to use his or her thumb. For nonoperative treatment a cast or splint might provide adequate protection for return to play. Once the athlete is medically cleared to play, a protective splint or taping (Figure 21-43) to prevent reinjury from extension and abduction should be fabricated by a hand therapist or athletic trainer. Protective splinting during sports should continue for at least 8 weeks until pain and swelling subside and patient has complete pain-free ROM.[30]

If surgical repair is performed, the athlete will be out for a minimum of 2 weeks while the incision heals. After that the position and sport determine the length of time until return. If the athlete does not have to use his or her thumb, follow protective splinting guidelines for nonoperative conditions above. For either treatment where active thumb movement is necessary (e.g., in the throwing hand of the quarterback), the athlete will be out at least 4 to 6 weeks.[36]

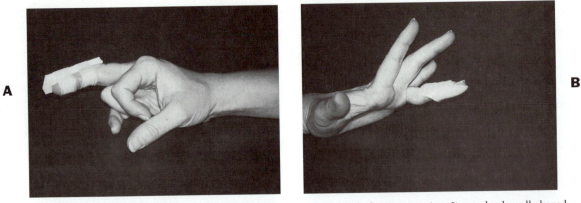

Figure 21-44   A mallet finger splint must hold the DIP in neutral to slight hyperextension. It may be dorsally based, volarly based, or circumferential. **A,** A dorsal splint made from Alumafoam, or **B,** a stack-type splint are usually preferred, as they rarely impede PIP motion.

Finger Joint Dislocations

Pathomechanics.   Dislocation of the MCP joint is very infrequent. The force is dissipated by joint mobility.[49] These injuries can be a simple dorsal subluxation, in which the proximal phalanx rotates on the metacarpal head and locks the joint in 60 degrees of hyperextension; or an irreducible dorsal dislocation where the volar plate is interposed dorsally to the metacarpal head and prevents reduction. For a simple dislocation, after reduction some physicians splint the MCP joints in 50 degrees of flexion for 7 to 10 days.[49] Others buddy tape and allow full motion immediately. If the fracture is irreducible, it must be openly reduced with the volar plate retracted. The MCP joints are then splinted at 50 degrees or greater of flexion.

Dislocation of the PIP joint volarly is very rare and is usually a grade III irreducible fracture. It requires open reduction. Because it is very complex and rare in athletes, it will not be covered in depth in this chapter.

Dorsal dislocations are much more common in sports. The athlete might not even bring the injury to the attention of the trainer, but might instead just pull the finger back into place independently. If a finger PIP is dorsally dislocated, immediate reduction (usually by physician) is preferred. X rays should be taken to be sure there is no fracture. If there is no fracture, and the PIP joint is reduced and stable, the finger should be wrapped in Coban for edema control and buddy taped to the adjacent finger. ROM is begun immediately (Figures 21-14 through 21-17). These injuries do not need to be splinted, and should not be overtreated.

DIP joint dislocations are more rare than PIP dislocations.[13] Dorsal dislocations occur more frequently than volar. If the injury is closed, it is usually reducible. X rays should be taken to rule out fracture. If the joint is reduced

and there is no fracture, splint the DIP only in neutral for 1 to 2 weeks (Figure 21-44). If the DIP dislocation is open (and it frequently is) or is irreducible, it needs to be surgically addressed.[49] With all finger dislocations in a gloved athlete, the glove must be removed to determine whether the injury is open or closed.

Injury Mechanism.   The mechanism for all finger dislocations is a hyperextension force or a compressive load force.[7]

Rehabilitation Concerns.   The initial concern is to rule out a fracture and relocate the injured joint. If the joint is not reducible, appropriate surgical intervention is needed. Once reduced, Coban (Figure 21-45) should be applied to decrease edema. Protective splinting or buddy taping is also applied. In PIP dorsal dislocations without fracture, immediate ROM is important to decrease stiffness. Complications of finger dislocations include pain, swelling, stiffness, or loss of reduction.

Rehabilitation Progressions.   Simple dorsal subluxation of the MCP joints are reduced and splinted in 50 degrees of flexion for 7 to 10 days. Following splinting, AROM is begun. Because the joints are immobilized in flexion, the collateral ligaments remain taut and full MCP flexion should be maintained. Extension is not lost at the MCP joints with this injury. Progression is from full ROM to gentle strengthening to more aggressive strengthening.

If the MCP joint dislocation is irreducible, it will require open reduction. Pins may be placed holding MCP joints in flexion. If not, the hand needs to be splinted with MCP joints in flexion. Once motion is allowed, active flexion and extension are initiated. Stiffness can be a problem, as can tendon adherence in the scar. Rehabilitation might be difficult and require consultation with a hand therapist for splinting to regain motion. ROM is pro-

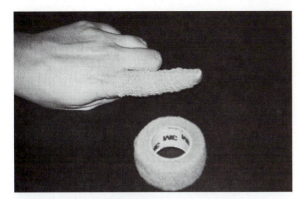

Figure 21-45 Coban is similar to Ace wrap in that it is elastic. It sticks to itself, so there is no need for clips. It comes in varying widths from 1 to 3 inches. One inch is perfect for fingers. Start wrapping from distal to proximal, pulling slightly but still leaving some wrinkles. Check circulation following application. Coban is perfect to help prevent swelling in finger injuries, especially PIP dislocations, immediately following injury.

gressed to ADLs, strengthening, and functional return to sport activities.

PIP dislocations without fractures, once reduced, need to be wrapped in Coban for edema control (Figure 21-45) and started on early motion. Exercises include composite flexion and extension, and blocked PIP and DIP flexion exercises (Figures 21-14 through 21-16). Buddy taping is often helpful to encourage ROM and provide protection. This is frequently enough to maintain motion and strength. If stiffness does occur, a referral to a hand therapist may be necessary for dynamic splinting or an aggressive strength and motion program.

If the DIP is dislocated, closed, and easily reduced, it should be splinted in neutral to slight flexion for 1 to 2 weeks. AROM begins at 2 to 3 weeks, with protective splinting continued between exercise sessions for 4 to 6 weeks.[49] At that time putty for strengthening (Figure 21-7) and blocked DIP exercises (Figure 21-16) may begin.

Open or irreducible fractures require surgical wound care with debridement to prevent infection. These injuries are then treated like mallet fingers and progressed accordingly.[49]

Criteria for Return.   Return to play for all finger joint dislocations is dependent upon the complexity of the dislocation and whether a fracture has occurred. If the MCP joints have a simple dislocation and are easily reduced, and remain reduced, the affected finger may be buddy taped, Coban wrapped for edema control, and protective splinted for pain control if necessary, with return to sport immediately or within the first few days after injury. If it is a complex dislocation and surgery is

necessary, the athlete will be out a minimum of 2 to 3 weeks.

For PIP joint dorsal dislocations without fracture, once the joint is reduced and stable, the finger should be Coban wrapped and buddy taped. A dorsal Alumafoam splint is optional for pain control during sport activity. The athlete may return to activity immediately. If the joint is not reducible, or there is a fracture, the length of time lost from sport will vary depending on the sport and severity of injury.

For DIP joint dislocations that are easily reduced, the athlete may return immediately with Coban and splint. If the dislocation is open or irreducible, the athlete can usually return once sutures are removed after surgery, at about 10 days, with protective splinting. The criteria for the DIP joint is very similar to criteria for mallet finger.

Flexor Digitorum Profundus Avulsion (Jersey Finger)

Pathomechanics.   Jersey finger is a rupture of the flexor digitorum profundus (FDP) tendon from its insertion on the distal phalanx. It most frequently occurs in the ring finger. It may be avulsed with or without bone. If avulsed with bone, depending on the size of the fragment, the tendon will usually not retract back into the palm, as it gets "caught" on the pulley system of the finger. If no bone, or only a very small fleck of bone, is avulsed, the tendon will retract back into the palm. This is the most common.[50] Each time the athlete tries to flex his or her finger, the muscle is contracting but the insertion is not attached. This brings the insertion closer to its origin.

The way to isolate the FDP to evaluate function and integrity is to hold the MCP and PIP joints of the affected finger in full extension, then have the athlete attempt to flex the DIP joint. If it flexes, it is intact. If it does not, it is ruptured (Figure 21-16).

If the tendon is ruptured, there are two options. The first is do nothing. If the tendon is not repaired, the athlete will be unable to flex the DIP joint, might have decreased grip strength, and might have tenderness at the site of tendon retraction, but functionally should not have difficulty.[50] The second option is to have the tendon surgically repaired. If it is repaired, the athlete should be informed that this is a labor-intensive operation and rehabilitation, there is a risk of scarring with poor tendon glide, and there is a risk of tendon rupture. The athlete will not have full activity level for approximately 12 weeks after surgery. The repair should be done within 10 days of injury for the best results.

Injury Mechanism.   Forceful hyperextension of the fingers while tightly gripping into flexion is the injury mechanism. It most frequently happens in football when

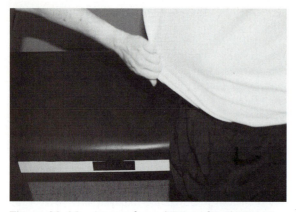

Figure 21-46 A jersey finger (FDP avulsion) injury is named for the injury mechanism—forced hyperextension with finger flexion, as in trying to grab a shirt during a tackle. The position of the DIP joint after injury will be extension or hyperextension.

a shirt is grabbed to try to make a tackle and the finger gets caught[50] (Figure 21-46).

Rehabilitation Concerns. This can be a very difficult injury to treat if surgically repaired. The surgery should be done by an experienced hand surgeon[11] with rehabilitation by an experienced hand therapist. Close communication between hand surgeon, hand therapist, and athletic training staff is a must. All protocols are guidelines and as such may need to be altered if complications such as infection, poor tendon glide, or excellent tendon glide occur. With this injury, unlike most others, the better a person is doing (i.e., full active tendon glide) the more they are held back and protected. Good tendon glide is indicative of less scar, which means there is less scar holding the repaired tendon together, thus less tensile strength and increased chance of rupture. If a tendon is ruptured, it must be repaired again and the prognosis is poorer.

Proper patient education is a must. Instruction in what to expect, reasons for specific exercises, and consequences must be conveyed.

Rehabilitation Progressions. The following are guidelines. They are not all-inclusive, nor are they an indication that just anyone can treat this injury. For more specific information on the protocol, readers are encouraged to read and review the Roslyn Evans article on zone I flexor tendon rehabilitation.[14]

Between 2 and 5 days postoperative, the bulky dressing should be removed and a dorsal splint fabricated to hold the wrist in neutral, MCP joints in 30 degrees of flexion, and IP joints in full extension with the hood extending to the fingertips for protection (Figure 21-47). The affected DIP joint is splinted at 45 degrees

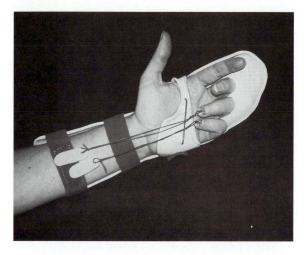

Figure 21-47 A flexor tendon splint—usually applied within 5 days postsurgery—is dorsally based and includes the wrist in neutral to slight flexion, MCP joint flexion, and IP joint extension. Depending on the location of injury, the amount of flexion may be increased or decreased, and rubberband traction may be applied from fingernails to forearm strap.

of flexion with a second dorsal splint that extends from the PIP joint to the fingertip, held on with tape at the middle phalanx only. Exercises for the first 3 weeks are (1) passive DIP flexion; (2) full composite passive flexion, then extend MCP joints passively to a modified hook position; (3) hyperflexion of MCP joints with active extension of PIP joints to 0 degrees; (4) strap or hold noninvolved fingers to the top of the splint. Position PIP joint in flexion passively then actively hold the joint in flexion (Figure 21-18). All exercises should be done with the splint on, at a frequency of ten repetitions every waking hour. The patients should not use the injured hand for anything, extend the wrist or fingers with the splint off, or actively flex the fingers—all of these could cause tendon rupture. In addition, during the first weeks Coban (Figure 21-45) can be used for edema control and scar control. Scar massage may be performed in the splint. The dressing may be changed at home, but the DIP splint should remain in place at all times for 3 weeks.

Between 3 and 4 weeks post repair the digital splint is discontinued, passive fist and hold is begun for composite flexion, and dorsal protective splinting is continued. Between 4 and 6 weeks active hook fist and active composite fisting is begun, wrist ROM is begun, and gentle isolated profundus exercises are initiated (Figures 21-14 through 21-16). The splint may be discontinued if poor tendon glide is present.

At 6 to 8 weeks the splint is discontinued, ADLs may be done with the injured hand, and tendon-gliding exercises and blocked DIP exercises are continued. Light resistive exercises (putty) (Figure 21-7) may be initiated. Graded resistive exercises are begun if there is poor tendon glide. Be very careful during this time—it is a prime time for tendon ruptures. Patients are excited to be out of their splints and might overdo. Graded resistive exercises and dynamic splinting, if necessary, are initiated at 8 to 10 weeks.

Between 10 and 12 weeks strengthening is begun. By 12 weeks patients should be back with full tendon glide and good tendon strength to return to all normal activities. Activities and sports in which a sudden surprise force might pull on flexed fingers, such as rock climbing, windsurfing, water skiing, or dog walking, should not be done until 14 to 16 weeks postoperative.

Criteria for Return. Return to activity is dependent on sport and position played, and the decision must be made with physician, hand therapist, and training staff involved. It will be 10 to 12 weeks before the athlete can play without protection and with little risk of tendon reinjury. There are instances where a non-ball-handling athlete may return sooner if cleared by the physician. In these cases the athlete's affected hand must be tightly taped into a fist and then casted with wrist in flexion, padded according to sport rules. Nothing hard should be placed in the athlete's hand—if they squeeze against resistance, they might rupture. The athlete and coaching staff must be made aware of the possibility of rupture with early return to sport.

Mallet Finger

Pathomechanincs. A mallet finger is the avulsion of the terminal extensor tendon,[37] which is responsible for extension of the DIP joint. It can occur with or without fracture of bone. If there is a large fracture fragment, where the fracture fragment is displaced greater than 2 mm, or the DIP joint has volar subluxation on X ray, the injury will require ORIF.

There is no other mechanism for extending the DIP joint. The presenting complaint is inability to extend the DIP joint (Figure 21-48).

Treatment is splinting the DIP joint in neutral to slight hyperextension (Figure 21-44) for 6 to 8 weeks with no flexion of the DIP joint.[12,42] If the DIP joint is flexed even once during that time, the 6 weeks starts again.

Injury Mechanism. Injury mechanism is forced flexion of the DIP joint while it is held in full extension.[49] It frequently happens when the end of the finger is struck by a ball.

Rehabilitation Concerns. Rehabilitation of the mallet finger is minimal. A splint may be custom made or

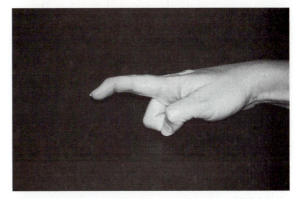

Figure 21-48 A mallet finger deformity with DIP flexion. There might or might not be redness dorsally.

prefabricated, such as a stack splint or Alumafoam. It should hold the DIP joint in neutral to slight hyperextension. Skin integrity needs to be monitored, and the splint modified or redesigned if breakdown occurs. ROM of noninvolved fingers and joints should be maintained. PIP flexion with the DIP splinted will not put tension on the injury and should be encouraged.

Rehabilitation Progressions. Once the tendon is healed, at approximately 6 to 8 weeks, splinting may be discontinued. If an extensor lag is present, splinting may be continued longer. Night splinting is often continued for 2 weeks after full-time splinting is discontinued. AROM to DIP joint following splint removal. No attempts to passively flex the finger to regain ROM should be attempted for 4 weeks. Blocked DIP flexion exercises are most important. Full ROM is usually gained through blocked exercises (Figure 21-16) and regular functional hand use.

Criteria for Return. Return to sports is permitted immediately with the DIP joint splinted in full extension. If the sport does not permit playing with the finger splint on, the athlete will be out of competition for 8 weeks.

Boutonniere Deformity

Pathomechanics. The posture of a finger with a boutonniere deformity is PIP joint flexion and DIP joint hyperextension (Figure 21-49). It is caused by interruption of the central slip. Normally the central slip will initiate extension of flexed PIP joints. The lateral bands cannot initiate PIP joint extension but can maintain extension if passively positioned, because they are dorsal to the axis of motion. When the central slip is disrupted, the extensor muscle displaces proximally and shifts the lateral bands volarly. The FDS is unopposed without an intact central slip and will flex the PIP joint. As the length of time postinjury increases, the lateral bands displace

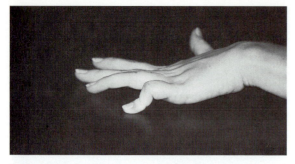

Figure 21-49   A boutonniere deformity might start as a PIP contracture. In time it will cause hyperextension of the DIP joint.

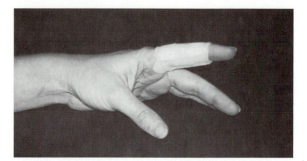

Figure 21-50   A boutonniere splint needs to immobilize the PIP joint in full extension, leaving the MCP and DIP joint free. The author makes these in two pieces, overlapping slightly, held on with tape.

volarly and might become fixed to the joint capsule or collateral ligament. This makes passive correction very difficult. The DIP joint hyperextends because all the force to extend the PIP is transmitted to the DIP joint.[37]

Once a fixed deformity is present, it is much more difficult to treat. However, many athletes do not seek immediate medical attention, feeling that the finger was "jammed" and will be fine in several days or weeks.

Treatment for the acute injury is uninterrupted splinting of the PIP joint in full extension for 6 weeks (Figure 21-50). The DIP joint is left free with motion encouraged. This will synergistically relax the extrinsic and intrinsic extensor tendon muscles and also exercises the oblique retinacular ligament.[37]

Following 6 weeks of immobilization, gentle careful flexion of the PIP joint is begun. Continue splinting for 2 to 4 weeks when not exercising. When full PIP joint extension can be maintained throughout the day, then night splinting only is appropriate. Length of treatment and splinting may be several months.

Injury Mechanism.   Injury occurs when the extended finger is forcibly flexed, as when being hit by a ball or striking the finger on another player during a fall.[50]

Rehabilitation Concerns.   Of primary concern is early and proper diagnosis and treatment. X rays should be taken to rule out fracture or PIP joint dislocation. It is

also very important to splint the PIP in full extension. If edema is present when initially splinted, as edema decreases the splint gets loose and full extension is no longer achieved. Passive flexion should not be performed to the PIP joint following removal of the splint. Blocked PIP ROM exercises are appropriate to isolate flexion (Figure 21-15). If diagnosis is made late and there is a fixed PIP flexion contracture, serial casting may be necessary to restore extension. Following return of full extension, the finger is then splinted for 8 weeks. One other factor to keep in mind is that initially a central slip injury does not present as a boutonniere, but rather a PIP flexor contracture. DIP hyperextension comes later.

Rehabilitation Progressions.   The progression is increasing ROM following splint removal. Strengthening of grip may also be performed, if needed, at 10 to 12 weeks following acute injury (approximately 4 weeks following splinting).

Criteria for Return.   The athlete may return to activity when the finger is comfortable. The affected finger must be splinted at all times in full extension. If the sport does not allow for the finger to be splinted, the athlete will be out approximately 8 weeks.

The author wishes to thank Dr. Wallace Andrew of Raleigh Orthopaedic Clinic for his support, knowledge, and willingness to answer my countless questions.

Summary

1. Flexor tendon injuries are very labor-intensive, significant injuries. An experienced hand surgeon and hand therapist must be involved in the care, and the athlete must be made aware of what to expect.

2. The goal in the treatment of ulnar collateral ligament injuries (gamekeeper's thumb) is stability of the MCP joint. Athletes will be stiff following immobilization—the sports therapist should not passively push motion initially.

3. Early treatment of the boutonniere deformity is essential, as is proper splint position. The PIP joint should be fully extended with the DIP joint free.

4. The mallet finger must be splinted in full extension uninterrupted for 6 to 8 weeks. If the DIP joint is flexed, even once, any healing is disrupted and the 6 to 8 weeks begins again.

5. Dislocations of the MCP joints are very rare and are often complicated. Dorsal PIP dislocations without fracture are common and need early range of motion and edema control. Splinting for comfort during competition is acceptable, but does not need to continue off-field unless the dislocation is unstable. DIP dislocations are frequently open and require surgery. They are treated like a mallet finger.

6. Boxer's fractures tend to heal without incident with full return of motion in 4 to 6 weeks. Splint immobilization should leave the PIP joint and wrist free to move.

7. Tendinitis and DeQuervain's tenosynovitis should be immobilized for 2 to 3 weeks with gentle pain-free range of motion performed daily to maintain mobility. Activity should be increased as pain decreases.

8. Carpal tunnel syndrome is very rare in athletes.

9. Ganglion cysts need to be treated only if symptomatic. Multiple aspirations may be performed during the season with excision postseason if necessary. There are usually few rehabilitation needs.

10. Wrist sprains are a diagnosis of exclusion. All other pathology must be ruled out prior to return to sport.

11. Lunate dislocations are serious injuries that require ORIF and possible lengthy rehabilitation.

12. Hamate hook fractures are not seen on regular X ray views. A carpal tunnel view will confirm the diagnosis, and the fracture should be treated symptomatically.

13. Scaphoid fractures might not be seen on initial X ray. If suspected, but the X ray is negative, the athlete should be treated as if a fracture is present, with X rays repeated in 2 weeks to confirm diagnosis. Early proper immobilization is important to the long-term outcome.

14. Distraction of the wrist while performing passive range of motion after fracture can help increase motion and decrease pain during stretching.

References

1. Baxter-Petralia, P., and V. Penney. 1992. Cumulative trauma. In *Concepts in hand rehabilitation,* edited by B. G. Stanley and S. M. Tribuzi. Philadelphia: F. A. Davis.

2. Bishop, A. T., and R. D. Beckenbaugh. 1988. Fracture of the hamate hook. *Journal of Hand Surgery* 13A:135–39.

3. Bohler, L. 1942. *The treatment of fractures.* 4th ed. Baltimore: William Wood.

4. Bryan, R. S., and J. H. Dobyns. 1980. Less commonly fractured carpal bones. *Clinical Orthopaedics and Related Research* 149:108–9.

5. Bush, D. C. 1995. Soft-tissue tumors of the hand. In *Rehabilitation of the hand: surgery and therapy,* 4th ed., edited by J. M. Hunter, E. J. Mackin, and A. D. Callahan. St. Louis: Mosby.

6. Butler, D. S. 1991. *Mobilization of the nervous system.* Melbourne: Churchill Livingstone.

7. Cahalan, T. D., and W. P. Cooney. 1996. Biomechanics. In *Operative techniques in upper extremity sports injuries,* edited by F. W. Jobe, M. M. Pink, R. E. Glousman, R. S. Kvitne, and N. P. Zemel. St. Louis: Mosby.

8. Campbell, C. S. 1955. Gamekeeper's thumb. *Journal of Bone and Joint Surgery* 37B:148–49.

9. Cooney, W. P. 1984. Sports injuries in the upper extremity. *Postgrad Med* 76:45–50.

10. Crosby, E. B., and R. L. Linscheid. 1974. Rupture of the flexor profundus tendon of the ring finger secondary to ancient fracture of the hook of the hamate: review of the literature and report of two cases. *Journal of Bone and Joint Surgery* 56A:1076–78.

11. Culp, R. W., and J. S. Taras. 1995. Primary care of flexor tendon injuries. In *Rehabilitation of the hand: Surgery and therapy,* 4th ed., edited by J. M. Hunter, E. J. Mackin, and A. D. Callahan. St. Louis: Mosby.

12. Doyle, J. R. 1988. Extensor tendons: Acute injuries. In *Operative hand surgery,* 2d ed., edited by D. P. Green. New York: Churchill Livingstone.

13. Dray, G. J., and R. G. Eaton. 1993. Dislocations and ligament injuries in the digits. In *Operative hand surgery,* 3d ed., vol. 1, edited by D. P. Green. New York: Churchill Livingstone.

14. Evans, R. 1990. A study of the zone I flexor tendon injury and implications for treatment. *Journal of Hand Therapy* 3:133.

15. Finklestein, H. 1930. Stenosing tendovaginitis at the radial styloid process. *Journal of Bone and Joint Surgery* 12:509.

16. Frykman, G. 1967. Fracture of the distal radius including sequelae-shoulder-hand-finger syndrome, disturbance in the distal radioulnar joint, and impairment of nerve function: A clinical and experimental study. *Acta Orthop Scand Suppl* 108:1.

17. Frykman, G. K., and W. E. Kropp. 1995. Fractures and traumatic conditions of the wrist. In *Rehabilitation of the*

hand: Surgery and therapy, 4th ed., edited by J. M. Hunter, E. J. Mackin, and A. D. Callahan. St. Louis: Mosby.

18. Gartland, J. J., and C. W. Werley. 1961. Evaluation of healed colles' fractures. *Journal of Bone and Joint Surgery* 43B:245.

19. Hunter, J. M., L. B. Davlin, and L. M. Fedus. 1995. Major neuropathies of the upper extremity: The median nerve. In *Rehabilitation of the hand: Surgery and therapy,* 4th ed., edited by J. M. Hunter, E. J. Mackin, and A. D. Callahan. St. Louis: Mosby.

20. Husband, J. B., and S. A. McPherson. 1996. Bony skier's thumb injuries. *Clinical Orthopaedics and Related Research* 327:79–84.

21. Jupiter, J. B., and M. R. Belsky. 1992. Fractures and dislocations of the hand. In *Skeletal trauma,* edited by B. D. Browner, J. B. Jupiter, A. M. Levine, and P. G. Trafton. Philadelphia: W. B. Saunders.

22. Kaplan, E. M. 1965. *Joints and ligaments in functional and surgical anatomy of the hand.* Philadelphia: Lippincott.

23. Kauer, J. M. 1980. Functional anatomy of the wrist. *Clinical Orthopaedics and Related Research* 149:9–20.

24. Kirkpatrick, W. H., and S. Lisser. 1995. Soft-tissue conditions: Trigger fingers and DeQuervain's disease. In *Rehabilitation of the hand: Surgery and therapy,* 4th ed., edited by J. M. Hunter, E. J. Mackin, and A. D. Callahan. St. Louis: Mosby.

25. Korman, J., R. Pearl, and V. R. Hentz. 1992. Efficacy of immobilization following aspiration of carpal and digital ganglion. *Journal of Hand Surgery* 17:1097.

26. Kozin, S. H., and M. B. Wood. 1993. Early soft tissue complications after fractures of the distal part of the radius. *Journal of Bone and Joint Surgery* 75A:144.

27. London, P. S. 1961. The broken scaphoid bones: The case against pessimism. *Journal of Bone and Joint Surgery* 42B:237.

28. Mazet, R., and M. Hohl. 1967. Fractures of the carpal navicular: Analysis of 91 cases and review of the literature. *Journal of Bone and Joint Surgery* 45A:82.

29. McCue, F. C. 1988. The elbow, wrist and hand. In *The injured athlete,* 2d ed., edited by D. Kulund. Philadelphia: Lippincott.

30. McCue, F. C., and W. E. Nelson. 1993. Ulnar collateral ligament injuries of the thumb. *Physician and Sports Medicine* 21(9):67–80.

31. McCue, F. C. et al. 1979. Hand and wrist injuries in the athlete. *American Journal of Sports Medicine* 7:275–86.

32. Meyer, F. N., and R. L. Wilson. 1995. Management of nonarticular fractures of the hand. In *Rehabilitation of the hand: Surgery and therapy,* 4th ed., edited by J. M. Hunter, E. J. Mackin, and A. D. Callahan. St. Louis: Mosby.

33. Mosher, F. J. 1986. Peripheral nerve injuries and entrapments of the forearm and wrist. In *American Academy of Orthopaedic Surgeons: Symposium on upper extremity injuries in athletes,* edited by F. A. Pettrone. St. Louis: Mosby.

34. Palmer, A. K., J. H. Dobyns, and R. L. Linscheid. 1978. Management of post-traumatic instability of the wrist secondary to ligament rupture. *Journal of Hand Surgery* 3:507.

35. Pianka, G., and E. B. Hershman. 1990. Neurovascular injuries. In *Upper extremity in sports medicine,* edited by J. A. Nicholas and E. B. Hershman. St. Louis: Mosby.

36. Rettig, A. C. 1991. Current concepts in management of football injuries of the hand and wrist. *Journal of Hand Therapy* 4 (April–June).

37. Rosenthal, E. A. 1995. The extensor tendons: Anatomy and management. In *Rehabilitation of the hand: Surgery and therapy,* 4th ed., edited by J. M. Hunter, E. J. Mackin, and A. D. Callahan. St. Louis: Mosby.

38. Sarrafian, S., J. L. Melamed, and G. M. Goshgarian. 1977. Study of wrist motion in flexion and extension. *Clinical Orthopaedics* 126:153.

39. Smith, R. J. 1977. Posttraumatic instability of the metacarpophalangeal joint of the thumb. *Journal of Bone and Joint Surgery* 59:14–21.

40. Stark, H. H. et al. 1977. Fracture of the hook of the hamate in athletes. *Journal of Bone and Joint Surgery* 59A:575–82.

41. Stark, H. H. et al. 1989. Fracture of the hook of the hamate. *Journal of Bone and Joint Surgery* 71A:1202–7.

42. Stark, H. H., J. H. Bayer, and J. N. Wilson. 1962. Mallet finger. *Journal of Bone and Joint Surgery* 44:1061.

43. Stener, B. 1962. Displacement of the ruptured ulnar collateral ligament of the metacarpophalangeal joint of the thumb. *Journal of Bone and Joint Surgery* 44B:869–79.

44. Vender, M. I. 1987. Degenerative changes in symptomatic scaphoid non-union. *Journal of Hand Surgery* 12A:514.

45. Viegas, S. F. et al. 1991. Simulated scaphoid proximal pole fracture. *Journal of Hand Surgery* 16A:485–500.

46. Volz, R. G., M. Lieb, and J. Benjamin. 1980. Biomechanics of the wrist. *Clinical Orthopaedics and Related Research* 149:112–17.

47. Watson, H. K., and W. D. Rogers. 1989. Nonunion of the hook of the hamate: An argument for bone grafting the nonunion. *Journal of Hand Surgery* 14A:486–90.

48. Weinstein, S. M., and S. A. Herring. 1992. Nerve problems and compartment syndromes in the hand, wrist, and forearm. *Clinics in Sports Medicine* 11(1).

49. Wilson, R. L., and J. Hazen. 1995. Management of joint injuries and intraarticular fractures of the hand. In *Rehabilitation of the hand: Surgery and therapy,* 4th ed., edited by J. M. Hunter, E. J. Mackin, and A. D. Callahan. St. Louis: Mosby.

50. Wright, H. H., and A. C. Rettig. 1995. Management of common sports injuries. In *Rehabilitation of the hand: Surgery and therapy,* 4th ed., edited by J. M. Hunter, E. J. Mackin, and A. D. Callahan. St. Louis: Mosby.

51. Zemel, N. P. Anatomy and surgical approaches: Hand, wrist and forearm. In *Operative techniques in upper extremity sports injuries,* edited by F. W. Jobe, M. M. Pink, R. E. Glousman. R. S. Kvitne, and N. P. Zemel. St. Louis: Mosby.

52. Zemel, N. P. Fractures and ligament injuries of the wrist. *Operative techniques in upper extremity sports injuries,* edited by F. W. Jobe, M. M. Pink, R. E. Glousman. R. S. Kvitne, and N. P. Zemel. St. Louis: Mosby.

53. Zubowicz, V. N., and C. H. Ishii. 1987. Management of ganglion cysts by simple aspiration. *Journal of Hand Surgery* 12:618.

CHAPTER 22

Rehabilitation of Groin, Hip, and Thigh Injuries

Bernie DePalma

After completion of this chapter, the student should be able to do the following:

- Discuss the functional anatomy and biomechanics of the groin, hip, and thigh.

- Discuss athletic injuries to the groin, hip, and thigh and describe the biomechanical changes occurring during and after injury.

- Discuss and describe functional injury evaluation, utilizing biomechanical changes, to the groin, hip, and thigh.

- Recognize abnormal gait patterns as they relate to specific groin, hip, and thigh injuries and utilize this knowledge during the evaluation process and rehabilitation program.

- Discuss the various rehabilitative techniques used for specific groin, hip, and thigh injuries, including open- and closed-kinetic-chain strengthening

exercises, stretching exercises, and plyometric, isokinetic, and PNF exercises.

- Discuss the role of functional evaluation in determining when to return an athlete to competition, based on rehabilitation progression.

This chapter describes functional rehabilitation programs that follow groin, hip, and thigh injuries. The sports therapist and athlete, together, should develop the rehabilitation program with an emphasis on injury mechanism, the sports therapist's functional and biomechanical evaluation, and clinical findings. Each exercise program should be presented to the athlete in terms of short-term goals. One objective for the sports therapist is to make the rehabilitation experience challenging for the athlete, to promote adherence to the rehabilitation program.

FUNCTIONAL ANATOMY AND BIOMECHANICS

The pelvis and hip are made up of the pelvic girdle and the articulation of the femoral head to the bony socket of the pelvic girdle, the acetabulum, forming a ball-in-socket joint.[14] This joint connects the lower extremity to the pelvic girdle.[6] The angle of inclination and angle of declination are used to describe the position of the femoral head and neck with respect to the shaft of the femur.[6] The frontal projection of the angle formed by the femoral shaft and neck is the angle of inclination. The angle of declination is sometimes referred to as the angle of anteversion.[6] This is the angle formed between the femoral neck down through the femur to the femoral condyles. Changes in both these angles could cause changes in rotation of the femoral head within the acetabulum that predispose the athlete to stress fractures and overuse hip injuries, as well as hip subluxation.

The pelvis itself moves in three directions: anteroposterior tilting, lateral tilting, and rotation. The iliopsoas muscle and other hip flexors, as well as extensors of the lumbar spine, perform anterior tilting in the sagittal plane and facilitates, lumbar lordosis. The rectus abdominus, obliques, gluteus maximus, and hamstrings posteriorly tilt the pelvis and cause a decrease in lumbar lordosis.[6] During lateral tilting in the frontal plane the hip joint acts as the center of rotation.[6] Hip abduction or adduction is a result of pelvic lateral tilting. The hip abductors control lateral tilting by contracting isometrically or eccentrically.[6] Pelvic rotation occurs in the transverse plane, again using the hip joint as the axis of rotation. The gluteal muscles, external rotators, adductors, pectineus, and iliopsoas all act together to perform this movement in the transverse plane.[6] These movements of the pelvis are important when analyzing gait, injury evaluation, and teaching correct gait.

The hip joint is a true ball-in-socket joint and has intrinsic stability not found in other joints.[6] This intrinsic stability does not prevent the hip joint from retaining great mobility.[6] During normal gait, the hip joint moves in all three planes: sagittal, frontal, and transverse. To participate in athletic activities, a greater range of motion is needed. With the increased range of motion, the hip is capable of performing a wide range of combined movements. Forces at the hip joint have been increased to five times the body weight during running. These forces can also contribute to injuries, both muscular and bony.

The most frequently injured structures of the groin, hip, pelvis, and thigh are the muscles and tendons that perform the movements. The majority of these muscles originate on the pelvis or the proximal femur. The iliac crest serves as the attachment site for the abdominal muscles, the ilium serves as the attachment for the gluteals and then the gluteals insert to the proximal femur. The pubis serves as the attachment for the adductors, and the iliopsoas inserts distally to the lesser trochanter of the proximal femur.[6] Due to all the attachments in a small area, injury to these structures can be very disabling and difficult to distinguish.[6]

The quadriceps inserts by a common tendon to the proximal patella. The rectus femoris is the only quadriceps muscle that crosses the hip joint, which not only extends the knee but also flexes the hip. This is very important in differentiating hip flexor strains (e.g., iliopsoas vs. rectus femoris) and the ensuing treatment and rehabilitation programs.

The hamstrings all cross the knee joint posteriorly, and all except the short head of the biceps cross the hip joint. These biarticular muscles produce forces dependent upon the position of both the knee joint and the hip joint. The positions of the hip and knee during movement and injury mechanism play a very important role and provide information to utilize when rehabilitating and preventing hamstring injuries.

REHABILITATION TECHNIQUES FOR THE GROIN, HIP, AND THIGH

Strengthening Exercises

Isotonic Open-Kinetic-Chain Strengthening Exercises.

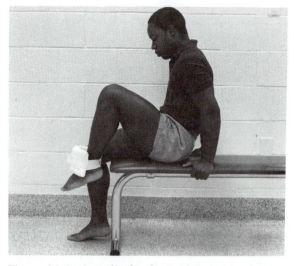

Figure 22-1   Pain-free hip flexion iliopsoas progressive resistive strengthening exercises: 4 sets of 10 to 15 repetitions daily.

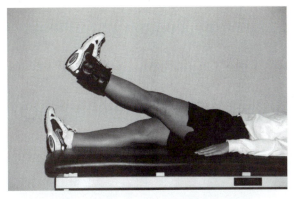

Figure 22-2 Straight leg raises (quadriceps and iliopsoas), 4 sets of 10 repetitions, daily.

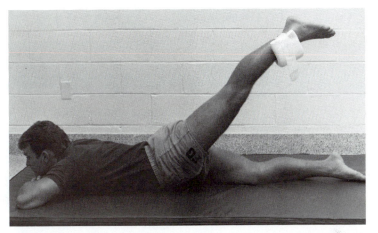

Figure 22-3 Pain-free hip extension (gluteus maximus and hamstring) progressive resistive strengthening exercises: 4 sets of 10 to 15 repetitions daily.

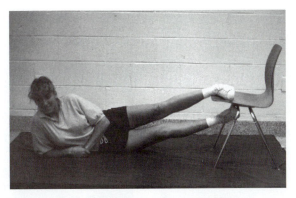

Figure 22-4 Pain-free hip adduction (adductor magnus, brevis, longus, pectineus, and gracilis) progressive resistive strengthening exercises: 4 sets of 10 to 15 repetitions daily.

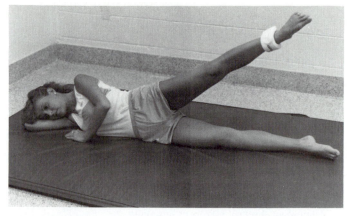

Figure 22-5　Pain-free hip abduction (gluteus medius, maximus, and tensor facia latae) progressive resistive strengthening exercises: 4 sets of 10 to 15 repetitions daily.

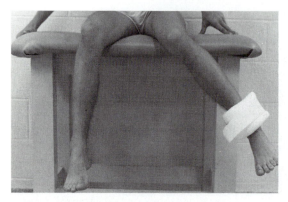

Figure 22-6　Pain-free hip internal rotation (gluteus minimus, tensor facia latae, semitendinosus, and semimembranosus) progressive resistive strengthening exercises: 4 sets of 10 to 15 repetitions daily.

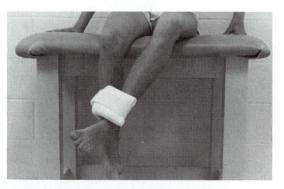

Figure 22-7　Pain-free hip external rotation (piriformis and gluteus maximus) progressive resistive strengthening exercises: 4 sets of 10 to 15 repetitions daily.

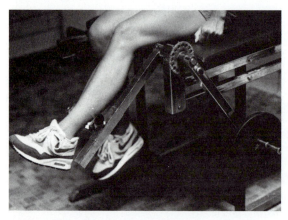

Figure 22-8　Pain-free seated hamstring progressive resistive strengthening exercises (maintain lordotic lumbar curve). Isotonics performed on the NK table, 4 sets of 10 repetitions, 2 to 3 days/week.

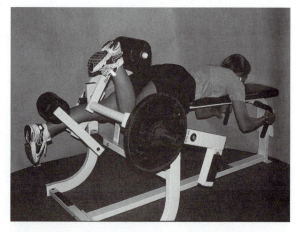

Figure 22-9　Pain-free prone hamstring single-leg progressive resistive strengthening exercises: 4 sets of 12 repetitions, 2 to 3 days/week.

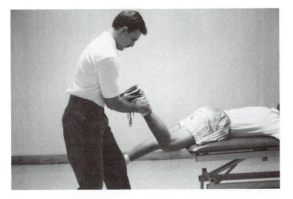

Figure 22-10   Manual resistance hamstring strengthening to fatigue. Athlete lies prone with knee over the edge of treatment table. With the athlete in full knee extension, resistance is applied to the back of the heels as the athlete contracts concentrically to full knee flexion for a count of 5 seconds. After a 2-second pause at full flexion, resistance is applied into extension for a count of 5 as the athlete contracts the hamstrings eccentrically. This is repeated, contracting as fast as possible for 2 to 3 sets of 10 to 12 repetitions or until failure, 1 to 2 days/week.

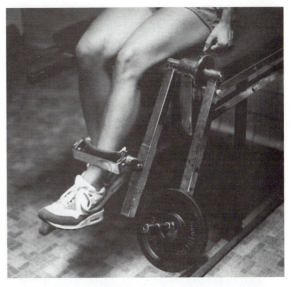

Figure 22-11   Pain-free seated quadriceps progressive resistive strengthening exercises. Isotonics using the NK table, 4 sets of 10 repetitions, 2 to 3 days/week.

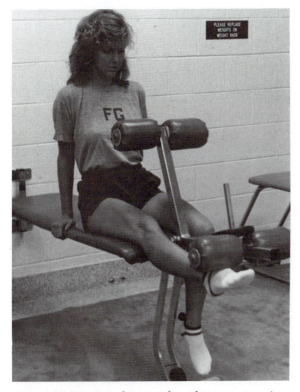

Figure 22-12   Pain-free seated quadriceps progressive resistive strengthening exercises, single leg, 3 to 4 sets of 10 to 12 repetitions, 1 to 2 days/week.

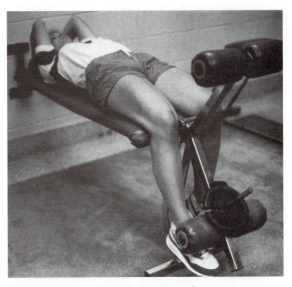

Figure 22-13   Pain-free supine quadriceps progressive resistive strengthening exercises, single leg (lying supine), to isolate rectus femoris, 2 to 3 sets of 10 to 12 repetitions, 1 to 2 days/week.

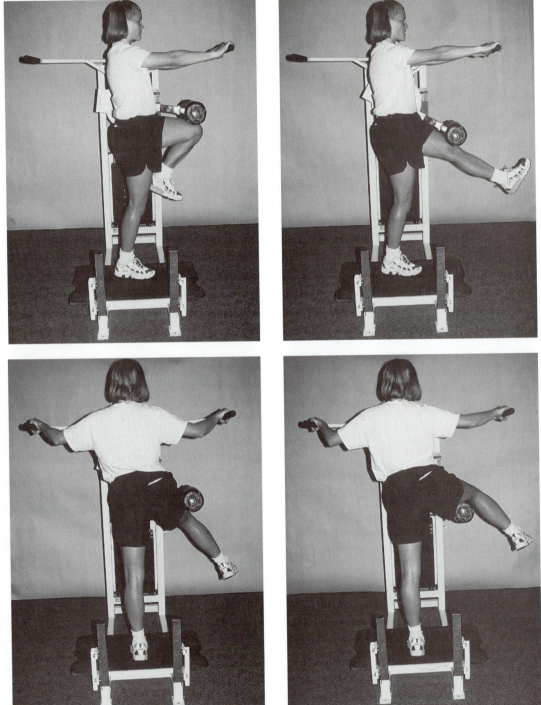

Figure 22-14 Pain-free multi-hip progressive resistive strengthening exercises in all four directions, 2 sets of 15 repetitions, 1 to 2 days/week **A,** flexion with knee flexed (rectus femoris) and **B,** knee extended (iliopsoas), **C,** abduction, **D,** adduction, **E,** extension with knee extended start position to knee bent terminal position (semimembranosus, tendinosis, and gluteus maximus) and knee bent start position to knee extended terminal position (biceps femoris and gluteus maximus).

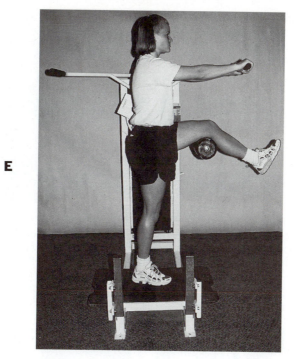

Figure 22-14 *continued*

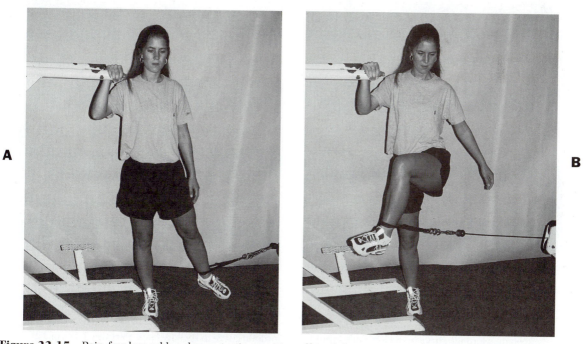

Figure 22-15 Pain-free low cable column starting position of hip abduction, extension, and external rotation to terminal position of adduction, flexion, and internal rotation, 3 sets of 15 repetitions, 1 to 2 days/week.

Closed-Kinetic-Chain Strengthening Exercises.

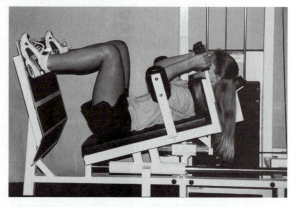

Figure 22-16   Leg press with feet high on the foot plate and shoulder-width apart to work the upper hamstring while keeping knees over the feet (not over the toes or in front of the toes). Seat setting should be close so that at the bottom of the motion the hips are lower than the knees (quadriceps, upper hamstrings, and gluteus maximus). Perform 3 sets of 12 repetitions, 2 days/week.

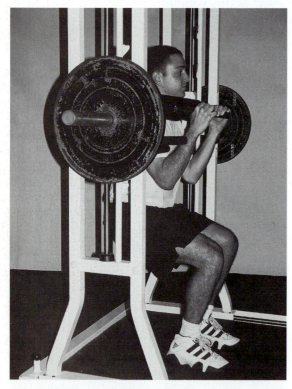

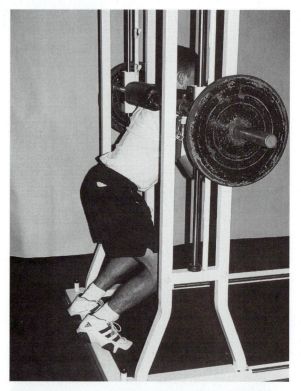

Figure 22-17   Smith press squats with feet placement forward of the athlete's center of gravity and close (within 1 to 2 inches of each other) or hack squat (quadriceps, upper hamstrings, and gluteus maximus). The athlete descends, keeping a lordotic curve in the low back, until the hip joints break parallel (lower than the knee joints). Perform 3 sets of 12 repetitions, 2 days/week.

Figure 22-18   Smith press squats with feet behind the athlete's center of gravity and hip in extension (as on a hip sled) (quadriceps, lower lateral hamstring, and gluteus maximus). The athlete descends while keeping a lordotic curve in the low back. Perform 3 sets of 12 repetitions, 2 days/week.

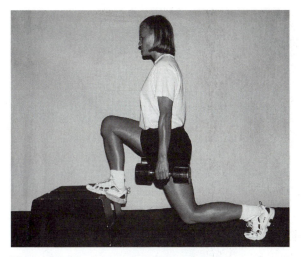

Figure 22-19   Lunges (quadriceps, hamstrings, gluteus maximus, groin muscles, and iliopsoas) stepping onto 4- to 6-inch step height. Once the foot hits the step, the athlete should bend the back knee straight down toward the floor to work the upper hamstring of the front leg and the hip flexors of the back leg. Perform 2 sets of 12 to 15 repetitions, 2 days/week.

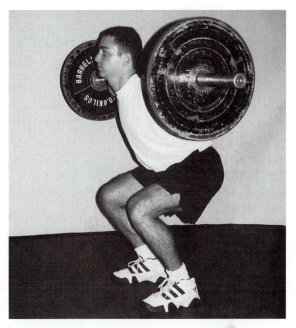

Figure 22-20   Standard squats below parallel (quadriceps, upper hamstrings, groin muscles, and gluteus maximus). 3 sets of 12 repetitions, 2 days/week.

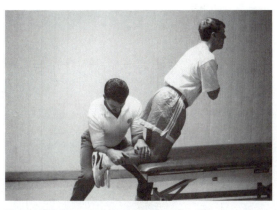

Figure 22-21   Hamstring leans—kneeling eccentric hamstring lowering exercises. With the athlete kneeling on a treatment table and feet hanging over the end, the sports therapist stabilizes the lower legs as the athlete lowers the body to the prone position, eccentrically contracting the hamstrings. The athlete should maintain a lumbar lordotic curve and stay completely erect, avoiding any hip flexion. The athlete should perform 2 sets of 8 to 10 repetitions or until failure, 1 to 2 days/week.

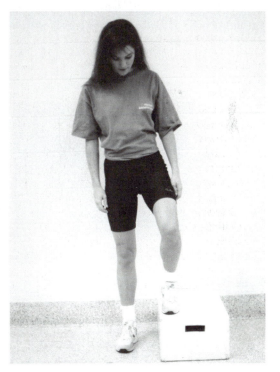

Figure 22-22   Lateral step-ups (quadriceps, hamstrings, gluteus maximus, gluteus medius, and tensor facia latae) using repetitions and sets, or time, 2 to 3 days/week.

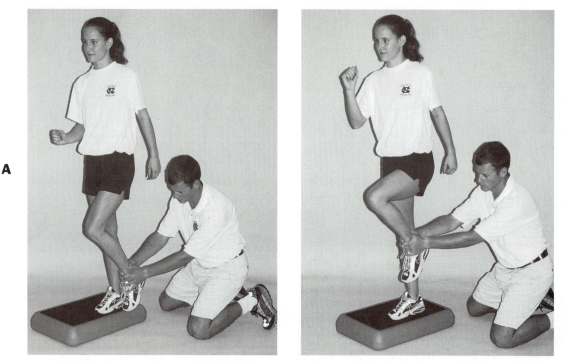

Figure 22-23 Standing running pattern, manual resistance starting position, 2 sets of 20 repetitions, 1 to 2 days/week. Resistance is applied to the back of the heel, resisting hip flexion and knee flexion to terminal position, then resisting hip extension and knee extension back down to starting position. **A,** The athlete contracts as fast as possible through the entire range of running motion. **B,** Standing running pattern, terminal position.

Isokinetic Exercises.

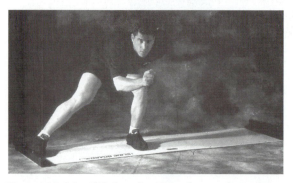

Figure 22-24 Slide board or Fitter, keeping knees bent and maintaining a squat position for the entire workout (increases hamstring activity). Utilize sets and repetitions, or time, 1 to 2 days/week.

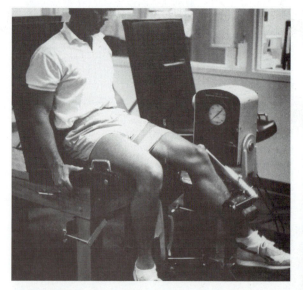

Figure 22-25 Seated isokinetic hamstring and quadriceps strengthening. 3 speed settings, 2 sets of 15 to 20 repetitions each setting, each leg, 1 to 2 days/week.

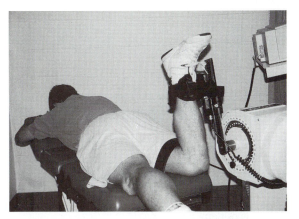

Figure 22-26 Prone-lying single-leg isokinetic hamstring and quadriceps strengthening. 3 speed settings, 2 sets of 15 to 20 repetitions each setting, for each leg, 1 to 2 days/week.

Plyometric Exercises.

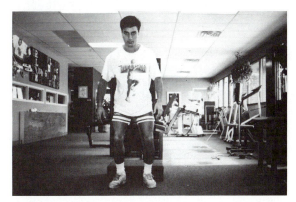

Figure 22-27 Jump-down exercises (sets and repetitions, or time), 1 to 2 days/week.

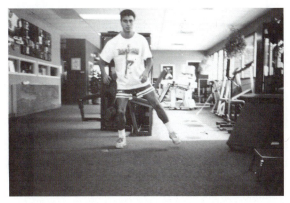

Figure 22-28 Lateral bounding (sets and repetitions, or time), 1 to 2 days/week.

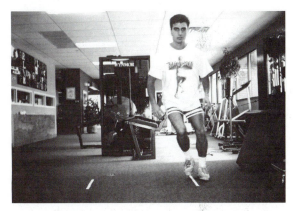

Figure 22-29 Lateral sliding (sets and repetitions, or time), 1 to 2 days/week.

PNF Strengthening Exercises.

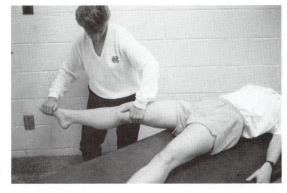

Figure 22-30A D1 movement pattern into flexion, starting position, 2 sets of 12 to 15 repetitions, 2 to 3 days/week.

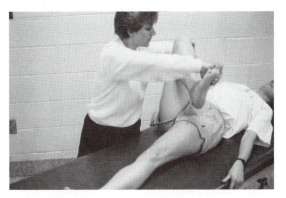

Figure 22-30B D1 movement pattern into flexion, terminal position.

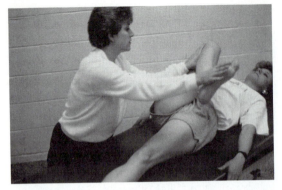

Figure 22-31A D1 movement pattern into extension, starting position, 2 sets of 12 to 15 repetitions, 2 to 3 days/week.

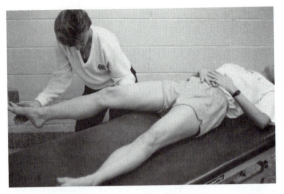

Figure 22-31B D1 movement pattern into extension, terminal position.

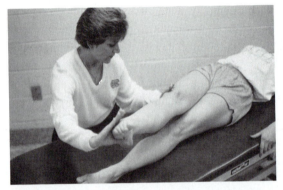

Figure 22-32A D2 movement pattern into flexion, starting position, 2 sets of 12 to 15 repetitions, 2 to 3 days/week.

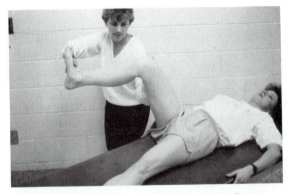

Figure 22-32B D2 movement pattern into flexion, terminal position.

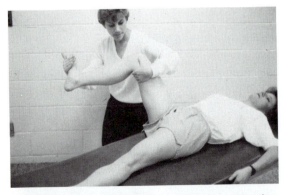

Figure 22-33A D2 movement pattern into extension, starting position, 2 sets of 12 to 15 repetitions, 2 to 3 days/week.

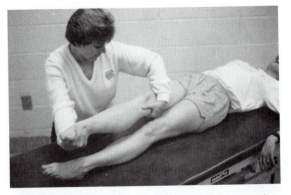

Figure 22-33B D2 movement pattern into extension, terminal position.

Stretching Exercises.

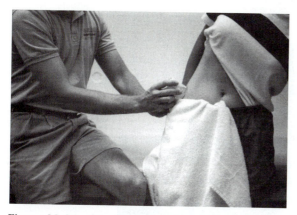

Figure 22-34 Hip pointer stretching with ice.

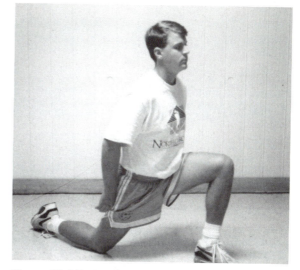

Figure 22-35 Hip flexor stretch.

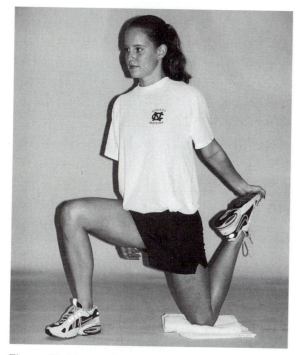

Figure 22-36 Hip flexor stretch with knee flexed to isolate the rectus femoris.

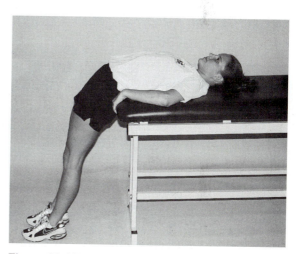

Figure 22-37 Passive static stretch over end of table with hip extended (using ice or heat for 15 to 20 minutes).

A

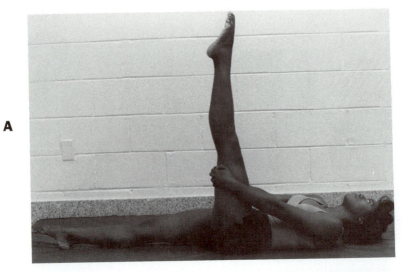

B

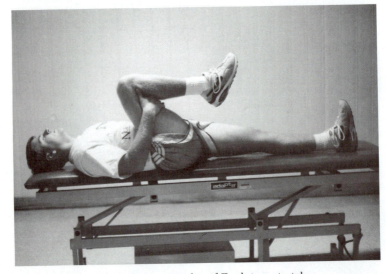

Figure 22-38 **A,** Hamstring stretch and **B,** gluteus stretch.

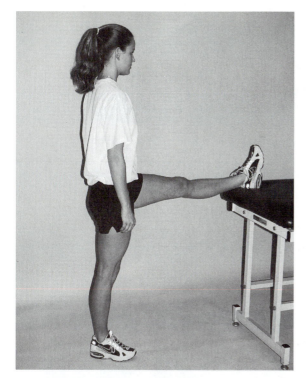

Figure 22-39 Hamstring stretch maintaining lordotic curve.

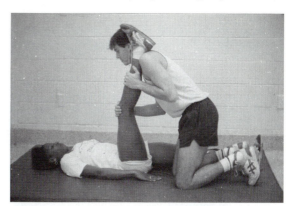

Figure 22-40 PNF hamstring stretching.

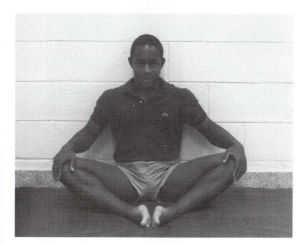

Figure 22-41 Hip adductor stretch.

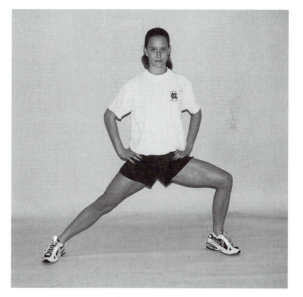

Figure 22-42 Standing hip adductor stretch.

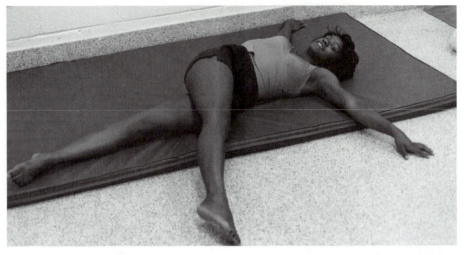

Figure 22-43   Hip abductor stretch.

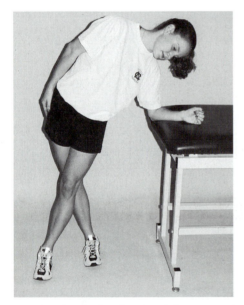

Figure 22-44   Standing hip abductor stretch.

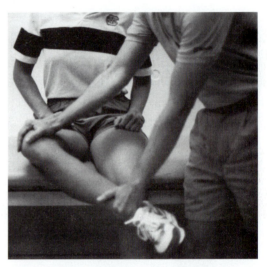

Figure 22-45   Hip internal rotator stretch.

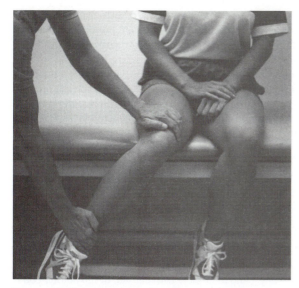

Figure 22-46 Hip external rotator stretch.

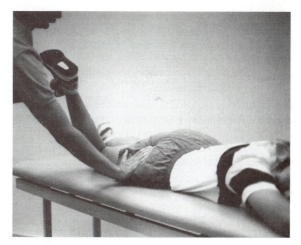

Figure 22-47 Piriformis evaluation stretch test.

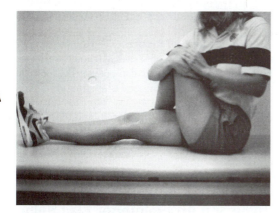

Figure 22-48 Piriformis stretches.

REHABILITATION TECHNIQUES FOR SPECIFIC INJURIES

Preferred treatment and rehabilitation of these injuries are broken down into phases. During the early phase of rehabilitation, ice, compression, and modalities are utilized with pain-free active range of motion as early as possible. Try to avoid any movement that causes pain, especially passive range of motion started too early. After the acute phase, the sports therapist should utilize modalities in combination with active range of motion and the beginning of active resistive pain-free strengthening exercises, both open- and closed-kinetic-chain, as well as concentric and eccentric contractions. Pain-free stretching is also started in this phase. During the late phase the sports therapist should progress the athlete into plyometric ac-

tivities, sport-specific functional training with agility, and ground/power-based activities. Keep in mind that the time sequences for programs and phases are approximations and should be adjusted depending upon the degree of injury, the sport, and the athlete.

Hip Pointer

Pathomechanics. A hip pointer can best be described as a subcutaneous contusion. In most cases, the contusion can cause separation or tearing of the origins or insertions of the muscles that attach to the prominent bony sites.[18] Usually the athlete has no immediate concern, but within hours of the injury, bleeding, swelling, and pain can severely limit the athlete's movement. In rare cases, a fracture of the crest may occur.[1] More serious injuries must be ruled out. One athlete who reported the signs and symptoms of a hip pointer on the field later was determined to have a ruptured spleen.

Injury Mechanism.   A hip pointer is usually caused by a direct blow to the iliac crest or the anterosuperior iliac spine. A strain of the abdominal muscles at their attachment to the anterior and inferior iliac crest can be differentiated from a contusion by obtaining a good history of the mechanism of injury at the time it occurs. A forceful contraction of the abdominal muscles while the trunk is being passively forced to the opposite side can cause a strain of the muscles at their insertion to the iliac bone.[32]

Rehabilitation Concerns.   An X ray film should be taken to rule out iliac crest fractures or avulsion fractures, especially in younger athletes.[18] If the hip pointer is not treated early, within approximately 2 to 4 hours, the athlete may experience severe pain and limited range of motion of the trunk because of the muscle attachments involved.

As in most contusions, the hip pointer is graded. An athlete with a grade I hip pointer might have both normal gait cycle and normal posture. The athlete might complain of slight pain on palpation with little or no swelling. This athlete might also present with full range of motion of the trunk, especially when checking for lateral side bending to the opposite side of the injury.

An athlete with a grade II hip pointer might have moderate to severe pain on palpation, noticeable swelling, and an abnormal gait cycle. The gait cycle might be changed because of a short swing-through phase on the affected side; the athlete might take a short step and be reluctant to keep the foot off the ground. The athlete's pelvis and therefore posture might be slightly tilted to the side of the injury. Active hip and trunk flexion might cause pain, especially if the anterosuperior iliac spine is involved because of the insertion of the sartorius muscle. Range of motion might be limited, especially lateral side bending to the opposite side of the injury and trunk rotation in both directions.

An athlete with a grade III hip pointer might have severe pain on palpation, noticeable swelling, and possible discoloration. The athlete's gait cycle could be abnormal, with very slow, deliberate ambulation and extremely short stride length and swing-through phase. The athlete's posture might present a severe lateral tilt to the affected side. Trunk range of motion could be limited in all directions. Active hip and trunk flexion might reproduce pain.

With all hip pointers, continue with ice, compression, and rest. Subcutaneous steroid injection has been known to decrease inflammation and enable early range of motion exercises. Oral anti-inflammatory medication is also beneficial in the early stages to reduce pain and inflammation and facilitate early range of motion. Transcutaneous electrical nerve stimulation (TNS) may be helpful on the day of injury to decrease pain and allow early range of motion exercises. To regain normal function and speed recovery, use ice massage with pain-free trunk range of motion exercises at the same time. Concentrate on lateral side bending to the side opposite to the injury (Figure 22-34). Other modalities such as ultrasound and electric stimulation are beneficial for increasing range of motion and functional movement. Pain-free active motion and active resistance range of motion exercises are vital to the functional recovery process. Active motion helps promote healing and decreases the time the athlete is prohibited from practice and competition. Exercises as shown in Figures 22-1 through 22-7, 22-14, and 22-15 should be utilized to progress the athlete. Trunk-strengthening exercises may also be added.

Rehabilitation Progression.   A grade I hip pointer usually does not prevent the athlete from competing. An athlete with a grade II hip pointer could miss 5 to 14 days, and an athlete with a grade III hip pointer could miss 14 to 21 days of competition. An athlete with a grade II or III hip pointer can progress to active resistive strengthening exercises, if pain-free, after the initial 2 days of ice, compression, and active range of motion.

Criteria for Full Return.   The athlete is capable of returning to competition when full trunk range of motion is obtained and the athlete can perform all sport-specific activities, such as cutting and changing directions (see Figures 17-4 through 17-14). Compression should be maintained throughout the period, and on returning to competition the athlete should wear a custom-made protective relief doughnut pad with a hard protective shell over the top.

Injury to the Anterosuperior Iliac Spine and Anteroinferior Iliac Spine

Pathomechanics.   Pain at the site of the anterosuperior iliac spine might indicate contusion or apophysitis, an inflammatory response to overuse.[1] Severe pain associated with disability requires an X-ray to rule out an avulsion fracture.[1]

As with the anterosuperior iliac spine, the anteroinferior iliac spine can also present with apophysitis or a contusion. An avulsion fracture should also be ruled out with severe pain. These injuries are seen more often in younger athletes.[34]

Injury Mechanism.   The anterosuperior iliac spine serves as an attachment for the sartorius, and the anteroinferior iliac spine serves as an attachment for the rectus femoris. In both cases a violent, forceful passive stretch of the hip into extension or a violent, forceful active contraction into flexion can cause injury to these sites.[38] Apophysitis or a contusion to these two sites may accompany a hip pointer to the iliac crest.

Rehabilitation Concerns and Progression.
After ruling out an avulsion fracture, rehabilitation for these injuries should follow the same guidelines as for a hip pointer.

Posterosuperior Iliac Spine Contusion

Pathomechanics. Contusions to the posterosuperior iliac spine must be differentiated from vertebral fractures and more serious internal organ injuries.[1] Depending upon the athlete's pain and range of motion, an X ray should be taken to rule out vertebral fractures, vertebral transverse process fractures, and fractures of the posterosuperior iliac spine. Other injuries to this area are not common because of the lack of muscle attachments.[23] Avulsion fractures are rare in this area, although a fracture of the posterosuperior iliac spine should be ruled out. The injury can be painful but usually does not cause disability.

Injury Mechanism and Rehabilitation Concerns. A contusion to the posterosuperior iliac spine is usually caused by a blow or fall. An athlete with a contusion might complain of pain on palpation and have swelling that is usually not extensive. The athlete's gait cycle may look normal except in severe cases, when the athlete may take short, choppy steps to avoid the pain associated with landing at heel strike. In severe cases, the athlete's posture may show a slight forward flexion tilt of the trunk. This athlete might show full active range of motion of the trunk, with mild discomfort. In moderate to severe cases, up to 3 days of rest may be needed before return to competition.

Rehabilitation Progression and Criteria for Full Return. The same treatment can be followed that is used for hip pointers. Pain-free active and passive range of motion exercises of the trunk and hip can be utilized in sets and repetitions, with stretches held for 20 to 30 seconds for each repetition. Guidelines for return to competition are the same as for a hip pointer, and protective padding is recommended.

Piriformis Syndrome (Sciatica)

Pathomechanics. The sciatic nerve is a continuation of the sacral plexus as it passes through the greater sciatic notch and descends deeply through the back of the thigh.[25] Hip and buttock pain is often diagnosed as sciatic nerve irritation. The sciatic nerve can be irritated by a low back problem, but it is also subject to trauma where the nerve passes underneath or through the piriformis muscle, in which case sciatic nerve irritation is also called piriformis syndrome.[1,20] In approximately 15 percent of the population, the sciatic nerve passes through the piriformis muscle, separating it into two. This condition is seen in more women than men, and the cause of piriformis syndrome might be a tight piriformis muscle.[22]

Injury to the hamstring muscles can also cause sciatic nerve irritation, as can irritation from ischial bursitis.[22] In a traumatic accident that causes posterior dislocation of the femoral head, the sciatic nerve might be crushed or severed and require surgery.[22]

Injury Mechanism. The most common cause of sciatic nerve irritation in athletics, especially contact sports, is a direct blow to the buttock. Because of the large muscle mass, this injury is not usually disabling when the sciatic nerve is not involved. When the sciatic nerve is involved, however, the athlete may experience pain in the buttock, extending down the back of the thigh, possibly into the lateral calf and foot. Sciatic pain is usually a burning sensation.[32]

Rehabilitation Concerns. With sciatica, the sports therapist must rule out disk disease before starting any exercise rehabilitation program. Stretching exercises that are indicated for sciatica, such as trunk and hip flexion, might be contraindicated for disk disease. To differentiate low back problems (disk disease) from piriformis syndrome as the cause of sciatica, determine whether the athlete has low back pain with radiation into the extremity. Back pain is most likely midline, exacerbated by trunk flexion and relieved by rest.[13] Coughing and straining may also increase back pain and possibly the radiation. Muscle weakness and sensory numbness may also be found in an athlete with disk disease.[13] Athletes with piriformis syndrome may have the same symptoms without the low back pain and without the low back pain being reproduced with coughing and straining. If, after treatment and rehabilitation, the athlete still maintains neurological deficits, further evaluation to rule out disk disease is necessary.

In the case of piriformis syndrome, the athlete might report a deep pain in the buttock without low back pain and possibly radiating pain in the back of the thigh, lateral calf, and foot, also indicating sciatica.[22] The sports therapist's evaluation should include the low back, as well as the hip and thigh. The athlete's gait cycle could include lack of heel strike, landing in the foot-flat phase, a shortening of the stride, and possible ambulation with a flexed knee to relieve the stretch on the sciatic nerve. The athlete's posture, in severe cases, shows a flexed knee with the leg externally rotated. Palpation in the sciatic notch could also produce pain.

With the athlete lying prone and the hip in a neutral position with the knee in flexion, active resistive external rotation and passive internal rotation of the hip might reproduce the pain[22] (Figure 22-47). Straight leg raises performed passively or actively might also cause symptoms. With the athlete in the same position as above and the knee in extension and relaxed, a decrease in passive internal rotation of the hip joint as compared to the uninjured side may indicate piriformis tightness.

Rehabilitation Progression.   Severe sciatica caused by piriformis syndrome can keep the athlete out of competition for 2 to 3 weeks or longer. If the sciatic nerve is irritated and the athlete complains of radiation into the extremity, the first 3 to 5 days should consist of rest and modalities to decrease the pain associated with sciatica.

After the acute pain has been controlled, the athlete may perform pain-free stretching exercises for the low back and hamstring muscles, as long as disk disease has been ruled out. Stretching exercises (Figures 22-38 through 40, 22-45, 22-48) can be used to treat piriformis syndrome. Piriformis strengthening may be accomplished through resistive external rotation of the hip (Figure 22-7).

Reviewing a normal gait cycle can also aid in gaining range of motion if the athlete has been ambulating with a flexed knee. The hamstrings, as well as the sciatic nerve, may have shortened in this case.

Criteria for Full Return.   The athlete should be capable of performing pain-free activity, such as running and cutting, without neurological symptoms, before returning to competition (see Figures 17-4 through 17-14). Participating with constant radiation into the extremity poses a risk for developing chronic problems. The best method of treatment is prevention by instituting a good flexibility program for all athletes.

Trochanteric Bursitis

Pathomechanics.   The most commonly diagnosed hip bursitis is greater trochanteric bursitis. The greater trochanteric bursa lies between the gluteus maximus and the surface of the greater trochanter.[22,37]

Bursitis and other disorders of the bursa are often mistaken for other injuries because of the location of numerous other structures around the bursa. The bursa is a structure that normally lies within the area of a joint and produces a fluid that lubricates the two surfaces between which it lies.[16] It also may attach, very loosely, to the joint capsule, tendons, ligaments, and skin. Therefore, it is indirectly involved with other close structures.[16] The function of the bursa is to dissipate friction caused by two or more structures moving against one another.

Bursitis associated with bleeding into the bursa is the most disabling form. With hemorrhagic bursitis, swelling and pain may limit motion.[27] The sports therapist must also consider the possibility of an infected bursa. If it is suspected, the athlete should be referred for a medical evaluation.

Injury Mechanism.   Bursitis in general is usually caused by direct trauma or overuse stress. One possible cause for trochanteric bursitis may be irritation caused by the iliotibial band at the insertion of the gluteus maximus.[22] Repetitive irritation such as running with one leg slightly adducted (as on the side of a road), can cause trochanteric bursitis on the adducted side.

Trochanteric bursitis caused by overuse is mostly seen in women runners who have an increased Q angle with or without a leg-length discrepancy.[1] Tight adductors can cause a runner's feet to cross over the midline, resulting in excessive tilting of the pelvis in the frontal plane, and consequently place an exceptional amount of force on the trochanteric bursa.[18]

Lateral heel wear in running shoes can also cause excessive hip adduction, which may indirectly result in trochanteric bursitis. In contact sports, a direct blow may result in a hemorrhagic bursitis, which could be extremely painful to the athlete.[16]

Rehabilitation Concerns.   Traumatic trochanteric bursitis is more easily diagnosed than overuse trochanteric bursitis. Palpation produces pain over the lateral hip area and greater trochanter. In both cases the athlete's gait cycle may be slightly abducted on the affected side to relieve pressure on the bursa. An athlete's attempt to remove weight from the affected extremity may cause a shortened weight-bearing phase. The athlete might report an increase in pain on activity, and active resistive hip abduction might also reproduce the pain.

A complete history must be taken to determine the cause of trochanteric bursitis. The athlete's gait cycle, posture, flexibility, and running shoes should be examined. Oral anti-inflammatory medication usually helps decrease pain and inflammation initially. After the initial treatment of ice, compression, and modalities the athlete can utilize various stretching exercises (Figures 22-35, 22-38 through 46, 22-48).

Rehabilitation Progression.   An orthotic evaluation should be performed to check for any malalignment that may have caused dysfunction, excessive adduction, or leg-length discrepancy. Progressive resistive strengthening exercises in hip abduction may be performed when the athlete is free of pain. Also see treatment for all hip bursitis injuries.

Criteria for Full Return.   This athlete could miss 3 to 5 days of competition, depending on the severity of the bursitis. For contact sports, a protective pad should be worn upon return to competition after the athlete can perform the sport-specific functional tests (see Figures 17-4 through 17-14).

Ischial Bursitis

Pathomechanics and Injury Mechanism.   The ischial bursa lies between the ischial tuberosity and the gluteus maximus (also see Bursitis of the Hip, Pathomechanics). Ischial bursitis is often seen in people who sit for long periods.[22] In athletes, ischial bursitis is more commonly caused by direct trauma, such as falling or a direct hit when the hip is in a flexed position that exposes the ischial area.

Rehabilitation Concerns. The athlete might report trauma to the area. With the hip in a flexed position, palpation over the ischial tuberosity might reproduce the pain. The athlete might experience pain on ambulation when the hip is flexed during the gait cycle. Also, stair climbing and uphill walking and running may reproduce pain.

Rehabilitation Progression. Treatment for ischial bursitis consists of positioning the athlete with the hip in a flexed position to expose the ischial area. After the initial phase of treatment with ice and anti-inflammatory medication, the athlete may begin a pain-free stretching program (Figures 22-38 through 46, 22-48).

Criteria for Full Return. Depending on injury severity, this athlete need not miss competition time. Avoiding direct trauma to the area usually allows healing within 3 to 5 days. For contact sports, a protective pad should be worn (see treatment for all hip bursitis injuries). Sport-specific functional testing and exercises should be performed as described above before the athlete returns to competition.

Iliopectineal Bursitis

Pathomechanics and Injury Mechanism. Iliopectineal bursitis is often mistaken for a strain of the iliopsoas muscle and can be difficult to differentiate. Rarely seen in athletes, iliopectineal bursitis could potentially be caused by a tight iliopsoas muscle.[22] Osteoarthritis of the hip can also cause iliopectineal bursitis.[22]

Rehabilitation Concerns. Resistive hip flexion—sitting with the knee bent or lying supine with the knee extended—may reproduce the pain associated with iliopectineal bursitis. Also, passive hip extension with the knee extended may produce pain. Palpable pain in the inguinal area may also help in evaluating the athlete. In some cases, the nearby femoral nerve may become inflamed and cause radiation into the front of the thigh and knee.[22] Osteoarthritis must be ruled out in evaluating iliopectineal bursitis.

Rehabilitation Progression. Oral anti-inflammatory medication may be helpful initially. A form of deep heat or ice massage may be used to aid in decreasing inflammation and pain. The iliopsoas tendon must be stretched (Figures 22-35 through 22-37), and hip flexion strengthening exercises are performed pain-free with the knee straight (Figures 22-2, 22-3, 22-14B).

Snapping or Clicking Hip Syndrome

Pathomechanics and Injury Mechanism. Clinically, snapping hip syndrome is secondary to what could be a number of causes.[6] Excessive repetitive movement has been linked to snapping hip syndrome in dancers, gymnasts, hurdlers, and sprinters where a muscle imbalance develops.[1] The most common causes of the "snapping," when muscle is involved, is the iliotibial band over the greater trochanter resulting in trochanteric bursitis (see Trochanteric Bursitis) and the iliopsoas tendon over the iliopectineal eminence.[6] Other extra-articular causes of the "snapping" are the iliofemoral ligaments over the femoral head, and the long head of the biceps femoris over the ischial tuberosity.[6] Extra-articular causes commonly occur when the hip is externally rotated and flexed. Other causes or anatomical structures that can predispose "snapping hip" are a narrow pelvic width, abnormal increases in abduction range of motion, and lack of range of motion into external rotation or tight internal rotators.[1] Intra-articular causes are less likely but may consist of loose bodies, synovial chondromatosis, osteocartilaginous exostosis, and possibly subluxation of the hip joint itself.[6]

Rehabilitation Concerns, Progression, and Criteria for Full Return. Due to the extra-articular causes, the hip joint capsule, ligaments, and muscles become loosened and allow the hip to become unstable. The athlete will complain of a "snapping," and this snapping might be accompanied by severe pain and disability upon each "snap."

The key to treating and rehabilitating the snapping hip syndrome is to decrease pain and inflammation with ice, anti-inflammatory medication, and other modalities such as ultrasound. This could significantly decrease the pain initially so that the athlete can begin a stretching and strengthening program. The most important aspect of the evaluation process is to find the source of the imbalance (which muscles are tight and which are weak).

In the case of the iliopsoas muscle snapping over the iliopectineal eminence, the following stretches should be utilized (Figures 22-35 through 37, 22-48). Strengthening should take into account the entire hip, especially the hip extensors and internal and external rotators (Figures 22-3, 22-6, 22-7).

After pain has subsided and the athlete can actively flex the hip pain-free, the athlete can begin strengthening exercises for the hip flexor (Figures 22-1, 22-2, and 22-14) flexion with the knee straight. After the first 3 to 5 days, the athlete can begin jogging and sport-specific functional drills (see Figures 17-4, 17-7 through 17-14) and progress to exercises shown in Figures 17-5 and 17-6, if all are pain-free.

Osteitis Pubis

Pathomechanics. Pain in the area of the pubic symphysis may be difficult to diagnose. Unless the athlete reports being hit or experiencing some kind of direct trauma, pubic pain might be caused by osteitis pubis, fractures of the inferior ramus (stress fractures and avulsion fractures), or a groin strain.[1]

Because an overuse situation and rapid repetitive changes of direction predispose an athlete to this injury, osteitis pubis is seen mostly in distance running, football, wrestling, and soccer. Constant movement of the symphysis in sports such as football and soccer produces inflammation and pain.

Injury Mechanism. Repetitive stress on the pubic symphysis, caused by the insertion of muscles into the area, creates a chronic inflammation.[1] Direct trauma to the symphysis can also cause periostitis. Symptoms develop gradually, and might be mistaken for muscle strains. Exercises that aid muscle strains might cause more irritation to the symphysis; thus early active exercises are contraindicated.[18]

Rehabilitation Concerns. Referral to a physician to rule out hernia problems, infection, and prostatitis may be helpful in evaluating osteitis pubis.[18] Changes in X ray films can take 4 to 6 weeks to show. The athlete should be treated symptomatically.

An athlete with osteitis pubis may have pain in the groin area and might complain of an increase in pain with running, sit-ups, and squatting.[1] The athlete might also complain of lower abdominal pain with radiation into the inner thigh. Differentiating osteitis pubis from a muscle strain is difficult.

Palpation over the pubic symphysis may reproduce pain. In severe cases the athlete may show a waddling gait because of the shear forces at the symphysis.[1] Rest is the main course of treatment, with modalities and anti-inflammatory medication to ease pain. As soon as pain permits, the athlete should begin pain-free adductor stretching exercises as shown in Figure 22-41 and 22-42. Also, pain-free abdominal strengthening, low back strengthening, and open-chain hip abductor, adductor, flexor, and extensor strengthening can be started (Figures 22-1 through 22-5). Because excessive movement that causes shear forces at the symphysis is the main cause of pain, stabilization exercises that concentrate on tightening the muscles around the pubic symphysis are recommended. The athlete is asked to concentrate on tightening the buttock, groin, abdomen, and low back (the entire pelvic area) while performing a closed-chain exercise such as the leg press (Figure 22-16) and lunges (Figure 22-19). This stabilization technique helps to control excessive movement at the pubic symphysis while the athlete performs movements at other joints. These closed-chain exercises may be started, for stabilization purposes, and might actually be pain-free before the start of open-chain exercises.

Rehabilitation Progression and Criteria for Full Return. The lower body must be protected from shear forces to the symphysis area. Most athletes will miss 3 to 5 days of competition. In severe cases, from 3 weeks up to 3 months and possibly 6 months of rest and treatment may be necessary. In severe cases, the athlete should not participate until able to perform pain-free plyometric exercises (Figures 22-27 through 22-29). Sport-specific functional drills may be started as soon as the athlete can perform them pain-free (see Figures 17-4 through 17-14).

Fractures of the Inferior Ramus

Pathomechanics. Stress and avulsion fractures should be ruled out before treating the pubic area for injury. The extent of an avulsion fracture must be diagnosed by X ray. In some cases, a palpable mass may be detected under the skin. Stress fractures may be diagnosed with the same symptoms as in osteitis pubis. With a stress fracture an X ray might appear normal until the third or fourth week. Obtaining a good history can aid in diagnosing a stress fracture.

Injury Mechanism. Avulsion fracture of the inferior ramus is usually caused by a violent, forceful contraction of the hip adductor muscles or forceful passive movement into hip abduction, as in a split. Stress fractures can occur from overuse (see treatment for Femoral Stress Fractures).

Rehabilitation Concerns, Progression, and Criteria for Full Return. Rest is the key in treating fractures of the inferior ramus. Hip stretching and strengthening exercises may be performed, as in pubic injuries, within a pain-free range of motion. An avulsion fracture might keep an athlete out of competition for up to 3 months. An athlete with a stress fracture may miss 3 to 6 weeks of competition. Rest from the activities that cause muscle contraction forces at the inferior ramus should be avoided, and closed-chain stabilization exercises as described in pubic symphysis injury rehabilitation should be utilized. Return to activity should be gradual and deliberate, and must be pain-free.

Groin and Hip Flexor Strain

Pathomechanics. A groin strain can occur to any muscle in the inner hip area. Whether it is to the sartoris, rectus femoris, the adductors, or the iliopsoas, the muscle and degree of injury must be determined and the injury treated accordingly.[5]

Discomfort may start as mild but develop into moderate to severe pain with disability if not treated correctly. A chronic strain can cause bleeding into the groin muscles, resulting in myositis ossificans (see the section on myositis ossificans). If a groin strain is treated acutely, myositis ossificans can be avoided.

Injury Mechanism and Rehabilitation Concerns. A groin strain can develop from overextending and externally rotating the hip or from forcefully contracting the muscles into flexion and internal rotation as involved in running, jumping, twisting, and kicking. Differential diagnosis and treatment may be difficult because of the number of muscles in the area.

With a grade 1 groin strain, the athlete may complain of mild discomfort with no loss of function and full range of motion and strength. Point tenderness may be minimal, with negative swelling. The gait cycle may be normal.

With a grade 2 groin strain, palpation may reproduce pain and show a minimal to moderate defect. Swelling might also be detected. This athlete may show an abnormal gait cycle. Ambulation may be slow, and the stride length may be shortened on the affected side. The athlete may tend to hike the hip and tilt the pelvis in the frontal plane rather than drive the knee through during the swing-through phase. Range of motion may be severely limited, and resistance could cause an increase in pain. When the iliopsoas is involved, the athlete may experience severe pain after the initial injury. This is thought to be caused by spasm of the iliopsoas muscle, which tilts the pelvis in the frontal plane. The athlete will walk with a flexed hip and knee and will be unable to extend the hip during the push-off phase of the gait cycle because the muscle spasm does not allow hip extension and active hip flexion during swing-through. This athlete will also externally rotate the hip in order to utilize the hip adductors for the swing-through phase.

An athlete with a grade 3 groin strain may need crutches to ambulate. A moderate to severe defect may be detected in the involved muscle or tendon. Point tenderness may be severe, with noticeable swelling. Range of motion is severely limited, especially if the iliopsoas is involved. The athlete might splint the legs together and be apprehensive about allowing movement in abduction. Resistance might not be tolerated.

Differentiating a hip adductor strain from a hip flexor strain is the first step in treating this injury. Resistive adduction while lying supine with the knee in extension may significantly increase pain if the hip adductors are involved. Flexing the hip and knee and resisting hip adduction may also increase pain. If the injury is a pure hip adductor strain, the supine position with the knee extended may reproduce more discomfort than flexing the hip and knee. If resistive adduction with the hip and knee flexed produces more discomfort, the hip flexor may also be involved.

With the athlete lying supine, more pain on resistive hip flexion with the knee in extension (straight leg raise)

tests for iliopsoas involvement. More pain on resistive hip flexion with the knee flexed tests for rectus femoris involvement. After determining the muscle or muscle groups involved and the degree of the injury, treatment and rehabilitation is the next step.

Rehabilitation Progression and Criteria for Full Return. With a grade 1 strain, modalities and pain-free hip stretching exercises can begin immediately (Figures 22-35 through 22-37, 22-41, 22-42, 22-45, 22-46). Pain-free progressive strengthening exercises may also be performed (Figures 22-1, 22-2, 22-4, 22-6, 22-7, 22-14), progressing to flexion with knee straight and bent and adduction (Figures 22-15, 22-19, 22-22, 22-23), and PNF exercises (Figures 22-30A,B, 22-32A,B). Depending upon the severity of the injury, this athlete need not miss competition time and can be progressed to the slide board (Figure 22-24), plyometrics (Figures 22-27 through 22-29), and sport-specific functional drills (see Figures 17-4 through 17-14) as soon as pain allows.

An athlete with a grade 2 strain should be started immediately, with gentle, pain-free, active range-of-motion exercises of the hip. When the iliopsoas is involved, it has been found that lying supine on a treatment table with the leg and hip hanging over the end of the table, with the hip in a passively extended position, while applying ice for 15 to 20 minutes, can help eliminate muscle spasm and pain (Figure 22-37). Electrical muscle stimulation modalities can be very useful in the early stages to decrease inflammation, pain, and spasm and to promote range of motion.[29] Isometrics should also be performed as soon as they can be managed without pain. If crutches are used, a normal gait cycle is taught. The athlete can begin pain-free stretching as soon as possible (Figures 22-35, through 22-37, 22-41, 22-42, 22-45, 22-46). As soon as pain allows, the athlete can begin pain-free strengthening exercises (Figures 22-1, 22-2, 22-4, 22-6, 22-7, 22-13, 22-14), flexion and adduction strengthening exercises (Figures 22-15, 22-19, 22-22, 22-23), and PNF (Figures 22-30A,B, 22-32A,B). After approximately 1 week the athlete can begin pain-free slide board exercises (Figure 22-24) and plyometrics (Figures 22-27 through 22-29), as well as sport-specific functional drills (see Figures 17-4 through 17-14). This athlete may miss 3 to 14 days of competition, depending on the severity of injury. Hip adductor strains usually take longer to treat and rehabilitate than hip flexor strains of the same grade, especially if the muscle spasm involved with a hip flexor is eliminated as soon as possible. Treatment and rehabilitation should be modified accordingly.

An athlete with a grade 3 strain should be iced, compressed, immobilized, and non-weight-bearing. Electrical muscle stimulation modalities are useful in the acute stage to decrease inflammation and pain and to promote range of motion. Rest for 1 to 3 days is recommended, with compression at all times. If the iliopsoas is involved, passive stretching with ice (Figure 22-37) can be started after the third day.

If surgery is ruled out, the athlete may perform pain-free isometric exercises between days 3 and 5. Slow, pain-free, active range of motion exercises may also be performed between days 3 and 5. A normal gait cycle should be emphasized using crutches. Crutches should not be eliminated until the athlete can ambulate with a normal, pain-free gait cycle. Between days 7 and 10, the athlete may perform pain-free stretching exercises (Figures 22-35 through 22-37, 22-41, 22-42, 22-45, 22-46) and can begin progressive resistive strengthening exercises without pain, progressing in weight and motion (Figures 22-1, 22-2, 22-4, 22-6, 22-7, 22-13, 22-14), flexion and adduction (Figures 22-15, 22-19, 22-22, 22-23), and PNF (Figures 22-30A,B, 22-32A,B). The athlete needs to achieve a good strength level, usually within 10 days after starting progressive resistive strengthening exercises, to perform pain-free slide board exercises (Figure 22-24) and plyometrics (Figures 22-27 through 22-29), as well as sport-specific functional activities (see Figures 17-4 through 17-14).

Treatment and rehabilitation timetables may be modified. The modifications should be based on the degree of injury within the grade presented. This athlete could potentially miss 3 weeks to 3 months of competition.

Hip Dislocation

Pathomechanics. Dislocation of the hip joint is extremely rare in athletics and takes a considerable amount of force because of the deep-seated ball-in-socket joint.[26,33] Fractures and avascular necrosis, which is a degenerative condition of the head of the femur caused by a disruption of blood supply during dislocation, should always be considered.[1,12,19] Dislocation should be treated as a medical emergency. The athlete should be checked for distal pulses and sensation. The sciatic nerve should be examined to see if it has been crushed or severed.[1] Do this by checking sensation and foot and toe movements. If the sciatic nerve is damaged, knee, ankle, and toe weakness may be pronounced.

Injury Mechanism. A hip dislocation is generally a posterior dislocation that takes place with the knee and hip in a flexed position. The athlete may be totally disabled, in severe pain, and usually unwilling to allow movement of the extremity. The trochanter may appear larger than normal with the extremity in internal rotation, flexed, and adducted.[32] X-ray studies should be performed before anesthetized reduction.[26]

Rehabilitation Concerns, Progression, and Criteria for Full Return. Two or 3 weeks (and in some

cases, a longer period) of immobilization is initially needed. Rehabilitation of the thigh, knee, and ankle may be included at this time. Pain-free hip isometric exercises should be performed. Electrical muscle stimulation modalities may be used initially to promote muscle reeducation and retard muscle atrophy.[32] At approximately 3 to 6 weeks, pain-free active range of motion exercises can be performed (Figures 22-1 through 22-7) with no resistance/weight. Crutch walking is progressed and performed until the athlete can ambulate with a normal gait cycle and without pain. At approximately 6 weeks, the athlete may perform gentle progressive resistive strengthening exercises with a weight cuff or weight boot. All six movements of the hip should be included in the progressive resistive strengthening exercises (hip flexion, abduction, extension, adduction, internal rotation, and external rotation, (Figures 22-1 through 22-7, 22-14) and PNF exercises (Figures 22-30A,B through 22-33A,B). Pain-free stretching exercises should not be performed for 8 to 12 weeks (Figures 22-35, 22-36, 22-38 through 22-48). At approximately 12 weeks, the athlete may begin closed-chain exercises (Figures 22-16 through 22-22A,B), as well as open-chain exercises (Figure 22-15). At 16 to 20 weeks, the athlete may progress to pain-free slide board (Figure 22-24), plyometric exercises (Figures 22-27 through 22-29), and sport-specific functional activities (see Figures 17-4, 17-7 through 17-14) and then progress to the functional exercises (Figures 17-5, 17-6). If pain returns, the athlete must eliminate plyometrics and functional activities until they can be performed pain-free. This athlete may return to competition in 6 to 12 months if there have been no delays and the athlete is pain-free with all activity.

Hamstring Strain and Avulsion Fracture of the Ischial Tuberosity

Pathomechanics. The ischial tuberosity is a common site of injury to the hamstring muscle group (the biceps femoris, semitendinosus, and semimembranosus). All three hamstring muscles originate from the ischial tuberosity. The most common ischial injury, as it relates to the hamstring group, is an avulsion fracture of the tuberosity.[2,28]

Injury Mechanism. This injury usually results from a violent, forceful flexion of the hip, with the knee in extension.[1] A less severe irritation of the hamstring origin at the ischial tuberosity may also develop.

Rehabilitation Concerns, Rehabilitation Progression, and Criteria for Full Return (Strain). An athlete with a less severe injury or irritation of the hamstring origin at the ischial tuberosity may complain of discomfort on sitting for extended periods and discomfort on palpation. This athlete may also complain of pain while walking up stairs or uphill. The athlete may ambulate with a normal gait cycle. Also, the athlete may be able to jog normally, but pain may be present with attempts at sprinting. Resistive knee flexion and resistive hip extension with the knee in an extended position may reproduce the pain. Passive hip flexion with the knee in extension may also cause discomfort.

After the initial treatment phase of ice and other modalities, the athlete may begin gentle, pain-free hamstring stretching exercises (Figures 22-38, 22-39, 22-40). To isolate the hamstring muscle while stretching, the athlete should maintain a lordotic curve in the lumbar back area while flexing at the trunk to stretch the hamstrings (Figure 22-39). Pain-free hamstring muscle progressive resistive strengthening exercises may also be performed, as soon as possible, (Figures 22-3, 22-8, through 22-10, 22-14), closed-chain extension exercise (Figures 22-16 through 22-22), and PNF exercises (Figures 22-31A,B, and 22-33A,B). This athlete might not miss competition time and can be progressed functionally as tolerated.

Rehabilitation Concerns (Avulsion Fracture). The more severe ischial tuberosity avulsion fracture presents a different clinical picture. Palpation may produce moderate to severe pain, and the athlete may be in moderate to severe pain with a very abnormal gait cycle. The athlete's gait cycle may lack a heel-strike phase and have a very short swing-through phase.[2] The athlete may attempt to keep the injured extremity behind or below the body to avoid hip flexion during the gait cycle. Resistive knee flexion and hip extension with the knee in an extended or flexed position may reproduce the pain. Passive hip flexion with the knee extended and with the knee flexed may cause moderate to severe pain at the ischial tuberosity. X-rays might or might not show the injury.[32]

After week 3 and the initial acute phase of treatment with modalities, the athlete may begin pain-free active range of motion lying prone and supine. Pain-free hamstring stretching exercises (Figures 22-38 through 22-40) may also be performed. Regaining full range of motion during the rehabilitation program is very important. Many athletes never gain full hip flexion range of motion after this injury.

Weeks 6 through 12 are a progressive phase for pain-free hamstring progressive resistive strengthening exercises (Figures 22-3, 22-8 through 22-10, 22-14), closed-chain extension exercises (Figures 22-16, 22-17, 22-20, 22-22), isokinetics (Figures 22-25, 22-26), and PNF exercises (Figures 22-31A,B, and 22-33A,B). After 2 to 3 weeks the athlete may progress to the exercises as shown in Figures 22-19, 22-21, 22-23A,B.

Rehabilitation Progression and Criteria for Full Return (Avulsion Fracture). Surgery is usually not necessary. Immobilization and limiting physical activity are usually enough to allow healing. Ice and limited physical activity that involves hip flexion and forceful hip extension and knee flexion for the first 3 weeks are usually all that is necessary. Crutches should be used until normal gait is taught. During weeks 6 to 12, the athlete will begin activities such as swimming, biking, and jogging, but the athlete should avoid forceful knee and hip flexion and forceful hip extension. After week 12 the athlete, without pain, may progress to the slide board (Figure 22-24), plyometrics (Figures 22-27 through 22-29), and sport-specific functional drills (see Figures 17-4, 17-7 through 17-14) and then progress to the exercises shown in Figures 17-5 and 17-6.

Hamstring Strains

Pathomechanics. Hamstring strains are common, and the causes are numerous.[40] The ability of the hamstring muscles and quadriceps muscles to work together is very complex because the hamstrings cross two joints.[20] This produces forces and therefore stresses on the hamstrings dependent upon the positions of the hip and knee.[6] Some dissection research has shown that there is consistent overlap of tendon vertically, over the course of the muscle, with the exception of the semitendinosus.[6] With research showing the musculotendinous junction as the main injury site, anywhere along the muscle/tendon is susceptible to injury.[6]

The athlete might report a "pop." Palpation is the easiest way to identify the site and extent of injury. Even though bleeding (ecchymosis) may be present, some people believe that this isn't associated with the degree or severity of injury.[6]

An athlete with a grade 1 hamstring strain will complain of sore hamstring muscles, with some pain on palpation and possibly minimal swelling. An athlete with a grade 2 hamstring strain may report having heard or felt a "pop" during the activity. At the first or second day, moderate ecchymosis may be observed. Palpation may produce moderate to severe pain, and even though a defect and noticeable swelling in the muscle belly may be evident, the grade 2 hamstring strain most likely occurs at the musculotendinous junction either mid to high semimembranosus/tendinosis or lower lateral biceps femoris. An athlete with a grade 3 strain may report having heard or felt a "pop' during the activity. The sports therapist may detect swelling and severe pain on palpation. A noticeable defect may be present, again at the musculotendinous junction as described above. After the first through third days, moderate to severe ecchymosis may be observed.

Injury Mechanism. A quick, explosive contraction that involves a "rapid activity" could lead to a strain of the hamstring muscles. Many theories try to explain the cause of hamstring strains. Imbalance with the quadriceps is one theory, according to which the hamstring muscles should have 60 to 70 percent of the quadriceps muscles' strength. Other possibilities are hamstring muscle fatigue, running posture and gait, leg-length discrepancy, decreased hamstring range of motion, and an imbalance between the medial and lateral hamstring muscle.[1]

Another factor that plays a role in injury, as well as rehabilitation, is that the semitendinosus, semimembranosus, and long head of the biceps femoris are innervated from the tibial branch of the sciatic nerve, while the short head of the biceps femoris is innervated by the peroneal branch of the sciatic nerve.[6] This innervation difference makes the short head a completely separate muscle—"a factor implicated in the etiology of hamstring muscle strains" as described by DeLee and Drez.[6]

Two phases of the running gait described by DeLee and Drez show that the support phase and the recovery phase may predispose the athlete to hamstring strains. During the support phase, foot strike, mid-support, and take-off occurs.[6] During recovery phase, follow-through, forward swing, and foot descent occurs.[6] The two portions of these two phases that are implicated in hamstring strains are the late forward swing segment of the recovery phase and the take-off phase of the support phase. EMG data show that the semimembranosus is very active during the late forward swing segment and that the biceps femoris is inactive.[6] At take-off of the support phase, the biceps femoris shows maximal activity.[6] This shows that the mid to high semimembranosus and semitendinosus strains may occur during the deceleration portion of the running cycle while the lower lateral biceps femoris strains are occurring at the take-off or push-off portion of the running cycle. The rehabilitation implications are connected to the position of the hip and knee while rehabilitating in order to isolate and identify the specific muscle involved.[4] Utilizing the correct biomechanical positions during rehabilitation, based on the EMG findings presented above, will enhance rehabilitation and improve preventive programs.

Rehabilitation Concerns. An athlete with a grade 1 hamstring strain may have a normal gait cycle. Hip flexion range of motion is probably normal, with a tight feeling reported at the extreme range of hip flexion. Resistive knee flexion and hip extension with the knee extended are probably free of pain or possibly produce a tight feeling with good strength present.

An athlete with a grade 2 hamstring strain usually ambulates with an abnormal gait cycle. The athlete may lack heel strike and land during the foot-flat phase of the gait cycle. The swing-through phase may be limited because of the athlete's unwillingness to flex the hip and knee. The athlete may tend to ambulate with a flexed knee. Resistive knee flexion and hip extension with the knee extended may cause moderate to severe pain. The athlete may also have a noticeable weakness on resistive knee flexion and hip extension with the knee extended and flexed. Resistive hip extension with the knee flexed also tests the strength of the gluteus maximus muscle. Passive hip flexion with the knee extended may also produce moderate to severe pain. The athlete's range of motion may be moderately to severely limited in hip flexion with the knee extended and moderately limited in hip flexion with the knee flexed.

An athlete with a grade 3 hamstring strain may be unable to ambulate without the aid of crutches. The athlete may have poor strength and be unable to resist knee flexion and hip extension with the knee extended. The athlete may have fair strength upon resistive hip extension with the knee flexed because of the gluteus maximus muscle. Resisting these motions usually causes pain. Passive hip flexion, with the knee extended, might not be tolerated because of pain. Passive hip flexion, knee flexed, may be moderately to severely limited.

Because most hamstring injuries occur due to a "rapid activity" that involves an explosive concentric contraction during toe-off or a strong eccentric contraction during deceleration swing-through, it is this author's belief that the hamstring should be rehabilitated in a "rapid activity" fashion with high intensity and a high volume of exercises. After the initial treatment of ice, rest, compression, and active range of motion, the following exercises, in the order given and with a load that doesn't produce pain, should be instituted. Alternating a single-joint open-chain exercise with a multijoint closed-chain exercise, with 30 seconds rest between sets and actual exercises, has shown to facilitate rapid healing and earlier return to activity, as well as present preventive advantages (all exercises are performed pain-free and in the order given): Bike, Stair Master, and stretch (Figures 22-38, through 22-42, 22-45, 22-46, 22-48). Stretching is followed by pain-free progressive strengthening exercises in the following order: extension knee straight to bent for mid/high semimembranosus/tendinosis strains and knee bent to straight for lower/lateral biceps femoris strains (Figures 22-9, 22-14E, 22-16); followed by heavy negatives (two legs up, one leg down), 1 set of 8 each leg (Figure 22-19); feet in front for mid/high strain (Figure 22-17); feet in back for lower/lateral strain (Figure 22-18); for mid/high strain (Figures 22-10, 22-21, 22-23A,B, 22-25); for lower/lateral strain (Figure 22-26); and PNF stretching (Figures 22-31A,B and 22-33A,B).

Rehabilitation Progression. Each exercise done in the order given and sets, reps, and suggested rest periods should be progressed based on daily evaluation that involves pain, range of motion, muscle strength from previous workout session, and how the athlete subjectively feels. Days between strengthening workout sessions should be utilized for aerobic conditioning such as biking, Stair Master, and aquatic therapy, as well as slide board activity (Figure 22-24) followed by stretching as described above.

A pain-free normal gait cycle should be taught as soon as possible, and crutches should be used to accomplish a normal gait cycle. Ice, compression, and gentle, pain-free hamstring stretching exercises, making sure the athlete maintains a lumbar lordotic curve to isolate the hamstring muscles, are performed on day 1. Electrical muscle stimulation modalities may be used to promote range of motion and to decrease pain and spasm.[20] Active knee and hip range of motion while lying prone may also be performed on days 1 through 3, if the athlete can do so without pain. Hamstring isometric exercises are taught as soon as possible, again within pain-free limits. Starting pain-free active range of motion, as soon as possible, is very important and usually decreases the length of time an athlete misses competition. At approximately day 3, the athlete may begin heat in the form of hot packs and whirlpool, combined with pain-free stretching exercises described earlier. If pain-free, the above strengthening program may be started between days 3 and 7.

Criteria for Full Return. An athlete with a grade 1 hamstring strain might not miss competition but should be watched closely for further injury. The rehabilitation program described should begin immediately to avoid further injury. An athlete with a grade 2 hamstring strain could miss 5 to 21 days of competition. An athlete with a grade 3 hamstring strain could miss 3 to 12 weeks of competition. In all situations the athlete should not return to competition until plyometrics (Figures 22-27 through 22-29) and sport-specific functional drills (see Figures 17-4 through 17-14) are accomplished pain-free. Once you begin sport-specific drills, it is advised to warm up the athlete's core body temperature. This can be accomplished by utilizing hamstring functional activities such as backpedals, side shuffles, carioca, plyometrics, and straight-ahead pain-free strides up to 100 yards in length.

Hamstring Tendon Strains

Pathomechanics. Another injury that occurs to the hamstring muscles is a strain of the hamstring tendons near their attachments to the tibia and fibula. This injury has also been diagnosed as tendinitis. Injury to the gastrocnemius muscle tendons in the same area must be ruled out.

Injury Mechanism. The athlete might report pain but might not experience disability. An athlete with a hamstring tendon strain or tendinitis may present a history of overuse and chronic pain for a few days with no specific mechanism of injury.

Rehabilitation Concerns, Rehabilitation Progression, and Criteria for Full Return. Palpation helps to isolate which tendon or tendons are involved, and resistive knee flexion, with the tibia in internal and external rotation, aids in the evaluation. If resistive ankle plantar flexion with the knee in extension does not reproduce symptoms, gastrocnemius involvement may be ruled out.

An athlete who presents with this condition responds nicely to 1 to 2 days of rest with oral anti-inflammatory medication. Ice massage and ultrasound help decrease inflammation and pain. Gentle hamstring stretching exercises (Figures 22-38, 22-39) with the hip in internal and external rotation help to isolate the tendon or tendons involved, and PNF stretching (Figure 22-40) should be performed on day 1. Hamstring progressive resistive strengthening exercises that isolate the hamstring muscles can be performed on day 1 (Figures 22-3, 22-9, 22-10, 22-14E), along with extensions (Figures 22-21), if they can be performed without pain.

Femoral Stress Fractures

Pathomechanics and Injury Mechanism. A stress fracture, often described as a partial or incomplete fracture of the femur, may be seen because of repetitive microtrauma or cumulative stress overload to a localized area of the bone.[9,41] Young athletes are more likely to develop this injury. The athlete may complain of pinpoint pain that increases during activity. The initial X-ray film is usually negative. Obtaining a good history is very important and should include activities, change in activities and surfaces, and running gait analysis.[41]

The basic biomechanics and biodynamics of normal bone are very important to understanding the mechanism of stress fractures. A process of bone resorption, followed by new bone formation, in normal bone, is constantly occurring through turning over and remodeling by the dynamic organ itself.[41] This remodeling occurs in response to stress, weight-bearing, and muscular contractions that cause stresses. Responses by the bone to these loads allow the bone to become as strong as it has to be to withstand the stresses placed upon it during the required activity.[10,41] Because bone is a dynamic tissue, there is a cell system in place that carries out the process of constant bone breakdown and bone repair for the task at hand.[41] There are two types of bone cells responsible for this dynamic procedure—osteoclasts, which resorb bone, and osteoblasts, which produce new bone to fill the areas that have been resorbed.[41] When stress is applied, the osteoblasts produce new bone at a rate comparable to the osteoclasts. When the stress is applied over time, as in overuse, the osteoclasts work at a faster rate than the osteoblasts and a stress fracture occurs. Some studies have shown that this stress reaction occurs approximately during the third week of a workout session.[11] This becomes very important when developing a rehabilitation program in reference to utilizing the advantages of bone physiology within the rehabilitation program to facilitate new bone formation.

Rehabilitation Concerns, Progression, and Criteria for Full Return.   As with all stress fractures, finding the cause is the first step in treatment and rehabilitation.[35] The athlete may perform pain-free thigh strengthening and stretching exercises and progress as shown in the sections on hamstring and quadriceps rehabilitation programs.

The most important treatment for stress fractures is rest, especially from the sport or activity that caused the fracture. In a period of 6 to 12 weeks, most femoral stress fractures heal clinically if the specific cause is discontinued.[41] The resorptive process will slow down, and the reparative process will catch up, with simple rest from the activity that caused the problem. Rest should be "active." This allows the athlete to exercise pain-free and helps prevent muscle atrophy and deconditioning. Except in special "problem" fractures, immobilization in a cast or brace is usually unnecessary. When there is excessive pain or motion of the part, casts or braces may be used. In unreliable patients, a cast or some form of immobilization may be recommended. Non-weight-bearing or partial-weight-bearing with crutches is highly recommended as the process of ambulating with a normal gait, while utilizing crutches, can facilitate bone formation at the fracture site.[24]

Until ordinary, "normal" activities are pain-free with no tenderness or edema over the fracture site and no abnormal gait patterns during ambulation, the athlete is held back from sport activities. Pain-free rehabilitation should start immediately and continue throughout the recovery period with a slow progressive return to activity. Immediately discontinue all activity with recurrence of any symptoms.[41]

The first phase of the rehabilitation program begins when the stress fracture is diagnosed. This phase consists of modalities to decrease pain and swelling and to increase or maintain active range of motion to the hip, knee, and ankle joints.[41] The second phase of rehabilitation begins as acute pain subsides. This phase consists of functional rehabilitation and conditioning in a progression of sport-specific training. Keeping in mind bone physiology as described, the athlete who has begun sport-specific training is advised not to run, jump, or force activity during the third week after 2 weeks of vigorous "normal" exercise or rehabilitation and conditioning. This cycle is repeated—2 weeks of vigorous "normal" activity, followed by 1 week of either eliminating running and jumping or at least cutting it back to half the "normal" activity level. This cycling of activities, every third week, facilitates osteoblast function (bone formation) and, therefore, new bone growth at the fracture site as the osteoblasts are able to keep pace with and actually work faster than the osteoclasts.

Rehabilitation and treatment should be an ongoing process as described above, with general physical conditioning as part of the "active rest" period. Aquatic exercise and conditioning, such as swimming, treading water, running in a swimming pool, biking, Stair Master, and the slide board, (Figure 22-24), should be started as soon as they are pain-free. These activities could come under the umbrella of "normal" exercise or rehabilitation and conditioning. Upper-body ergometers may also be utilized. An athlete with a femoral stress fracture should also be evaluated for lower-extremity deformities and foot malalignments.[41] Orthotics can be very useful in treating a femoral stress fracture if a malalignment is found.

Avulsion Fracture of the Femoral Trochanter

Pathomechanics and Injury Mechanism.   Athletes might suffer an isolated avulsion fracture of the femoral trochanters. When the greater trochanter is involved, the cause is usually a violent, forceful contraction of the hip abductor muscles. An avulsion fracture of the lesser trochanter occurs because of a violent, forceful contraction of the iliopsoas muscle.[30]

Palpation may produce pain and possibly a noticeable defect of the greater trochanter. Resistive movements and passive range of motion of the hip may reproduce pain. X rays must be taken to confirm the injury. Immobilization may be the treatment of choice for a incomplete avulsion fracture. With a complete avulsion fracture, internal fixation is usually required.

Rehabilitation Concerns, Progression, and Criteria for Full Return.   During the initial immobilization period, as prescribed by the physician, the athlete with a femoral avulsion fracture should perform isometric hip exercises on the first day of rehabilitation, with isometric quadriceps and hamstring exercises and ankle-strengthening exercises. Crutches should be used for the first 6 weeks until a pain-free normal gait cycle can be accomplished. After 6 weeks, the athlete may perform pain-free active range of motion exercises, as well as pain-free stretching exercises (Figures 22-35 through 22-42, 22-48). When pain allows, the athlete may add stretching (Figures 22-43 through 22-46, 22-48). The athlete may also begin pain-free straight-leg-raise exercises, (Figures 22-2 through 22-4), and progress to hip abduction and rotation (Figures 22-5 through 22-7). During approximately week 8, the athlete may perform hip progressive resistive exercises in all four directions (Figure 22-14). Swimming can be added as soon as pain allows, and biking is performed when sufficient range of motion is attained. The athlete is then progressed to closed-chain weight-bearing lifting activities (Figures 22-16, 22-17, 22-19, 22-20, 22-22, 22-23). Jogging, plyometrics (Figures 22-27 through 22-29), slide board (Figure 22-24), and sport-specific functional drills (see Figures 17-4 through 17-14) can be started as soon as the athlete is pain-free and has the necessary strength base.

Traumatic Femoral Fractures

Pathomechanics and Injury Mechanism. A femoral neck fracture is often associated with osteoporosis and is rarely seen in athletics.[16,36] However, a twisting motion combined with a fall can produce this fracture. Because the femoral neck fracture can disrupt the blood supply to the head of the femur, avascular necrosis is often seen later. This injury must receive proper treatment.

Rehabilitation Concerns, Progression, and Criteria for Full Return. After surgery or during immobilization, isometric hip exercises are started immediately. Athletes, especially younger athletes, are progressed slowly. A normal gait cycle should be taught to the athlete as soon as possible. In some cases where osteoporosis has been known to be involved, exercise has been shown to increase bone density and reverse the rate of osteoporosis. Progress the athlete with functional range of motion and functional strength, aquatic therapy, and biking, if pain-free. Within 6 to 8 weeks, gentle active hip range of motion exercises with no weight can be performed (Figures 22-1 through 22-7). Stretching exercises are performed at approximately week 8 (Figures 22-35 through 22-44, 22-49) and progress to stretches for hip rotation and the piriformis (Figures 22-45, 22-46, 22-48). Progressive resistive muscle-strengthening exercises should be started after 2 to 4 weeks of active range of motion and stretching exercises. At approximately week 12, weight can be added to the exercises shown in Figures 22-1 through 22-7, and the exercises shown in Figures 22-9, 22-12, 22-14 can be added, along with

closed-chain exercises (Figures 22-16, 22-17, 22-19, 22-20, 22-22, 22-23A,B).

After the athlete's strength level has reached the "norms," the athlete may begin pain-free slide board (Figure 22-24), plyometrics (Figures 22-27 through 22-29), and sport-specific functional drills (see Figures 17-4, 17-7 through 17-14), and then progress to the exercises shown in Figures 17-5 and 17-6.

Quadriceps Muscle Strain

Pathomechanics. A strain to the large quadriceps muscles in the front of the thigh can be very disabling, especially when the rectus femoris muscle is involved due to its involvement at two joints.[17] The four quadriceps muscles share the same innervation and tendon of insertion.[6] The rectus femoris is the only quadriceps muscle that crosses the hip joint, therefore it is considered a biarticular muscle. The quadriceps muscles are very similar to the hamstrings in that they produce a great deal of force and contract in a "rapid" fashion.[6] Most strains occur at the musculotendinous junctions. A strain shows acute pain, possibly after a workout has been completed, swelling to a specific area, and loss of knee flexion. If the rectus femoris is involved, knee flexion range of motion lying prone (hip in extended position) will be severely limited and painful. Rectus femoris involvement is more disabling than a strain to any of the other quadriceps muscles.

Injury Mechanism. With no history of direct contact to the quadriceps area, the injury can be treated as a muscle strain. A quadriceps strain, with the biceps femoris involved, usually occurs because of a sudden, violent, forceful contraction of the hip and knee into flexion, with the hip initially extended. An overstretch of the quadriceps, with the hip in extension and the knee flexed, can also cause a quadriceps strain. Tight quadriceps, imbalance between quadriceps muscles, and leg-length discrepancy can predispose someone to a quadriceps strain.[1]

An athlete with a grade 1 quadriceps strain may complain of tightness in the front of the thigh. The athlete may be ambulating with a normal gait cycle and present with a history of the thigh feeling fatigued and tight. Swelling might not be present, and the athlete usually has very mild discomfort on palpation. With the athlete sitting over the edge of a table, resistive knee extension might not produce discomfort. If the athlete is lying supine with the knee flexed over the edge of a table, resistive knee extension may produce mild discomfort, if the rectus femoris is involved. With the athlete lying prone, active knee flexion may produce a full pain-free range of motion, with some tightness at extreme flexion.

An athlete with a grade 2 quadriceps strain may have an abnormal gait cycle. The knee may be splinted in extension. The athlete may present an externally rotated hip to use the adductors to pull the leg through and avoid hip extension, during the swing-through phase from push-off, especially when the rectus femoris is involved. In severe cases, it may also be accompanied by hiking the hip during the swing-through phase, which causes a tilting of the pelvis in the frontal plane. The athlete may have felt a sudden twinge and pain down the length of the rectus femoris during activity.[1] Swelling may be noticeable, and palpation may produce pain. A defect in the muscle may also be evident in a grade 2 strain. Resistive knee extension, both when sitting and when lying supine, may reproduce pain. Lying supine and resisting knee extension may be more painful when the rectus femoris is involved. With the athlete lying prone, active knee flexion range of motion may present a noticeable decrease, in some cases a decrease up to 45 degrees. With a quadriceps strain, any decrease in knee flexion range of motion should classify the injury as a grade 2 or 3 strain.

An athlete with a grade 3 quadriceps strain may be unable to ambulate without the aid of crutches and will be in severe pain, with a noticeable defect in the quadriceps muscle. Palpation will usually not be tolerated, and swelling will be present almost immediately. The athlete may not be able to extend the knee actively and against resistance. An isometric contraction will be painful and may produce a bulge or defect in the quadriceps muscle, especially the rectus femoris. With the athlete lying prone, active knee flexion range of motion may be severely limited and might not be tolerated.

Rehabilitation Concerns and Progression. An athlete with a grade 1 quadriceps strain should start ice, compression, active range of motion, and isometric quadriceps exercises immediately. Pain-free quadriceps progressive resistive strengthening exercises may be performed within the first 2 days, in the order given (Figures 22-2, 22-11 through 22-14A,B), flexion with knee both extended and flexed (Figures 22-16 through 22-20, 22-22), and isokinetics (Figures 22-25 and 22-26). The NK table (Figure 22-11) is utilized because of its ability to change the force on the quadriceps muscles by changing the lever arm, and therefore the torque and forces placed upon the injured muscle(s). It is very important that this athlete be able to stretch pain-free and begin pain-free stretching as described in Figures 22-35 and 22-36. Compression should be used at all times until the athlete is free of pain and no longer complaining of tightness.

An athlete with a grade 2 quadriceps strain should begin ice, 24-hour compression, and crutches immediately and for the first 3 to 5 days. Electrical muscle stimulation modalities may be used acutely to decrease swelling, inflammation, and pain and promote range of motion.[20] At approximately day 3, or sooner if pain-free, the athlete may perform quadriceps isometric exercises and pain free quadriceps active range of motion exercises, both sitting and lying prone. These active range of motion exercises are then progressed to the supine position with the knee bent over the end of a table to allow more efficiency to the rectus femoris muscle (Figure 22-13), but with no resistance or weight. Ice used in conjunction with active range of motion, as described above, is very helpful in regaining motion, and strengthening the quadriceps muscles without pain. Passive stretching exercises to the quadriceps muscles are not recommended in the rehabilitation program until later phases, because a passive stretch might have been the cause of the strain. Twenty-four-hour compression is continued throughout the rehabilitation period. A pain-free normal gait cycle is reviewed and emphasized, with and without crutches.

At approximately days 3 to 7, the athlete may begin heat before exercise even though ice is still preferred if the athlete has not obtained full pain-free range of motion. During this phase of rehabilitation, pain-free straight-leg raises without weight, progressing to straight-leg raises with weight, are performed (Figure 22-2).

Continue pain-free quadriceps progressive resistive strengthening exercises on days 7 through 14. The athlete should be progressed, in the order given and pain-free, through the exercises shown in Figures 22-2 and 22-11 through 22-14A,B, flexion with knee both extended and flexed (Figures 22-16 through 22-23), and isokinetics (Figures 22-25, 22-26). Swimming and biking can also be performed as long as the athlete avoids forceful kicking. The bike seat should be adjusted to accommodate a pain-free range of motion. Pain-free passive quadriceps stretching exercises are not performed until days 7 to 14 (Figures 22-35, 22-36). All exercises should be pain-free.

An athlete with a grade 3 quadriceps strain should be on crutches for 7 to 14 days to allow for rest and normal gait before walking without crutches. Twenty-four-hour compression, ice, and electrical muscle stimulation modalities should be used immediately. Quadriceps stretching exercises are not performed until later phases. Twenty-four-hour compression is maintained until the athlete has full pain-free range of motion. When pain-free, the athlete may begin quadriceps isometric exercises. Gentle pain-free quadriceps active range of motion exercises, while the athlete is lying prone and/or sitting, should be performed if special attention is paid to avoiding overstretching the quadriceps muscles. Ice, in conjunction with active range of motion while sitting over the end of a table, is very useful in regaining range of motion. Heat (hot packs, whirlpool, ultrasound) may be used if the athlete is approaching full range of motion. Pain-free straight-leg raises without weight may be performed. Weight may be added after days 10 to 14 (Figure 22-2).

Depending upon active range of motion, swimming and biking may be added to the rehabilitation program. The bicycle seat height should be adjusted to accommodate the athlete's available range of motion. Also, depending upon active range of motion, pain-free quadriceps active progressive resistive strengthening exercises may be performed after the third week, in the order given (Figures 22-2, 22-11 through 22-14), flexion with knee both extended and flexed (Figures 22-16 through 22-20, 22-22), and isokinetics (Figures 22-25, 22-26).

Depending on the severity of the injury, the athlete should have full active range of motion by the fourth week. Only when full active range of motion is accomplished should quadriceps stretching exercises be added (Figures 22-35 and 22-36).

Criteria for Full Return. An athlete with a grade 1 quadriceps strain might not miss competition but should be watched closely and started on a rehabilitation and strengthening program immediately.

An athlete with a grade 2 quadriceps strain might miss 7 to 21 days of competition, depending upon the amount of active range of motion present. The lack of range of motion and the number of competition days missed are usually directly correlated. At approximately days 5 to 7 and within pain-free limits, this athlete may begin the slide board (Figure 22-24), plyometrics (Figures 22-27 through 22-29), and sport-specific functional drills (see Figures 17-4 through 17-14).

An athlete with a grade 3 quadriceps strain might miss 3 to 12 weeks of competition. In severe cases, surgery may be a consideration. At approximately day 14, and within pain-free limits, this athlete may begin the slide board (Figure 22-24), plyometrics (Figures 22-27 through 22-29), and sport-specific functional drills (see Figures 17-4 through 17-14).

Quadriceps Contusion

Pathomechanics. Because the quadriceps muscle is in the front of the thigh, a direct blow to the area that causes the muscle to compress against the femur can be very disabling.[1,31] A direct blow to the anterior portion of the muscle is usually more serious and disabling than a direct blow to the lateral quadriceps area because of the differences in muscle mass present in the two areas. Blood vessels that break cause bleeding in the area where muscle tissue has been damaged.[3] If not treated correctly or if treated too aggressively, a quadriceps contusion can lead to the formation of myositis ossificans (see Myositis Ossificans).

At the time of injury, the athlete may develop pain, loss of function to the quadriceps mechanism, and loss of knee flexion range of motion. How relaxed the quadriceps were at the time of injury, and how forceful the blow was, determine the grade of injury.

Injury Mechanism. An athlete with a grade 1 contusion may present a normal gait cycle, negative swelling, and only mild discomfort on palpation. The athlete's active knee flexion range of motion while lying prone should be within normal limits. Resistive knee extension while sitting and lying supine with the knee bent over the end of a table might not cause discomfort.

An athlete with a grade 2 contusion may have a normal gait cycle, but before notifying the medical staff of the injury might attempt to continue to participate while the injury progressively becomes disabling. If the gait cycle is abnormal, the athlete will splint the knee in extension and avoid knee flexion while bearing weight because the knee feels like it will give out. This athlete might also externally rotate the extremity to use the hip adductors to pull the leg through during the swing-through phase. This move might be accompanied by hiking the hip at push-off, which causes tilting of the pelvis in the frontal plane. Swelling may be moderate to severe, with a noticeable defect and pain on palpation. While the athlete is lying prone, active range of motion in the knee may be limited, with possibly 30 to 45 degrees of motion lacking. Resistive knee extension while sitting and lying supine with the knee bent over the end of a table may be painful, and a noticeable weakness in the quadriceps mechanism may be evident.

A grade 2 quadriceps contusion to the lateral thigh area is usually less painful because of the lack of muscle mass involved at the injury site. The athlete might experience pain on palpation but not have disability. While the athlete is lying prone, knee flexion, range of motion will be within normal limits, with possibly a small decrease in range present. Resistive knee extension while the athlete is sitting and lying supine with the knee bent over the end of a table may cause mild discomfort with good strength present.

An athlete with a grade 3 contusion might herniate the muscle through the fascia to cause a marked defect, severe bleeding, and disability. The athlete may not be able to ambulate without crutches. Pain, severe swelling, and a bulge of muscle tissue may be present on palpation. When the athlete is lying prone, knee flexion active range of motion may be severely limited. Active resistive knee extension while the athlete is sitting and lying supine with the knee bent over the end of a table might not be tolerated, and severe weakness may be present.

Rehabilitation Concerns and Progression. An athlete with a grade 1 quadriceps contusion should begin ice and 24-hour compression immediately. Twenty-four hour compression should be continued until all signs and symptoms are absent. Gentle, pain-free quadriceps stretching exercises (Figures 22-35, 22-36) may be performed on the first day. Quadriceps progressive resistive strengthening exercises may also be performed as soon as possible, usually on the second day, in the order given and pain-free (Figures 22-2, 22-11 through 22-14), flexion with knee both extended and flexed (Figures 22-16 through 22-20, 22-22), and isokinetics (Figures 22-25, 22-26). This athlete's active range of motion should be carefully monitored. If motion decreases, the injury should be updated to a grade II contusion and treated as such.

An athlete with a grade 2 contusion should be treated very conservatively. Crutches should be used until a normal gait can be accomplished free of pain. Ice, 24-hour compression, and electrical muscle stimulation modalities may be started immediately to decrease swelling, inflammation, and pain and to promote range of motion.[29] Compression should be applied at all times to counteract bleeding into the area. Pain-free quadriceps isometric exercises may be performed as soon as possible, usually within the first 3 days. Between days 3 and 5, ice is continued with pain-free active range of motion, while the athlete is sitting and lying prone. Active range of motion lying supine with the knee bent over the end of a table can be added. Passive stretching is not used until the later phases of rehabilitation. Massage and heat modalities are also contraindicated in the early phases because of the possibility of promoting bleeding and eventually myositis ossificans. At approximately day 5, the athlete may perform straight-leg raises without weights and then progress to weights, pain-free (Figure 22-2). As active range of motion increases and approaches 95 to 100 degrees of knee flexion, swimming, aquatic therapy, and biking may be performed if the bicycle seat height is adjusted to the athlete's available range of motion. Between days 7 and 10, heat in the form of hot packs, ultrasound, or whirlpool may be used, as long as swelling is negative and the athlete is approaching full active range

of motion while lying prone. Pain-free quadriceps progressive resistive strengthening exercises may be performed in the order given (Figures 22-2, 22-11 through 22-14), flexion with knee both extended and flexed, (Figures 22-16 through 22-20, 22-22), and isokinetics (Figures 22-25, 22-26). Ice or heat modalities, with active range of motion, should be continued before all exercises as a warm-up. Pain-free quadriceps stretching exercises should not be rushed and can be started between 10 and 14 days (Figures 22-35, 22-36).

An athlete with a grade 3 quadriceps contusion should use crutches, rest, ice, 24-hour compression, and electrical muscle stimulation modalities immediately to decrease pain, bleeding, and swelling and counteract atrophy.[29] After surgery has been ruled out, the athlete may begin pain-free isometric quadriceps exercises between days 5 and 7. Ice and 24-hour compression should be continued from day 1 through day 7. Pain-free active range of motion exercises, while the athlete is sitting and lying prone, are added about day 7. Active range of motion lying supine with the knee bent over the end of a table can also be added. At approximately day 10, the athlete may perform straight leg raises without weights and then progress to weights by day 14 (Figure 22-2). Electrical muscle stimulation modalities may be very helpful in this phase to counteract muscle atrophy and reeducate muscle contraction. Again, as active range of motion increases and approaches 95 to 100 degrees of knee flexion, swimming, aquatic therapy, and biking may be performed if the bicycle seat height is adjusted to the athlete's available range of motion. After day 14, the athlete may use heat in the form of hot packs or whirlpool, as long as the swelling has decreased and the athlete has gained active range of motion. At approximately the third week of rehabilitation, pain-free quadriceps progressive resistive strengthening exercises may be performed in the order presented (Figures 22-2, 22-11 through 22-14), flexion with knee both extended and flexed (Figures 22-16 through 22-20, 22-22), and isokinetics (Figures 22-25, 22-26). Pain-free quadriceps stretching may also be performed (Figures 22-35, 22-36, 22-49) if the athlete is careful not to overstretch the quadriceps muscles. The rehabilitation timetables presented for grades 2 and 3 quadriceps contusions may be modified, depending upon the severity of the injury within its grade.

Criteria for Full Return. An athlete with a grade I quadriceps contusion might not miss competition, but compression and protective padding should be worn until the athlete is symptom-free.

An athlete with a grade 2 quadriceps contusion might miss 3 to 21 days of participation, depending upon the severity of the injury. Jogging, slide board (Figure 22-24), plyometrics (Figures 22-27 through 22-29), and sport-specific functional drills (see Figures 17-4 through 17-14) may be used after the fourteenth day. Compression and protective padding should be worn during all competition until the athlete is symptom-free.

An athlete with a grade 2 quadriceps contusion to the lateral thigh area might not miss competition but should wear compression and protective padding during participation.

An athlete with a grade 3 quadriceps contusion might miss 3 weeks to 3 months of competition time. In general, at approximately week 3, the athlete may begin jogging, slide board (Figure 22-24), plyometrics (Figures 22-27, 22-29), and sport-specific functional drills (Figures 7-4 through 7-14). Again, compression and protective padding should be worn during all competition until the athlete is symptom-free.

Grade 3 lateral quadriceps contusions are very rare due to the lack of muscle belly tissue. If a grade III lateral quadriceps contusion is diagnosed, a femoral contusion and possible fracture should be ruled out.

Myositis Ossificans

Pathomechanics and Injury Mechanism. With a severe direct blow or repetitive direct blows to the quadriceps muscles that cause muscle tissue damage, bleeding, and injury to the periosteum of the femur, ectopic bone production may occur.[1,21] In 3 to 6 weeks, calcium formation may be seen on X-ray films. If the trauma was to the quadriceps muscles only and not the femur, a smaller bony mass may be seen on X-ray films.[1]

If quadriceps contusion and strain are properly treated and rehabilitated, myositis ossificans can be prevented. Myositis ossificans can be caused by trying to "play through" a grade 2 or 3 quadriceps contusion or strain and by early use of massage, stretching exercises into pain, ultrasound, and other heat modalities.[1]

Rehabilitation Concerns and Progression. After 1 year, surgical removal of the bony mass may be helpful. If the bony mass is removed too early, the trauma caused by the surgery can actually enhance the condition.

After diagnosis by X-ray film, treatment and rehabilitation should follow the guidelines for a grade 2 or 3 quadriceps contusion or quadriceps strain (see treatment and rehabilitation for grade 2 and 3 quadriceps contusions and strains). The bony mass usually stabilizes after the sixth month.[18] If the mass does not cause disability, the athlete should be closely monitored and follow the treatment and rehabilitation programs outlined in grade 2 and 3 quadriceps contusions and strains. It has also been recommended that myositis be treated using acetic acid with iontophoresis.[39]

The author would like to thank Jim Case, M.A., A.T. C., Assistant Athletic Trainer at Cornell University, for his contribution to various portions of this chapter.

Summary

1. Injuries to the groin, hip, and thigh can be extremely disabling and often require a substantial amount of time for rehabilitation.
2. Hip pointers are contusions of the soft tissue in the area of the iliac crest and must be treated aggressively during the first 2 to 4 hours after injury.
3. Piriformis syndrome sciatica should be specifically differentiated from other problems that produce low back pain or radiating pain in the buttocks and leg. Rehabilitation programs are extremely variable for different conditions and can even be harmful if used inappropriately.
4. Trochanteric bursitis is relatively common in athletes, as is ischial bursitis. Treatment involves efforts directed at protection and reduction of inflammation in the affected area.
5. Snapping or clicking hip syndrome most often occurs when the iliotibial band snaps over the greater trochanter, causing trochanteric bursitis.
6. Osteitis pubis and fractures of the inferior ramus both produce pain at the pubic symphysis and are best treated with rest.
7. Hip dislocations are rare in athletes and requires 6 to 12 months of rehabilitation before the athlete can return to full activity.
8. Strains of the groin musculature, the hamstring, and the quadriceps muscles can require long periods of rehabilitation for the athlete. Early return often exacerbates the problem.
9. The femur is subject to stress fractures, avulsion fractures of the lesser trochanter, and traumatic fractures of the femoral neck.
10. Protection is the key to treatment and rehabilitation of quadriceps contusions and accompanying myositis ossificans.

References

1. Arnheim, D. D., and W. E. Prentice. 1997. *Principles of athletic training.* Madison, WI: Brown & Benchmark.

2. Berry, J. M. 1992. Fracture of the tuberosity of the ischium due to muscular action. Journal of American Medical Association 59:1450.

3. Brunet, M., and R. Hontas. 1994. The thigh. In *Orthopaedic sports medicine,* vol. 2, edited by J. C. DeLee and D. Drez. Philadelphia: W. B. Saunders.

4. Coole, W. G., and J. H. Gieck. 1987. An analysis of hamstring strains and their rehabilitation. *Journal of Orthopaedic and Sports Physical Therapy* 9(2): 77–85.

5. Daniels, L., and C. Worthingham. 1996. *Muscle testing: Techniques of manual examination.* Philadelphia: W. B. Saunders.

6. DeLee, J. C., and D. Drez. 1994. *Orthopaedic sports medicine.* Vol. 2. Philadelphia: W. B. Saunders.

7. DeLorme, T. I., and A. L. Watkins. 1952. *Progressive resistive exercise technique and medical application.* New York: Appleton-Century-Crofts.

8. DePalma, B. F., and R. R. Zclko. 1986. Knee rehabilitation following anterior cruciate ligament injury or surgery. *Athletic Training* 21:3.

9. Devas, M. B. 1975. *Stress fractures.* New York: Longman.

10. Frost, H. 1964. *Laws of bone structures.* Springfield, IL: Charles C. Thomas.

11. Gilbert, R. S., and H. A. Johnson. 1966. Stress fractures in military recruits: A review of 12 years' experiences. *Military Medicine* 131: 716–21.

12. Gordon, E. J. 1981. Diagnosis and treatment of common hip disorders. *Med Tra Tech Q* 28(4): 443.

13. Harvey, J. 1985. ed. *Rehabilitation of the injured athlete: Clinics in sports medicine.* Philadelphia: W. B. Saunders.

14. Hollinshead, W. H. 1976. *Functional anatomy of the limbs and back.* Philadelphia: W. B. Saunders.

15. Hoppenfield, S. 1976. *Physical examination of the spine and extremities.* New York: Appleton-Century-Crofts.

16. Hunter-Griffen, L. 1987. ed. *Overuse injuries: Clinics in sports medicine.* Philadelphia: W. B. Saunders.

17. Jaivin, J., and J. Fox. 1995. Thigh injuries. In *The lower extremity and spine in sports medicine,* edited by J. Nicholas and E. Hershman. St. Louis: Mosby.

18. Kuland, D. N. 1982. *The injured athlete.* Philadelphia: Lippincott.

19. Lewinneck, G. 1980. The significance and comparison analysis of the epidemiology of hip fractures. *Clin Orthop* 152:35.

20. Lewis, A. 1977. Normal human locomotion. Hamden, CT: Quinnipiac College.

21. Lipscomb, A. B. 1976. Treatment of myositis ossificans traumatic in athletes. *Journal of Sports Medicine* 4:61.

22. Malone, T., et al. 1996. *Orthopedic and sports physical therapy.* St Louis: Mosby.

23. Magee, D. J. 1997. *Orthopedic physical assessment.* Philadelphia: W. B. Saunders.

24. Mendez, A., and R. Eyster. 1992. Displaced nonunion stress fracture of the femoral neck treated with internal fixation and bone graft. *American Journal of Sports Medicine* 20(2): 220–23.

25. Moore, K. L. 1985. *Clinical oriented anatomy.* Baltimore: Williams & Wilkins.

26. Nadkarni, J. 1991. Simultaneous anterior and posterior dislocation of the hip. *J Postgrad Ed* 37(2): 117–18.

27. Norkin, L., and P. LeVange. 1983. *Joint structure and function.* Philadelphia: F. A. Davis.

28. Orava, S., and U. Kujala. 1995. Rupture of the ischial origin of the hamstrings. *American Journal of Sports Medicine* 22(6): 702–5.

29. Prentice, W. E. 1998. *Therapeutic modalities in sports medicine.* Dubuque, IA: WCB/McGraw-Hill.

30. Pruner, R., and C. Johnston. 1991. Avulsion fracture of the ischial tuberosity. *Ped Ortho* 13(3): 357–58.

31. Ryan, J. J. Wheeler, and W. Hopkinson. 1991. Quadriceps contusion: West Point update. *American Journal of Sports Medicine* 19:299–303.

32. Sanders, B., and W. Nemeth. 1996. Hip and Thigh injuries. In *Athletic injuries and rehabilitation,* edited by J. Zachazewski, D. Magee, and S. Quillen. Philadelphia: W. B. Saunders.

33. Schlickewei, W., and B. Elsasser. 1993. Hip dislocation without fracture. *Injury* 24(1): 27–31.

34. Sim, F., M. Rock, and S. Scott. 1995. Pelvis and hip injuries in athlete: Anatomy and function. In *The lower extremity and spine in sports medicine,* edited by J. Nicholas and E. Hershman. St. Louis: Mosby.

35. Stanitski, C. L., J. H. McMaster, and P. E. Scranton. 1978. On the nature of stress fractures. *American Journal of Sports Medicine* 6:391–96.

36. Stevens, J. 1962. The incidence of osteoporosis in patients with femoral neck fractures. *Journal of Bone and Joint Surgery* 44:520.

37. Tinker, R. ed. 1979. *Ramamurti's orthopaedics in primary care.* Baltimore: Williams & Wilkins.

38. Torg, J., J. Vegso, and P. Torg. 1987. *Rehabilitation of athletic injuries: A guide to therapeutic exercise.* St. Louis: Mosby.

39. Wieder, D. 1992. Treatment of traumatic myositis ossificans with acetic acid and iontophoresis. *Physical Therapy* 72:133–37.

40. Worrell, T., and D. Perrin. 1992. Hamstring muscle injury: The influence of strength, flexibility, warmup and fatigue. *Journal of Orthopaedic and Sports Physical Therapy* 16:12–18.

41. Zelko, R. R., and B. F. DePalma. 1986. Stress fractures in Athletes: Diagnosis and treatment. *Forum Medicus: Postgraduate Advances in Sports Medicine* I-XI.

CHAPTER 23

Rehabilitation of Knee Injuries

William E. Prentice
J. Marc Davis

After completion of this chapter, the student should be able to do the following:

- Discuss the functional anatomy and biomechanics associated with normal function of the knee joint.

- Discuss the various rehabilitative strengthening techniques for the knee, including both open- and closed-kinetic-chain isotonic, plyometric, isokinetic, and PNF exercises.

- Identify the various techniques for regaining range of motion, including stretching exercises and joint mobilizations.

- Discuss exercises that may be used to reestablish neuromuscular control.

- Discuss the rehabilitation progressions for various ligamentous and meniscal injuries.

- Describe and explain the rationale for various treatment techniques in the management of injuries to the patellofemoral joint and the extensor mechanism.

FUNCTIONAL ANATOMY AND BIOMECHANICS

The knee is part of the kinetic chain and is directly affected by motions and forces occurring in and being transmitted from the foot, ankle, and lower leg. In turn, the knee must transmit forces to the thigh, hip, pelvis, and spine.[86] Abnormal forces that cannot be distributed must be absorbed by the tissues. In a closed kinetic chain, forces must be either transmitted to proximal segments or absorbed in a more distal joint. The inability of this closed system to dissipate these forces typically leads to a breakdown in some part of the system. Certainly, as part of the kinetic chain, the knee joint is susceptible to injury resulting from absorption of these forces.

The knee is commonly considered a hinge joint because its two principal movements are flexion and extension (Figure 23-1). However, because rotation of the tibia is an essential component of knee movement, the knee is not a true hinge joint. The stability of the knee joint depends primarily on the ligaments, the joint capsule, and muscles that surround the joint. The knee is designed primarily to provide stability in weight bearing and mobility in locomotion; however, it is especially unstable laterally and medially.

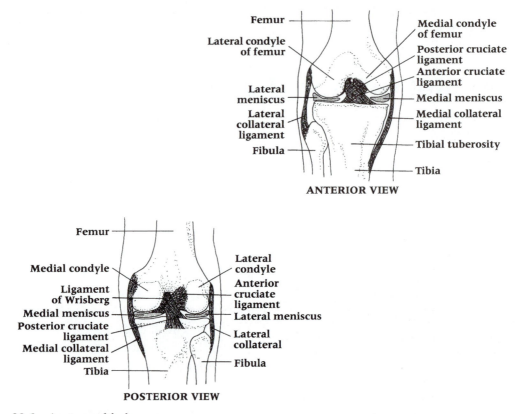

Figure 23-1 Anatomy of the knee.

Movement between the tibia and the femur involves the physiological motions of flexion, extension, and rotation, as well as arthrokinematic motions including rolling and gliding. As the tibia extends on the femur, the tibia glides and rolls anteriorly. If the femur is extending on the tibia, gliding occurs in an anterior direction, whereas rolling occurs posteriorly.

Axial rotation of the tibia relative to the femur is an important component of knee motion. In the "screw home" mechanism of the knee, as the knee extends, the tibia externally rotates. Rotation occurs because the medial femoral condyle is larger than the lateral condyle. Thus, when weight bearing, the tibia must rotate externally to achieve full extension. The rotational component gives a great deal of stability to the knee in full extension. When weight bearing, the popliteus muscle must contract and externally rotate the femur to "unlock" the knee so that flexion can occur.

Collateral Ligaments

The medial collateral ligament (MCL) is divided into two parts, the stronger superficial portion and the thinner and weaker "deep" medial ligament or capsular ligament,

with its accompanying attachment to the medial meniscus.[85] The superficial position of the MCL is separate from the deeper capsular ligament at the joint line. The posterior aspect of the ligament blends into the deep posterior capsular ligament and semimembranous muscle. Fibers of the semimembranous muscle go through the capsule and attach to the posterior aspect of the medial meniscus, pulling it backward during knee flexion. The MCL functions as the primary static stabilizer against valgus stress. The MCL is taut at full extension and begins to relax between 20 to 30 degrees of flexion and comes under tension again at 60 to 70 degrees of flexion, although a portion of the ligament is taut throughout the range of motion.[42,85] Its major purpose is to prevent the knee from valgus and external rotating forces.

The medial collateral ligament was thought to be the principal stabilizer of the knee in a valgus position when combined with rotation. In the normal knee, valgus loading is greatest during the push-off phase of gait when the foot is planted and the tibia is externally rotated relative to the femur. It is now known that the anterior cruciate ligament plays an equal or greater part in this function.[82]

The lateral (fibular) collateral ligament is a round, fibrous cord about the size of a pencil. It is attached to the lateral epicondyle of the femur and to the head of the fibula. The lateral collateral ligament (LCL) functions with the iliotibial band, the popliteous tendon, the arcuate ligament complex, and the biceps tendons to support the lateral aspect of the knee. The LCL is under constant tensile loading, and the thick, firm configuration of the ligament is well designed to withstand this constant stress.[42] The lateral collateral ligament is taut during knee extension but relaxed during flexion.

Capsular Ligaments

The deep medial capsular ligament is divided into three parts: the anterior, medial, and posterior capsular ligaments. The anterior capsular ligament connects with the extensor mechanism and the medial meniscus through the coronary ligaments. It relaxes during knee extension and tightens during knee flexion. The primary purposes of the medial capsular ligaments are to attach the medial meniscus to the femur and to allow the tibia to move on the meniscus inferiorly. The posterior capsular ligament is called the posterior oblique ligament. It attaches to the posterior medial aspect of the meniscus and intersperses with the semimembranous muscle. Along with the MCL, the pes anserinus tendons, and the semimembranosus, the posterior oblique ligament reinforces the posteromedial joint capsule.

The arcuate ligament is formed by a thickening of the posteriorlateral capsule. Its posterior aspect attaches to the fascia of the popliteal muscle and the posterior horn of the lateral meniscus. This arcuate ligament and the iliotibial band, the popliteus, the biceps femoris, and the LCL reinforce the posteriorlateral joint capsule.

The iliotibial band becomes taut during both extension and flexion. The popliteal muscle stabilizes the knee during flexion and, when contracting, protects the lateral meniscus by pulling it posteriorly. The biceps femoris muscle also stabilizes the knee laterally by inserting into the fibular head, iliotibial band, and capsule.

Cruciate Ligaments

The anterior cruciate ligament prevents the femur from moving posteriorly during weight bearing, stabilizes the knee in full extension, and prevents hyperextension. It also stabilizes the tibia against excessive internal rotation and serves as a secondary restraint for valgus/varus stress with collateral ligament damage. The anterior cruciate ligament works in conjunction with the thigh muscles, especially the hamstring muscle group, to stabilize the knee joint.

During extension there is external rotation of the tibia during the last 15 degrees of the anterior cruciate

ligaments unwinding. In full extension the anterior cruciate ligament is tightest, and it loosens during flexion. When the knee is fully extended, the posterolateral portion of the anterior cruciate ligament is tight. In flexion the posterolateral fibers loosen and the anteromedial fibers tighten.

Some portion of the posterior cruciate ligament is taut throughout the full range of motion. As the femur glides on the tibia, the posterior cruciate ligament becomes taut and prevents further gliding. In general, the posterior cruciate ligament prevents excessive internal rotation. Hyperextension of the knee guides the knee in flexion, and acts as a drag during the initial glide phase of flexion.

Menisci

The medial and lateral menisci function to improve the stability of the knee, increase shock absorption, and distribute weight over a larger surface area. The menisci help to stabilize the knee, especially the medial meniscus, when the knee is flexed at 90 degrees. The menisci transmit one-half of the contact force in the medial compartment and even a higher percentage of the contact load in the lateral compartment.

During flexion the menisci move posteriorly, and during extension they move anteriorly, primarily due to attachments of the medial meniscus to the semimembranosus, and the lateral meniscus to the popliteus tendon. During internal rotation the medial meniscus moves anteriorly relative to the medial tibial plateau, and the lateral meniscus moves posteriorly relative to the lateral tibial plateau. In internal rotation the movements are reversed.

Function of Patella

Collectively the quadriceps muscle group, the quadriceps tendon, the patella, and the patellar tendon form the extensor mechanism. The patella aids the knee during extension by lengthening the lever arm of the quadriceps muscle. It distributes the compressive stresses on the femur by increasing the contact area between the patellar tendon and the femur.[65] It also protects the patellar tendon against friction. Tracking within this groove depends on the pull of the quadriceps muscle, patellar tendon, depth of the femoral condyles, and shape of the patella.

During full extension the patella lies slightly lateral and proximal to the trochlea. At 20 degrees of knee flexion there is tibial rotation, and the patella moves into the trochlea. At 30 degrees the patella is most prominent. At 30 degrees and more the patella moves deeper into the trochlea. At 90 degrees the patella again becomes positioned laterally. When knee flexion is 135 degrees, the patella has moved laterally beyond the trochlea.[65]

Muscle Actions

For the knee to function properly, a number of muscles must work together in a highly complex fashion. The following is a list of knee actions and the muscles that initiate them.

- Knee flexion is executed by the biceps femoris, semitendinous, semimembranous, gracilis, sartorius, gastrocnemius, popliteus, and plantaris muscles.
- Knee extension is executed by the quadriceps muscle of the thigh, consisting of three vasti—the vastus medialis, vastus lateralis, and vastus intermedius—and by the rectus femoris.
- External rotation of the tibia is controlled by the biceps femoris. The bony anatomy also produces external tibial rotation as the knee moves into extension.
- Internal rotation is accomplished by the popliteus, semitendinous, semimembranous, sartorius, and gracilis muscles. Rotation of the tibia is limited and can occur only when the knee is in a flexed position.
- The iliotibial band on the lateral side primarily functions as a dynamic lateral stabilizer.

REHABILITATION TECHNIQUES

Strengthening Exercises

A primary goal in knee rehabilitation is the return of normal strength to the musculature surrounding the knee. Along with the return of muscular strength, it is also important to improve muscular endurance and power.[71]

It is critically important to understand that strength will be gained only if the muscle is subjected to overload. However, it is also essential to remember that healing tissues can be further damaged by overloading the injured structure too aggressively. Especially during the early phases of rehabilitation, muscular overload needs to be carefully applied to protect the damaged structures. The recovering knee needs protection, and the high-resistance, low-repetition program designed to strengthen a healthy knee can compromise the integrity of the injured knee.[49] The strengthening phase of rehabilitation must be gently progressive and will generally

progress from isometric to isotonic to isokinetic to plyometric to functional exercise.

For years, open-kinetic-chain exercises were the treatment of choice. However, more recently closed-kinetic-chain exercises have been widely used and recommended in the rehabilitation of the injured knee. Closed-kinetic-chain exercises may be safely introduced early in the rehabilitation process for virtually all types of knee injury.[11,22,76,77,84] Closed-kinetic-chain activities may involve isometric, isotonic, plyometric, and even isokinetic techniques.

Isotonic Open-Kinetic-Chain Exercises.

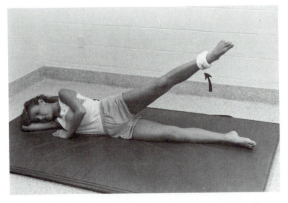

Figure 23-2 Hip abduction. Used to strengthen the gluteus medius and tensor fascia lata, which share a common tendon, the iliotibial band. The iliotibial band serves as a weak knee flexor and helps to provide stability laterally.

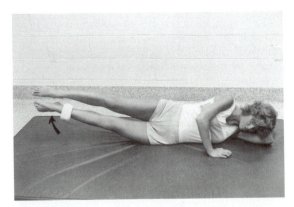

Figure 23-3 Hip adduction. Used to strengthen the adductor magnus, longus, and brevis; pectineus, gracilis. The gracilis is the only one of the hip adductors to cross the knee joint.

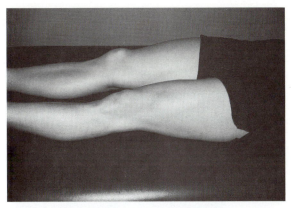

Figure 23-4 Quad sets are done isometrically with the knee in full extension to help the athlete relearn how to contract the quadriceps following injury or surgery.

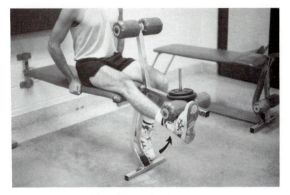

Figure 23-7 Knee extension. Primary muscles: rectus femoris, vastus lateralis, vastus intermedialis, vastus medialis.

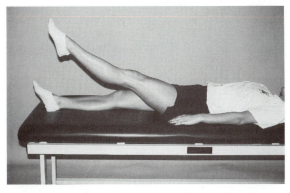

Figure 23-5 Straight leg raising is done early in the rehabilitation for active contraction of the quadriceps.

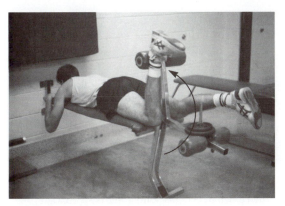

Figure 23-6 Knee flexion. Primary muscles: biceps femoris, semimembranous, semitendinous. Secondary muscles: gracilis, gastrocnemius, sartorius, popliteus. Note: Biceps femoris is best strengthened with tibia rotated externally; semimembranous and semitendinous muscles are best strengthened with tibia rotated internally.

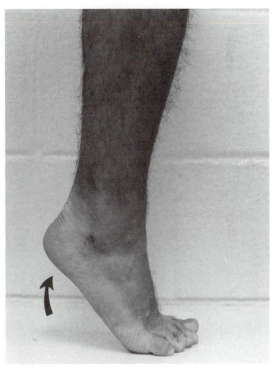

Figure 23-8 Ankle plantarflexion. Used to strengthen the gastrocnemius, which serves as a knee flexor.

Closed-Kinetic-Chain Strengthening Exercises.

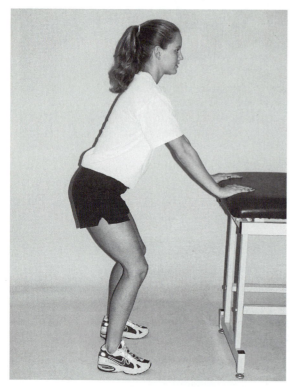

Figure 23-9 Minisquat performed in 0 to 40 degrees range.

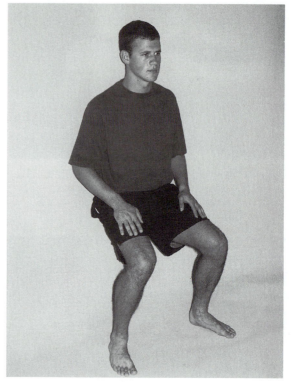

Figure 23-10 Standing wall slides are done to strengthen the quadriceps.

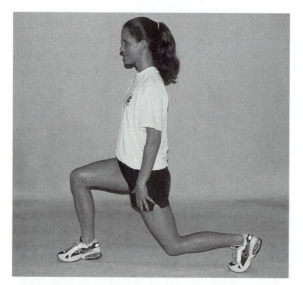

Figure 23-11 Lunges are done to strengthen quadriceps eccentrically.

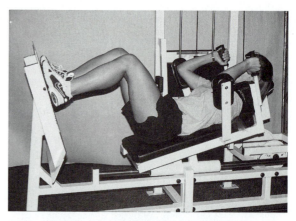

Figure 23-12 Leg-press exercise. The seat may be adjusted to whatever knee joint angle is appropriate.

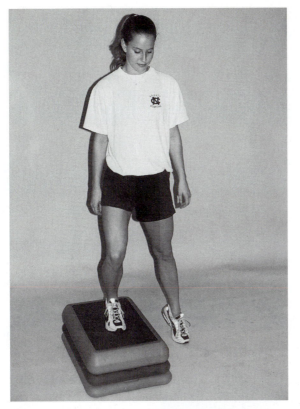

Figure 23-13   Lateral step-ups as well as forward step-ups may be done using different stepping heights.

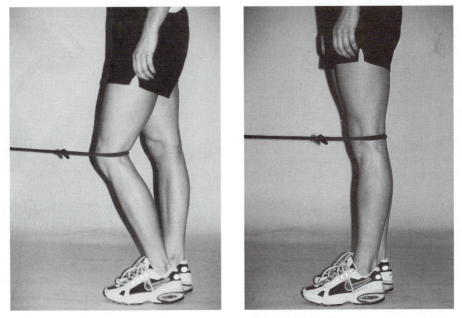

Figure 23-14   Terminal knee extensions using surgical tubing resistance for strengthening primarily the vastus medialis.

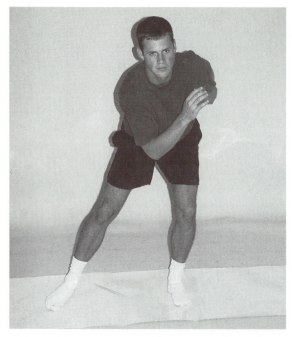

Figure 23-15 Slide board exercises are used in side-to-side training.

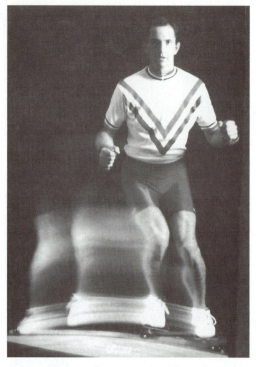

Figure 23-16 The Fitter is useful in side-to-side functional training.

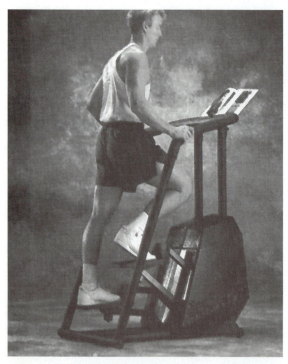

Figure 23-17 Stair Master stepping machine allows the athlete to maintain constant contact with the step.

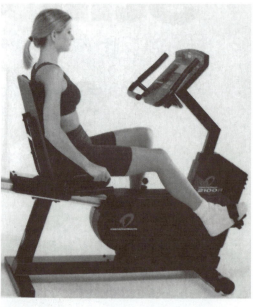

Figure 23-18 Stationary bicycling is good for regaining ROM, with seat adjusted to the appropriate height, and also for maintaining cardiorespiratory endurance.

Plyometric Strengthening Exercises.

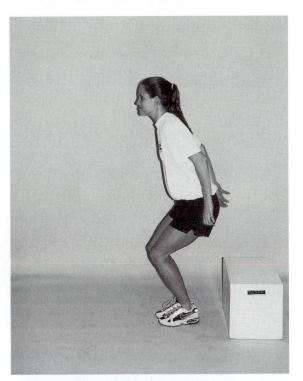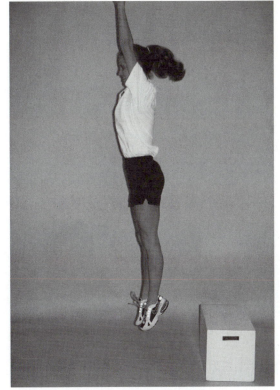

Figure 23-19 Box jumps. The athlete should jump off a box at heights ranging from 6 to 24 inches and then immediately jump again as soon as contact is made with the floor.

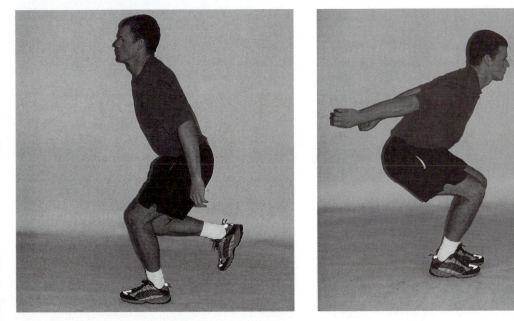

Figure 23-20 Single-leg and double-leg bounding hops.

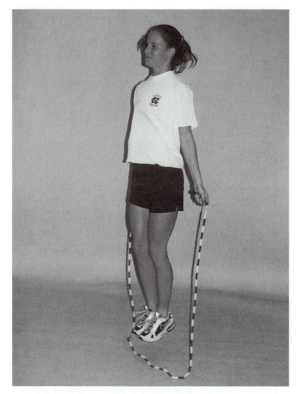

Figure 23-21 Rope skipping is a plyometric exercise that is also good for improving cardiorespiratory endurance.

Isokinetic Strengthening Exercises.

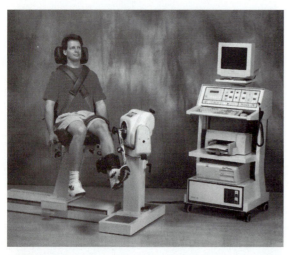

Figure 23-22 Knee extension set-up to strengthen the quadriceps.

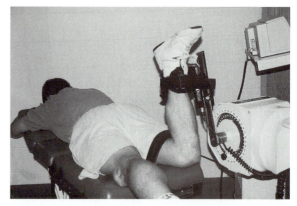

Figure 23-23 Knee flexion set-up to strengthen the hamstrings.

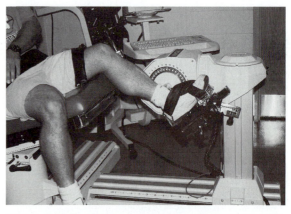

Figure 23-24 Tibial rotation is done with resistance at the ankle joint and is an extremely important, though often neglected, aspect of knee rehabilitation.

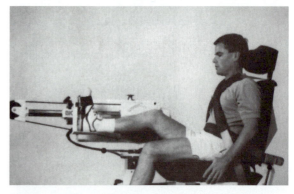

Figure 23-25 Biodex manufactures an isokinetic closed-chain exercise device.

PNF Strengthening Exercises.

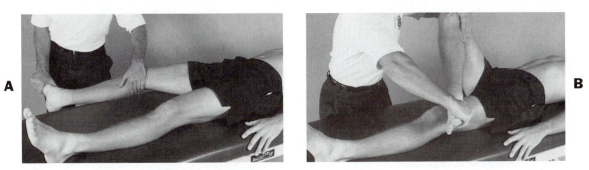

Figure 23-26 D1 lower-extremity movement pattern moving into flexion. **A,** Starting position. **B,** Terminal position.

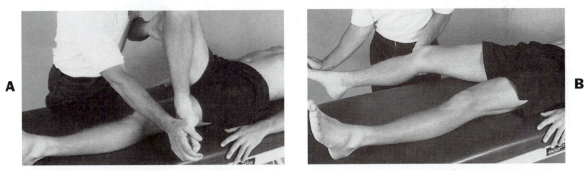

Figure 23-27 D1 lower-extremity movement pattern moving into extension. **A,** Starting position. **B,** Terminal position.

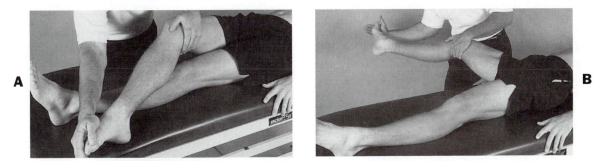

Figure 23-28 D2 lower-extremity movement pattern moving into flexion. **A,** Starting position. **B,** Terminal position.

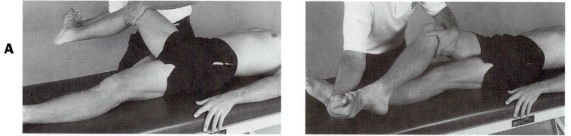

Figure 23-29 D2 lower-extremity movement pattern moving into extension. **A,** Starting position. **B,** Terminal position.

Range-of-Motion Exercises

After injury to the knee, some loss of motion is likely. This loss can be caused by the effects of the injury, the trauma of surgery, or the effects of immobilization. Waiting for ligaments to heal completely is a luxury that cannot be afforded in an effective rehabilitation program. Ligaments do not heal completely for 18 to 24 months, yet periarticular tissue changes can begin within 4 to 6 weeks of immobilization.[40] This is marked histologically by a decrease in water content in collagen and by an increase in collagen cross-linkage.[40] The initiation of an early range of motion program can minimize these harmful changes. Controlled movement should be initiated early in the recovery process and progress based on healing constraints and patient tolerance toward a normal range of approximately 0 to 130 degrees.

Pitfalls that can slow or prevent regaining normal range of motion include imperfect surgical technique (improper placement of an anterior cruciate replacement), development of joint capsule or ligament contracture, and muscular resistance caused by pain.[32,40,45] The surgeon must address motion lost from technique, but the sports therapist can successfully deal with motion lost from soft tissue contracture or muscular resistance.

To effectively alleviate lost motion, the cause of the limitation must be identified. An experienced sports therapist can detect soft-tissue resistance to motion by the quality of the feel of the resistance at the end of the range. Muscular resistance, which restricts normal physiological movement, has a firm end feel and can best be treated by using PNF stretching techniques in combination with appropriate therapeutic modalities (heat, ice, electrical stimulation, etc.).[66]

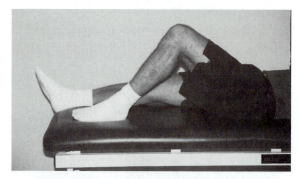

Figure 23-30 Knee slides are done on a treatment table by sliding a foot in a sock forward and backward, flexing and extending the knee through a pain-free range.

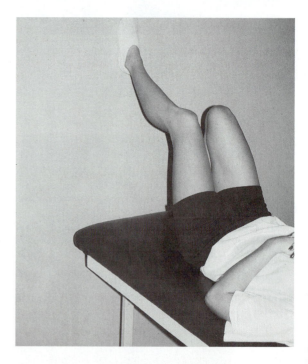

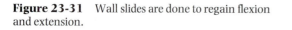

Figure 23-31 Wall slides are done to regain flexion and extension.

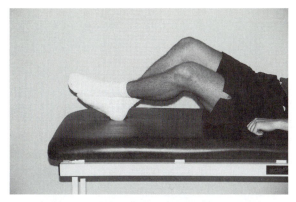

Figure 23-32 Active assistive knee slides use the good leg supporting the injured knee to regain flexion and extension.

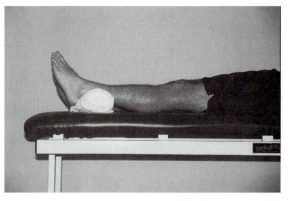

Figure 23-33 Knee extension with the foot supported on a rolled-up towel is used to regain knee extension.

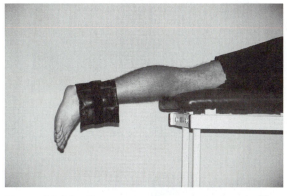

Figure 23-34 Knee extension in prone with an ankle weight around the foot is used to regain extension.

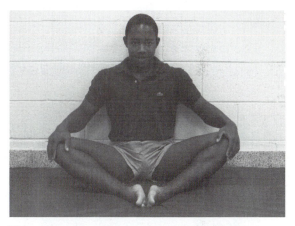

Figure 23-35 Groin stretch. Muscles: adductor magnus, longus, and brevis; pectineus; gracilis.

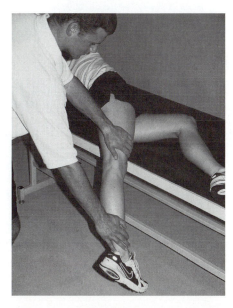

Figure 23-36 Iliotibial band stretch. The iliotibial band may be stretched in a variety of ways that use a scissoring position with extreme hip adduction. The major problem with these techniques is the lack of stabilization of the pelvis and therefore loss of stretch force transmission to the iliotibial band. To maximize the stretch, the pelvis must be manually stabilized to prevent lateral pelvic tilt. If the tensor fascia lata portion is tight, the hip should be flexed, abducted, extended, and adducted, in sequence, to position the tensor fascia lata fibers directly over the trochanter (rather than anterior to it) to produce maximal stretch.[9]

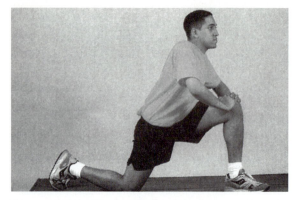

Figure 23-37 Kneeling thrusts. Muscles: rectus femoris.

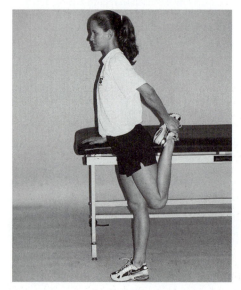

Figure 23-38 Knee extensors stretch. Muscles: quadriceps.

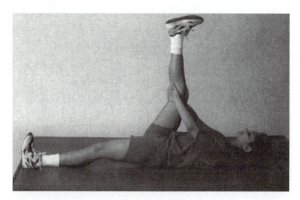

Figure 23-39 Knee flexors stretch. Muscles: hamstrings. Note: Externally rotated tibia stretches the semimembranous and semitendinous; internally rotated tibia stretches the biceps femoris.

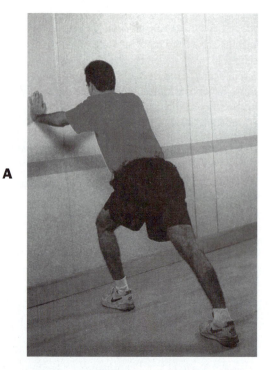

A

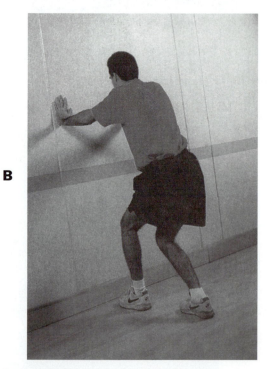

B

Figure 23-40 Ankle plantarflexors stretch. **A,** Muscles: gastrocnemius, **B,** soleus.

Joint Mobilization Techniques

Joint capsule or ligamentous contractures have a leathery end feel and might not respond to conventional simple passive, active-assistive, and active motion exercises.[32] These contractures can limit the accessory motions of the joint, and until the accessory motions are restored, conventional exercises will not produce positive results. Accessory motions in the knee joint must occur between the patella and femur, the femur and tibia, and the tibia and fibula. Restriction in any or all of these ac-

cessory motions must be addressed early in the rehabilitation program.

Mobilization of a knee that is restricted by soft-tissue constraints may be accomplished by specifically applying graded oscillations to the restricted soft tissue as discussed in Chapter 12. In doing so, the sports therapist is addressing a specific limiting structure rather than assaulting the entire joint with a "crank till you cry" technique. After the release of the soft-tissue contracture, accessory motion should improve, and so should physiological motion.

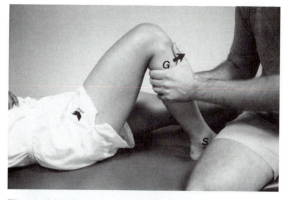

Figure 23-41   Anterior tibial glides are appropriate for the patient who lacks full extension. Anterior glides should be done in prone position with the femur stabilized. Pressure is applied to the posterior tibia to glide anteriorly.

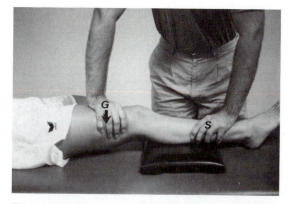

Figure 23-42   Posterior femoral glides are appropriate for the patient who lacks full extension. Posterior femoral glides should be done in supine position with the tibia stabilized. Pressure is applied to the anterior femur to glide posteriorly.

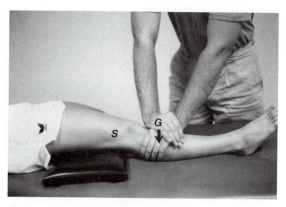

Figure 23-43   Posterior tibial glides increase flexion. With the patient in supine position, stabilize the femur, and glide the tibia posteriorly.

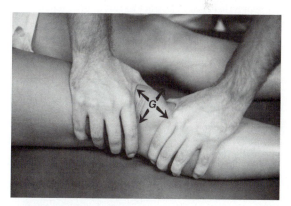

Figure 23-44   Patellar glides. Superior patellar glides increase knee extension. Inferior glides increase knee flexion. Medial glides stretch the lateral retinaculum. Lateral glides stretch tight medial structures.

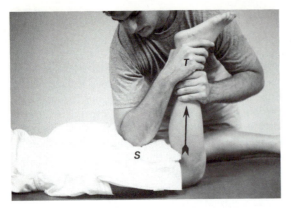

Figure 23-45 Tibiofemoral joint traction reduces pain and hypomobility. It may be done with the patient prone and the knee flexed at 90 degrees. The elbow should stabilize the thigh while traction is applied through the tibia.

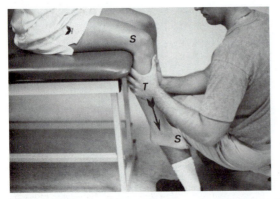

Figure 23-46 Alternative techniques for tibiofemoral joint traction. In very large individuals, an alternative technique for tibiofemoral joint traction uses body weight of the sports therapist to distract the joint, once again for reducing pain and hypomobility.

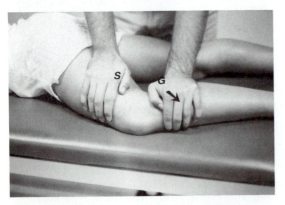

Figure 23-47 Anterior and posterior glides of the fibula may be done proximally. They increase mobility of the fibular head and reduce pain. The femur should be stabilized. With the knee slightly flexed, grasp the head of the femur, and glide it both anteriorly and posteriorly.

Exercises to Reestablish Neuromuscular Control.

A

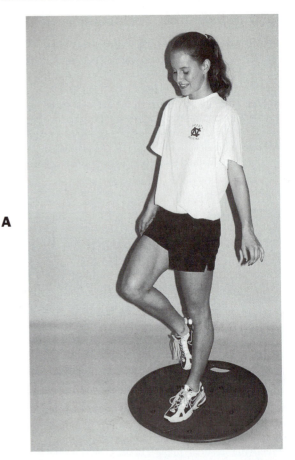

B

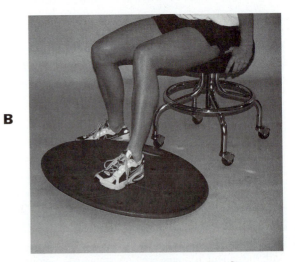

Figure 23-48 BAPS board exercise. **A,** Standing. **B,** Sitting.

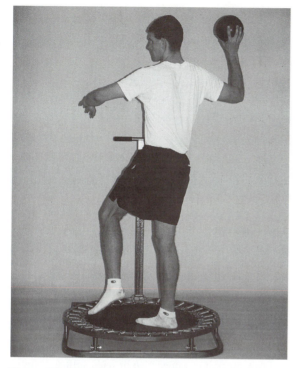

Figure 23-49   Minitramp provides an unstable base of support to which other functional plyometric activities may be added.

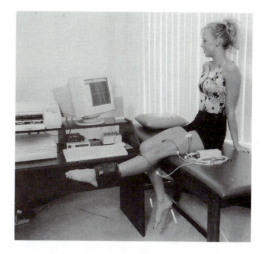

Figure 23-51   Biofeedback units can be used to help the athlete learn how to fire a specific muscle or muscle group.

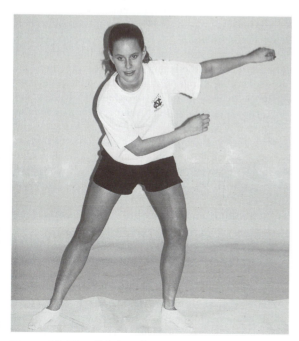

Figure 23-50   Slide board training.

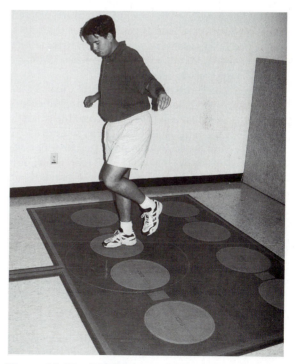

Figure 23-52   FASTEX is a useful device for functional neuromuscular training.

REHABILITATION TECHNIQUES FOR LIGAMENTOUS AND MENISCAL INJURIES

Medial Collateral Ligament Sprain

Pathomechanics.   The MCL is the most commonly injured ligament in the knee.[57] About 65 percent of MCL sprains occur at the proximal insertion site on the femur. Individuals with proximal injuries tend to have more stiffness but less residual laxity than those with injuries nearer the tibial insertion. Tears of the medial meniscus are occasionally associated with grades 1 and 2 MCL sprains but almost never occur with grade 3 sprains.

Diagnosis of MCL sprains can usually always be made by physical evaluation and do not generally require MRI. The grade of ligament injury is usually determined by the amount of joint laxity. In a grade 1 sprain the MCL is tender due to microtears, but has no increased laxity and there is a firm end point. A grade 2 sprain involves an incomplete tear with some increased laxity with valgus stress at 30 degrees of flexion and minimal laxity in full extension, yet there is still a firm end point. There is tenderness to palpation, hemorrhage, and pain on valgus stress test. A grade 3 sprain is a complete tear with significant laxity on valgus stress in full extension. No end point is evident, and pain is generally less than with grades 1 or 2. Significant laxity with valgus stress testing in full extension indicates injury to the medial joint capsule and to the cruciate ligaments.[37]

Injury Mechanism.   An MCL sprain usually always occurs with contact from a laterally applied valgus force to the knee that is sufficient to exceed the strength of the ligament. This is especially true with grade 3 sprains. Very rarely, an MCL sprain can occur with noncontact and result in an isolated MCL tear. It has also been suggested that the majority of grade 2 sprains occur through indirect rotational forces associated with valgus movement of the knee.[76] The athlete will usually explain that the knee was hit on the lateral side with the foot planted, and that there was immediate pain on the medial side of the knee that felt more like a "pulling" or "tearing" than a "pop." Swelling occurs immediately, and some ecchymosis likely will appear over the site of injury within 3 days.

Rehabilitation Concerns.   Since the early 1990s, the treatment of MCL sprains has changed considerably. Typically grade 3 MCL sprains were treated surgically to repair the torn ligament and then immobilized for 6 weeks. However, several studies have demonstrated

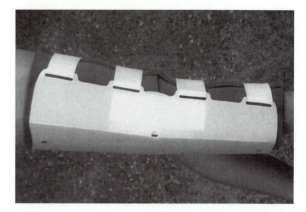

Figure 23-53   A knee immobilizer can be used for comfort following injury.

that treating patients with isolated MCL sprains nonoperatively with immobilization is as effective as treating them surgically, regardless of the grade of injury, the age of the patient, or the activity level.[36] This is especially true with isolated MCL tears where the ACL is intact.[1,83] Patients with a combined MCL-ACL injury will most likely have an ACL reconstruction without MCL repair, and this procedure appears to provide sufficient functional stability. Three conditions must be met for healing to occur at the MCL: (1) the ligament fibers must remain in continuity or within a well-vascularized soft-tissue bed, (2) there must be enough stress to stimulate and direct the healing process, and (3) there must be protection from harmful stresses.[85]

With grade 2 and 3 sprains there will be some residual laxity because the ligament has been stretched, but this does not seem to have much effect on knee function. Patients with grade 1 and 2 sprains may be treated symptomatically and may be fully weight-bearing as soon as tolerated. It is possible that an athlete with a grade 1 and occasionally even a grade 2 sprain can continue to play. With grade 3 sprains the athlete should not be allowed to play and a rehabilitative brace should be worn for 4 to 6 weeks set from 0 to 90 degrees to control valgus stress (Figure 23-53).

Rehabilitation Progression.   Initially, cold, compression, elevation, and electrical stimulation can be used to control swelling, inflammation, and pain. It may be necessary to have the athlete on crutches initially, progressing to full weight bearing as soon as tolerated. The athlete should use crutches until (1) full extension without an extension lag can be demonstrated, and (2) the athlete can walk normally without gait deviation. For patient comfort, a knee immobilizer may be worn for a few days to a week following injury with grade 2 sprains requiring 7 to 14 days in either an immobilizer or a brace.

The athlete with a grade 1 sprain can, on the second day following injury, begin quad sets (Figure 23-4) and straight leg raising (Figure 23-5). Early pain-free range-of-motion exercises should be incorporated with grade 1 sprains, whereas grade 2 sprains may require 4 to 5 days for inflammation to subside. With grade 1 and 2 sprains, the athlete may begin by doing knee slides on a treatment table (Figure 23-30), wall slides (Figure 23-31), active assistive slides (Figure 23-32), or riding an exercise bike with the seat adjusted to the appropriate height to permit as much knee flexion as can be tolerated (Figure 23-15).

As pain subsides and ROM improves, the athlete may incorporate isotonic open-chain flexion and extension exercises (Figures 23-4, 23-5), but the athlete should concentrate on closed-chain strengthening exercises, as tolerated, throughout the rehabilitation process (Figures 23-9 through 23-18). Functional PNF patterns stressing tibial rotation should be incorporated for strengthening, with resistance increasing as the athlete becomes stronger (Figures 23-26 through 23-29). As strength improves the athlete should engage in plyometric exercises (Figures 23-16 through 23-18) and functional activities to enhance the dynamic stability of the knee (see Chapter 17). With a grade 1 sprain the athlete should be able to return to full activity in 3 to 5 weeks.

With a grade 3 sprain the athlete will be in a brace for 2 to 3 weeks with the braced locked from 0 to 45 degrees, and at 0 to 90 degrees for another 2 or 3 weeks, during which time isometric quad sets and SLR strengthening exercises may be performed as tolerated.[12] The athlete should remain non-weight-bearing with crutches for 3 weeks. The strengthening program should progress as with grade 1 and 2 sprains, with return to activity at about 3 months.[12,81]

Criteria for Return.   The athlete may return to activity when (1) they have regained full ROM, (2) they have equal bilateral strength in knee flexion and extension, (3) there is no tenderness, and (4) they can successfully complete functional performance tests such as hopping, shuttle runs, carioca, and co-contraction tests.

Lateral Collateral Ligament Sprains

Pathomechanics.   Fortunately, the lateral aspect of the knee is well supported by secondary stabilizers. Isolated injury to the LCL is rare in athletics, and when it does occur it is critical to rule out other ligamentous injuries.[76] Most LCL sprains in the athletic population re-

sult from a stress placed on the lateral aspect of the knee. Isolated sprain of the LCL is the least common of all knee ligament sprains.[57] LCL sprains result in disruption at the fibular head either with or without avulsion in approximately 75 percent of cases, with 20 percent occurring at the femur, and only 5 percent as midsubstance tears.[82] It is not uncommon to see associated injuries of the peroneal nerve, because the nerve courses around the head of the fibula. A complete disruption of the LCL often involves injury to the posterolateral joint capsule as well as the PCL and occasionally the ACL.[19,42,49]

The extent of laxity determines the severity of the injury. In a grade 1 sprain the LCL is tender due to microtears with some hemorrhage and tenderness to palpation. However, there is no increased laxity and there is a firm end point. A grade 2 sprain involves an incomplete tear with some increased laxity with varus stress at 30 degrees of flexion and minimal laxity in full extension, yet there is still a firm end point. There is tenderness to palpation, hemorrhage, and pain on a varus stress test. A grade 3 sprain is a complete tear with significant laxity on varus stress in 30 degrees of flexion and in full extension when compared to the opposite knee. No end point is evident, and pain is generally less than with grades 1 or 2. Significant laxity with varus stress testing in full extension indicates injury to the posterolateral joint capsule, the PCL, and perhaps the ACL.

Injury Mechanism.   An isolated MCL injury is almost always the result of a varus stress applied to the medial aspect of the knee. Occasionally a varus stress may occur during weight bearing when weight is shifted away from the side of injury, creating stress on the lateral structures.[39] Athletes who sustain an LCL sprain will report that they heard or felt a "pop" and that there was immediate lateral pain. Swelling will be immediate and extra-articular with no joint effusion unless there is an associated menicus or capsular injury.

Rehabilitation Concerns.   Athletes with grade 1 and 2 sprains that exhibit stability to varus stress may be treated symptomatically and may be full weight bearing as soon as tolerated. For patient comfort a knee immobilizer may be worn for a few days to a week following injury. However, the use of a brace is not necessary. It is possible that an athlete with a grade 1 and occasionally even a grade 2 sprain can continue to play. With grade 2 and 3 sprains there will be some residual laxity, because the ligament has been stretched. Grade 3 sprains may be managed nonoperatively with bracing for 4 to 6 weeks limited to 0 to 90 degrees of motion. However, grade 3 MCL tears with associated ligamentous injuries that result in rotational instabilities are usually managed by surgical repair or reconstruction. This is certainly the case if the athlete has chronic varus laxity and intends to continue participation in athletics, or if there is a displaced avulsion.

Rehabilitation Progression. The rehabilitation progression following LCL sprains should follow the same course as was previously described for MCL sprains. In the case of a grade 3 LCL sprain that involves multiple ligamentous injury with associated instability that is surgically repaired or reconstructed, the athlete should be placed in a postoperative brace with partial weight bearing for 4 to 6 weeks. At 6 weeks a rehabilitation program involving a carefully monitored, gradual, sport-specific functional progression should begin. In general the athlete may return to full activity at about 6 months.[39]

Criteria for Return. The athlete may return to activity when (1) they have regained full ROM, (2) they have equal bilateral strength in knee flexion and extension, and (3) they can successfully complete functional performance tests such as hopping, shuttle runs, carioca, and co-contraction tests, as described in Chapter 17.

Anterior Cruciate Ligament Sprain

Pathomechanics. The ACL is perhaps the most commonly injured ligament in the knee. In simple terms, the ACL functions as a primary stabilizer to prevent anterior translation of the tibia on the fixed femur and posterior translation of the femur if the tibia is fixed as in a closed chain. It also serves as a secondary stabilizer to prevent external and internal rotation as well as valgus and varus stress. It works in conjunction with the posterior cruciate ligament to control the gliding and rolling of the tibia on the femur during normal flexion and extension, limiting hyperextension. The twisted configuration of the fibers of the ACL causes the ligament to be under some degree of tension in all positions of knee motion, with lesser tension present at 30 to 90 degrees[39,40,42]

Injury to the ACL most often occurs as a result of sport-related activities that place significant stress on the knee joint, as in cutting or jumping.[39] It appears that females tend to have a higher incidence of ACL injury than males.[51] Recently there seems to be increasing evidence that individuals with a narrow intracondylar notch width may be at greater risk for ACL injury.[46,79] This is particularly evident in athletes with noncontact injuries. It has also been suggested that poor conditioning results in increased physiological laxity, although this has never been demonstrated experimentally.

Tears of the ACL occur in the midsubstance of the ligament about 75 percent of the time, with 20 percent of the tears at the femur and 5 percent at the tibia.[38] As

with MCL and LCL sprains, the severity of the injury is indicated by the degree of laxity or instability. A grade 1 sprain of the ACL results in partial microtears with some hemorrhage, but there is no increased laxity and there is a firm end point. A grade 2 sprain involves an incomplete tear with hemorrhage, some loss of function, and increased anterior translation, yet there is still a firm end point. A grade 2 sprain is painful, and pain increases with Lachman's and anterior drawer stress tests.

A grade 3 sprain is a complete tear with significant laxity with Lachman's and anterior drawer stress tests. There is also rotational instability as indicated by a positive pivot shift. No end point is evident. The athlete will most often report feeling and hearing a "pop" and a feeling that the knee "gave out." There is significant pain initially, but pain decreases substantially within several minutes. With a complete ACL tear, insignificant hemarthrosis occurs within 1 to 2 hours.

The term *anterior cruciate deficient knee* refers to a grade 3 sprain in which there is a complete tear of the ACL. It is generally accepted that a torn ACL will not heal.[78] An ACL-deficient knee will exhibit rotational instability that may eventually cause functional disability in the athlete. Additionally, rotational instability can lead to tears of the meniscus and subsequent degenerative changes in the joint.

Injury Mechanism. The ACL can be injured in several different ways. By far the most common mechanism of injury involves a noncontact injury twisting motion in which the foot is planted and the athlete is attempting to change direction, creating deceleration, valgus stress, and external rotation of the knee. Occasionally the mechanism of injury involves deceleration, valgus stress, and internal rotation.[87] Knee hyperextension combined with internal rotation can also produce a tear of the ACL.

It is possible that the ACL can be torn with contact involving a valgus force that can produce a tear of the ACL and MCL, and possibly a detachment of the medial meniscus, originally described by O'Donohue as the "unhappy triad."[60]

Rehabilitation Concerns. After the diagnosis of injury to the ACL, the athlete, the physician, the sports therapist, and the athlete's family are faced with various treatment options. The conservative approach is to allow the acute phase of the injury to pass and to then implement a vigorous rehabilitation program. If it becomes apparent that normal function cannot be recovered with rehabilitation, and if the knee remains unstable even with normal strengthening and hamstring retraining, then reconstructive surgery is considered. For a sedentary individual, this approach may be acceptable, but most athletes prefer a more aggressive approach.

The older and more sedentary the individual, the less appropriate a reconstruction. This individual may not have the inclination or the time for an extensive rehabilitation program and may not be greatly inconvenienced by some degree of knee instability. Conversely, the ideal patient is a young, motivated, and skilled athlete who is willing to make the personal sacrifices necessary to successfully complete the rehabilitation process. Wilk and Andrews state that any active individual with a goal of returning to stressful pivoting activities should undergo surgical ACL reconstruction.[84] Thus, successful surgical repair/reconstruction of the ACL-deficient knee largely depends upon patient selection.[40] The following would be indications for deciding to surgically repair/reconstruct the injured knee:

- The ACL-injured individual is highly athletic.
- The injured person is unwilling to change their active lifestyle.
- There is rotational instability and a feeling of the knee "giving way" in normal activities.
- There is injury to other ligaments and/or the menisci.
- There are recurrent effusions.
- There is failure at rehabilitation and instability after 6 months of intensive rehabilitation.[40]
- Surgery is necessary to prevent the early onset of degenerative changes within the knee.[42]

In the case of a partially torn ligament, the medical community is split on a treatment approach. Some feel that a partially damaged ACL is incompetent, and the knee should be viewed as if the ligament were completely gone. Others prefer a prolonged initial period of immobilization and limited motion, hoping that the ligament will heal and remain functional. Decisions to treat a patient nonoperatively should be based on the individual's preinjury status and willingness to engage only in activities such as jogging, swimming, or cycling that will not place the knee at high risk.[58] This is clearly a case where the athlete may wisely seek several opinions before choosing the treatment course.

The most widely accepted opinion seems to be that when more than one major ligament is disrupted and there is functional disability, surgery is indicated. The surgical approach to ACL pathology is either repair or reconstruction. With a surgical repair, the damaged ligament is sutured if the tear is in the midsubstance of the ligament, or the bony fragment is reattached in the case of an avulsion injury. However, it is generally felt that direct repair of an isolated ACL tear will tend to have a poor result.[1] In the case of suturing, the repair may be augmented with an internal splint or an extra-articular reconstruction, which seems to be more successful than a direct repair.[73]

Surgical reconstruction is performed using either an extra-articular or an intra-articular technique. An extra-articular reconstruction involves taking a structure that lies outside of the joint capsule and moving it so that it can affect the mechanics of the knee in a manner that mimics normal ACL function. The iliotibial band is the most commonly used structure. This procedure is effective in reducing the pivot shift phenomena that is found in anterolateral rotational instability but cannot match the normal biomechanics of the ACL.[40,49] Isolated extra-articular reconstructions can be effective in patients with mild to moderate instability. Also it may be the treatment of choice in patients who cannot afford the commitment of time and resources for an intra-articular reconstruction.[40] The rehabilitation after an extra-articular reconstruction is aggressive and permits an earlier return to functional activities, but as an isolated procedure it is not recommended for high-level athletes.

Intra-articular reconstruction involves placing a structure within the knee that will roughly follow the course of the ACL and will functionally replace the ACL. Bone-patellar tendon-bone grafts are the current state of the art, using human autografts/allografts,[22,25,40,71,84] while semitendinosis or gracilis autografts and Achilles tendon allografts have been used.[41] Procedures that use synthetic replacements have generally not produced favorable results. The major problem with an autograft is avascularity of the tissue, which results in a progressive decrease in strength of the graft, resulting in possible failure.[25] The main problems with allografts are disease transmission, and rejection of the tissue. It has been demonstrated that at 6 months postsurgery, allografts show a prolonged inflammatory response and a more significant decrease in their structural properties.[41] Rehabilitation following an allograft reconstruction should be less aggressive than with an autograft reconstruction.[39]

Surgical technique is crucial to a successful outcome. Improper placement of the tendon graft by only a few millimeters can prevent the return of normal motion.

In cases where there is reconstruction of the ACL along with a repair of a torn meniscus, the time required for rehabilitation will be slightly longer. This will be discussed in detail under the section dealing with meniscus tears.

Rehabilitation Progression.
Nonoperative rehabilitation. If the ACL-deficient knee is to be treated nonoperatively, it is critical to rule out any other existing problems (torn meniscus, loose bodies, etc.) and correct those problems before proceeding with rehabilitation.[58] Initial treatment should involve controlling swelling, pain, and inflammation through the use of cold, compression, and electrical stimulation. If

necessary, the knee can be placed in an immobilizer for the first few days for comfort and minimal protection, with the athlete ambulating on crutches until they regain full extension and can walk without an extension lag. The athlete can begin immediately following injury with quad sets (Figure 23-4) and straight leg raising (Figure 23-5) to regain motor control and minimize atrophy. Early pain-free range of motion exercises using knee slides on a treatment table (Figure 23-30), wall slides (Figure 23-31), active assistive slides (Figure 23-32), or riding an exercise bike with the seat adjusted to the appropriate height to permit as much knee flexion as can be tolerated (Figure 23-15).

As pain subsides and ROM improves, the athlete may incorporate isotonic open-chain flexion and extension exercises (Figures 23-6, 23-7). With open-chain strengthening exercises, it has been recommended that extension be restricted initially to 0 to 45 degrees for as long as 8 to 12 weeks (6 to 9 weeks being a minimum) to minimize stress on the ACL.[58] Strengthening exercises should be emphasized for both the hamstrings and the gastrocnemius muscles (Figure 23-8), which act to translate the tibia posteriorly, minimizing anterior translation. Closed-chain strengthening exercises (Figures 23-9 through 23-18) are thought to be safer because they minimize anterior translation of the tibia. Closed-chain exercises are used to regain neuromuscular control by enhancing dynamic stabilization through co-contraction of the hamstrings and quadriceps (Figures 23-48 to 23-51). Closed-chain exercises also minimize the possibility of developing patellofemoral pain. A goal of these strengthening exercises should be to achieve a quadriceps/hamstring strength ratio of 1:1.

It is important to incorporate PNF strengthening patterns that stress tibial rotation (Figures 23-26 through 23-29). These manually resisted PNF patterns are essentially the only way to concentrate on strengthening the rotational component of knee motion, which is essential to normal function of the knee. Unfortunately many of the more widely known and used rehabilitation protocols fail to address this critical rotational component.

The use of functional knee braces for an athlete with either a partial ACL tear or an ACL-deficient knee is controversial (Figure 23-54). These braces have not been shown to control translation, especially at functional loads.[6,67] However, there may be some benefit in terms of increased joint position sense, through stimulation of cutaneous sensory receptors, that may enhance both conscious and subconscious awareness of the existing injury.[47]

It is incumbent on the sports therapist to counsel the patient with regard to the precautions that must be exer-

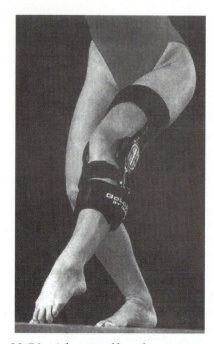

Figure 23-54   A functional knee brace can provide some protection to the injured knee.

cised when engaging in physical activity with an ACL-deficient knee. Nonoperative treatment is appropriate for an individual who does not plan on engaging in the types of activities that can potentially create stresses that can further damage the supporting structures of that joint. If the patient is not willing to make lifestyle changes relative to those activities, then surgical intervention may be a better treatment alternative.

Surgical reconstruction.   There is great debate as to the course of rehabilitation following ACL reconstruction. Traditionally, rehabilitation has been conservative, and there are a great number of physicians and sports therapists who maintain this basic traditional philosophy.[20,63] However, in recent years the trend has been to become more aggressive in rehabilitation of the reconstructed ACL, primarily as a result of the reports of success by Shelbourne and Nitz.[77] This has been referred to as an accelerated protocol. They have demonstrated that this program returns the patient to normal function early, results in fewer patellofemoral problems, and reduces the number of surgeries to obtain extension, all without compromising stability.[77] The accelerated rehabilitation protocol is not without its detractors. Some clinicians feel that it places too much stress on vulnerable tissues and that there are not sufficient scientific data to justify the protocol.[25,59,64,84]

The traditional protocol emphasizes the following:
- Slow progression to regain flexion and extension
- Partial- or nonweight-bearing postoperatively
- Closed-chain exercises at 3 to 4 weeks postoperatively
- Return to activity at 6 to 9 months[20,25,84]

The accelerated protocol emphasizes the following:
- Immediate motion, including full extension
- Immediate weight bearing within tolerance
- Early closed-chain exercise for strengthening and neuromuscular control
- Return to activity at 2 months and to competition at 5 to 6 months[77]

Preoperative period. Regardless of the various recommended time frames for rehabilitation, the rehabilitative process begins immediately following injury in what has been referred to as the preoperative phase. There is general agreement that surgical reconstruction be delayed until pain, swelling, and inflammation have subsided and range of motion, quadriceps muscle control, and a normal gait pattern have been regained during this preoperative phase. This appears to occur at about 2 to 3 weeks postinjury.[33,75] It also appears that delaying surgery decreases the incidence of postoperative arthrofibrosis.[75]

Postoperative Period. Perhaps the single most important rehabilitation consideration postoperatively has to do with the initial strength of the graft and how the graft heals and matures. It has been demonstrated that the tensile strength of a 10 mm central third patellar tendon graft is approximately 107 percent of the normal ACL initially, and it has been predicted that the strength is at 57 percent at 3 months, 56 percent at 6 months, and 87 percent at 9 months.[15] Stress on the graft should be minimized during the period of graft necrosis (6 weeks), revascularization (8–16 weeks), and remodeling (16 weeks).[84] Assuming that the surgical technique for reconstruction is technically sound, the graft is at its strongest immediately following surgery, so rehabilitation can be very aggressive early in the process. Also it appears that an aggressive rehabilitation program minimizes complications and maximizes restoration of function following ACL reconstruction.[39]

Controlling Swelling. Immediately following surgery, the goal is to minimize pain and swelling by using cold, compression, and electrical stimulation. A Cryo-cuff is widely used for this purpose. Significant swelling can initially inhibit firing of the quadriceps.

Bracing. The athlete is placed in a rehabilitative brace and most often locked in either full extension,[77] or 0 to 90 degrees passive with 40 to 90 degrees active ROM, for the first 2 weeks (Figure 23-55). The brace will be worn for 4 to 6 weeks, or until knee flexion exceeds the limits of

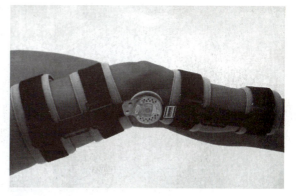

Figure 23-55   In a rehabilitative brace the range of movement can be restricted and changed whenever appropriate.

the brace, and may be removed for exercise and for bathing. Shellbourne and Nitz recommend that a knee immobilizer be used for the first 2 weeks but that at the end of the first week the athlete be fitted for a functional brace, which should be worn for protection throughout the rehabilitation process.[77] There does not appear to be a general consensus among physicians as to the value of wearing a functional brace during return to activity. This decision should be made on an individual basis.

Weight bearing. Generally the athlete is placed on crutches either with 50 percent weight bearing,[64] or progressed to full weight bearing as tolerated[77] for the first 2 weeks. The athlete can get off the crutches when there is minimal swelling, no extension lag, and sufficient quadriceps strength to allow for nearly normal gait. This may take anywhere from 2 to 6 weeks.

Range of motion. Range-of-motion exercises can begin immediately. Some clinicians advocate the judicious use of continuous passive motion (CPM) machines, which may be applied immediately after surgery (Figure 23-56),[53,59,61,72] while others prefer that the athlete engage in active range-of-motion exercises as soon as possible (Figures 23-30 through 23-32). Certainly, current research is sparse regarding the efficacy of CPM.

In their accelerated rehabilitation program, Shellbourne and Nitz emphasize the importance of early restoration of full knee extension.[77] Full extension can be achieved using knee extension on a rolled-up towel (Figure 23-33) or prone leg hangs (Figure 23-34). Exercises to maintain full extension should be emphasized throughout the rehabilitation process. Active knee extension should be limited to 60 to 90 degrees to minimize anterior tibial translation, whereas knee flexion should reach 90 degrees by the end of the second week. Full flexion (135 degrees) should be achieved at 5 to 6 weeks.

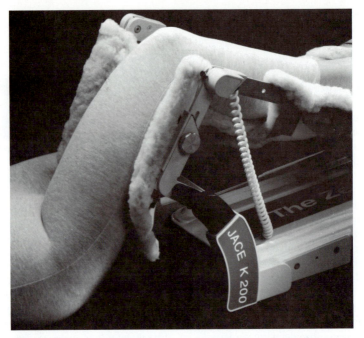

Figure 23-56   A CPM device may be used to help regain ROM.

Once knee flexion reaches 100 to 110 degrees, the athlete may begin stationary cycling to help with regaining ROM (Figure 23-18).

During the second week the sports therapist should teach the athlete self-mobilization techniques for the patella (Figure 23-44). Restriction of patellar motion can interfere with regaining both flexion and extension. The grade of mobilization used should be based on the degree of inflammation, and should avoid creating additional pain and swelling.[68]

Strengthening. Initially, strengthening exercises should avoid placing high levels of stress on the graft. Quad sets (Figure 23-4) and straight leg raises (Figure 23-5) using co-contraction of the hamstrings should begin immediately to prevent shutdown of the quadriceps. Progressive resistive exercise can begin during the second week for hamstrings (Figure 23-6), hip adductors (Figure 23-3), hip abductors (Figure 23-2), and gastrocnemius muscles (Figure 23-8). Strengthening exercises for all of these muscle groups, particularly emphasizing strengthening of the hamstrings, should continue throughout rehabilitation.

The rationale and biomechanical advantages for using closed-kinetic-chain strengthening exercises in the rehabilitation of various knee injuries was discussed in detail in Chapter 11. When using the different closed-kinetic-chain exercises, it is essential to emphasize co-

contraction of the hamstrings, both to stabilize the knee and to provide a posterior translational force to counteract the anterior shear force created by the quadriceps during knee extension. Once flexion reaches 90 degrees, which should generally be in 1 to 2 weeks, the athlete can begin closed-kinetic-chain minisquats in the 40 to 90 degrees range (Figure 23-9), lateral step-ups (Figure 23-13), standing wall slides (Figure 23-8) or leg press (Figure 23-12).

Open-kinetic-chain quadriceps strengthening exercises should be completely avoided in the early stages of rehabilitation, due to the anterior shear forces, which are greatest from 30 degrees of flexion to full extension. However, at some point in the later stages of rehabilitation, open-kinetic-chain quadriceps strengthening exercises may be safely incorporated (Figure 23-7).

It should be reemphasized that the graft is at its weakest between weeks 8 to 14, during the period of revascularization. Therefore caution should be exercised relative to strengthening exercises during this period. The accelerated program has recommended that isokinetic testing begin at about 2 months. Other programs recommend that testing be delayed until 4 or 5 months. This should be done only using an antishear device with a 20-degree terminal extension block.[44,76] Isokinetic strengthening exercises may be safely incorporated at about 4 months (Figures 23-22 to 23-24).

PNF strengthening patterns that stress tibial rotation may also be used. These manually resisted PNF patterns are essentially the only way to concentrate on strengthening the rotational component of knee motion, which is essential to normal function of the knee. Because the PNF patterns are done in an open kinetic chain, they should involve only active contraction through the functional movement pattern. Progressively resisted patterns can be used beginning at about 5 months (Figures 23-26 through 23-29).

Reestablishing neuromuscular control. Along with the early controlled weight bearing and closed-chain exercises that act to stimulate muscle and joint mechanoreceptors, seated BAPS board exercises to reestablish balance and neuromuscular control should also begin early in the rehabilitation process (Figure 23-48B). Balance training using a standing BAPS board (Figure 23-48A), and lateral shifting for strengthening and agility using the Fitter (Figure 23-51), may be incorporated at 6 weeks.

Cardiorespiratory endurance. Cycling on an upper-extremity ergometer may begin during the first week. Cycling on a stationary bike can begin as early as possible when the athlete achieves about 100 to 110 degrees of flexion (Figure 23-18). Walking with full weight bearing on a treadmill can usually begin at about 3 weeks, using forward walking initially then progressing to retro walking. Swimming is considered to be a safe activity at 4 to 5 weeks. Stair climbing (Figure 23-17) or cross-country skiing can begin as early as week 6 or 7. Recommendations for progressing to jogging/running are as early as 4 months in the accelerated program but are more often closer to 6 months.

Functional training. Functional training should progressively incorporate the stresses, strains, and forces that occur during normal running, jumping, and cutting activities in a controlled environment.[12,23] Exercises such as single- and double-leg hopping, carioca, shuttle runs, vertical jumping, rope skipping, and co-contraction activities, most of which were described in Chapter 17, should be incorporated. In the more traditional programs these activities may begin at about 4 months, although in the accelerated program they may begin as early as 5 or 6 weeks.

Criteria for Return. Physicians typically have varying criteria for full return of the athlete following injury to the anterior cruciate. Perhaps the greatest variability exists in the recommended time frames for full return. Among the more widely used protocols are the following recommendations:

- Shellbourne and Nitz—4 to 6 months
- Andrews and Wilk—5 to 6 months
- Fu and Irrgang—6 to 9 months
- Campbell Clinic—6 to 12 months
- Paulos and Stern—9 months
- Kerlan and Jobe—9 months

In general the following criteria appear to be the most widely accepted: (1) No joint effusion, (2) full ROM, (3) isokinetic testing indicates that strength of the quadriceps and hamstrings are at 85 to 100 percent of the uninvolved leg, (4) satisfactory ligament stability testing using a KT-1000 arthrometer,[2] (5) successful progression from walking to running, and (6) successful performance during functional testing (hop tests, agility runs, etc.).

Posterior Cruciate Ligament Sprains

Pathomechanics. Isolated tears of the posterior cruciate ligament (PCL) are not common but certainly do occur in athletes. It is more likely that the PCL is injured concurrently with the ACL, MCL, LCL, or menisci. The PCL is the strongest ligament in the knee and functions with the ACL to control the rolling and gliding of the tibiofemoral joint and has been called the primary stabilizer of the knee. More specifically the PCL prevents 85 to 90 percent of the posterior translational force of the tibia on the femur. This is evident in the PCL-deficient knee when, upon descending an incline, the force of gravity works to increase the anterior glide of the femur on the tibia; without the PCL the femur will sublux on the tibia from midstance to toe-off, where the quadriceps are less effective in controlling the anterior motion of the femur on the tibia.[50,52]

The majority (70 percent) of PCL tears occur on the tibia, while 15 percent occur on femur and 15 percent are midsubstance tears.[82] In the PCL-deficient knee there is an increased likelihood of meniscus lesions and chondral defects, most often involving the medial side.[29]

The extent of laxity determines the severity of the injury. In a grade 1 sprain the PCL is tender due to microtears with some hemorrhage and tenderness to palpation. However, there is no increased laxity and there is a firm end point. A grade 2 sprain involves an incomplete tear with some increased laxity in a positive posterior drawer test, yet there is still a firm end point. There is tenderness to palpation, hemorrhage, and pain on posterior drawer test. A grade 3 sprain is a complete tear with significant posterior laxity in posterior drawer, posterior sag, and reverse pivot shift tests when compared to the opposite knee. No end point is evident, and pain is generally less than with grades 1 or 2.

Injury Mechanism. In athletics, the most common mechanism of injury to the PCL is with the knee in a position of forced hyperflexion with the foot plantar flexed. The PCL can also be injured when the tibia is forced posteriorly on the fixed femur or the femur is forced anteriorly on the fixed tibia.[49] It is also possible to injure the PCL when the knee is hyperflexed and a downward force is applied to the thigh.

Forced hyperextension will usually result in injury to both the PCL and the ACL. If an anteromedial force is applied to a hyperextended knee, the posterolateral joint capsule may also be injured. If enough valgus or varus force is applied to the fully extended knee to rupture either collateral ligament, it is possible that the PCL may also be torn.

The athlete will indicate that they felt and heard a "pop" but will often feel that the injury was minor and that they can return to activity immediately. There will be mild to moderate swelling within 2 to 6 hours.

Rehabilitation Concerns. Perhaps the greatest concern in rehabilitating an athlete with an injured PCL is the fact that the arthrokinematics of the joint are altered, and this change can eventually lead to degeneration of both the medial compartment and the patellofemoral joint.[39]

The decision as to whether the PCL-deficient knee is best treated nonoperatively or surgically is controversial. This is primarily due to the relative lack of data-based information in the literature regarding the normal history of PCL tears. Many athletes with an isolated PCL tear do not seem to exhibit any functional performance limitations and can continue to compete athletically, while others occasionally are limited in performing normal daily activities.[29]

Parolie and Bergfeld reported a more than 80 percent success rate with nonoperative treatment.[62] On the other hand, Clancy reported a high incidence of femoral condylar articular injury involving degenerative changes that may eventually result in arthritis in patients 4 years after PCL injury. Thus surgical reconstruction has been advocated.[16,52]

It is generally felt that the surgical treatment of PCL tears is technically difficult. Surgery to reconstruct a PCL-deficient knee is most often indicated with avulsion injuries. Reconstructive procedures using the semitendinous tendon, the tendon of the medial gastrocnemius, the Achilles tendon, the patellar tendon, or synthetic material to replace the lost PCL have been recommended.[39] Both autografts and allografts have been used.

Rehabilitation Progression.
Nonoperative rehabilitation. If the PCL-deficient knee is to be treated nonoperatively, initial treatment should involve controlling swelling, pain, and inflammation through the use of cold, compression, and electrical stimulation. If necessary, the knee can be placed in an immobilizer for the first few days for comfort and minimal protection, with the athlete ambulating on crutches until

they regain full extension and they can walk without an extension lag. Because there is often little functional limitation, the athlete may progress rapidly through the rehabilitative process, the rate of progression limited only by pain and swelling.

The athlete can begin immediately following injury with quad sets (Figure 23-4) and straight leg raising (Figure 23-5) to regain motor control and minimize atrophy. Early pain-free range-of-motion exercises can begin using knee slides on a treatment table (Figure 23-30), wall slides (Figure 23-31), active assistive slides (Figure 23-32), or riding an exercise bike with the seat adjusted to the appropriate height to permit as much knee flexion as can be tolerated (Figure 23-15). Hamstring exercises should be avoided initially to minimize posterior laxity.

Nonoperative rehabilitation should focus primarily on quadriceps strengthening. As pain subsides and ROM improves, the athlete may incorporate isotonic open-chain extension exercises (Figure 23-7). With open-chain quadriceps strengthening exercises, it has been recommended that extension be restricted initially in the 45 to 20 degrees range to avoid developing patellofemoral pain.[35] It has also been recommended that quadriceps strength in the PCL-deficient knee be greater than 100 percent of the uninjured knee, particularly in athletes attempting to fully return to sport activity.[62]

Open-chain hamstring strengthening exercises using knee flexion that increase posterior translation of the tibia should be avoided. Posterior tibial translation can be minimized by strengthening the hamstrings using open-chain hip extension with the knee fully extended (see Figure 22-3). Closed-chain exercises (Figures 23-9 through 23-18) that use a co-contraction of the quadriceps to reduce posterior tibial translation and also to minimize the possibility of developing patellofemoral pain may safely be used to strengthen the hamstrings.

The use of functional knee braces for an athlete with a PCL-deficient knee is generally not recommended, because functional braces are designed primarily for ACL-deficient knees. However, there may be some benefit in terms of increased joint position sense, through stimulation of cutaneous sensory receptors, that may enhance both conscious and subconscious awareness of the existing injury.[47]

Because of the tendency toward progressive degeneration of the medial aspect of the knee with a PCL-deficient knee, it is incumbent on the sports therapist to counsel the patient to avoid repetitive activities that produce pain or swelling.[39]

Surgical rehabilitation. The time frame for the maturation and healing process for a PCL graft has not been documented in the literature, as it has been for ACL grafts. The course of rehabilitation following surgical reconstruction of the PCL is not well defined, and recommended rehabilitation protocols are difficult to find. Clancy has perhaps the largest study of operative PCL reconstructions using a patellar tendon graft.[16]

Immediately following surgery, the goal is to minimize pain and swelling by using cold, compression, and electrical stimulation. A Cryo-cuff may be used to accomplish this. The athlete is placed in a rehabilitative brace and locked in 0 degrees of extension at all times for the first week (Figure 23-54). During the second week the brace may be unlocked for ambulation and passive ROM exercises. The brace will be worn for 4 to 6 weeks until the athlete can achieve 90 to 100 degrees of flexion. Generally the athlete is placed on crutches with full weight bearing as soon as possible, but they should stay on crutches for 4 to 6 weeks until they can achieve full extension.

Quad sets (Figure 23-4) and straight leg raises (Figure 23-5) done in the brace can begin at 2 to 4 weeks. Resisted exercise can begin during the second week for hip adductors (Figure 23-3) and hip abductors (Figure 23-2). After surgical reconstruction of the PCL, it is important to limit hamstring function to reduce the posterior translational forces.[50] Strengthening exercises for the hamstrings should be avoided initially because they tend to place stress on the graft. At 4 to 6 weeks, closed-chain exercises from 0 to 45 degrees of flexion are initiated. Resisted terminal knee extensions in a closed chain should also be used (Figure 23-14).

Along with the early controlled weight bearing and closed-chain exercises begun at about 6 weeks which act to stimulate muscle and joint mechanoreceptors, seated BAPS board exercises to reestablish balance and neuromuscular control should also begin early in the rehabilitation process (Figure 23-48B).

Cycling on a stationary bike can begin at 6 weeks when the athlete achieves about 100 to 110 degrees of flexion (Figure 23-18). Walking with full weight bearing on a treadmill can begin when the athlete has no extension lag and has sufficient quadriceps strength to allow for nearly normal gait. Progressing to jogging/running is generally not recommended until 9 months. Functional training should progressively incorporate the stresses, strains, and forces that occur during normal running, jumping, and cutting activities in a controlled environment.

Criteria for Return. In general the following criteria for return appear to be the most widely accepted: (1) There is no joint effusion. (2) There is full ROM. (3) Isokinetic testing indicates that strength of the quadriceps greater than 100 percent of the uninvolved leg. (4) The athlete has made successful progression from walking to running. (5) The athlete has successful performance during functional testing (hop tests, agility runs, etc.).

Meniscal Injury

Pathomechanics. The menisci aid in joint lubrication, help distribute weight-bearing forces, help increase joint congruency (which aids in stability), act as a secondary restraint in checking tibiofemoral motion, and act as a shock absorber.[13,48]

The medial meniscus has a much higher incidence of injury than the lateral meniscus. The higher number of medial meniscal lesions may be attributed to the coronary ligaments that attach the meniscus peripherally to the tibia and also to the capsular ligament. The lateral meniscus does not attach to the capsular ligament and is more mobile during knee movement. Because of the attachment to the medial structures, the medial meniscus is prone to disruption from valgus and torsional forces.

A meniscus tear can result in immediate joint-line pain localized to either the medial or the lateral side of the knee. Effusion develops gradually over 48 to 72 hours, although a tear at the periphery might produce a more acute hemarthrosis. Initially pain is described as a "giving-way" feeling, but the knee may be "locked" near full extension due to displacement of the meniscus. A knee that is locked at 10 to 30 degrees of flexion may indicate a tear of the medial meniscus, while a knee that is locked at 70 degrees or more may indicate a tear of the posterior portion of the lateral meniscus.[18] A positive McMurray's test usually indicates a tear in the posterior horn of the meniscus. The knee that is locked by a displaced meniscus may require unlocking with the athlete under anesthesia so that a detailed examination can be conducted. If discomfort, disability, and locking of the knee continue, arthroscopic surgery may be required to remove a portion of the meniscus. If the knee is not locked but shows indications of a tear, the physician might initially obtain an MRI. A diagnostic arthroscopic examination may also be performed. Diagnosis of meniscal injuries should be made immediately after the injury has occurred and before muscle guarding and swelling obscure the normal shape of the knee.

Injury Mechanism. The most common mechanism of meniscal injury is weight bearing combined with internal or external rotation while extending or flexing the knee.[14] A valgus or varus force sufficient to cause disruption of the MCL or LCL also might produce an ACL tear as well as a meniscus tear. A large number of medial meniscus lesions are the outcome of a sudden, strong, internal rotation of the femur with a partially flexed knee while the foot is firmly planted, as would occur in a cutting motion. As a result of the force of this action, the medial meniscus is detached and pinched between the femoral condyles.

Meniscal lesions can be longitudinal, oblique, or transverse. Stretching of the anterior and posterior horns of the meniscus can produce a vertical-longitudinal or "bucket-handle" tear. A longitudinal tear can also result from forcefully extending the knee from a flexed position while the femur is internally rotated. During extension the medial meniscus is suddenly pulled back, causing the tear. In contrast, the lateral meniscus can sustain an oblique tear by a forceful knee extension with the femur externally rotated.

Rehabilitation Concerns.   Quite often in the athletic population, the choice is to initially treat meniscus tears conservatively, taking a "wait and see" approach. Occasionally the athlete will be able to complete the competitive season by simply "dealing" with the associated symptoms of a torn meniscus, with the idea that the problem will be taken care of surgically at the end of the season. In some individuals the symptoms may resolve so that there is no longer a need for surgery.

The problem is that once a meniscal tear occurs, the ruptured edges harden and can eventually atrophy. On occasion, portions of the meniscus may become detached and wedge themselves between the articulating surfaces of the tibia and femur, imposing a chronic locking, "catching," or "giving way" of the joint. Chronic meniscal lesions can also display recurrent swelling and obvious muscle atrophy around the knee. The athlete might complain of an inability to perform a full squat or to change direction quickly when running without pain, a sense of the knee collapsing, or a "popping" sensation. Displaced meniscal tears can eventually lead to serious articular degeneration with major impairment and disability. Such symptoms and signs usually warrant surgical intervention.

Three surgical treatment choices are possible for the athlete with a damaged meniscus: partial meniscectomy, meniscal repair, and meniscal transplantation. It was not too long ago that the accepted surgical treatment for a torn meniscus involved total removal of the damaged meniscus. However, total meniscectomy has been shown to cause premature degenerative arthritis. With the advent of arthroscopic surgery, the need for total meniscectomy has been virtually eliminated. In surgical management of meniscal tears, every effort should be made to minimize loss of any portion of the meniscus.

The location of the meniscal tear often dictates whether the surgical treatment will involve a partial meniscectomy or a meniscal repair. Tears that occur within the inner third of the meniscus will have to be re-

sected because they are unlikely to heal, even with surgical repair, due to avascularity. Tears in the middle third of the meniscus and, particularly, in the outer third, may heal well following surgical repair because they have a good vascular supply. Partial meniscectomy of a torn meniscus is much more common than meniscal repair.

Rehabilitation Progressions.

Nonoperative management.   If a consensus decision is made by the physician, the athlete, and the sports therapist to treat a meniscus tear nonoperatively, the athlete may return to full activity as soon as the initial signs and symptoms resolve. Rehabilitation efforts should be directed primarily at minimizing pain and controlling swelling in addition to getting the athlete back to functional activities as soon as possible. Generally the athlete may require 3 to 5 days of limited activity to allow for resolution of symptoms.

Partial meniscectomy.   Postsurgical management for a partial meniscectomy that is not accompanied by degenerative change or injury to other ligaments initially involves controlling swelling, pain, and inflammation through the use of cold, compression, and electrical stimulation. The athlete should ambulate on crutches for 1 to 3 days, progressing to full weight bearing as soon as tolerated until regaining full extension and walking without a limp or an extension lag. Early pain-free range-of-motion exercises using knee slides on a treatment table (Figure 23-30), wall slides (Figure 23-31), active assistive slides (Figure 23-32), and stationary cycling (Figure 23-18) can begin immediately along with quad sets (Figure 23-4) and straight leg raising (Figure 23-5), which are used to regain motor control and minimize atrophy. As pain subsides and ROM improves, the athlete may incorporate isotonic open- and closed-chain exercises (Figures 23-6, 23-7, 23-9 through 23-18). Functional activity training may begin as soon as the athlete feels ready. It is not uncommon in the athletic population for functional activity training to begin within 3 to 6 days after a partial meniscectomy, although it is more likely that full return will require about 2 weeks.

Meniscal repair.   The repair of a damaged meniscus involves the use of absorbable sutures, vascular access channels drilled from vascular to nonvascular areas, and the insertion of a fibrin clot.[14] Rehabilitation after arthroscopic surgery for a partial meniscectomy with no associated capsular damage is rapid, and the likelihood of complications is minimal.

Rehabilitation after either meniscal repair or meniscus transplant requires that joint motion be limited and thus is more prolonged than for a partial meniscectomy. For the athlete it is essential that some type of cardiorespiratory endurance conditioning be incorporated throughout the period of immobilization. Because of the limitation of the rehabilitative brace, use of an upper-extremity ergometer is perhaps the most effective way to maintain endurance.

The athlete is placed in a rehabilitative brace locked in full extension for the first 2 weeks, both for protection and to prevent flexion contractures (Figure 23-54). During this period, there is partial weight bearing on crutches. Submaximal isometric quad sets are performed in the brace along with hip abduction and adduction strengthening exercises (Figures 23-2, 23-3).

For weeks 2 to 4, motion in the brace is limited to 20 to 90 degrees of flexion, and for weeks 4 to 6, motion is limited in the 0 to 90 degrees range. Hip exercises and isometric quad sets should continue. Range-of-motion exercises using knee slides (Figure 23-30), wall slides (Figure 23-31), and active assistive slides (Figure 23-32), should all be done in the brace within the protected range. Partial weight bearing on crutches should progress to full weight bearing after 6 weeks.

At 6 weeks the brace can be removed and the knee rehabilitation progressions described above may be incorporated, as tolerated by the athlete, to regain full range of motion and normal muscle strength. Generally the athlete can return to full activity at about 3 months.

If an athlete has had an ACL reconstruction in addition to a meniscal repair, the healing constraints associated with meniscal repair must be taken into consideration in the rehabilitation plan.[81] Range-of-motion exercises, strengthening exercises, and weight bearing all have some mechanical impact on the meniscus. If the rehabilitation protocols for other ligament injuries are more aggressive or accelerated, the guidelines for meniscus repair healing must be incorporated into the treatment plan.

Meniscal transplant. Meniscal transplants using either allografts or synthetic material have been recommended.[28,80] Although reports of the efficacy of these procedures have been inconsistent,[18] generally the preference seems to be an allograft using bone plugs and suturing to the capsule at the periphery of the graft.[28] Meniscal transplants are markedly less common than either meniscectomy or repair.

It is recommended that following transplantation, a rehabilitative brace be locked in full extension for 6 weeks. The brace may be unlocked during this period to allow passive range-of-motion exercises in the 0 to 90 degrees range. Isometric quad sets and hip exercises are performed throughout this 6-week period. Also only partial weight bearing on crutches is allowed.

At 6 weeks the brace is unlocked, and there should be progression to full weight bearing. Use of the brace may be discontinued at 8 weeks or whenever the athlete can achieve full extension, flexion to 100 degrees, and a

normal gait.[39] At that point progressive strengthening, range of motion, and functional training techniques as described previously can be incorporated when appropriate. Full return is expected in 9 to 12 months.

Criteria for Return. Time frames required for full return following nonoperative management, partial menisectomy, meniscal repair, and meniscal transplant were discussed previously. Generally, with meniscus injury, the athlete may return to activity when (1) swelling does not occur with activity, (2) full ROM has been regained, (3) there is equal bilateral strength in knee flexion and extension, and (4) the athlete can successfully complete functional performance tests such as hopping, shuttle runs, carioca, and co-contraction tests.

REHABILITATION TECHNIQUES FOR PATELLOFEMORAL AND EXTENSOR MECHANISM INJURIES

Complaints of pain and disability associated with the patellofemoral joint and the extensor mechanism are exceedingly common among the athletic population. The terminology used to describe this anterior knee pain has been a source of some confusion and thus requires some clarification. Until recently, it was not uncommon for every athlete who walked into a sports medicine clinic complaining of anterior knee pain to be diagnosed as having *condromalacia patella.* However, there can be many other causes of anterior knee pain, and chondromalacia patella is only one of these causes. The term *patellofemoral arthralgia* is a catchall term used to describe anterior knee pain. Chondromalacia patella, along with patellofemoral stress syndrome, patellar tendinitis, patellar bursitis, chronic patellar subluxation, acute patellar dislocation, and a synovial plica, are all conditions that can cause anterior knee pain. The treatment and rehabilitation of athletes complaining of anterior knee pain can be very frustrating for the sports therapist. The more conservative approach to treatment of patellofemoral pain described below should be used initially. If this approach fails, surgical intervention may be required.

Patellofemoral Stress Syndrome

Pathomechanics. Athletes presenting with patellofemoral pain typically exhibit relatively common symptoms.[27] They complain of nonspecific pain in the anterior portion of the knee. It is difficult to place one finger on a specific spot and be certain that the pain is there. Pain seems to be increased when either ascending or descending stairs or when moving from a squatting to a standing position. Athletes also complain of pain when

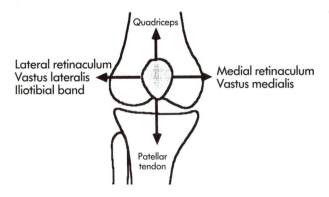

Figure 23-57 Static and dynamic patellar stabilizers.

sitting for long periods of time—this has occasionally been referred to as the "moviegoer's sign." Reports of the knee "giving away" are likely, although typically no instability is associated with this problem. When evaluating the pathomechanics of the patellofemoral joint, the sports therapist must assess static alignment, dynamic alignment, and patellar orientation.

Static alignment. Static stabilizers of the patellofemoral joint act to maintain the appropriate alignment of the patella when no motion is occurring (Figure 23-57). The superior static stabilizers are the quadriceps muscles (vastus lateralis, vastus intermedius, vastus medialis, rectus femoris). Laterally, static stabilizers include the lateral retinaculum, vastus lateralis, and iliotibial band. Medially, the medial retinaculum and the vastus medialis are the static stabilizers. Inferiorly, the patellar tendon stabilizes the patella.

Dynamic alignment. Dynamic alignment of the patella must be assessed during functional activities. It is critical to look at the tracking of the patella from an anterior view during normal gait. Muscle control should be observed while the athlete engages in other functional activities, including stepping, bilateral squats, or one-legged squats.

A number of different anatomical factors can affect dynamic alignment. It is essential to understand that both static and dynamic structures must create a balance of forces about the knee. Any change in this balance might produce improper tracking of the patella and patellofemoral pain.

Increased Q-angle. The Q-angle (Figure 23-58) is formed by drawing a line from the anterosuperior iliac spine to the center of the patella. A second line drawn from the tibial tubercle to the center of the patella that intersects the first line forms the Q-angle. A normal Q-angle falls between 10 to 12 degrees in the male and 15 to

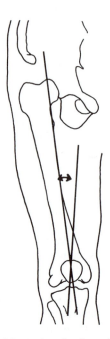

Figure 23-58 Measuring the Q-angle.

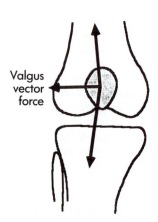

Figure 23-59 A lateral valgus vector force is created when the quadriceps is contracted.

17 degrees in the female. Q-angle can be increased by lateral displacement of the tibial tubercle, external tibial torsion, or femoral neck anteversion. The Q-angle is a static measurement and might have no direct correlation with patellofemoral pain.[26] However, dynamically this increased Q-angle may increase the lateral valgus vector force, thus encouraging lateral tracking, resulting in patellofemoral pain[45] (Figure 23-59).

A-angle. The A-angle (Figure 23-60) measures the patellar orientation to the tibial tubercle. It is created by

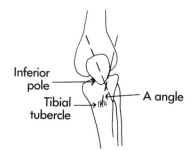

Figure 23-60   Measurement of the A-angle.

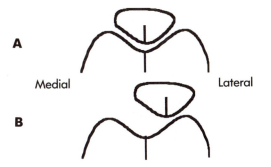

Figure 23-61   Positive lateral glide. **A,** Normal positioning, **B,** positive lateral glide component.

the intersection of lines drawn bisecting the patella longitudinally and from the tibial tubercle to the apex of the inferior pole of the patella. An angle of 35 degrees or greater has been correlated with patellofemoral pathomechanics, resulting in patellofemoral pain.[3]

Iliotibial band. The distal portion of the iliotibial band interdigitates with both the deep transverse retinaculum and the superficial oblique retinaculum. As the knee moves into flexion, the iliotibial band moves posteriorly, causing the patella to tilt and track laterally.[27]

Vastus medialis oblique insufficiency. The vastus medialis oblique (VMO) functions as an active and dynamic stabilizer of the patella. Anatomically it arises from the tendon of the adductor magnus.[10] Normally, the VMO is tonically active electromyographically throughout the range of motion. In individuals with patellofemoral pain, it is phasically active, and it tends to lose fatigue-resistant capabilities.[70] The VMO is innervated by a separate branch of the femoral nerve; therefore it can be activated as a single motor unit.[4] In normal individuals the VMO to vastus lateralis (VL) ratio has been shown to be 1:1.[69] However, in individuals who complain of patellofemoral pain the VMO:VL ratio is less than 1:1.

Vastus lateralis. The vastus lateralis interdigitates with fibers of the superficial lateral retinaculum. Again, if this retinaculum is tight or if a muscle imbalance exists between the vastus lateralis and the vastus medialis with the lateralis being more active, lateral tilt or tracking of the patella may occur dynamically.[26]

Excessive pronation. Excessive pronation may result from existing structural deformities in the foot. With overpronation there is excessive subtalar eversion and adduction with an obligatory internal rotation of the tibia, increased internal rotation of the femur, and thus an increased lateral valgus vector force at the knee that encourages lateral tracking.[32] Various structural deformities in the feet that can cause knee pain should be corrected biomechanically according to techniques recommended in Chapter 25.

Tight hamstring muscles. Tight hamstring muscles cause an increase in knee flexion. When the heel strikes the ground, there must be increased dorsiflexion at the talocrural joint. Excessive subtalar joint motion may occur to allow for necessary dorsiflexion. As stated previously, this produces excessive pronation with concomitant increased internal tibial rotation and a resultant increase in the lateral valgus vector force.

Tight gastrocnemius muscle. A tight gastrocnemius muscle will not allow for the 10 degrees of dorsiflexion necessary for normal gait. Once again this produces excessive subtalar motion, increased internal tibial rotation, and increased lateral valgus vector force.[32]

Patella alta. In patella alta, the ratio of patellar tendon length to the height of the patella is greater than the normal 1:1 ratio. In patella alta the length of the patellar tendon is 20 percent greater than the height of the patella. This creates a situation where greater flexion is necessary before the patella assumes a stable position within the trochlear groove, and thus there is an increased tendency toward lateral subluxation.[38]

Patellar orientation.   Patellar orientation is the positioning of the patella relative to the tibia. Assessment should be done with the athlete in supine position. Four components should be assessed when looking at patellar orientation: glide, tilt, rotation, and anteroposterior tilt.

Glide component. This component assesses the lateral or medial deviation of the patella relative to the trochlear groove of the femur. Glide should be assessed both statically and dynamically. Figure 23-61 provides an example of a positive lateral glide.

Tilt component. Tilt is determined by comparing the height of the medial patellar border with the lateral patellar border. Figure 23-62 shows an example of a positive lateral tilt.

Rotational component. Rotation is identified by assessing the deviation of the longitudinal axis (a line drawn

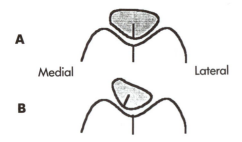

Figure 23-62   Positive lateral tilt. **A,** Normal positioning, **B,** positive lateral tilt component.

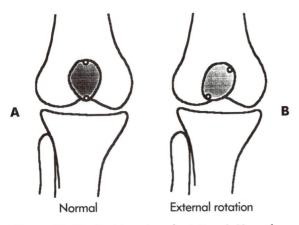

Figure 23-63   Positive external rotation. **A,** Normal positioning **B,** positive external rotation.

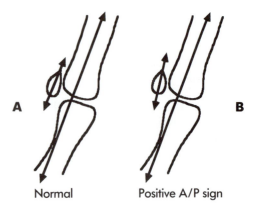

Figure 23-64   Positive inferior anteroposterior tilt. **A,** Normal positioning, **B,** positive inferior anteroposterior tilt component.

from superior pole to inferior pole) of the patella relative to the femur. The point of reference is the inferior pole. If the inferior pole is more lateral than the superior pole, a positive external rotation exists (Figure 23-63).

Anteroposterior tilt component. This must be assessed laterally to determine if a line drawn from the inferior patellar pole to the superior patellar pole is parallel to the long axis of the femur. If the inferior pole is posterior to the superior pole, the athlete has a positive anteroposterior tilt component (Figure 23-64).

Rehabilitation Concerns.   Traditionally, rehabilitation techniques for athletes complaining of patellofemoral pain tended to concentrate on avoiding those activities that exacerbated pain (for example, squatting or stair climbing), occasional immobilization, and strengthening of the quadriceps group using open-kinetic-chain exercises. The current treatment approach has a new direction and focus that includes strengthening of the quadriceps through closed-kinetic-chain exercise, regaining optimal patellar positioning and tracking, and regaining neuromuscular control to improve lower-limb mechanics.

Strengthening techniques.   Earlier in this chapter, closed-kinetic-chain exercises were recommended for strengthening in the rehabilitation of ligamentous knee injuries. These same exercises are also useful in the rehabilitation of patellofemoral pain, not because anterior shear is reduced but because of how they affect patellofemoral joint reaction force (PFJRF).

More traditional rehabilitation techniques focused on reducing the compressive forces of the patella against the femur and reducing PFJRF. PFJRF increases when the angle between the patellar tendon and the quadriceps tendon decreases (Figure 23-65). PFJRF also increases when the quadriceps tension increases to resist the flexion moment created by the lever arms. PFJRF can be minimized by maximizing the area of surface contact of the patella on the femur. As the knee moves into greater degrees of flexion, the area of surface contact increases, distributing the forces associated with increased compression over a larger area (Figure 23-66), minimizing the compressive forces per unit area.[31]

Rehabilitation techniques involving closed-kinetic-chain exercises try to maximize the area of surface contact. With closed-kinetic-chain exercises, as the angle of knee flexion decreases, the flexion moment acting on the knee increases. This requires greater quadriceps and patellar tendon tension to counteract the effects of the increased flexion moment arm, resulting in an increase in PFJRF as flexion increases. However, the force is distributed over a larger patellofemoral contact area, minimizing the increase in contact stress per unit area. Therefore it appears that closed-kinetic-chain exercises may be better tolerated by the patellofemoral joint than open-kinetic-chain exercises.

Closed-kinetic-chain exercises were discussed in detail in Chapter 11. In the case of patellofemoral rehabili-

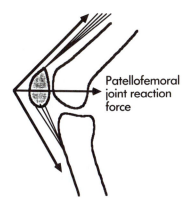

Figure 23-65   Patellofemoral joint reaction forces (PFJRF).

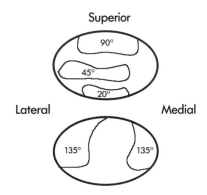

Figure 23-66   Compression force and contact stress. Even though compression forces increase with increasing knee flexion, the amount of contact stress per unit area decreases.

tation, minisquats from 0 to 40 degrees (Figure 23-9), leg press from 0 to 60 degrees (Figure 23-12), lateral step-ups using an 8-inch step (Figure 23-13), a stepping machine (Figure 23-17), a stationary bike (Figure 23-18), slide board exercises (Figure 23-15), and a Fitter (Figure 23-16) are all examples of closed-kinetic-chain strengthening exercises that may be used in patellofemoral rehabilitation.

Regaining optimal patellar positioning and tracking.   This second goal in our current treatment approach is based on the work of an Australian physiotherapist, Jenny McConnell.[30,55] This goal can be accomplished by stretching the tight lateral structures, correcting patellar orientation, and improving the timing and force of the VMO contraction.

Stretching. Successfully stretching the tight lateral structures involves a combination of both active and passive stretching techniques. Active stretching techniques include mobilization techniques as discussed in Chapter 12. Specific techniques should involve medial patellar glides and medial patellar tilts along the longitudinal axis of the patella (Figure 23-44). Passive stretch is accomplished through a long-duration stretch created by the use of very specific taping techniques to alter patellar alignment and orientation.

Correcting patellar orientation. After a thorough assessment of patellofemoral mechanics as described earlier, the sports therapist should have the athlete perform an activity that produces patellofemoral pain, such as step-ups or double- or single-leg squats to establish a baseline for comparison.

It should be stressed that not all individuals who complain of patellofemoral pain exhibit a positive patellar orientation component. In athletes who do, patellofemoral orientation can be corrected to some degree by using tape.

Correction of patellar positioning and tracking is accomplished by using passive taping of the patella in a more biomechanically correct position. In addition to correcting the orientation of the patella, the tape provides a prolonged stretch to the soft-tissue structures that affect patellar movement.

Taping should be done using two separate types of highly adhesive tape available from several different manufacturers. A base layer using white tape is applied directly to the skin from the lateral femoral condyle to just posterior to the medial femoral condyle, making certain that the patella is completely covered by the base layer (Figure 23-67). This tape is used as a base to which the other tape is adhered to correct patellar alignment. The glide component should always be corrected first, followed by the component found to be the most excessive. If no positive glide exists, begin with the most pronounced component found.

The glide component should always be corrected with the knee in full extension. To correct a positive lateral glide, attach the tape one thumb's breadth from the lateral patellar border, push the patella medially, gather the soft tissue over the medial condyle, push toward the condyle, and adhere to the medial condyle (Figure 23-68).

The tilt component should be corrected with the knee flexed 30 to 45 degrees. To correct a positive lateral tilt, from the middle of the patella pull medially to lift the lateral border. Again, gather the skin underneath, and adhere to the medial condyle (Figure 23-69).

The rotational component is corrected in 30 to 40 degrees of flexion. To correct a positive external rotation, from the middle of the inferior border pull upward and medially while rotating the superior pole externally (Figure 23-70).

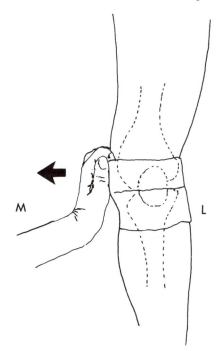

Figure 23-67 Application of base tape.

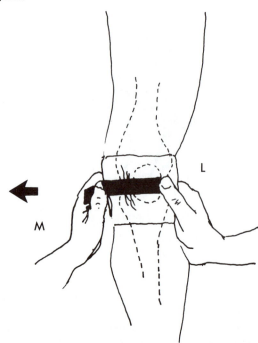

Figure 23-68 Taping to correct positive lateral glide.

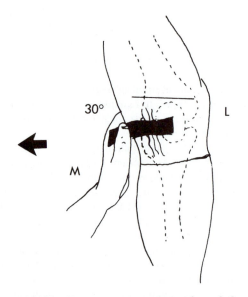

Figure 23-69 Taping to correct positive lateral tile.

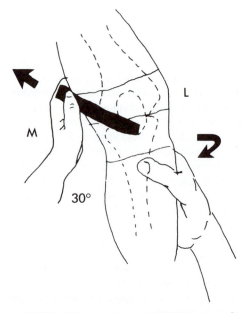

Figure 23-70 Taping to correct positive external rotation.

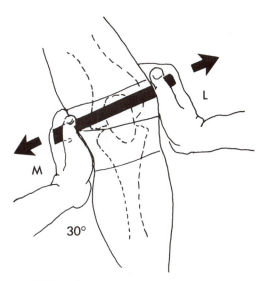

Figure 23-71 Taping to correct positive inferior anteroposterior tilt.

To correct a positive anteroposterior inferior tilt, place the knee in full extension. Adhere a 6-inch strip of tape over the upper half of the patella, and press directly posterior, adhering with equal pressure on both sides (Figure 23-71).

One piece of tape can be used to correct two components simultaneously. For example, when correcting a lateral glide along with an anteroposterior inferior tilt, follow the same taping procedure for the glide component except that the tape should be applied to the upper half of the patella.

After this taping procedure, the sports therapist should reassess the activity that caused the athlete's pain. In many cases the athlete will indicate improvement almost immediately. If not, the order of the taping or the way the patella is taped may have to be changed considerably. The tape should be worn 24 hours a day initially, and the sports therapist should instruct the athlete in how to adjust and tighten the tape as necessary.

It is important to understand that taping changes the forces acting on the patella and thus the kinematics of the knee joint. Taping essentially attempts to decrease the lateral pull on the patella. When combined with an increase in the force and timing of the VMO contraction, this will result in alteration of the balance of forces on the patella. Interestingly, a study by Bockrath et al. demonstrated that patellar taping reduced pain in patients with anterior knee pain, but radiographic studies before and after taping revealed no change in patellofemoral congruency or patellar rotational angles. Hence the reduction in pain was not associated with positional change of the patella.[8]

Reestablishing neuromuscular control. Establishing neuromuscular control involves improving the timing and force of VMO contraction. It is perhaps most important for the sports therapist to emphasize the quality rather than the quantity of the contraction. This means that training the VMO should concentrate more on motor skill acquisition than on strengthening activities. Strengthening should occur concomitantly with improvement in motor skill.

As mentioned previously the VMO:VL strength ratio should be 1:1. In athletes who have a VMO:VL ratio of less than 1:1 with patellofemoral pain, training efforts should focus on selectively strengthening the VMO. Isolating and training the VMO selectively requires concentration on the part of the athlete. Techniques of facilitation, such as manually stroking or taping the VMO or the use of biofeedback, are recommended. The use of a dual-channel biofeedback unit capable of monitoring both VMO and VL electromyographic activity can help the athlete gain neuromuscular control over both the force of contraction and timing for the firing of the VMO.

The VMO is a tonic muscle that acts to stabilize the patella both statically and dynamically, so it should be active throughout the range of motion. Training goals should be directed toward increasing the force of the VMO contraction both concentrically and eccentrically throughout the range of motion. Because the VMO arises from the adductor magnus tendon, adduction exercises may be used to facilitate VMO contraction. The VMO should be trained to respond to a new length-tension relationship between the agonist (VMO) and the antagonist (VL).

Several sources have indicated that the VMO has a separate nerve supply from the rest of the quadriceps, although this is in our opinion somewhat debatable.[4,10,24] Nevertheless, assuming this is the case, then the athlete should be taught to fire the VMO before the VL. Neuromuscular control of the VMO firing should help the athlete maintain appropriate patellar alignment.

VMO exercises should concentrate on controlling the firing of the VMO. Exercises should be performed slowly and with concentration to selectively activate muscles. The sports therapist should address concentric and eccentric control in a variety of functional tasks and positions. Minisquats, step-ups or step-downs, and leg presses are good exercises for establishing concentric and eccentric control. Training on a BAPS board is useful for proprioceptive training (Figure 23-48). It is extremely important to concentrate on VMO control during gait-training activities.

Criteria for Return. Taping should continue throughout the VMO training period. Again, tape should initially be worn 24 hours a day. The athlete may be weaned from tape progressively when he or she demonstrates VMO control. Examples of functional criteria for weaning would be when the athlete can keep the VMO activated for 5 minutes during a walking gait and when the athlete can fire the VMO either before or simultaneously with the vastus lateralis consistently in step-downs for 1 minute. At this point, tape may be left off every third day for 1 week, then every second day for 1 week, then worn only during activity, and finally worn only if pain is present. Taping can be eliminated altogether when the athlete can perform step-downs for 5 minutes with appropriate timing and when she or he can sustain a quarter to a half squat for 1 minute without VMO loss.

Chondromalacia Patella

Pathomechanics and Injury Mechanism. Chondromalacia patella can occur either as a consequence of patellofemoral stress syndrome or from a direct impact to the patella. It is a softening and deterioration of the articular cartilage on the back of the patella that has been described as undergoing three stages: swelling and softening of the articular cartilage, fissuring of the softened articular cartilage, and deformation of the surface of the articular cartilage caused by fragmentation.[13]

The exact cause of chondromalacia is unknown. As indicated previously, abnormal patellar tracking could be a major etiological factor. However, individuals with normal tracking have acquired chondromalacia, and some individuals with abnormal tracking are free of it.[9]

The athlete may experience pain in the anterior aspect of the knee while walking, running, ascending and descending stairs, or squatting. There may be recurrent swelling around the kneecap and a grating sensation when flexing and extending the knee. There may also be crepitation and pain during a patellar grind test. During palpation there may be pain on the inferior border of the patella or when the patella is compressed within the femoral groove while the knee is passively flexed and extended. Degenerative arthritis occurs on the lateral facet of the patella, which makes contact with the femur when the athlete performs a full squat.[9] Degeneration first occurs in the deeper portions of the articular cartilage, followed by blistering and fissuring that stems from the subchondral bone and appears on the surface of the patella.[9,13]

Rehabilitation Concerns. Chondromalacia patella is initially treated conservatively using the same rehabilitation plan as was described for patellofemoral stress syndrome.[54] If conservative measures fail to help, surgery may be the only alternative. Some of the following surgical measures have been recommended:[9] realignment procedures such as lateral release of the retinaculum; moving the insertion of the vastus medialis muscle forward; shaving and smoothing the irregular surfaces of the patella and/or femoral condyle; in cases of degenerative arthritis, removing the lesion through drilling; elevating the tibial tubercle; or, as a last resort, completely removing the patella.

Rehabilitation Progression. Chondromalacia patella is a degenerative process that unfortunately does not tend to get better or resolve with time. There are times when the knee is painful and other times when it feels all right. Perhaps the key to managing chondromalacia is to maintain strength of the quadriceps muscle group and in particular the VMO. Closed-chain exercises are recommended because they tend to decrease the patellofemoral joint reaction forces. The athlete must be consistent in these strengthening efforts.

Irritating activities that tend to exacerbate pain, such as stair climbing, squatting. and long periods of sitting, should be avoided. Isometric exercises or closed-chain isotonics performed through a pain-free arc to strengthen the quadriceps and hamstring muscles should be routinely done. The use of oral anti-inflammatory agents and small doses of aspirin may help to modulate pain. Wearing a neoprene knee sleeve helps certain athletes but does absolutely nothing for others. Use of an orthotic device to correct pronation and reduce tibial torsion is helpful in many instances.

Criteria for Return. As long as the athlete can tolerate the pain and discomfort that occurs with chondromalacia patella, they can continue to train and compete. Again the key is essentially to "play games" with this condition, training normally when there is no pain and backing off when the knee is painful.

Acute Patellar Subluxation or Dislocation

Pathomechanics. The patella, as it tracks superiorly and inferiorly in the femoral groove, can be subject to direct trauma or degenerative changes, leading to chronic pain and disability.[34] Of major importance among athletes are those conditions that stem from abnormal patellar tracking within the femoral groove. Improper patellar tracking leading to patellar subluxation or dislocation can result from a number of biomechanical factors, including femoral anteversion with increased internal femoral rotation; genu valgum with a concomitant increase in the Q-angle; a shallow femoral groove; flat lateral femoral condyles; patella alta; weakness of the vastus medialis muscle relative to the vastus lateralis; ligamentous laxity with genu recurvatum; excessive external rotation of the tibia; pronated feet; a tight lateral retinaculum; and a patella with a positive lateral tilt. Each of these factors was discussed in detail earlier in this chapter.

Injury Mechanism. When the athlete plants the foot, decelerates, and simultaneously cuts in an opposite direction from the weight-bearing foot, the thigh rotates internally while the lower leg rotates externally, causing a forced knee valgus. The quadriceps muscle attempts to pull in a straight line and as a result pulls the patella laterally, creating a force that can sublux the patella. As a rule, displacement takes place laterally, with the patella shifting over the lateral condyle.

A chronically subluxing patella places abnormal stress on the patellofemoral joint and the medial restraints. The knee may be swollen and painful. Pain is a result of swelling but also results because the medial capsular tissue has been stretched and torn. Because of the associated swelling the knee is restricted in flexion and extension. There may also be a palpable tenderness over the adductor tubercle where the medial retinaculum (patellar femoral ligament) attaches.

Acute patellar dislocation most often occurs when the foot is planted and there is contact with another athlete on the medial surface of the patella, forcing it to dislocate laterally. The athlete reports a painful "giving way" episode. The athlete experiences a complete loss of knee function, pain, and swelling, with the patella remaining in an abnormal lateral position. A physician should immediately reduce the dislocation by applying mild pressure on the patella with the knee extended as much as possible. If a period of time has elapsed before reduction, a general anesthetic may have to be used. After aspiration of the joint hematoma, ice is applied, and the joint is immobilized. A first-time patellar dislocation is sometimes associated with loose bodies from a chondral or osteochondral fracture as well as articular cartilage lesions. Thus some physicians advocate arthroscopic examination following patellar dislocation.[74]

Rehabilitation Progression.

Chronic patellar subluxation. Rehabilitation for a chronically subluxing patella should focus on addressing each of the potential biomechanical factors that either individually or collectively contribute to the pathomechanics. It is important to regain a balance in strength of all musculature associated with the knee joint. Postural malalignments must be corrected as much as possible. Shoe orthotic devices may be used to reduce foot pronation and tibial internal rotation, and subsequently to reduce stress to the patellofemoral joint.

Particular attention should be given to strengthening the quadriceps through closed-kinetic-chain exercises; strengthening the hip abductors (Figure 23-2),

hip adductors (Figure 23-3), and gastrocnemius (Figure 23-8); stretching the tight lateral structures using a combination of patellar mobilization glides (Figure 23-44) and medial patellar tilts along the longitudinal axis of the patella as well as stretching for the iliotibial band (Figure 23-36) and biceps femoris (Figure 23-39); correcting patellar orientation; and establishing neuromuscular control by improving the timing and force of the VMO contraction.

If the athlete does not respond to extensive efforts by the sports therapist to correct the pathomechanics and subluxation remains a recurrent problem, surgical intervention may be necessary. However, a surgical release of the lateral retinacular ligaments does not appear to be a particularly effective procedure and should be done only after failure of more conservative treatment.

Acute patellar dislocation. In the case of acute patellar dislocation, following reduction the knee should be placed in an immobilizer immediately, and it is recommended that it remain in place for 3 to 6 weeks with the athlete ambulating on crutches until regaining full extension and walking without an extension lag. The athlete can begin immediately following the dislocation with isometric quad sets (Figure 23-4) and straight leg raising (Figure 23-5), always paying close attention to achieving a good contraction of the VMO. Early pain-free range-of-motion exercises including knee slides on a treatment table (Figure 23-30), wall slides (Figure 23-31), or active assistive slides (Figure 23-32) can be used.

As pain subsides and ROM improves, the athlete should incorporate closed-chain strengthening exercises (Figure 23-9 through 23-18) to minimize stress on the patellofemoral joint. Strengthening should be directed toward increasing the force of the VMO contraction both concentrically and eccentrically throughout the range of motion. Neuromuscular control of the VMO firing should help the athlete maintain appropriate patellar alignment. It is also important to concentrate on VMO control during gait-training activities.

After 3 to 6 weeks when immobilization is discontinued, the athlete should wear a neoprene knee sleeve with a lateral horseshoe-shaped felt pad that helps the patella track medially (Figure 23-72). This support should be worn while running or performing in sports.

Criteria for Return. The athlete should have good quadriceps strength and should be able to demonstrate VMO control during functional activities. Examples of functional criteria would be when the athlete can keep the VMO activated for 5 minutes during a walking gait and when the athlete can fire the VMO either before or simultaneously with the vastus lateralis consistently in step-downs for 1 minute. The athlete should be able to

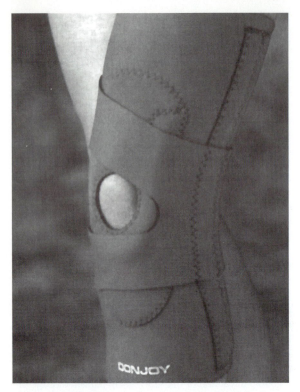

Figure 23-72 A brace that can help limit patellar dislocation and/or subluxation should have a felt horseshoe applied laterally.

perform step-downs for 5 minutes with appropriate timing and sustain a quarter to a half squat for 1 minute without VMO loss.

Patellar Tendinitis (Jumper's Knee)

Pathomechanics and Injury Mechanism. Jumper's knee occurs when chronic inflammation develops in the patellar tendon either at the superior patellar pole (usually referred to as quadriceps tendinitis), the tibial tuburcle, or most commonly at the distal pole of the patella (patellar tendinitis). It usually develops in athletes involved in activities that require repetitive jumping; hence the name. Point tenderness on the posterior aspect of the inferior pole of the patella is the hallmark of patellar tendinitis. This condition is felt to be related to the shock-absorbing function (an eccentric contraction) that the quadriceps provides upon landing from a jump. Initially the athlete complains of a dull aching pain after jumping or running following repetitive jumping activities. Pain usually disappears with rest but returns with activity. Pain becomes progressively worse until the ath-

lete is unable to continue. There are also reports of difficulty in stair climbing and an occasional feeling of "giving way."

Rehabilitation Concerns. Because jumper's knee involves a chronic inflammation, rehabilitation strategies may take one of two courses. The sports therapist may choose to use traditional techniques designed to reduce the inflammation, which include rest, anti-inflammatory medication, ice, and ultrasound. Another, more aggressive approach would be to use a transverse friction massage technique designed to exacerbate the acute inflammation, so that the healing process is no longer "stuck" in the inflammatory-response phase and can move on to the fibroblastic-repair phase. The technique involves a 5- to 7-minute friction massage at the inferior pole of the patella in a direction perpendicular to the direction of the tendon fibers, performed every other day for approximately 1 week. During this treatment, all other medicative or modality efforts to reduce inflammation should be eliminated. It is our experience that if pain is not decreased after 4 or 5 treatments it is unlikely that this technique will resolve the problem.

Ruptures of the patellar tendon are rare in young athletes but increase in incidence with age. A sudden powerful contraction of the quadriceps muscle with the weight of the body applied to the affected leg can cause a rupture of the patellar tendon.[86] The rupture may occur to the quadriceps tendon or to the patellar tendon. Usually rupture does not occur unless there has been a prolonged period of inflammation of the patellar tendon that has weakened the tendon. Seldom does a rupture occur in the middle of the tendon; usually the tendon is torn from its attachment. The quadriceps tendon ruptures from the superior pole of the patella, whereas the patellar tendon ruptures from the inferior pole of the patella. A rupture of the patellar tendon usually requires surgical repair.

Rehabilitation Progression. Regardless of which of the two treatment approaches is used, once the problem begins to resolve, the athlete should engage in a thorough warm-up prior to activity. Initially, jumping and running activities should be restricted. Strengthening of the quadriceps is critical during rehabilitation. Success has been reported using eccentric strengthening exercises for both the quadriceps and the ankle dorsiflexors.[17,42,56] Curwin and Stanish have theorized that a graded program of eccentric stress will stimulate the tendon to heal.[17] They feel that rest does not stimulate healing, while low- to moderate-level eccentric exercise will. Their program consists of five parts: warm-up, stretching, eccentric squatting, stretching, and ice.[5,17] The eccentric squats, called drop squats, are performed

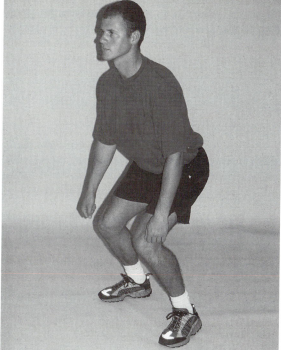

Figure 23-73 Drop squats are performed with the athlete moving slowly from standing to a squat position and return.

with the athlete moving slowly from standing to a squat position and return. To increase stress, the speed of the drop is increased until a mild level of pain is experienced (Figure 23-73). The goal is to perform 3 sets of 10 repetitions at a speed that causes mild pain during the last set. The presence of mild pain is indicative of the mild stress.

Jensen and DiFabio have suggested treating patellar tendinitis with a program of isokinetic eccentric quadriceps training[43] (Figure 23-22). The program begins with 6 sets of 5 repetitions at 30 degrees per second 3 times per week, progressing over an 8-week period to 4 sets of 5 repetitions each at 30, 50, and 70 degrees per second.[43] Vigorous quadriceps and hamstring stretching precede and follow each workout (Figures 23-38, 23-39).

The use of a tenodesis strap or brace worn about the patellar tendon has also been recommended for patellar tendinitis (Figure 23-74). It appears that the effectiveness of this strap in reducing pain varies from one athlete to another.

Injection of cortisone into the tendon to reduce inflammation is not recommended because it will tend to weaken the tendon and can predispose the athlete to patellar tendon rupture.

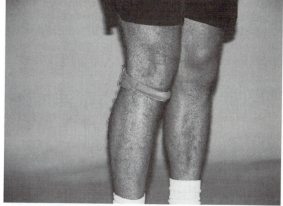

Figure 23-74 A tenodesis strap can be used to help control patellar tendinitis.

Criteria for Return. The athlete may return to full activity when pain has subsided to the point where he or she is capable of performing jumping and running activities without increased swelling or exacerbation of pain. There should be normal strength in the quadriceps bilaterally.

Bursitis

Pathophysiology. Bursitis in the knee can be acute, chronic, or recurrent. Although any one of the numerous knee bursae can become inflamed, anteriorly the prepatellar, deep infrapatellar, and suprapatellar bursae have the highest incidence of irritation in sports. The pathophysiological reaction that occurs with bursitis follows the normal course of the inflammatory response as described in Chapter 2.

Swelling patterns can often help differentiate bursitis from other conditions in the injured knee. With bursitis, swelling is localized to the bursa. For example, prepatellar bursitis results in localized swelling above the knee that is ballottable. In the more severe cases it may seem to extend over the lower portion of the vastus medialis. Swelling is not intra-articular, and there may be some redness and increased temperature. In acute prepatellar bursitis the range of motion of the knee is not restricted except in the last degrees of flexion when pain-producing pressure is felt in the bursa, whereas a true hemarthrosis or synovitis of the knee joint most frequently shows a more significant limitation of terminal flexion and extension of the joint.[9]

Injuries to the ligaments of the knee and also fractures of the patella may occur along with acute prepatellar bursitis. Patellar fractures can occur from a direct blow to the patella with the knee held in flexion. A violent contraction of the quadriceps mechanism can also produce transverse patellar fractures, which should be ruled out with radiographs. Infection of the infrapatellar bursa can be similarly difficult to diagnosis because of its deep location. It is a rare condition and requires aspiration for diagnosis.

Swelling posteriorly in the popliteal fossa does not necessarily indicate bursitis but could instead be a sign of Baker's cyst. A Baker's cyst is connected to the joint, which swells because of a problem in the joint and not due to bursitis. A Baker's cyst is often asymptomatic, causing little or no discomfort or disability.

Injury Mechanism. The cause of prepatellar bursitis can involve either a single trauma, as would occur in falling on a flexed knee, or it can result from repetitive crawling or kneeling on the knee, as would occur in wrestling. Acute or posttraumatic inflammation is not uncommon. The prepatellar bursa is more likely to become inflamed from continued kneeling, whereas the deep infrapatellar becomes irritated from repetitive stress to the patellar tendon, as is the case in jumper's knee.

Rehabilitation Concerns and Progression. Acute prepatellar bursitis should be treated conservatively, and rehabilitation should begin with ice, compression, anti-inflammatory medication, and possibly a brief period of immobilization in a knee splint. If necessary the athlete should walk on crutches until they have regained quadriceps control and can ambulate without a limp. The compression wrap should be applied from the foot upward to the middle of the thigh in a manner that maintains constant pressure on the bursa. The leg should be elevated as much as possible. The athlete should begin with quad sets (Figure 23-4) and straight leg raising (Figure 23-5), both to maintain function of the quadriceps and to use active muscle contractions to help facilitate resorption of fluid. On the second day, the athlete may begin ROM exercises doing knee slides on a treatment table (Figure 23-30), wall slides (Figure 23-31), or active assistive slides (Figure 23-32). The compression wrap should be left in place until there is no evidence of fluid reaccumulation.

Occasionally, a physician may choose to aspirate the bursa to relieve the pressure and speed up the recovery period. If so it is essential to take necessary precautions to prevent contamination and subsequent infection. If infection does occur, it should be treated with antibiotics.

In cases of chronic bursitis, the techniques for controlling swelling listed above should be used. A compression wrap needs to be worn constantly. Unfortunately there will generally not be complete resolution. Chronic bursitis becomes a recurrent problem with thickening of

the bursa and reaccumulation of fluid. In these cases injection with a corticosteroid or surgical excision of the bursa may be necessary.

Criteria for Return. The athlete may return to full activity when there is no reaccumulation of fluid following their exercises, when there is full ROM, and when there is normal quadriceps control.

Iliotibial Band Friction Syndrome

Pathomechanics. The iliotibial band is a tendinous extension of the fascia covering the gluteus maximus and tensor fasciae latae muscles proximally; it attaches distally at Gerdy's tubercle on the proximal portion of the lateral tibial. As the athlete flexes and extends the knee, the tendon glides anteriorly and posteriorly over the lateral femoral condyle. This repetitive motion, as typically occurs in runners, may produce irritation and inflammation of the tendon.

Iliotibial band friction syndrome involves localized pain about 2 cm above the joint line over the lateral femoral condyle when the knee is in 30 degrees of flexion. Pain appears to radiate toward the lateral joint line and down toward the proximal tibia, becoming increasingly severe as the athlete continues to run. Eventually it becomes so symptomatic that the activity must be discontinued. The athlete has tenderness, crepitus, and an area of swelling over the lateral condyle. In some instances athletes with iliotibial band friction syndrome also have a history of trochanteric bursitis and pain along the iliac crest at the origin at the tensor fasciae latae.

Leg length discrepancies, contractures of the tensor fasciae latae and gluteus maximus, tightness of the hamstrings and quadriceps, genu varum, excessive pronation leading to increased internal tibial torsion, and a tight heel cord can individually or collectively increase the tension of the iliotibial band across the femoral condyle. Ober's test to detect tightness in this muscle group will be positive.

Injury Mechanism. As is the case in many injuries associated with running, there is often a history of poor training techniques that may include running on irregular surfaces (such as on the side of the road), downhill running, or running long distances without gradually building up to that level. Symptoms frequently develop in athletes who do not have an adequate stretching program.

Rehabilitation Concerns and Progression. Initial treatment for iliotibial band friction syndrome is directed at reducing the local inflammatory reaction by using rest, ice, ultrasound, and oral anti-inflammatory medications. Rehabilitation should focus on correcting the underlying biomechanical factors that may cause the problem. If Ober's test is positive, stretching exercises to correct this static contracture should be used (Figure 23-36). Some athletes also have hip flexion contractures with a positive Thomas test and require stretching of the iliopsoas and the anterior capsule, as well as the tensor fasciae latae.

During normal gait, pronation leads to an obligatory internal rotation of the tibia. Orthotics may help reduce this pronation and relieve symptoms at the knee. Generally 4 to 6 weeks of conservative treatment is required to control the symptoms of iliotibial band syndrome. While conservative treatment is usually effective in controlling symptoms, occasionally cases of iliotibial band syndrome do not respond and require surgical treatment.

As was the case with patellar tendinitis, transverse friction massage used to increase the inflammatory response appears to be effective in treating iliotibial band friction syndrome. A 5- to 7-minute friction massage to the iliotibial band over the lateral femoral condyle in a direction perpendicular to the direction of the tendon fibers, should be done every other day for approximately 1 week. During this treatment, all other medicative or modality efforts to reduce inflammation should be eliminated.

Criteria for Return.   When the local tenderness over the lateral epicondyle has subsided, the athlete may resume running but should avoid prolonged workouts and running on hills and irregular surfaces. If it is necessary to run on the side of the road, it is essential that the patient alternate sides of the road during workouts. Shortening the stride and applying ice after running may also be beneficial.

Patellar Plica

Pathomechanics.   A plica is a fold in the synovial lining of the knee that is a remnant from the embryological development within the knee. The most common synovial fold is the infrapatellar plica, which originates from the infrapatellar fat pad and extends superiorly in a fanlike manner. The second most common synovial fold is the suprapatellar plica, located in the suprapatellar pouch. The least common, but most subject to injury, is the mediopatellar plica, which is bandlike, begins on the medial wall of the knee joint, and extends downward to insert into the synovial tissue that covers the infrapatellar fat pad.[7] The medipatellar plica can bowstring across the anteromedial femoral condyle, impinging between the articular cartilage and the medial facet of the patella with increasing flexion. A plica is often associated with a torn meniscus, patellar malalignment, or osteoarthritis. Because most synovial plicae are pliable, most are asympto-

matic; however, the mediopatellar plica may be thick, nonyielding, and fibrotic, causing a number of symptoms.

Injury Mechanism.   The athlete may or may not have a history of knee injury. If symptoms are preceded by trauma, it is usually one of blunt force such as falling on the knee or of twisting with the foot planted, either of which can lead to inflammation and hemorrhage. Inflammations leads to fibrosis and thickening with a loss of extensibility.

As the knee passes 15 to 20 degrees of flexion, a snap may be felt or heard. Internal and external tibial rotation can also produce this snapping. The mediopatellar plica can snap over the medial femoral condyle, contributing to the development of chondromalacia.[7] A major complaint is recurrent episodes of painful pseudolocking of the knee when sitting for a period of time. Such characteristics of locking and snapping could be misinterpreted as a torn meniscus. The athlete complains of pain while ascending or descending stairs or when squatting. Unlike meniscal injuries, there is little or no swelling and no ligamentous laxity.

Rehabilitation Concerns and Progression.   Initially, a plica should be treated conservatively to control inflammation with rest, anti-inflammatory agents, and local heat. If the plica is associated with improper patellar tracking, the pathomechanics should be corrected as previously discussed. If conservative treatment is unsuccessful, the plica may be surgically excised, usually with good results.[21]

Criteria for Return.   The athlete can return to full activity when she or he can perform normal functional activities with minimal or no pain and without a recurrence of swelling.

Osgood-Schlatter Disease

Pathomechanics and Injury Mechanism.   Two conditions common to the immature adolescent's knee are Osgood-Schlatter disease and Larsen-Johansson disease. Osgood-Shlatter disease is characterized by pain and swelling over the tibial tuberosity that increases with activity and decreases with rest. Traditionally Osgood-Schlatter disease was described as either a partial avulsion of the tibial tubercle or an avascular necrosis of the same. Current thinking views it more as an apophysitis characterized by pain at the attachment of the patellar tendon at the tibial tubercle with associated extensor mechanism problems. The most commonly accepted cause of Osgood-Schlatter disease is repeated stress of the patellar tendon at the apophysis of the tibial tubercle. Complete avulsion of the patellar tendon is a uncommon complication of Osgood-Schlatter disease.

This condition first appears in adolescents and usually resolves when the athlete reaches the age of 18 or 19. The only remnant is an enlarged tibial tubercle. Repeated irritation causes swelling, hemorrhage, and gradual degeneration of the apophysis as a result of impaired circulation. The athlete complains of severe pain when kneeling, jumping, and running. There is point tenderness over the anterior proximal tibial tubercle.

Larsen-Johansson disease, although much less common, is similar to Osgood-Schlatter disease, but it occurs at the inferior pole of the patella. As with Osgood-Schlatter disease, the cause is believed to be excessive repeated strain on the patellar tendon. Swelling, pain, and point tenderness characterize Larsen-Johansson disease. Later, degeneration can be noted during X-ray examination.

Rehabilitation Concerns and Progression. Management is usually conservative and includes the following: Stressful activities are decreased until the apophyseal union occurs, usually within 6 months to 1 year; ice is applied to the knee before and after activities; isometric strengthening of quadriceps and hamstring muscles is performed; and severe cases may require a cylindrical cast.

Treatment is symptomatic with emphasis on icing, quadriceps strengthening, hamstring stretching, and activity modification. Only in extreme cases is immobilization necessary.

Summary

1. To be effective in a knee rehabilitation program, the sports therapist must have a good understanding of the functional anatomy and biomechanics of knee joint motion.

2. Techniques of strengthening involving closed-kinetic-chain, isometric, isotonic, isokinetic, and plyometric exercises are recommended after injury to the knee because of their safety and because they are more functional than open-chain exercises.

3. Range of motion may be restricted either by lack of physiological motion, which may be corrected by stretching, or by lack of accessory motions, which may be corrected by patellar mobilization techniques. Constant passive motion may be used postoperatively to assist the athlete in regaining range of motion.

4. PCL, MCL, and LCL injuries are generally treated nonoperatively, and the athlete is progressed back into activity rapidly within their limitations.

5. The current surgical procedure of choice for ACL reconstruction uses an intra-articular patellar tendon graft.

6. Recent trends in rehabilitation after ACL reconstruction are toward an aggressive, accelerated program that emphasizes immediate motion, immediate weight bearing, early closed-chain strengthening exercises, and early return to activity.

7. The current trend in treating meniscal tears is to surgically repair the defect if possible or perform a partial meniscectomy arthroscopically. Repaired menisci should be immobilized NWB for 4 to 6 weeks.

8. It is critical to assess the mechanics of the patellofemoral joint in terms of static alignment, dynamic alignment, and patellar orientation to determine what specifically is causing pain.

9. Rehabilitation of patellofemoral pain concentrates on strengthening the quadriceps through closed-kinetic-chain exercises, regaining optimal patellar positioning and tracking, and regaining neuromuscular control to improve lower-limb mechanics.

References

1. Anderson, C., and J. Gillquist. 1992. Treatment of acute isolated and combined ruptures of the ACL: A long-term follow-up study. *American Journal of Sports Medicine* 20:7–12.

2. Anderson, A., R. Snyder, and C. Federspiel. 1992. Instrumented evaluation of knee laxity: A comparison of five arthrometers. *American Journal of Sports Medicine* 20:135–40.

3. Arno, S. 1990. The A-angle: A quantitative measurement of patellar alignment and realignment. *Journal of Orthopaedic and Sports Physical Therapy* 12[C]:237–42.

4. Basmajian, J., and C. DeLuca. 1985. *Muscles alive: Their functions revealed by electromyography.* Baltimore: Williams & Wilkins.

5. Bennet, J., and W. Stauber. 1986. Evaluation and treatment of anterior knee pain using eccentric exercise. *Medicine and Science in Sports and Exercise* 18(5).

6. Black, K., and W. Raasch. 1995. Knee braces in sports. In *The lower extremity and spine in sports medicine,* edited by J. Nicholas and E. Hershman. St. Louis: Mosby.

7. Blackburn, T. 1982. An introduction to the plica. *Journal of Orthopaedic and Sports Physical Therapy* 3:171.

8. Bockrath, K. 1993. *Effect of patellar taping on patellar position and perceived pain.* Poster presentation. APTA Combined Sections, San Antonio.

9. Boland, A., and M. Hulstyn. 1995. Soft tissue injuries of the knee. In *The lower extremity and spine in sports medicine,* edited by J. Nicholas, and E. Hershman. St. Louis: Mosby.

10. Bose, K., R. Kanagasuntheram, and M. Osman. 1980. Vastus medialis oblique: An anatomic and physiologic study. *Orthopaedics* 3:880–83.

11. Brewster, C., D. Moynes, and F. Jobe. 1983. Rehabilitation for the anterior cruciate reconstruction. *Journal of Orthopaedic and Sports Physical Therapy* 5:121–26.

12. Brotzman, B., and P. Head. 1996. The knee. In *Clinical Orthopedic rehabilitation,* edited by B. Brotzman. St. Louis: Mosby.

13. Calliet, R. 1983. *Knee pain and disability.* Philadelphia: F. A. Davis.

14. Cavenaugh, J. 1991. Rehabilitation following meniscal surgery. In *Knee ligament rehabilitation,* edited by R. Engle. New York: Churchill Livingstone.

15. Clancy, W., D. Nelson, and B. Reider. 1982. Anterior cruciate ligament reconstruction using one third of the patellar ligament augmented by extra-articular tendon transfers. *Journal of Bone and Joint Surgery* 62A:352.

16. Clancy, W., R. Narechania, and T. Rosenberg. 1981. Anterior and posterior cruciate ligament reconstruction in rhesus monkeys. *Journal of Bone and Joint Surgery* 63A:1270–84.

17. Curwin, S., and W. D. Stanish. 1984. *Tendinitis: Its etiology and treatment.* New York: Collamore Press.

18. DeHaven, K., and R. Bronstein. 1995. Injuries to the meniscii in the knee. In *The lower extremity and spine in sports medicine,* edited by J. Nicholas and E. Hershman. St. Louis: Mosby.

19. DeLee, J., M. Riley, and C. Rockwood. 1983. Acute straight lateral instability of the knee. *American Journal of Sports Medicine* 11:404–11.

20. DePalma, B., and R. Zelko. 1986. Knee rehabilitation following anterior cruciate injury or surgery. *JNATA* 21(3): 200–206.

21. Dorchak, J. 1991. Arthroscopic treatment of symptomatic synovial plica of the knee. *American Journal of Sports Medicine* 19:503.

22. Engle, R., and D. Giesen. 1991. ACL reconstruction rehabilitation. In *Knee ligament rehabilitation,* edited by R. Engle. New York: Churchill Livingstone.

23. Ferguson, D. 1988. Return to functional activities. *Sports Medicine Update* 3(3): 6–9.

24. Ficat, P., and D. Hungerford. 1977. *Disorders of the patellofemoral joint.* Baltimore: Williams & Wilkins.

25. Fu, F., S. Woo, J. Irrgang, et al. 1992. Current concepts for rehabilitation following ACL reconstruction. *Journal of Orthopaedic and Sports Physical Therapy* 15(6): 270–78.

26. Fulkerson, J. 1989. Evaluation of peripatellar soft tissues and retinaculum in patients with patellofemoral pain. *Clin Sports Med* 8(2): 197–202.

27. Fulkerson, J., and D. Hungerford. 1990. *Disorders of the patellofemoral joint.* Baltimore: Williams & Wilkins.

28. Garret, J., and R. Stevensen. 1991. Meniscal transplantation in the human knee: A preliminary report. *Arthroscopy* 7:57–62.

29. Geissler, W., and T. Whipple. 1993. Intraarticular abnormalities in association with PCL injuries. *American Journal of Sports Medicine* 21:846–49.

30. Gerrard, B. 1989. The patellofemoral pain syndrome: A clinical trial of the McConnell program. *Australian Journal of Physiotherapy* 35(2): 71–80.

31. Goodfellow, J., D. Hungerford, and C. Woods. 1976. Patellofemoral mechanics and pathology: II. Chondromalacia patella. *Journal of Bone and Joint Surgery* 58[B]: 287.

32. Gould, J., and G. Davies. 1990. *Orthopaedic and sports physical therapy.* St Louis: Mosby.

33. Harner, C., J. Irrgang, and L. Paul. 1992. Loss of motion after ACL reconstruction. *American Journal of Sports Medicine* 20:99–506.

34. Hughston, J., W. Walsh, and G. Puddu. 1984. *Patellar subluxation and dislocation.* Philadelphia: W. B. Saunders.

35. Hungerford, D., and M. Barry. 1979. Biomechanics of the patellofemoral joint. *Clin Ortho* 144:9–15.

36. Indelicato, P., J. Hermansdorfer, and M. Huegel. 1990. Non-operative management of incomplete tears of the MCL of the knee in intercollegiate football players. *Clin Orthop* 256:174–77.

37. Inoue, M. 1987. Treatment of MCL injury: The importance of the ACL ligament on varus-valgus knee laxity. *American Journal of Sports Medicine* 15:15.

38. Insall, J. 1979. Chondromalacia patella: Patellar malalignment syndromes. *Orthop Clin North Am* 10:117–25.

39. Irrgang, J., M. Safran, and F. Fu. 1995. The knee: Ligamentous and meniscal injuries. In *Athletic Injuries and rehabilitation,* edited by J. Zachazewski, D. Magee, and W. Quillen. Philadelphia: W. B. Saunders.

40. Jackson, D., and D. Drez. 1987. *The anterior cruciate deficient knee.* St Louis: Mosby.

41. Jackson, D., E. Grood, and J. Goldstein. 1993. A comparison of patellar tendon autograft and allograft used for ACL reconstruction in the goat model. *American Journal of Sports Medicine* 21:176–81.

42. Jenkins, D. 1985. *Ligament injuries and their treatment.* Rockville, MD: Aspen.

43. Jensen, J., and R. DiFabio. 1989. Evaluation of eccentric exercise in the treatment of patellar tendinitis. *Physical Therapy* 69(3): 211–16.

44. Johnson, D. 1982. Controlling anterior shear during isokinetic knee exercise. *Journal of Orthopaedic and Sports Physical Therapy* 4(1): 27.

45. Kramer, P. 1983. Patellar malalignment syndrome: Rationale to reduce lateral pressure. *Journal of Orthopaedic and Sports Physical Therapy* 8(6): 301.

46. LaPrade, R., and Q. Burnett. 1994. Femoral intercondylar notch stenosis and correlation to anterior cruciate ligament injuries: A prospective study. *American Journal of Sports Medicine* 22: 198–202.

47. Lephart, S., M. Kocher, and F. Fu. 1992. Proprioception following anterior cruciate ligament reconstruction. *Journal of Sport Rehabilitation* 1:188–96.

48. Lutz, G., and R. Warren. 1995. Meniscal injuries. In *Rehabilitation of the injured knee*, edited by L. Griffin. St. Louis: Mosby.

49. Mangine, R. 1988. *Physical therapy of the knee*. New York: Churchill Livingstone.

50. Mangine, R., and M. Eifert-Mangine. 1991. Postoperative PCL reconstruction rehabilitation. In *Knee ligament rehabilitation*, edited by R. Engle. New York: Churchill Livingstone.

51. Malone, T. 1992. *Relationship of gender in ACL injuries of NCAA Division I basketball players.* Paper presented at Specialty Day Meeting of the AOSSM, Washington, DC, February.

52. Mansmann, K. 1991. PCL reconstruction. In *Knee ligament rehabilitation*, edited by R. Engle. New York: Churchill Livingstone.

53. McCarthy, M., C. Yates, J. Anderson, et al. 1993. The effects of immediate CPM on pain during the inflammatory phase of soft tissue healing following ACL reconstruction. *Journal of Orthopaedic and Sports Physical Therapy* 17(2): 96–101.

54. McConnell, J. 1986. The management of chondromalacia patella: A long-term solution. *Australian Journal of Physiotherapy* 32(4): 215–23.

55. McConnell, J. and J. Fulkerson. 1995. The Knee: Patellofemoral and soft tissue injuries. In *Athletic injuries and rehabilitation*, edited by J. Zachazewski, D. Magee, and W. Quillen. Philadelphia: W. B. Saunders.

56. Mellion, M., ed. 1987. *Office management of sports injury and athletic problems*. Philadelphia: Hanley & Belfus.

57. Miyasaka, D. Danieal, and M. Stone. 1991. The incidence of knee ligament injuries in the population. *American Journal of Knee Surgery* 4:3–8.

58. Nichols, C., and R. Johnson. 1991. Cruciate ligament injuries: Non-operative treatment. In *Ligament and extensor mechanism injuries of the knee*, edited by N. Scott. St. Louis: Mosby.

59. Noyes, F., R. Mangine, and S. Barber. 1987. Early knee motion after open and arthroscopic anterior cruciate ligament reconstruction. *American Journal of Sports Medicine* 15:149.

60. O'Donohue, D. 1970. *Treatment of injuries to athletes.* Philadelphia: W. B. Saunders.

61. O'Driscoll, S., F. Keely, and R. Salter. 1986. The chondrogenic potential of free autogenous periosteal grafts for biological resurfacing of major full-thickness defects in joint surfaces under the influence of continuous passive motion: An experimental investigation in the rabbit. *Journal of Bone and Joint Surgery* 68A:1017.

62. Parolie, J., and J. Bergfeld. 1986. Long-term results of non-operative treatment of PCL injuries in the athlete. *American Journal of Sports Medicine* 14:35–38.

63. Paulos, L., F. Noyes, and E. Grood. 1981. Knee rehabilitation after anterior cruciate ligament reconstruction and repair, *American Journal of Sports Medicine* 9:140–49.

64. Paulos, L., and J. Stern. 1993. Rehabilitation after anterior cruciate ligament surgery, In *The anterior cruciate ligament*, edited by D. Jackson. New York: Raven Press.

65. Pittman, M., and V. Frankel. 1995. Biomechanics of the knee in athletics. In *The lower extremity and spine in sports medicine*, edited by J. Nicholas, and E. Hershman. St. Louis: Mosby.

66. Prentice, W. 1988. A manual resistance technique for strengthening tibial rotation. JNATA 23(3): 230–33.

67. Prentice, W., and T. Toriscelli. 1988. The effects of lateral knee stabilizing braces on running speed and agility. Ath Train 23(3): 230.

68. Quillen, W., and J. Gieck. 1988. Manual therapy: Mobilization of the motion restricted knee. JNATA 23(2): 123–30.

69. Reynold, L., T. Levin, J. Medoiros et al. 1983. EMG activity of the vastus medialis oblique and the vastus lateralis and their role in patellar alignment. *American Journal of Physical Medicine and Rehabilitation* 62(2): 61–71.

70. Richardson, C. 1985. The role of the knee musculature in high speed oscillating movements of the knee. *MTAA 4th Biennial Conference Proceedings*. Brisbane, Australia.

71. Saal, J., ed. 1987. *Physical medicine and rehabilitation: Rehabilitation of sports injuries*. Philadelphia: Hanley & Belfus.

72. Salter, R. 1983. Clinical applications for basic research on continuous passive motion for disorders and injuries of synovial joints: A preliminary report of a feasibility study. *Journal of Orthopaedic Research* 3:325.

73. Sgaglione, N., R. Warren, and T. Wickiewicz. 1990. Primary repair with semitendinosis augmentation of acute ACL injuries. *American Journal of Sports Medicine* 18:64–73.

74. Shea, K., and J. Fulkerson. 1995. Patellofemoral joint injuries. In *Rehabilitation of the knee*, edited by L. Griffin. St. Louis: Mosby.

75. Shelbourne, K., J. Wilckens, and A. Mollabashy. 1991. Arthrofibrosis in acute anterior cruciate ligament reconstruction: The effect of timing on reconstruction and rehabilitation. *American Journal of Sports Medicine* 19:322–36.

76. Shelbourne, K., T. Klootwyk, and M. DeCarlo. 1995. Ligamentous injuries. In *Rehabilitation of the knee*, edited by L. Griffin. St. Louis: Mosby.

77. Shelbourne, K., and P. Nitz. 1992. Accelerated rehabilitation after ACL reconstruction. *Journal of Orthopaedic and Sports Physical Therapy* 15(6): 256–64.

78. Sommerlath, K., J. Lysholm, and J. Gillquiost. 1991. The long-term course of treatment of acute ACL ruptures. A 9 to 16 year followup. *American Journal of Sports Medicine* 19:156–62.

79. Souryal, T., T. Freeman, and J. Evans. 1993. Intercondylar notch size and ACL injuries in athletes: A prospective study. *American Journal of Sports Medicine* 21:535–39.

80. Stone, K., and T. Rosenberg. 1993. Surgical technique of meniscal transplantation. *Arthroscopy* 9:234–37.

81. Sweitzer, R., D. Sweitzer, and A. Sarantini. 1991. Rehabilitation for ligament and extensor mechanism injuries. In *Ligament and extensor mechanism injuries of the knee*, edited by N. Scott. St. Louis: Mosby.

82. Tria, A., and K. Klein. 1991. *An illustrated guide to the knee.* New York: Churchill Livingstone.

83. Weiss, J., S. Woo, and K. Ohland. 1991. Evaluation of a new injury model to study MCL healing: Primary repair vs. non-operative treatment. J Orthop Res 9:516–28.

84. Wilk, K., and J. Andrews. 1992. Current concepts in treatment of ACL disruption. *Journal of Orthopaedic and Sports Physical Therapy* 15(6): 279–93.

85. Wilk, K., and W. Clancey. 1991. Medial collateral ligament injuries: Diagnosis, treatment, and rehabilitation. In *Knee ligament rehabilitation,* edited by R. Engle. New York: Churchill Livingstone.

86. Woodall, W., and J. Welsh. 1991. A biomechanical basis for rehabilitation programs involving the knee joint. *Journal of Orthopaedic and Sports Physical Therapy* 11(11): 535.

87. Zarins, B., and D. Fish. 1995. Knee ligament injury. In *The lower extremity and spine in sports medicine,* edited by J. Nicholas, and E. Hershman. St. Louis: Mosby.

CHAPTER 24

Rehabilitation of Lower-Leg Injuries

Christopher J. Hirth

After completion of this chapter, the student should be able to do the following:

- Discuss the functional anatomy and biomechanics of the lower leg during open-chain and weight-bearing activities such as walking and running.

- Identify the various techniques for regaining range of motion, including stretching exercises and joint mobilizations.

- Discuss the various rehabilitative strengthening techniques, including open- and closed-chain isotonic exercise, balance/proprioceptive exercises, and isokinetic exercise for dysfunction of the lower leg.

- Identify common causes of various lower-leg injuries and provide a rationale for treatment of these injuries.

- Discuss criteria for progression of the rehabilitation program for various lower-leg injuries.

- Describe and explain the rationale for various treatment techniques in the management of lower-leg injuries.

FUNCTIONAL ANATOMY AND BIOMECHANICS

The lower leg consists of the tibia and fibula and four muscular compartments that either originate on or traverse various points along these bones. Distally the tibia and fibula articulate with the talus to form the talocrural joint. Because of the close approximation of the talus within the mortise, movement of the leg will be dictated by the foot, especially upon ground contact. This becomes important when examining the effects of repetitive stresses placed upon the leg with excessive compensatory pronation secondary to various structural lower-extremity malalignments.[53,54] Proximally the tibia articulates with the femur to form the tibiofemoral joint as well as serving as an attachment site for the patellar tendon, the distal soft-tissue component of the extensor mechanism. The lower leg serves to transmit ground reaction forces to the knee as well as rotatory forces proximally along the lower extremity that may be a source of pain, especially with athletic activities.[54]

Compartments of the Lower Leg

The muscular components of the lower leg are divided anatomically into four compartments. In an open-kinetic-chain position, these muscle groups are responsible for movements of the foot primarily in a single plane. When the foot is in contact with the ground, these muscle-tendon units work both concentrically and eccentrically to absorb ground reaction forces, control excessive movements of the foot and ankle to adapt to the terrain, and, ideally, provide a stable base to propel the limb forward during walking and running.

The anterior compartment is primarily responsible for dorsiflexion of the foot in an open-kinetic-chain position. Functionally these muscles are active in early and midstance phase of gait, with increased eccentric muscle activity directly after heel strike to control plantarflexion of the foot and pronation of the forefoot.[11] EMG studies have noted that the tibialis anterior is active in more than 85 percent of the gait cycle during running.[35]

The deep posterior compartment is made up of the tibialis posterior and the long toe flexors and is responsible for inversion of the foot and ankle in an open kinetic chain. These muscles help control pronation at the subtalar joint and internal rotation of the lower leg.[11,35] Along with the soleus, the tibialis posterior will help decelerate the forward momentum of the tibia during midstance phase of gait.

The lateral compartment is made up of the peroneus longus and brevis, which are responsible for eversion of the foot in an open kinetic chain. Functionally the peroneus longus plantarflexes the first ray at heel off, while the peroneus brevis counteracts the supinating forces of the tibialis posterior to provide osseous stability of the subtalar and midtarsal joints during the propulsive phase of gait. EMG studies of running report an increase in peroneus brevis activity when the pace of running is increased.[35]

The superficial posterior compartment is made up of the gastrocnemius and soleus muscles, which in open-kinetic-chain position are responsible primarily for plantarflexion of the foot. Functionally these muscles are responsible for acting eccentrically controlling pronation of the subtalar joint and internal rotation of the leg in the midstance phase of gait and activated concentrically during the push-off phase of gait.[11,35]

REHABILITATION TECHNIQUES FOR THE LOWER LEG

Strengthening Techniques

Isotonic Open-Kinetic-Chain Exercises.

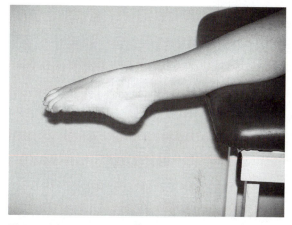

Figure 24-1   AROM ankle plantarflexion. Used to activate the primary and secondary ankle plantarflexor muscle-tendon units after a period of immobilization or disuse. This exercise can be performed in a supportive medium such as a whirlpool.

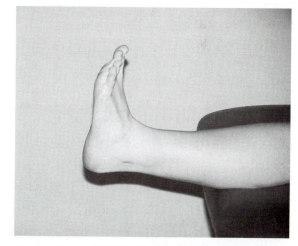

Figure 24-2   AROM ankle dorsiflexion. Used to activate the tibialis anterior, extensor hallicus longus, and extensor digitorum longus muscle-tendon units after a period of immobilization or disuse.

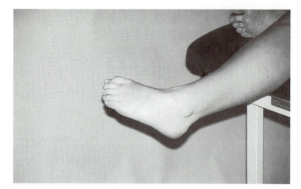

Figure 24-3   AROM ankle inversion start position/end position. Used to activate the tibialis posterior, flexor hallucis longus, and flexor digitorum longus muscle-tendon units after a period of immobilization or disuse.

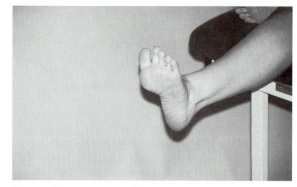

Figure 24-4   AROM ankle eversion start position/end position. Used to activate the peroneus longus and brevis muscle-tendon units after a period of immobilization or disuse.

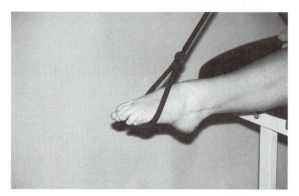

Figure 24-5   PROM ankle plantarflexion with rubber tubing. Used to strengthen the gastrocnemius, soleus, and secondary ankle plantarflexors, including the peroneals, flexor hallucis longus, flexor digitorum longus, and tibialis posterior, in an open-chain fashion. This exercise will also place a controlled concentric and eccentric load on the Achilles tendon.

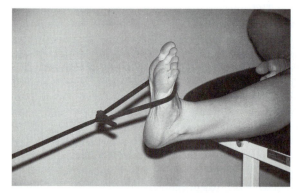

Figure 24-6   PROM ankle dorsiflexion with rubber tubing. Used to isolate and strengthen the ankle dorsiflexors, including the tibialis anterior, extensor hallucis longus, and extensor digitorum longus, in an open-chain fashion.

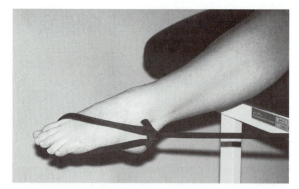

Figure 24-7   PROM ankle inversion with rubber tubing. Used to isolate and strengthen the ankle inverters, including the tibialis posterior, flexor hallucis longus, and flexor digitorum longus, in an open-chain fashion.

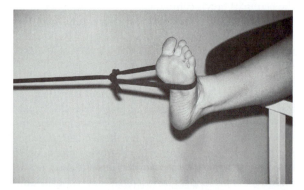

Figure 24-8   PROM ankle eversion with rubber tubing. Used to isolate and strengthen the ankle everters, including the peroneus longus and peroneus brevis, in an open-chain fashion.

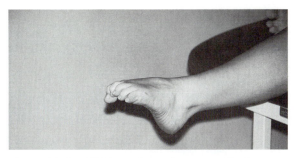

Figure 24-9 AROM toe flexion/extension. Used to activate the long toe flexers, extensors, and foot intrinsic musculature. This exercise will also help to improve the tendon-gliding ability of the extensor hallicus longus, extensor digitorum longus, flexor hallicus longus, and flexor digitorum longus tendons after a period of immobilization.

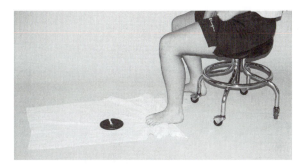

Figure 24-10 Towel-gathering exercise. Used to strengthen the foot intrinsics and long toe flexor and extensor muscle-tendon units. A weight can be placed on the end of the towel to require more force production by the muscle-tendon unit as ROM and strength improve.

Closed-Kinetic-Chain Strengthening Exercises.

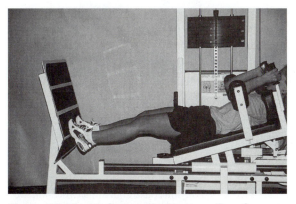

Figure 24-11 Heel raises. Used to strengthen the gastrocnemius musculature and will directly load the Achilles tendon with a percentage of the athlete's body weight depending on the angle of the carriage relative to the ground.

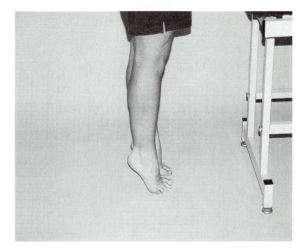

Figure 24-12 Two-legged heel raise. Used to strengthen the gastrocnemius when the knee is extended and the soleus when the knees are flexed. The flexor hallicus longus, flexor digitorum longus, tibialis posterior, and peroneals will also be activated during this activity. The athlete can modify concentric and eccentric activity depending on the type and severity of the condition. For example, if an eccentric load is not desired on the involved side, the athlete can raise up on both feet and lower down on the uninvolved side until eccentric loading is tolerated on the involved side.

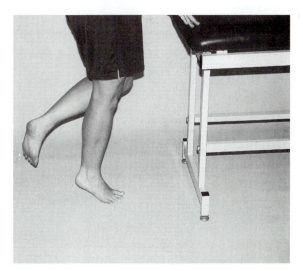

Figure 24-13 One-legged heel raise. Used to strengthen the gastrocnemius and soleus muscles when the knee is extended and flexed, respectively. This can be used as a progression from the two-legged heel raise.

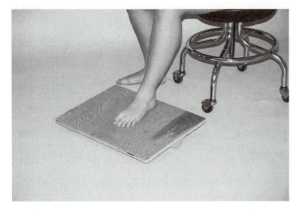

Figure 24-14 Seated closed-chain ankle dorsiflexion/plantarflexion AROM. Used to activate the ankle dorsiflexor/plantarflexor musculature in a closed-chain position.

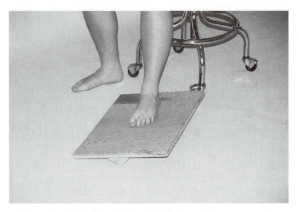

Figure 24-15 Seated closed-chain ankle inversion/eversion AROM. Used to activate the ankle inverter/everter musculature in a closed-chain position.

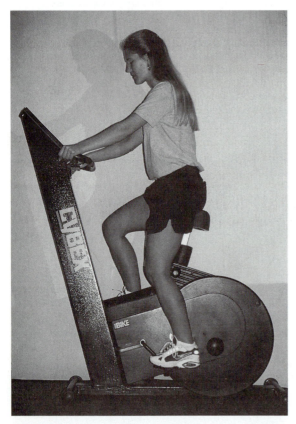

Figure 24-16 Stationary cycle. Used to reduce impact weight-bearing forces on the lower extremity while also maintaining cardiovascular fitness levels.

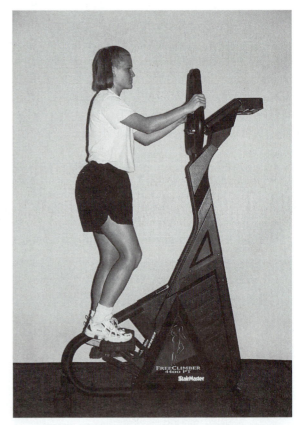

Figure 24-17 Stair-stepping machine. Used to progressively load the lower extremity in a closed-kinetic fashion as well as maintain and improve cardiovascular fitness.

Isokinetic Exercises.

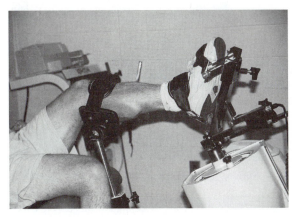

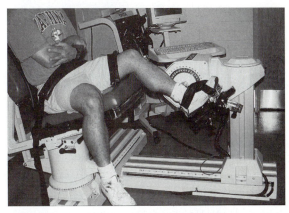

Figure 24-18 Isokinetic ankle inversion/eversion PROM. Used to improve the strength and endurance of the ankle inverters and everters in an open chain. Also can provide an objective measurement of muscular torque production.

Figure 24-19 Isokinetic ankle plantarflexion/ dorsiflexion PROM. Used to improve the strength and endurance of the ankle dorsiflexors and plantarflexors in an open chain. Also can provide an objective measurement of torque production.

Stretching Exercises

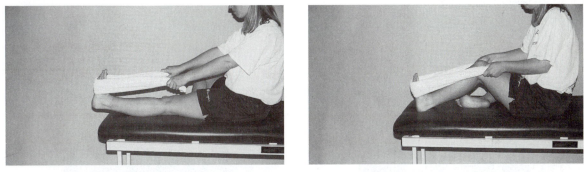

Figure 24-20 Ankle plantarflexion towel stretch. Used to stretch the gastrocnemius when the knee is extended and the soleus when the knee is flexed. The Achilles tendon will be stretched with both positions. The athlete can hold the stretch for 20 to 30 seconds.

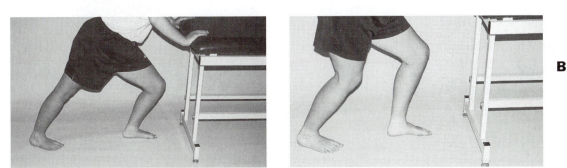

Figure 24-21 **A,** Standing gastrocnemius stretch. Used to stretch the gastrocnemius muscle. The Achilles tendon will also be stretched. The stretch is held for 20 to 30 seconds. **B,** Standing soleus stretch. Used to stretch the soleus muscle. The Achilles tendon will also be stretched. The stretch is held for 20 to 30 seconds.

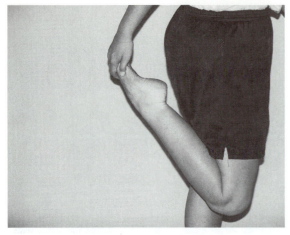

Figure 24-22　Standing ankle dorsiflexor stretch. Used to stretch the extensor hallicus longus, extensor digitorum longus, tibialis anterior, and anterior ankle capsule. The stretch is held for 20 to 30 seconds.

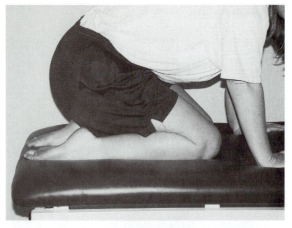

Figure 24-23　Kneeling ankle dorsiflexor stretch. Used to stretch the extensor hallicus longus, extensor digitorum longus, tibialis anterior, and anterior ankle capsule. This is an aggressive stretch that can be used in the later stages of rehabilitation to gain end-ROM ankle dorsiflexion.

Exercises to Reestablish Neuromuscular Control

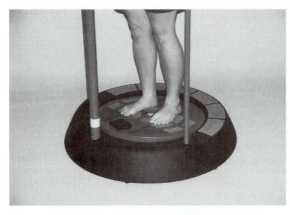

Figure 24-24　Standing double-leg balance board activity. Used to activate the lower-leg musculature and improve balance and proprioception in the lower extremity.

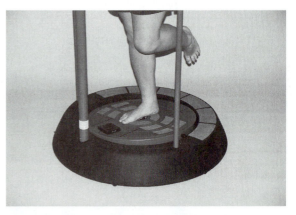

Figure 24-25　Standing single-leg balance board activity. Used to activate the lower-leg musculature and improve balance and proprioception in the involved extremity.

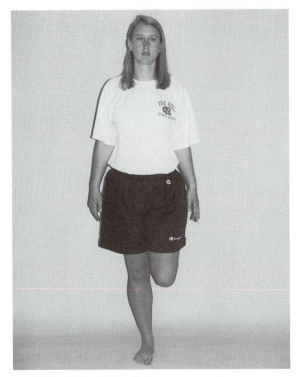

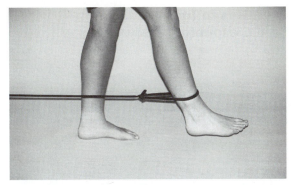

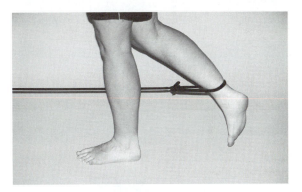

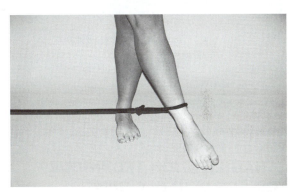

Figure 24-26   Static single-leg standing balance progression. Used to improve balance and proprioception of the lower extremity. This activity can be made more difficult with the following progression: (a) single-leg stand, eyes open; (b) single-leg stand, eyes closed; (c) single-leg stand, eyes open, toes extended so only the heel and metatarsal heads are in contact with the ground; (d) single-leg stand, eyes closed, toes extended.

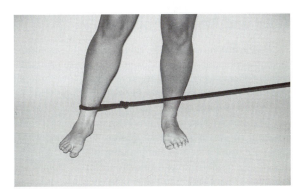

Figure 24-27   Single-leg standing rubber-tubing kicks. Used to improve muscle activation of the lower leg to maintain single-leg standing on the involved extremity while kicking against the resistance of the rubber tubing.

Exercises to Improve Cardiorespiratory Endurance

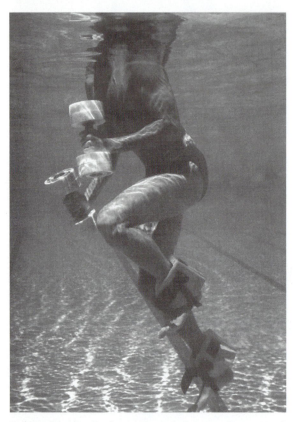

Figure 24-28 Pool running with flotation device. Used to reduce impact weight-bearing forces on the lower extremity while maintaining cardiovascular fitness level and running form.

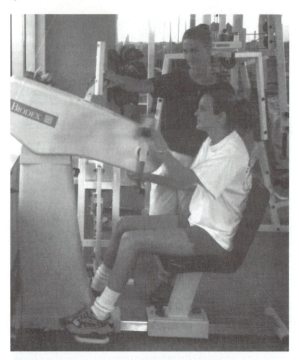

Figure 24-29 Upper-body ergometer. Used to maintain cardiovascular fitness when lower-extremity ergometer is contraindicated or too difficult for the athlete to use.

REHABILITATION TECHNIQUES FOR SPECIFIC INJURIES

Tibial and Fibular Fractures

Pathomechanics. The tibia and fibula constitute the bony components of the lower leg and are primarily responsible for weight bearing and muscle attachment. The tibia is the most commonly fractured long bone in the body, and fractures are usually the result of either direct trauma to the area or indirect trauma such as a combination rotatory/compressive force. Fractures of the fibula are usually seen in combination with a tibial fracture or as a result of direct trauma to the area. Tibial fractures will present with immediate pain, swelling, and pos-

sible deformity and can be open or closed in nature. Fibular fractures alone are usually closed and present with pain on palpation and with ambulation. These fractures should be treated with immediate medical referral and most likely a period of immobilization and restricted weight bearing for weeks to possibly months, depending on the severity and involvement of the injury. Surgery such as open reduction with internal fixation (ORIF) of the bone, usually of the tibia, is common.

Injury Mechanism. The two mechanisms of a traumatic lower-leg fracture are either a direct insult to the bone or indirectly through a combined rotatory/compressive force. Direct impact to the long bone, such as from a projectile object or the top of a ski boot, can produce enough damaging force to fracture a bone. Indirect trauma from a combination of rotatory and compressive forces can be manifested in sports when an athlete's foot is planted and the proximal segments are rotated with a large compressive force. An example of this could be a football running back attempting to gain more yardage while an opposing player is trying to tackle him from above the waist and applying a superincumbent compressive load. If the athlete's foot is planted and immovable and the lower extremity is rotated, the superincumbent weight of the defender may be enough to cause a fracture in the tibia. A fibular fracture may accompany the tibial fracture.

Rehabilitation Concerns. Tibial and fibular fractures are usually immobilized and placed on a restricted weight-bearing status for a period of time to facilitate fracture healing. Immobilization and restricted weight bearing of a bone, its proximal and distal joints, and surrounding musculature will lead to functional deficits once the fracture is healed. Depending on the severity of the fracture, there also may be postsurgical considerations such as an incision and hardware within the bone. Complications following immobilization include joint stiffness of any joints immobilized, muscle atrophy of the lower leg and possibly the proximal thigh and hip musculature, as well as an abnormal gait pattern. It is important that the sports therapist perform a comprehensive evaluation of the athlete to determine all potential rehabilitation problems, including range of motion, joint mobility, muscle flexibility, strength and endurance of the entire involved lower extremity, balance, proprioception and gait. The sports therapist must also determine the functional demands that will be placed on the athlete upon return to competition and set up short- and long-term goals accordingly. Upon cast removal it is important to address ROM deficits. This can be managed with PROM/AROM exercises in a supportive medium such as a warm whirlpool (see Figures 24-1 to 24-4, 24-9, 24-14, 24-15, 24-20, 24-22). Joint stiffness can be addressed via joint mobilization to any joint that was immobilized (see Chapter 25). It is possible to have post-traumatic edema in the foot and ankle after cast removal that can be reduced with massage. Strengthening exercises can help facilitate muscle firing, strength, and endurance (see Figures 24-5 to 24-8, 24-10 to 24-13). Balance and proprioception can be improved with single-leg standing activities and balance board activities (see Figures 24-24 to 24-27). Cardiovascular endurance can be addressed with pool activities including swimming and pool running with a flotation device, stationary cycling, and the use of an upper-body ergometer (see Figures 24-16, 24-17, 24-28, 24-29). A stair stepper is also an excellent way to address cardiovascular needs as well as lower-extremity strength, endurance, and weight bearing (see Figure 24-17).

Rehabilitation Progression. Management of a post-immobilization fracture will require good communication with the physician to determine progression of weight-bearing status, any assistive devices to be used during the rehabilitation process, such as a walker boot, and any other pertinent information that will influence

the rehabilitation process. It is important to address ROM deficits immediately with AROM, passive stretching, and skilled joint mobilization. Isometric strengthening can be initiated and progressed to isotonic exercises once ROM has been normalized. After weight-bearing status is determined, gait training to normalize walking should be initiated. Assistive devices should be utilized as needed. Strengthening of the involved lower extremity can be incorporated into the rehabilitation process, especially for the hip and thigh musculature. Balance and proprioceptive exercises can begin once there is full pain-free weightbearing on the involved lower extremity.

As ROM, strength, and walking gait are normalized, the athlete can be progressed to a walking/jogging progression and a sport-related functional progression. It must be realized that the rate of rehabilitation progression will depend on the severity of the fracture, any surgical involvement, and length of immobilization. The average healing time for uncomplicated nondisplaced tibial fractures is 10 to 13 weeks; for displaced, open, or comminuted tibial fracture, it is 16 to 26 weeks.[45]

Fibular fractures may be immobilized for 4 to 6 weeks. Again an open line of communication with the physician is required to facilitate a safe rehabilitation progression for the athlete.

Criteria for Full Return. The following criteria should be met prior to the return to full activity: (1) full ROM and strength, compared to the uninvolved side; (2) normalized walking, jogging, running gait; (3) ability to hop for endurance and 90 percent hop for distance as compared to the uninvolved side, without complaints of pain or observable compensation; and (4) successful completion of a sport-specific functional test.

Tibial and Fibular Stress Fractures

Pathomechanics. Stress fractures of the tibia and fibula are common in sports. Studies indicate that stress fractures of the tibia occur at a higher rate than those of the fibula.[3,4,32] Stress fractures in the lower leg are usually the result of the bone's inability to adapt to the repetitive loading response during training and conditioning of the athlete. The bone attempts to adapt to the applied loads initially through osteoclastic activity, which breaks down the bone. Osteoblastic activity, or the laying down of new bone, will soon follow.[34,52] If the applied loads are not reduced during this process, structural irregularities will develop within the bone, which will further reduce the bone's ability to absorb stress and will eventually lead to a stress fracture.[4,14,17] Stress fractures in the tibial shaft mainly occur in the midanterior aspect and the posteromedial aspect.[3,32,36,52] Anterior tibial stress fractures usually present in athletes involved in repetitive jumping activities with localized pain directly over the midanterior tibia. The athlete will complain of pain with activity that is relieved with rest. The pain can affect activities of daily living (ADLs) if activity is not modified. Vibration testing using a tuning fork will reproduce the symptoms, as will hopping on the involved extremity. A triple-phase technetium[99] bone scan can confirm the diagnosis faster than an X ray, as it can take a minimum of 3 weeks to demonstrate radiographic changes.[34,36,52] Posteromedial tibial pain usually occurs over the distal one-third of the bone with a gradual onset of symptoms.

Focal point tenderness on the bone will help differentiate a stress fracture from medial tibial stress syndrome (MTSS), which is located in the same area but is more diffuse upon palpation. The procedures listed above will be positive and will implicate the stress fracture as the source of pain. Fibular stress fractures usually occur in the distal one-third of the bone with the same symptomatology as for tibial stress fractures. Although less common, stress fractures of the proximal fibula are noted in the literature.[32,49,59]

Injury Mechanism.   Anterior tibial stress fractures are prevalent in athletes involved with jumping. Several authors have noted that the tibia will bow anteriorly with the convexity on the anterior aspect.[9,34,37,52] This places the anterior aspect of the tibia under tension, which is less than ideal for bone healing, which prefers compressive forces. Repetitive jumping will place greater tension on this area, which has minimal musculotendinous support and blood supply. Other biomechanical factors may be involved, including excessive compensatory pronation at the subtalar joint to accommodate lower-extremity structural alignments such as forefoot varus, tibial varum, and femoral anteversion. This excessive pronation might not affect the leg during ADLs or with moderate activity, but might become a factor with increases in training intensity, duration, and frequency, even with sufficient recovery time.[21,52] Increased training may affect the surrounding muscle-tendon unit's ability to absorb the impact of each applied load, which places more stress on the bone. Stress fractures of the distal posteromedial tibia will also arise from the same problems as listed above, with the exception of repetitive jumping. Excessive compensatory pronation may play a greater role with this type of injury. This hyperpronation can be accentuated when running on a crowned road, such is the case of the uphill leg.[40] Also, running on a track with a small radius and tight curves will tend to increase pronatory stresses on the leg that is closer to the inside of the track.[40] Excessive pronation may also play a role with fibular stress fractures. The repeated activity of

the ankle everters and calf musculature pulling on the bone may be a source of this type of stress fracture.[34] Training errors of increased duration and intensity along with worn out shoes will only accentuate these problems.[40] Other factors, including menstrual irregularities, diet, bone density, increased hip external rotation, tibial width, and calf girth, have also been identified as contributing to stress fractures.[4,20]

Rehabilitation Concerns.   Immediate elimination of the offending activity is most important. The athlete must be educated on the importance of this to prevent further damage to the bone. Many athletes will express concerns about fitness level with loss of activity. Stationary cycling and running in the deep end of the pool with a flotation device can help maintain cardiovascular fitness (Figures 24-16, 24-28). Eyestone et al. have demonstrated a small but statistically significant decrease in $\dot{V}O_2$max when water running was substituted for regular running.[13] This was also true with using a stationary bike.[13] These authors recommend that intensity, duration, and frequency be equivalent to regular training. Wilder et al. note that water provides a resistance that is proportional to the effort exerted.[56] These authors found that cadence, via a metronome, gave a quantitative external cue that with increased rate showed high correlation with heart rate.[56] Nonimpact activity in the pool or on the bike will help maintain fitness and allow proper bone healing. Proper footwear that matches the needs of the foot is also important. For example, a high arched or pes cavus foot type will require a shoe with good shock-absorbing qualities. A pes planus foot type or more pronated foot will require a shoe with good motion control characteristics. A detailed biomechanical exam of the lower extremity both statically and dynamically may reveal problems that require the use of a custom foot orthotic. Stretching and strengthening exercises can be incorporated in the rehabilitation process. The use of ice and electrical stimulation to control pain is also recommended. The utilization of an Aircast with athletes who have diagnosed stress fractures has produced positive results.[10] Dickson et al. speculate that the Aircast unloads the tibia and fibula enough to allow healing of the stress fracture with continued participation.[10] Fibular and posterior medial tibial stress fractures will usually heal without residual problems if the above-mentioned concerns are addressed. Stress fractures of the mid anterior tibia can take much longer, and residual problems might exist months to years after the initial diagnosis, with attempts at increased activity.[9,12,36,37] Initial treatment may include a short leg cast and non-weight-bearing for 6 to 8 weeks. Rettig et al. used rest from the offending activity as well as electrical stimulation in the form of a pulsed electromagnetic field for a period of 10 to 12 hours per day. The authors noted an average of 12.7 months from the onset of symptoms to return to full activity with this regimen.[37] They recommended using this program for 3 to 6 months before considering surgical intervention.[37] Chang et al. noted good to excellent results with a surgical procedure involving intramedullary nailing of the tibia with individuals with delayed union of this type of stress fracture.[9] Surgical procedures involving bone grafting have also been recommended to improve healing of this type of stress fracture.

Rehabilitation Progression.   After diagnosis of the stress fracture, the athlete may be placed on crutches, depending on the amount of discomfort with ambulation. Ice can be used to reduce local inflammation and pain. The athlete can immediately begin pool running with the same training parameters as their regular regimen. Stretching exercises for the gastrocnemius-soleus musculature can be performed 2 to 3 times per day (Figure 24-21). Isotonic strengthening exercises with rubber tubing can begin as soon as tolerated on an every-other-day basis, with an increase in repetitions and sets as the sports therapist sees fit (Figures 24-5 to 24-8). Strengthening of the gastrocnemius can be done initially in an open chain and eventually be progressed to a closed chain (Figures 24-5, 24-12, 24-13). The athlete should wear supportive shoes during the day and avoid shoes with a heel, which can cause adaptive shortening of the gastroc-soleus complex and increase strain on the healing bone. Custom foot orthotics can be fabricated for motion control in order to prevent excessive pronation for those athletes that need it. Foot orthotics can also be fabricated for a high arched foot to increase stress distribution throughout the plantar aspect of the whole foot versus the heel and the metatarsal heads. Shock-absorbing materials can augment these orthotics to help reduce ground reaction forces. As the symptoms subside over a period of 3 to 4 weeks and X rays confirm that good callus formation is occurring, the athlete may be progressed to a walking/jogging progression on a surface suitable to that athlete's needs. A quality track or grass surface may be the best choice to begin this progression. The athlete may be instructed to jog for 1 minute, then walk for 30 seconds for 10 to 15 repetitions. This can be performed on an every-other-day basis with high-intensity/long-duration cardiovascular training occurring daily in the pool or on the bike. The athlete should be reminded that the purpose of the walk/jog progression is to provide a gradual increase in stress to the healing bone in a controlled manner. If tolerated, the jogging time can be increased by 30 seconds every 2 to 3 training sessions until the athlete is running 5 minutes without walking. The

above progression is a guideline and can be modified based on individual needs. Experimentation with the use of an Aircast is recommended to determine its effectiveness with each individual. Initially it may be used with ADLs to allow pain relief and eventually for activity. As the athlete progresses without increased symptoms, a sport-specific functional progression should be initiated.

Criteria for Full Return.   The athlete can return to full activity when (1) there is no tenderness to palpation of the affected bone and no pain of the affected area with repeated hopping, (2) plain films demonstrate good bone healing, (3) there has been successful progression of a graded return to running with no increase in symptoms, (4) gastroc-soleus flexibility is within normal limits, and (5) hyperpronation has been corrected or shock-absorption problems have been decreased with proper shoes and foot orthotics if indicated.

Compartment Syndromes

Pathomechanics and Injury Mechanism.   Compartment syndrome is a condition in which increased pressure, within a fixed osseofascial compartment, causes compression of muscular and neurovascular structures within the compartment. As compartment pressures increase, the venous outflow of fluid decreases and eventually stops, which causes further fluid leakage from the capillaries into the compartment. Eventually arterial blood inflow also ceases secondary to rising intracompartmental pressures.[55] Compartment syndrome can be divided into three categories: acute compartment syndrome, acute exertional compartment syndrome, and chronic compartment syndrome. Acute compartment syndrome occurs secondary to direct trauma to the area and is a medical emergency.[26,50,55] The athlete will complain of a deep-seated aching pain, tightness, and swelling of the involved compartment. Reproduction of the pain will occur with passive stretching of the involved muscles. Reduction in pedal pulses and sensory changes of the involved nerve can be present but are not reliable signs.[55,58] Intracompartmental pressure measurements will confirm the diagnosis. Emergency fasciotomy is the definitive treatment. Acute exertional compartment syndrome occurs without any precipitating trauma. Cases have been cited in the literature in which acute compartment syndrome has evolved with minimal to moderate activity. If not diagnosed and treated properly, it can lead to a poor functional outcomes for the athlete.[14,58] Again intracompartmental pressures will confirm the diagnosis, with emergency fasciotomy being the treatment of choice. Chronic compartment syndrome (CCS) is activity-related in that the symptoms arise rather consistently at a certain point in the activity. The athlete complains of a sensation of pain, tightness, and swelling of the affected compartment, which resolves upon stopping the activity. Studies indicate that the anterior and deep posterior compartments are usually involved.[2,38,43,51,57] Upon presentation of these symptoms, intracompartmental pressure measurements will further define the severity of the condition. Pedowitz et al. have developed modified criteria using a slit catheter measurement of the intracompartmental pressures. These authors consider one or more of the following intramuscular pressure criteria as diagnostic of CCS: (1) preexercise pressure greater than 15 mm Hg, (2) 1 minute postexercise pressure of 30 mm Hg, (3) a 5-minute postexercise pressure greater than 20 mm Hg.[33]

Rehabilitation Concerns. Management of CCS is initially conservative with activity modification, icing, and stretching of the anterior compartment and gastrocsoleus complex (Figures 2421, 24-22, 24-23). A lower-quarter structural exam along with gait analysis might reveal a structural variation that is causing excessive compensatory pronation and might benefit from the use of foot orthotics and proper footwear. These measures will not address the issue of increased compartment pressures with activity, though. Cycling has been shown to be an acceptable alternative in preventing increased anterior compartment pressures when compared to running and can be utilized to maintain cardiovascular fitness.[2] If conservative measures fail, fasciotomy of the affected compartments has produced favorable results in a return to higher level of activity.[38,41,55,57]

Rehabilitation Progression. Following fasciotomy for CCS, the immediate goals are to decrease postsurgical pain, swelling with RICE, and assisted ambulation with the use of crutches. After suture removal and soft-tissue healing of the incision has progressed, AROM and flexibility exercises should be initiated (Figures 24-1 to 24-4, 24-20 through 24-23). Weight bearing will be progressed as ROM improves. Gait training should be incorporated to prevent abnormal movements in the gait pattern secondary to joint and soft-tissue stiffness or muscle guarding. AROM exercises should be progressed to open-chain exercises with rubber tubing (Figures 24-5 to 24-8). Closed-kinetic-chain activities can also be initiated to incorporate strength, balance, and proprioception that may have been affected by the surgical procedure (Figures 24-12, 24-13, 24-14, 24-15, 24-24 to 24-27). Lower-extremity structural variations that lead to excessive compensatory pronation during gait should be addressed with foot orthotics and proper shoeware after walking gait has been normalized. These measures should help control excessive movements at the subtalar joint/lower leg and thus theoretically decrease muscular

activity of the deep posterior compartment, which is highly active in controlling pronation during running.[35] Cardiovascular fitness can be maintained and improved with stationary cycling and running in the deep end of a pool with a flotation device (Figures 24-16, 24-28). When ROM, strength, and walking gait have normalized, a walking/jogging progression can be initiated.

Criteria for Returning to Full Activity. The athlete may return to full activity when (1) there is normalized ROM and strength of the involved lower leg, (2) there are no gait deviations with walking, jogging, and running, and (3) the athlete has completed a progressive jogging/running program with no complaints of CCS symptoms. It should be noted that athletes undergoing anterior compartment fasciotomy may not return to full activity for 8 to 12 weeks after surgery, while athletes undergoing deep posterior compartment fasciotomy may not return until 3 to 4 months post surgery.[28,41]

Muscle Strains

Pathomechanics. The majority of muscle strains in the lower leg occur in the medial head of the gastrocnemius at the musculotendinous junction.[19] The injury is more common in middle-aged athletes and occurs in activities requiring ballistic movement such as tennis and basketball. The athlete may feel or hear a pop as if being kicked in the back of the leg. Depending on the severity of the strain, the athlete may be unable to walk secondary to decreased ankle dorsiflexion in a closed kinetic chain which passively stretches the injured muscle and causes pain during the push-off phase of gait. Palpation will elicit tenderness at the site of the strain, and a palpable divot may be present, depending on the severity of the injury and how soon it is evaluated.

Injury Mechanism. Strains of the medial head of the gastrocnemius usually occur during sudden ballistic movements. A common scenario is the athlete lunging with the knee extended and the ankle dorsiflexed. The ankle plantarflexers, in this case the medial head of the gastrocnemius, are activated to assist in push-off of the foot. The muscle is placed in an elongated position and activated in a very short period of time. This places the musculotendinous junction of the gastrocnemius under excessive tensile stress. The muscle-tendon junction, a transition area of one homogeneous tissue to another, is not able to endure the tensile loads nearly as well as the homogeneous tissue itself, and tearing of the tissue at the junction occurs.

Rehabilitation Concerns. The initial management of a gastrocnemius strain is ICE. It is important for the athlete to pay special attention to compression and elevation of the lower extremity to avoid edema in the foot and ankle, which can further limit ROM and prolong the rehabilitation process. Gentle stretching of the muscle-tendon unit should be initiated early in the rehabilitation process (Figure 24-20). Ankle plantarflexor strengthening with rubber tubing can also be initiated when tolerated (Figure 24-5). Weight bearing may be limited to an as-tolerated status with crutches. The foot/ankle will prefer a plantarflexed position, and closed-kinetic-chain dorsiflexion of the foot and ankle, which is required during walking, will stress the muscle and cause pain. Pulsed ultrasound can be utilized early in the rehabilitation process and eventually progressed to continuous ultrasound for its thermal effects. A stationary cycle can be used for an active warm-up as well as cardiovascular fitness. A heel lift may be placed in each shoe to gradually increase dorsiflexion of the foot and ankle as the athlete is progressed off crutches. Standing, stretching and strengthening can be added as soft-tissue healing occurs and ROM and strength improve. Eventually the athlete can be progressed to a walking/jogging program and sport-specific activity. It is important that the athlete warm up and stretch properly before activity, to prevent reinjury.

Rehabilitation Progression. Early management of a medial head gastrocnemius strain focuses on reduction of pain and swelling with ICE and modified weight bearing. The athlete is encouraged to perform gentle towel stretching for the affected muscle group several times per day (Figure 24-20). AROM of the foot and ankle in all planes will also facilitate movement and act to stretch the muscle (Figures 24-1 to 24-4). With mild muscle strains, the athlete may be off crutches and performing standing calf stretches and strengthening exercises by about 7 to 10 days with a normal gait pattern (Figures 24-12, 24-13, 24-21). Moderate to severe strains may take 2 to 4 weeks before normalization of ROM and gait occur. This is usually due to the excessive edema in the foot and ankle. Strengthening can be progressed from open- to closed-chain activity as soft-tissue healing occurs (Figures 24-14, 24-15, 24-24 to 24-27). As walking gait is normalized, the athlete is encouraged to begin a graduated jogging program in which distance and speed are modulated throughout the progression. Most soft-tissue injuries demonstrate good healing by 14 to 21 days postinjury. In the case of mild muscle strain, as the athlete becomes more comfortable with jogging and running, plyometric activities can be added to the rehabilitation process. Plyometric activities should be introduced in a controlled fashion with at least 1 to 2 days of rest between activities to allow for muscle soreness to diminish. As the athlete adapts to the plyometric exercises, sport-specific training should be added. Care should be taken to save sudden, ballistic activities for when the athlete is warmed up and the gastrocnemius is well stretched.

Criteria for Full Return. The athlete may return to full activity when the following criteria have been met: (1) full ROM of the foot and ankle, (2) gastrocnemius strength and endurance that are equal to the uninvolved side, (3) ability to walk, jog, run, and hop on the involved extremity without any compensation, and (4) successful completion of a sport-specific functional progression with no residual calf symptoms.

Medial Tibial Stress Syndrome

Pathomechanics. Medial tibial stress syndrome (MTSS) is a condition that involves increasing pain about the distal two-thirds of the posterior medial aspect of the tibia.[17,47] The soleus and tibialis posterior have been implicated as muscular forces that can stress the fascia and periosteum of the distal tibia during running activities.[1,16,43] Pain is usually diffuse about the distal medial tibia and the surrounding soft tissues and can arise secondary to a combination of training errors, excessive pronation, improper shoeware, and poor conditioning level.[7,44] Initially, the area is diffusely tender and might hurt only after an intense workout. As the condition worsens, daily ambulation may be painful and morning pain and stiffness may be present. Rehabilitation of this condition must be comprehensive and address several factors, including musculoskeletal, training, and conditioning, as well as proper shoeware and orthotics intervention.

Injury Mechanism. Many sources have linked excessive compensatory pronation as a primary cause of MTSS.[7,16,43,47] Subtalar joint pronation serves to dissipate ground reaction forces upon foot strike in order to reduce the impact to proximal structures. If pronation is excessive or occurs too quickly or at the wrong time in the stance phase of gait, greater tensile loads will be placed on the muscle-tendon units that assist in controlling this complex triplanar movement.[22,53] Lower-extremity structural variations such as a rearfoot and forefoot varus can cause the subtalar joint to pronate excessively in order to get the medial aspect of the forefoot in contact with the ground for push-off.[47] The magnitude of these forces will increase during running, especially with a rearfoot striker. Sprinters may present with similar symptoms but with a different cause, that being overuse of the plantarflexors secondary to being on their toes during their event. Training surfaces including embankments and crowned roads can place increased tensile loads on the distal medial tibia, and modifications should be made whenever possible.

Rehabilitation Concerns. Management of this condition should include physician referral to rule out the possibility of stress fracture via the use of bone scan and plain films. Activity modification along with measures to maintain cardiovascular fitness are set in place immediately. Correction of abnormal pronation during walking and running must also be addressed with shoes and, if needed, custom foot orthotics. Ice massage to the area might help reduce localized pain and inflammation. A flexibility program for the gastroc-soleus musculature should be initiated.

Rehabilitation Progression. Running and jumping activities may need to be completely eliminated for the first 7 to 10 days after diagnosis. Pool workouts with a flotation device will help maintain cardiovascular fitness during the healing process. Gastrocnemius-soleus flexibility is improved with static stretching (Figure 24-21). Ice and electrical stimulation can be used to reduce inflammation and modulate pain in the early stages. As the condition improves, general strengthening of the ankle musculature with rubber tubing can be performed along with calf muscle strengthening (Figures 24-5 to 24-8, 24-12, 24-13). These exercises may cause muscle fatigue but should not increase the athlete's symptoms. An isokinetic strengthening program of the ankle inverters and everters can be utilized to improve strength and has been shown to reduce pronation during treadmill running[15] (Figure 24-18). As mentioned previously, it is imperative that all structural deviations that cause pronation be addressed with a foot orthotic or at least proper motion-control shoes. As pain to palpation of the distal tibia resolves, the athlete should be progressed to a jogging/running program on grass with proper footwear. This may involve beginning with a 10- to 15-minute run and progressing by 10 percent every week. In the case of track athletes, a pool or bike workout can be implemented for 20 to 30 minutes after the run to produce a fuller workout. The athlete needs to be compliant with a gradual progression and should be educated to avoid doing too much, too soon, which could lead to a recurrence of the condition or possibly a stress fracture.

Criteria for Returning to Full Activity. The athlete may return to full activity when (1) there is minimal to no pain to palpation of the affected area, (2) all causes of excessive pronation have been addressed with an orthotic and proper shoeware, (3) there is sufficient gastrocnemius-soleus musculature flexibility, and (4) the athlete has successfully completed the gradual running progression and a sport-specific functional progression without an increase in symptoms.

Achilles Tendinitis

Pathomechanics. Achilles tendinitis is an inflammatory condition that involves the Achilles tendon and/or its tendon sheath, the paratenon. Often there is excessive tensile stress placed on the tendon repetitively, as with running or jumping activities, that overloads the tendon, especially on its medial aspect.[29,42] This condition can be divided into Achilles paratenonitis or peritendinitis, which is an inflammation of the paratenon or tissue that surrounds the tendon, and tendinosus, which denotes tears within the tendon.[18,39] The athlete often complains of generalized pain and stiffness about the Achilles tendon region, which when localized is usually 2 to 6 cm proximal to the calcaneal insertion. Uphill running or hill workouts will usually aggravate the condition. There may be reduced gastrocnemius and soleus muscle flexibility in general that may worsen as the condition progresses and adaptive shortening occurs. Muscle testing of the above muscles may be within normal limits, but painful and a true deficit may be observed when performing toe raises to fatigue as compared to the uninvolved extremity.

Injury Mechanism. Achilles tendinitis will often present with a gradual onset over a period of time. Initially the athlete might ignore the symptoms, which might present at the beginning of activity and resolve as the activity progresses. Symptoms may progress to morning stiffness and discomfort with walking after periods of prolonged sitting. Repetitive weight-bearing activities, such as running or early-season conditioning in which the duration and intensity are increased too quickly with insufficient recovery time, will worsen the condition. Excessive compensatory pronation of the subtalar joint with concomitant internal rotation of the lower leg secondary to a forefoot varus, tibial varum, or femoral anterversion will increase the tensile load about the medial aspect of the Achilles tendon.[18,23,39] Decreased gastrocnemius and soleus complex flexibility can also increase subtalar joint pronation to compensate for the decreased closed-kinetic-chain dorsiflexion needed during early and midstance phase of running. If the athlete continues to train, the tendon will become further inflamed and the gastrocnemius-soleus musculature will become less efficient secondary to pain inhibition. The tendon may be warm and painful to palpation, as well as thickened, which may indicate the chronicity of the condition. Crepitace may be palpated with AROM plantar and dorsiflexion and pain will be elicited with passive dorsiflexion.

Rehabilitation Concerns. Achilles tendinitis can be resistant to a quick resolution secondary to the slower healing response of tendinous tissue. It has also been noted that an area of hypovascularity exists within the tendon that may further impede the healing response. It is important to create a proper healing environment by reducing the offending activity and replacing it with an activity that will reduce strain on the tendon. Addressing structural faults that may lead to excessive pronation or supination should be done through proper shoeware and foot orthotics as well as flexibility exercises for the gastrocnemius-soleus complex. Modalities such as ice can help reduce pain and inflammation early on, and ultrasound can facilitate an increased blood flow to the tendon in the later stages of rehabilitation. Cross-friction massage may be used to break down adhesions that may have formed during the healing response and further improve the gliding ability of the paratenon. Strengthening of the gastrocnemius-soleus musculature must be progressed carefully so as not to cause a recurrence of the symptoms. Lastly a gradual progression must be made for a safe return to activity to avoid the condition's becoming chronic.

Rehabilitation Progression. Activity modification is necessary to allow the Achilles tendon to begin the healing process. Swimming, pool running with a flotation device, stationary cycling, and use of an upper-body ergometer (UBE) are all possible alternative activities for cardiovascular maintenance (Figures 24-16, 24-28, 24-29). It is important to reduce stresses on the Achilles tendon that may occur with daily ambulation. Proper footwear with a slight heel lift, such as a good running shoe, can reduce stress on the tendon during gait. Structural biomechanical abnormalities that manifest with excessive pronation or supination should be addressed with a custom foot orthotic. Placing a heel lift in the shoe or building it into the orthotic can reduce stress on the Achilles tendon initially but should be gradually reduced so as not to cause an adaptive shortening of the muscle-tendon unit. Gentle pain-free stretching can be performed several times per day and can be done after an active or passive warm-up with exercise or modalities such as superficial heat or ultrasound (Figures 24-20, 24-21). Open-kinetic-chain strengthening with rubber tubing can begin early in the rehabilitation process and should be progressed to closed-kinetic-chain strengthening in a concentric and eccentric fashion utilizing the athlete's body weight with modification of sets, repetitions, and speed of exercise to intensify the rehabilitation session (Figures 24-5, 24-12, 24-13). A walking-jogging progression on a firm but forgiving surface can be initiated when the symptoms have resolved and ROM, strength, endurance, and flexibility have been normalized to the uninvolved extremity. The athlete must be reminded that

this progression is designed to improve the affected tendon's ability to tolerate stress in a controlled fashion and not to improve fitness level. Studies have shown that CV fitness can be maintained with biking and swimming.[13] Finally it is important to educate the athlete on the nature of the condition in order to set realistic expectations for a safe return without recurrence of the condition.

Criteria for Full Return. The athlete may return to full activity when (1) there has been full resolution of symptoms with ADLs and minimal or no symptoms with sport-related activity, (2) ROM, strength, flexibility, and endurance are equal to the opposite uninvolved extremity, and (3) all contributing biomechanical faults have been corrected during walking and running gait analysis with proper shoeware and/or custom foot orthotics.

Achilles Tendon Rupture

Pathomechanics. The Achilles tendon is the largest tendon in the human body. It serves to transmit force from the gastrocnemius and soleus musculature to the calcaneus. Rupture of the Achilles tendon usually occurs in an area 2 to 6 cm proximal to the calcaneal insertion, which has been implicated as an avascular site prone to degenerative changes.[8,25,27] The injury presents after a sudden plantarflexion of the ankle, as in jumping or accelerating with a sprint. The athlete will often feel or hear a pop and note a sensation of being kicked in the back of the leg. Plantarflexion of the ankle will be painful and limited but still possible with the assistance of the tibialis posterior and the peroneals. A palpable defect will be noted along the length of the tendon, and the Thompson test will be positive. The athlete will require the use of crutches to continue ambulation without an obvious limp.

Injury Mechanism. Achilles tendon rupture is usually caused by a sudden forceful plantarflexion of the ankle. It has been theorized that the area of rupture has undergone degenerative changes and is more prone to rupture when placed under higher levels of tensile loading.[25] The degenerative changes may be due to excessive compensatory pronation at the subtalar joint to accommodate for structural deviations of the forefoot, rearfoot, and lower leg during walking and running. This pronation can place an increased tensile stress on the medial aspect of the Achilles tendon. Also, a chronically inflexible gastrocnemius-soleus complex will reduce the available amount of dorsiflexion at the ankle joint, and excessive subtalar joint pronation will assist in accommodating this loss. The above mechanisms may result in tendinitis symptoms that precede the tendon rupture, but this is not always the case. Fatigue of the deconditioned athlete or weekend warrior may also contribute to tendon rupture, as well as improper warm-up prior to ballistic activities such as basketball or racquet sports.[24]

Rehabilitation Concerns. After an Achilles tendon rupture, the question of surgical repair versus cast immobilization will arise. Cetti et al. report that surgical repair of the tendon is recommended to allow the athlete to return to previous levels of activity.[8] Surgical repair of the Achilles tendon may require a period of immobilization for 6 to 8 weeks to allow for proper tendon healing.[6,25,31] The deleterious effects of this lengthy immobilization include muscle atrophy, joint stiffness including intra-articular adhesions and capsular stiffness of the involved joints, disorganization of the ligament substance, and possible disuse osteoporosis of the bone.[6] Isokinetic strength deficits for the ankle plantarflexors, especially at lower speeds, have been documented with periods of cast immobilization for 6 weeks.[30] Steele et al. noted significant deficits isokinetically of ankle plantarflexor strength after 8 weeks of immobilization.[48] These authors feel that the primary limiting factor that influences functional outcome might be the duration of postsurgical immobilization.[48] Several studies have been done using early controlled ankle motion and progressive weight bearing without immobilization.[6,25,31,46] It is important not only to regain full ROM without harming the repair, but also to regain normal muscle function through controlled progressive strengthening. This can be performed through a variety of exercises, including isometrics, isotonics, and isokinetics (Figures 24-1 to 24-13). Open- and closed-kinetic-chain activities can be incorporated into the progression to gradually increase weight-bearing stress on the tendon repair as well as to improve proprioception (Figures 24-11, 24-14, 24-15, 24-24 to 24-27). Cardiovascular endurance can be maintained with stationary biking and pool running with a flotation device. Gait normalization for walking and running can be performed using a treadmill.

Rehabilitation Progression. It is important for the sports therapist to have an open line of communication with the physician in charge of the surgical repair. Decisions about length and type of immobilization, weight-bearing progression, allowable ROM, and progressive strengthening should be thoroughly discussed with the physician. Recent literature reports excellent results with early and controlled mobilization with the use of a splint that allows early plantarflexion ROM and that slowly increases ankle dorsiflexion to neutral and full dorsiflexion over a 6- to 8-week period of time.[6,25] Controlled progressive weight bearing based on percentages of the athlete's body weight can be done over a 6 to 8 weeks postoperatively, with full weight bearing by the end of this time frame. During the early stages of rehabilitation, ICE is used to decrease swelling. A variety of ROM exercises are done to increase ankle ROM in all planes as well as initiate activation of the surrounding muscles (Figures 24-1 to 24-4, 24-9, 24-10, 24-14, 24-15, 24-20, 24-22). By 4 to 6 weeks postoperatively, strengthening exercises with rubber tubing can be progressed to closed-chain exercises utilizing a percentage of the athlete's body weight with heel raises on a Total Gym apparatus (Figures 24-5, 24-8, 24-11). It is important to do more concentric than eccentric loading initially, so as not to place excessive stress on the repair. Gradual increases in eccentric loading can occur from 10 to 12 weeks postoperatively. Also at this time, isokinetic exercise can be introduced with submaximal high-speed exercise and be progressed to lower concentric speeds gradually over time (Figure 24-19). By 3 months, full-weight-bearing heel raises can be performed (Figures 24-12, 24-13). At the same time a walking/jogging program can be initiated. Isokinetic strength testing can be done between 3 and 4 months to determine if any deficits in ankle plantarflexor strength exist (see Figure 24-19). The number of single-leg heel raises performed in a specified amount of time as compared to the uninvolved extremity can also be utilized to determine functional plantarflexor strength and endurance. Sport-related functional activities can be initiated at 3 months along with a progressive jogging program. A full return to unrestricted athletic activity can begin after 6 months, once the athlete successfully meets all predetermined goals.

Criteria for Full Return. The athlete can return to full activity after the following criteria have been met: (1) full AROM of the involved ankle as compared to the uninvolved side, (2) isokinetic strength of the ankle plantarflexors at 90 to 95 percent of the uninvolved side, (3) 90 to 95 percent of the number of heel raises throughout the full ROM in a 30-second period as compared to the uninvolved side, and (4) the ability to walk, jog, and run without an observable limp and successful completion of a sport-related functional progression without any Achilles tendon irritation.

Retrocalcaneal Bursitis

Pathomechanics. The retrocalcaneal bursae is a disc-shaped object that lies between the Achilles tendon and the superior tuberosity of the calcaneus.[5] The athlete will report a gradual onset of pain that may be associated with Achilles tendinitis. Careful palpation anterior to the Achilles tendon will rule out involvement of the tendon. Pain is increased with AROM/PROM ankle dorsiflexion and relieved with plantarflexion. Depending on the severity and swelling associated, it may be painful to walk, especially when attempting to attain full closed-kinetic-chain ankle dorsiflexion during the midstance phase of gait.

Injury Mechanism. Loading the foot and ankle in repeated dorsiflexion, as in uphill running, can be a cause of this condition. When the foot is dorsiflexed, the distance between the posterior/superior calcaneus and the Achilles tendon will be reduced, resulting in a repeated mechanical compression of the retrocalcaneal bursae. Also, structural abnormalities of the foot may lead to excessive compensatory movements at the subtalar joint, which may cause friction of the Achilles tendon on the bursae with running.

Rehabilitation Concerns. Because of the close proximity of other structures, it is important to rule out involvement of the calcaneus and Achilles tendon with careful palpation of the area. Rest and activity modification in order to reduce swelling and inflammation is necessary. If walking is painful, crutches with weight bearing as tolerated is recommended for a brief period. Gentle but progressive stretching and strengthening should be added as tolerated, with care being taken not to increase pain with gastrocnemius-soleus stretching (Figures 24-5, 24-12, 24-13, 24-20, 24-21). If excessive compensatory pronation is noted during gait analysis, recommendations on proper footwear should be made, especially in regard to the heel counter, and foot orthotics should be considered.

Rehabilitation Progression. The early management of this condition requires all measures to reduce pain and inflammation including ice, rest from offending activity, proper shoeware, and modified weight bearing with crutches if necessary. Cardiovascular fitness can be maintained with pool running with a flotation device. Gentle stretching of the gastrocnemius-soleus needs to be introduced slowly, because this will tend to increase compression of the retrocalcaneal bursae. As pain resolves and ROM and walking gait are normalized, the athlete may begin a progressive walking/jogging program. The athlete can progress back to activity as the condition allows. Heel lifts in both shoes may be necessary in the early return to activity, with gradual weaning away from them as AROM/PROM dorsiflexion improves. The condition may allow full return in 10 days to 2 weeks if treated early enough. If the condition persists, 6 to 8 weeks of rest, activity modification, and treatment may be needed before a successful result is attained with conservative care.

Criteria for Return to Full Activity. The following criteria need to met before return to full activity: (1) no observable swelling and minimal to no pain to palpation of the area at rest or after daily activity, (2) full ankle dorsiflexion AROM and normal pain-free strength of the gastrocnemius and soleus musculature, and (3) normal and pain-free walking and running gait.

Summary

1. Although some injuries in the region of the lower leg are acute, most injuries seen in an athletic population result from overuse, most often from running.

2. Tibial fractures can create long-term problems for the athlete if inappropriately managed. Fibular fractures generally require much shorter periods for immobilization. Treatment of these fractures involves immediate medical referral and most likely a period of immobilization and restricted weight bearing.

3. Stress fractures in the lower leg are usually the result of the bone's inability to adapt to the repetitive loading response during training and conditioning of the athlete and are more likely to occur in the tibia.

4. Chronic compartment syndromes can occur from acute trauma or repetitive trauma of overuse. They can occur in any of the four compartments, but are most likely in the anterior compartment or deep posterior compartment.

5. Rehabilitation of medial tibial stress syndrome must be comprehensive and address several factors, including musculoskeletal, training, and conditioning, as well as proper shoes and orthotics intervention.

6. Achilles tendinitis will often present with a gradual onset over a period of time and may be resistant to a quick resolution secondary to the slower healing response of tendinous tissue.

7. Perhaps the greatest question after an Achilles tendon rupture is whether surgical repair or cast immobilization is the best method of treatment. Regardless of treatment method, the time required for rehabilitation is significant.

8. With retrocalcaneal bursitis the athlete will report a gradual onset of pain that may be associated with Achilles tendinitis. Treatment should include rest and activity modification in order to reduce swelling and inflammation.

References

1. Andrish, J., and J. Work. 1990. How I manage shin splints. *Physician and Sports Medicine* 18(12): 113–14.

2. Beckham, S., W. Grana, and P. Buckley, et al. 1993. A comparison of anterior compartment pressures in competitive runners and cyclists. *American Journal of Sports Medicine* 21(1): 36–40.

3. Bennell, K., S. Malcolm, S. Thomas, et al. 1996. The incidence and distribution of stress fractures in competitive track and field athletes: A twelve-month prospective study. *American Journal of Sports Medicine* 24(2): 211–17.

4. Bennell, K., S. Malcolm, S. Thomas, et al. 1996. Risk factors for stress fractures in track and field athletes: A twelve-month prospective study. *American Journal of Sports Medicine* 24(6): 810–17.

5. Bordelon, R. 1994. The heel. In *Orthopaedic and sports medicine: Principles and practice,* edited by J. DeLee and D. Drez. Philadelphia: W. B. Saunders.

6. Carter, T., P. Fowler, and C. Blokker. 1992. Functional postoperative treatment of Achilles tendon repair. *American Journal of Sports Medicine* 20(4): 459–62.

7. Case, W. 1994. Relieving the pain of shin splints. *Physician and Sports Medicine* 22(4): 31–32.

8. Cetti, R., S. Christensen, R. Ejsted, et al. 1993. Operative versus nonoperative treatment of Achilles tendon rupture: A prospective randomized study and review of the literature. *American Journal of Sports Medicine* 21(6): 791–99.

9. Chang, P., and R. Harris. 1996. Intramedullary nailing for chronic tibial stress fractures: A review of five cases. *American Journal of Sports Medicine* 24(5): 688–92.

10. Dickson, T., and P. Kichline. 1987. Functional management of stress fractures in female athletes using a pneumatic leg brace. *American Journal of Sports Medicine* 15 (1): 86–89.

11. Donatelli, R. 1990. Normal anatomy and biomechanics. In *The biomechanics of the foot and ankle,* 1st ed., edited by R. Donatelli and S. Wolf. Philadelphia: F. A. Davis.

12. Ekenman, I., L. Tsai-Fellander, P. Westblad, et al. 1996. A study of intrinsic factors in patients with stress fractures of the tibia. *Foot and Ankle* 17(8): 477–82.

13. Eyestone, E., G. Fellingham, J. George, and G. Fisher. 1993. Effect of water running and cycling on maximum oxygen consumption and 2-mile run performance. *American Journal of Sports Medicine* 21(1): 41–44.

14. Fehlandt, A., and L. Micheli. 1995. Acute exertional anterior compartment syndrome in an adolescent female. *Medicine and Science in Sports and Exercise* 27(1): 3–7.

15. Feltner, M., H. Macrae, P. Macrae, et al. 1994. Strength training effects on rearfoot motion in running. *Medicine and Science in Sports and Exercise* 26(8): 102–7.

16. Fick, D., J. Albright, and B. Murray. 1992. Relieving painful shin splints. *Physician and Sports Medicine* 20(12): 105–13.

17. Fredericson, M., A. Bergman, K. Hoffman, and M. Dillingham. 1995. Tibial stress reaction in runners: A correlation of clinical symptoms and scintigraphy with a new magnetic resonance imaging grading system. *American Journal of Sports Medicine* 23(4): 472–81.

18. Galloway, M., P. Jokl, and W. Dayton. 1992. Achilles tendon overuse injuries. *Clin Sports Med* 11(4): 771–82.

19. Garrick, J., and G. Couzens. 1992. Tennis leg: How I manage gastrocnemius strains. *Physician and Sports Medicine* 20(5): 203–7.

20. Giladi, M., C. Milgrom, A. Simkin, et al. 1991. Stress fractures: Identifiable risk factors. *American Journal of Sports Medicine* 19(6): 647–52.

21. Goldberg, B., and C. Pecora. 1994. Stress fractures: A risk of increased training in freshmen. *Physician and Sports Medicine* 22(3): 68–78.

22. Gross, M. 1995. Lower quarter screening for skeletal malalignment: Suggestions for orthotics and shoeware. *Journal of Orthopaedic and Sports Physical Therapy* 21(6): 389–405.

23. Gross, M. 1992. Chronic tendinitis: Pathomechanics of injury factors affecting the healing response and treatment. *Journal of Orthopaedic and Sports Physical Therapy* 16(6): 248–61.

24. Hamel, R. 1992. Achilles tendon ruptures: Making the diagnosis. *Physician and Sports Medicine* 20(9): 189–200.

25. Heinrichs, K., and C. Haney. 1994. Rehabilitation of the surgically repaired Achilles tendon using a dorsal functional orthosis: A preliminary report. *Journal of Sport Rehabilitation* 3:292–303.

26. Kaper, B., C. Carr, and T. Shirreffs. 1997. Compartment syndrome after arthroscopic surgery of knee: A report of two cases managed nonoperatively. *American Journal of Sports Medicine* 25(1): 123–25.

27. Karjalainen, P., H. Aronen, H. Pihlajamaki, et al. 1997. Magnetic resonance imaging during healing of surgically repaired Achilles tendon ruptures. *American Journal of Sports Medicine* 25(2): 164–71.

28. Kohn, H. 1997. Shin pain and compartment syndromes in running. In *Running injuries,* edited by G. Guten. Philadelphia: W. B. Saunders.

29. Leach, R., A. Schepsis, and H. Takai. 1991. Achilles tendinitis: Don't let it be an athlete's downfall. *Physician and Sports Medicine* 19(8): 87–92.

30. Leppilahti, J., P. Siira, H. Vanharanta, et al. 1996. Isokinetic evaluation of calf muscle performance after Achilles rupture repair. *International Journal of Sports Medicine* 17(8): 619–23.

31. Mandelbaum, B., M. Myerson, and R. Forster. 1995. Achilles tendon ruptures: A new method of repair, early range of motion, and functional rehabilitation. *American Journal of Sports Medicine* 23(4): 392–95.

32. Matheson, G., B. Clement, C. McKenzie, et al. 1987. Stress fractures in athletes. A study of 320 cases. *American Journal of Sports Medicine* 15(1): 46–58.

33. Pedowitz, R., A. Hargens, S. Mubarek, et al. 1990. Modified criteria for the objective diagnosis of chronic compartment syndrome of the leg. *American Journal of Sports Medicine* 18(1): 35–40.

34. Puddu, G., G. Cerullo, A. Selvanetti, and F. DePaulis. 1994. Stress fractures. In *Oxford textbook of sports medicine*, edited by M. Harries, C. Williams, W. Stanish, and L. Micheli. New York: Oxford University Press.

35. Reber, L., J. Perry, and M. Pink. 1993. Muscular control of the ankle in running. *American Journal of Sports Medicine* 21(6): 805–10.

36. Reeder, M., B. Dick, J. Atkins, et al. 1996. Stress fractures: Current concepts of diagnosis and treatment. *Sports Med* 22(3): 198–212.

37. Rettig, A., K. Shelbourne, J. McCarrol, et al. 1988. The natural history and treatment of delayed union stress fractures of the anterior cortex of the tibia. *American Journal of Sports Medicine* 16(3): 250–55.

38. Rettig, A., J. McCarroll, and R. Hahn. 1991. Chronic compartment syndrome: Surgical intervention in 12 cases. *Physician and Sports Medicine* 19(4): 63–70.

39. Reynolds, N., and T. Worrell. 1991. Chronic Achilles peritendinitis: Etiology, pathophysiology, and treatment. *Journal of Orthopaedic and Sports Physical Therapy* 13(4): 171–76.

40. Sallade, J., and S. Koch. 1992. Training errors in long distance runners. *Journal of Athletic Training* 27(1): 50–53.

41. Schepsis, A., D. Martini, and M. Corbett. 1993. Surgical management of exertional compartment syndrome of the lower leg: Long term followup. *American Journal of Sports Medicine* 21(6): 811–17.

42. Schepsis, A., C. Wagner, and R. Leach. 1994. Surgical management of Achilles tendon overuse injuries: A long-term follow-up study. *American Journal of Sports Medicine* 22(5): 611–19.

43. Schon, L., D. Baxter. and T. Clanton. 1992. Chronic exercise-induced leg pain in active people: More than just shin splints. *Physician and Sports Medicine* 20(1): 100–114.

44. Shwayhat, A., J. Linenger, L. Hofher, et al. 1994. Profiles of exercise history and overuse injuries among United States Navy Sea, Air, and Land (SEAL) recruits. *American Journal of Sports Medicine* 22(6): 835–40.

45. Simon, R. 1995. The tibial and fibular shaft. In *Emergency orthopedics: The extremities*, 3d ed., edited by R. Simon and S. Koenigshnecht. Norwalk CT: Appleton-Lange.

46. Solveborn, S., and A. Moberg. 1994. Immediate free ankle motion after surgical repair of acute Achilles tendon ruptures. *American Journal of Sports Medicine* 22(5): 607–10.

47. Sommer, H., and S. Vallentyne. 1995. Effect of foot posture on the incidence of medial tibial stress syndrome. *Medicine and Science in Sports and Exercise* 27(6): 800–804.

48. Steele, G., R. Harter, and A. Ting. 1993. Comparison of functional ability following percutaneous and open surgical repairs of acutely ruptured tendons. *Journal of Sport Rehabilitation* (2): 115–27.

49. Strudwick, W., and G. Stuart. 1992. Proximal fibular stress fracture in an aerobic dancer: A case report. *American Journal of Sports Medicine* 20(4): 481–82.

50. Stuart, M., and T. Karaharju. 1994. Acute compartment syndrome: Recognizing the progressive signs and symptoms. *Physician and Sports Medicine* 22(3): 91–95.

51. Styf, J., M. Nakhostine, and D. Gershuni. 1992. Functional knee braces increase intramuscular pressures in the anterior compartment of the leg. *American Journal of Sports Medicine* 20(1): 46–49.

52. Taube, R., and L. Wadsworth. 1993. Managing tibial stress fractures. *Physician and Sports Medicine* 21(4): 123–30.

53. Tiberio, D. 1988. Pathomechanics of structural foot deformities. *Physical Therapy* 68 (12): 1840–49.

54. Tiberio, D. 1987. The effect of excessive subtalar joint pronation on patellofemoral mechanics: A theoretical model. *Journal of Orthopaedic and Sports Physical Therapy* 9(4): 160–65.

55. Vincent, N. 1994. Compartment syndromes. In *Oxford textbook of sports medicine*, edited by M. Harries, C. Williams, W. Stanish, and L. Micheli. New York: Oxford University Press.

56. Wilder, R., D. Brennan, and D. Schotte. 1993. A standard measure for exercise prescription for aqua running. *American Journal of Sports Medicine* 21(1): 45–48.

57. Wiley, J., D. Clement, D. Doyle, et al. 1987. A primary care perspective of chronic compartment syndrome of the leg. *Physician and Sports Medicine* 15(3): 111–20.

58. Willy, C., B. Becker, and H. Evers. 1996. Unusual development of acute exertional compartment syndrome due to delayed diagnosis: A case report. *International Journal of Sports Medicine* 17(6): 458–61.

59. Yasuda, T., K. Miyazaki, K. Tada, et al. 1992. Stress fracture of the right distal femur following bilateral fractures of the proximal fibulas: A case report. *American Journal of Sports Medicine* 20 (6): 771–74.

CHAPTER 25

Rehabilitation of Ankle and Foot Injuries

Skip Hunter
William E. Prentice

After completion of this chapter, the student should be able to do the following:

- Discuss the biomechanics and functional anatomy of the foot and ankle.

- Discuss the various injuries that occur at the ankle joint.

- Discuss the various treatment options for rehabilitating an ankle sprain.

- Discuss the effect of forefoot varus, forefoot valgus, and rearfoot varus on the foot and lower extremity.

- Describe the biomechanical examination of the foot.

- Describe techniques for orthotic fabrication.

- Identify problems associated with the foot and the treatment options for each.

FUNCTIONAL ANATOMY AND BIOMECHANICS

The Talocrural Joint

The ankle joint, or talocrural joint, is a hinge joint that is formed by an articular facet on the distal extremity of the tibia, which articulates with the superior articular surface (trochlea) of the talus; the medial malleolus, which articulates with the medial surface of the trochlea of the talus; and the lateral malleolus, which articulates with the lateral surface of the trochlea. The axis of motion of the talocrural joint passes transversely through the body of the talus. This bony arrangement forms what is referred to as the ankle mortise.[2]

The talus provides a link between the lower leg and the tarsus. The talus, the second largest tarsal and the main weight-bearing bone of the articulation, rests on the calcaneous and articulates with the lateral and medial malleoli. The relatively square shape of the talus allows the ankle only two movements; dorsiflexion and plantarflexion. Because the talus is wider anteriorly than posteriorly, the most stable position of the ankle is with the foot in dorsiflexion. In this position the wider anterior aspect of the talus comes in contact with the narrower portion lying between the malleoli, gripping it tightly. By contrast, as the ankle moves into plantarflexion, the wider portion of the tibia is brought in contact with the narrower posterior aspect of the talus, creating a less stable position than in dorsiflexion.[2]

The lateral malleolus of the fibula extends further distally so that the boney stability of the lateral aspect of the ankle is more stable than the medial. Motion at the talocrural joint ranges from 20 degrees of dorsiflexion to

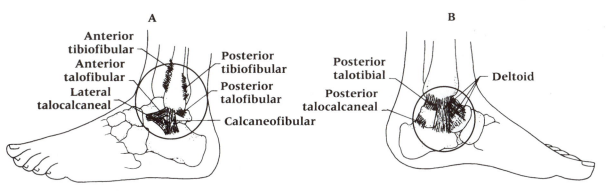

Figure 25-1   Ligaments of the talocrural joint. **A,** lateral aspect, **B,** Medial aspect.

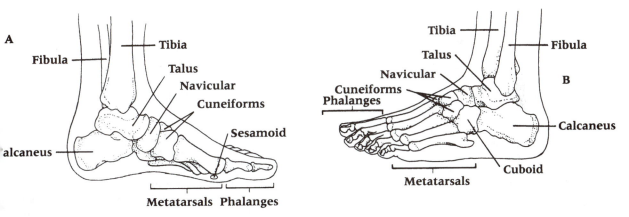

Figure 25-2   Bones of the foot. **A,** Medial aspect, **B,** Lateral aspect.

50 degrees of plantarflexion depending on the athlete. A normal foot requires 20 degrees of plantar flexion and 10 degrees of dorsiflexion with the knee extended for a normal gait.

Talocrural Joint Ligaments.   The ligamentous support of the ankle consists of the articular capsule, three lateral ligaments, two ligaments that connect the tibia and fibula, and the medial or deltoid ligament (Figure 25-1). The three lateral ligaments are the anterior talofibular, the posterior talofibular, and the calcaneofibular. The anterior and posterior tibiofibular ligaments hold the tibia and fibula and form the distal portion of the interrosseus membrane. The thick deltoid ligament provides primary resistance to foot eversion. A thin articular capsule encases the ankle joint.

Talocrural Joint Muscles.   The muscles passing posterior to the lateral malleolus will produce ankle plantar flexion along with toe extension. Anterior muscles serve to dorsiflex the ankle and to produce toe flexion.

The anterior muscles include the extensor hallucis longus, the extensor digitorum longus, the peroneus tertius, and the tibialis anterior. The posterior muscle group falls into three layers: at the superficial layer is the gastrocnemius; the middle layer includes the soleus and the plantaris; and the deep layer contains the tibialis posterior, the flexor digitorum longus, and the flexor hallucis longus.[2]

The Subtalar Joint

The subtalar joint consists of the articulation between the talus and the calcaneus[67] (Figure 25-2). Supination and pronation are normal movements that occur at the subtalar joint. These movements are triplanar movements, that is, movements that occur in all three planes simultaneously.[21,52,60] In weight bearing, the subtalar joint acts as a torque convertor to translate the pronation/supination into leg rotation.[74,84] The movements of the

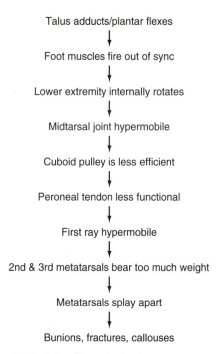

Talus adducts/plantar flexes

↓

Foot muscles fire out of sync

↓

Lower extremity internally rotates

↓

Midtarsal joint hypermobile

↓

Cuboid pulley is less efficient

↓

Peroneal tendon less functional

↓

First ray hypermobile

↓

2nd & 3rd metatarsals bear too much weight

↓

Metatarsals splay apart

↓

Bunions, fractures, callouses

Figure 25-3   The effects of a forefoot varus.

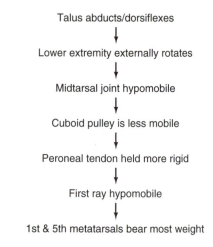

Talus abducts/dorsiflexes

↓

Lower extremity externally rotates

↓

Midtarsal joint hypomobile

↓

Cuboid pulley is less mobile

↓

Peroneal tendon held more rigid

↓

First ray hypomobile

↓

1st & 5th metatarsals bear most weight

Figure 25-4   The effects of a forefoot valgus.

talus during pronation and supination have profound effects on the lower extremity both proximally and distally.

When weight bearing, in supination the talus abducts and dorsiflexes on the calcaneus while the calcaneus inverts on the talus. The foot moves into adduction, plantarflexion, and inversion. Conversely, when weight bearing in pronation, the talus adducts and plantarflexes while the calcaneus everts on the talus. The foot moves into abduction, dorsiflexion, and eversion.[21,52]

The Midtarsal Joint

The midtarsal joint consists of two distinct joints: the calcaneocuboid and the talonavicular joint. The midtarsal joint depends mainly on ligamentous and muscular tension to maintain position and integrity. Midtarsal joint stability is directly related to the position of the subtalar joint. If the subtalar joint is pronated, the talonavicular and calcaneocuboid joints become hypermobile. If the subtalar joint is supinated, the midtarsal joint becomes hypomobile. As the midtarsal joint becomes more or less mobile, it affects the distal portion of the foot because of the articulations at the tarsometatarsal joint.[55]

Effects of Midtarsal Joint Position during Pronation.   During pronation, the talus adducts and plantarflexes and makes the joint articulations of the midtarsal joint more congruous. The long axes of the talonavicular and calcaneocuboid joints are more paral-

lel and thus allow more motion. The resulting foot is often referred to as a "loose bag of bones."[21,67]

As more motion occurs at the midtarsal joint, the lesser tarsal bones, particularly the first metatarsal and first cuneiform, become more mobile. These bones comprise a functional unit known as the *first ray*. With pronation of the midtarsal joint, the first ray is more mobile because of its articulations with that joint.[56] The first ray is also stabilized by the attachment of the long peroneal tendon, which attaches to the base of the first metatarsal. The long peroneal tendon passes posteriorly around the base of the lateral malleolus and then through a notch in the cuboid to cross the foot to the first metatarsal. The cuboid functions as a pulley to increase the mechanical advantage of the peroneal tendon. Stability of the cuboid is essential in this process. In the pronated position, the cuboid loses much of its mechanical advantage as a pulley; therefore the peroneal tendon no longer stabilizes the first ray effectively. This condition creates hypermobility of the first ray and increased pressure on the other metatarsals (Figure 25-3).

Effects of Midtarsal Joint Position during Supination.   During supination, the talus abducts and dorsiflexes, which raises the level of the talonavicular joint superior to that of the calcaneocuboid joint and allows lesser surface areas of both joint articulations to become congruous.[66] Also the long axes of the joints become more oblique. Both allow less motion to occur at this joint, making the foot very rigid and tight. Since less movement occurs at the calcaneocuboid joint, the cuboid becomes hypomobile. The long peroneal tendon has a greater amount of tension since the cuboid has less mobility and thus will not allow hypermobility of the first ray. In this case the majority of the weight is borne by the first and fifth metatarsals (Figure 25-4).

The Tarsometatarsal Joint

The tarsometatarsal joint is comprised of the cuboid; first, second, and third cuneiforms; and the bases of the metatarsal bones. These bones allow for rotational forces when engaged in weight-bearing activities. They move as a unit, depending on the position of the midtarsal and subtalar joints. Also known as the Lisfrancs' joint, the tarsometatarsal joint provides a locking device that enhances foot stability.

The Metatarsal Joints

Together with subtalar, talonavicular, and tarsometatarsal interrelationships, foot stabilization depends on the function of the metatarsal joints. The first metatarsal bone, along with the first cuneiform bone, forms the *first ray*. The first ray moves independently from the other metatarsal bones. As a main weight bearer, the first ray is concerned with body propulsion. Stabilization depends on the peroneus longus muscle that attaches on the medial aspect of the first ray. As with the other segments of the foot, stability of the first metatarsal bone depends on the relative position of the subtalar and talonavicular joints. The fifth metatarsal bone, like the first metatarsal bone, moves independently. In plantarflexion it moves into adduction and inversion; conversely, in dorsiflexion it moves the foot into abduction and eversion.[34]

Biomechanics of Normal Gait

The action of the lower extremity during a complete stride in running can be divided into two phases. The first is the stance, or support, phase, which starts with initial contact at heel strike and ends at toe-off. The second is the swing or recovery phase. This represents the time immediately after toe-off in which the leg is moved from behind the body to a position in front of the body in preparation for heel strike.

The foot's function during the support phase of running is twofold. At heel strike, the foot acts as a shock absorber to the impact forces and then adapts to the uneven surfaces. At push-off, the foot functions as a rigid lever to transmit the explosive force from the lower extremity to the running surface. In a heel-strike running gait, initial contact of the foot is on the lateral aspect of the calcaneus with the subtalar joint in supination.[5]

At initial contact, the subtalar joint is supinated. Associated with this supination of the subtalar joint is an obligatory external rotation of the tibia. As the foot is loaded, the subtalar joint moves into a pronated position until the forefoot is in contact with the running surface. The change in subtalar motion occurs between initial heel strike and 20 percent into the support phase of running. As pronation occurs at the subtalar joint, there is obligatory internal rotation of the tibia. Transverse plane rotation occurs at the knee joint because of this tibial rotation.[5] Pronation of the foot unlocks the midtarsal joint and allows the foot to assist in shock absorption and to adapt to uneven surfaces. It is important during initial impact to reduce the ground reaction forces and to distribute the load evenly on many different anatomical structures throughout the foot and leg. Pronation is normal and allows for this distribution of forces on as many structures as possible to avoid excessive loading on just a few structures. The subtalar joint remains in a pronated position until 55 to 85 percent of the support phase with maximum pronation is concurrent with the body's center of gravity passing over the base of support.[2]

The foot begins to resupinate and will approach the neutral subtalar position at 70 to 90 percent of the support phase. In supination the midtarsal joints are locked and the foot becomes stable and rigid to prepare for push-off. This rigid position allows the foot to exert a great amount of force from the lower extremity to the running surface.[39]

REHABILITATION TECHNIQUES

Strengthening Exercises

Isometric Strengthening Exercises.

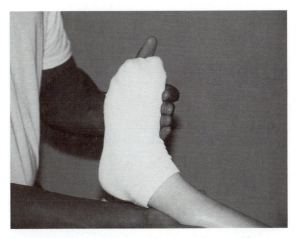

Figure 25-5   Isometric inversion against a stable resistance, used to strengthen the posterior tibialis, flexor digitorum longus, flexor hallucis longus.

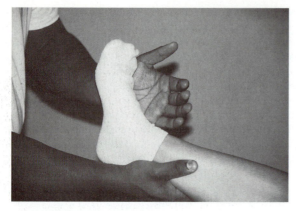

Figure 25-6   Isometric eversion against a stable resistance. Used to strengthen the peroneus longus, brevis, tertius, and extensor digitorum longus.

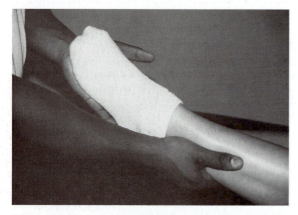

Figure 25-7   Isometric plantarflexion against a stable resistance. Used to strengthen the gastrocnemius, soleus, posterior tibialis, flexor digitorum longus, flexor hallicus longus, and plantaris.

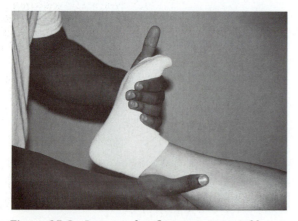

Figure 25-8   Isometric dorsiflexion against a stable resistance. Used to strengthen the anterior tibialis and peroneus tertius.

Isotonic Open-Chain Strengthening Exercises.

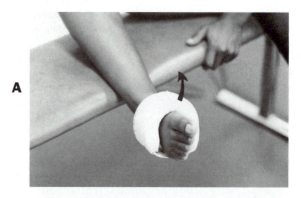

Figure 25-9   Inverion exercise. **A,** Using a weight cuff. **B,** Using resistive tubing. Used to strengthen the posterior tibialis, flexor digitorum longus, and flexor hallicus longus.

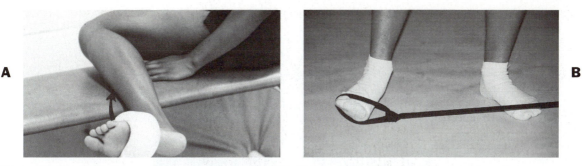

Figure 25-10 Eversion exercise. **A,** Using a weight cuff. **B,** Using resistive tubing. Used to strengthen the peroneus longus, brevis, tertius, and extensor digitorum longus.

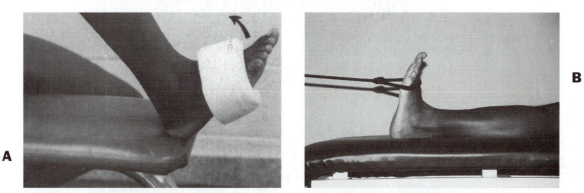

Figure 25-11 Dorsiflexion exercise. **A,** Using a weight cuff. **B,** Using resistive tubing. Used to strengthen the anterior tibialis and peroneus tertius.

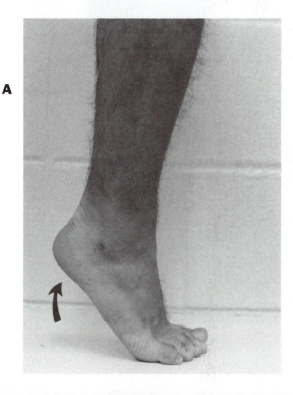

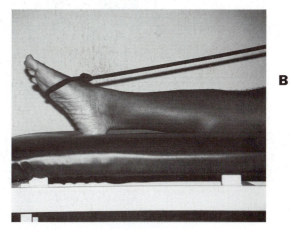

Figure 25-12 Plantarflexion exercise using surgical tubing. Used to strengthen the gastrocnemius, soleus, posterior tibialis, flexor digitorum longus, flexor hallicus longus, and plantaris.

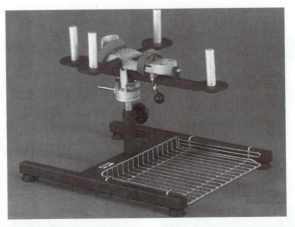

Figure 25-13   Multidirectional Elgin ankle exerciser.

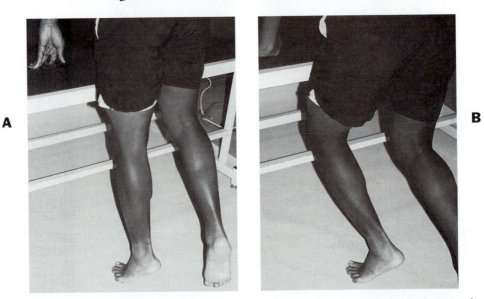

Figure 25-14   Toe raises. Used to strengthen the gastrocnemius, soleus, posterior tibialis, flexor digitorum longus, flexor hallicus longus, and plantaris. **A,** Extended knee strengthens the gastrocnemius, **B,** flexed knee strengthens the soleus.

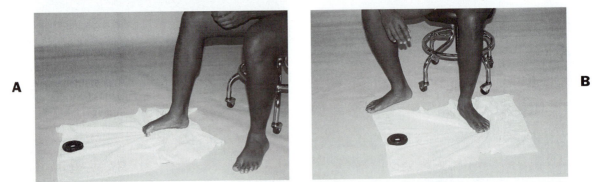

Figure 25-15   Towel-gathering exercise. **A,** Toe flexion. Used to strengthen the flexor digitorum longus and brevis, lumbricales, and flexor hallicus longus. **B,** Inversion/eversion exercises. Used to strengthen the posterior tibialis, flexor digitorum longus, flexor hallicus longus, peroneus longus, brevis, tertius, and extensor digitorum longus.

Closed-Chain Strengthening Exercises.

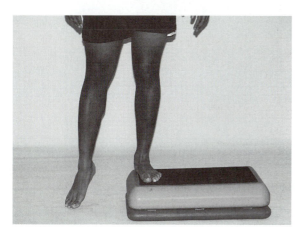

Figure 25-16 Lateral step-ups.

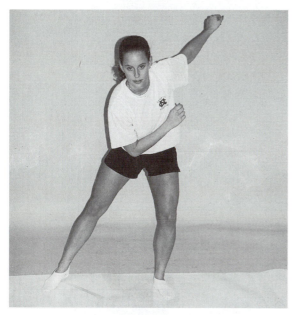

Figure 25-17 Slide board exercises.

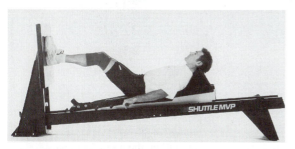

Figure 25-18 Fitter exercise machine.

Isokinetic Strengthening Exercises.

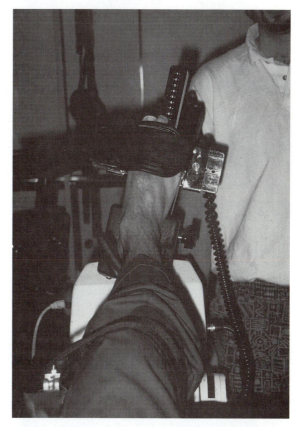

Figure 25-19 Isokinetic inversion/eversion exercise. Used to improve the strength and endurance of the ankle inverters and everters in an open chain. Also can provide an objective measurement of muscular torque production.

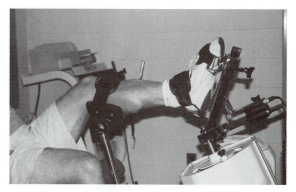

Figure 25-20 Isokinetic plantarflexion/dorsiflexion exercise. Used to improve the strength and endurance of the ankle dorsiflexors and plantarflexors in an open chain. Also can provide an objective measurement of torque production.

PNF Strengthening Exercises.

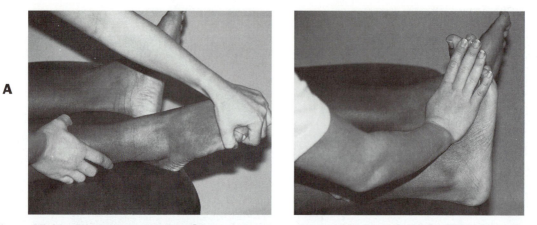

Figure 25-21 D1 pattern moving into flexion. **A,** Starting position, ankle plantarflexed, foot everted, toes flexed. **B,** Terminal position, ankle dorsiflexed, foot inverted, toes extended.

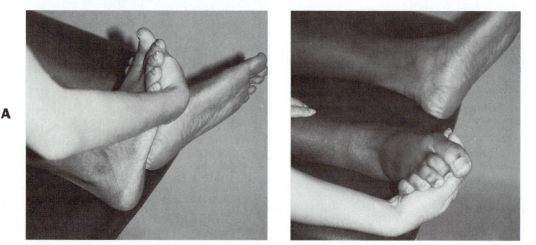

Figure 25-22 D1 pattern moving into extension. **A,** Starting position, ankle dorsiflexed, foot inverted, toes extended. **B,** Terminal position, ankle plantarflexed, foot everted, toes flexed.

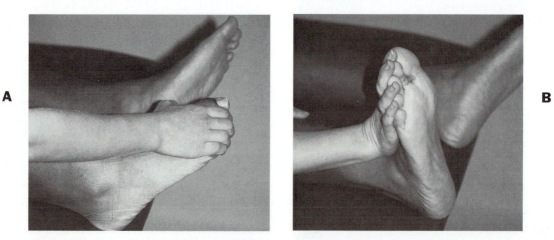

Figure 25-23 D2 pattern moving into flexion. **A,** Starting position, ankle plantarflexed, foot inverted, toes flexed. **B,** Terminal position, ankle dorsiflexed, foot everted, toes extended.

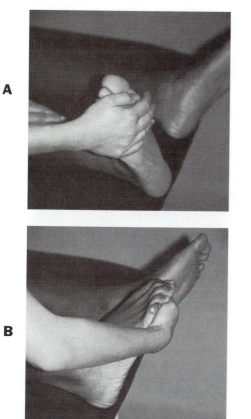

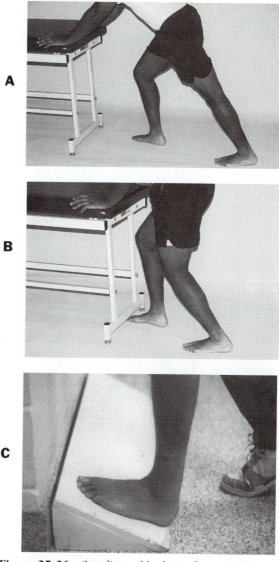

Figure 25-24   D2 pattern moving into extension.
A, Starting position, ankle dorsiflexed, foot everted, toes
extended. **B,** Terminal position, ankle plantarflexed, foot
inverted, toes flexed.

Figure 25-26   Standing ankle plantarflexors stretch.
A, Gastrocnemius. **B,** Soleus. **C,** Stretching may also be
done using a slant board.

Stretching Exercises.

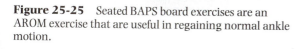

Figure 25-25   Seated BAPS board exercises are an
AROM exercise that are useful in regaining normal ankle
motion.

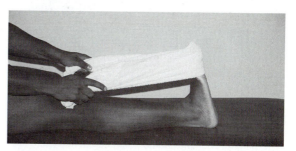

Figure 25-27   Seated ankle plantarflexors stretch
using a towel.

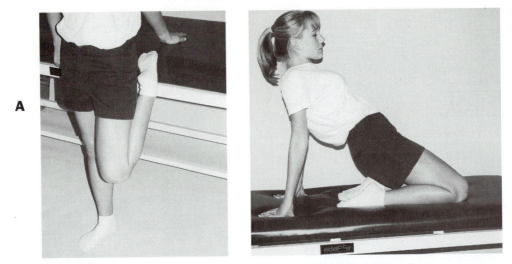

Figure 25-28 Ankle dorsiflexors stretch for the anterior tibialis. **A,** Standing. **B,** Kneeling.

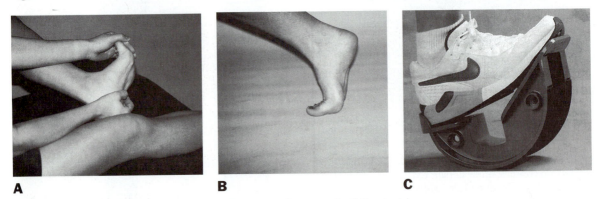

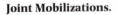

Figure 25-29 Plantar fascia stretches. **A,** Manual. **B,** Floor stretch. **C,** Prostretch.

Joint Mobilizations.

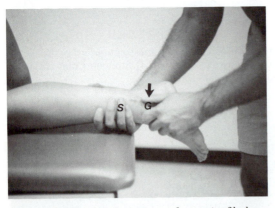

Figure 25-30 Distal anterior and posterior fibular glides. Anterior and posterior glides of the fibula may be done distally. The tibia should be stabilized, and the fibular malleolus is mobilized in an anterior or posterior direction.

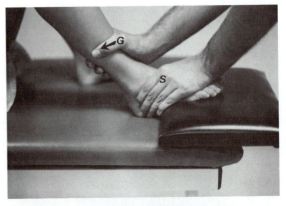

Figure 25-31 Posterior tibial glides increase plantarflexion. The foot should be stabilized, and pressure on the anterior tibia produces a posterior glide.

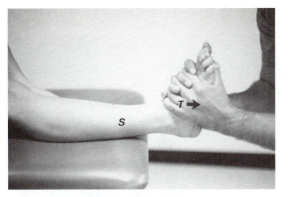

Figure 25-32 Talocrural joint traction is performed using the patient's body weight to stabilize the lower leg and applying traction to the midtarsal portion of the foot. Traction reduces pain and increases dorsiflexion and plantarflexion.

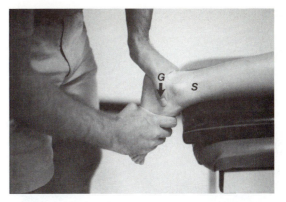

Figure 25-33 Anterior talar glides. Plantarflexion may also be increased by using an anterior talar glide. With the patient prone, the tibia is stabilized on the table, and pressure is applied to the posterior aspect of the talus to glide it anteriorly.

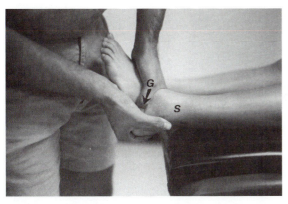

Figure 25-34 Posterior talar glides may be used for increasing dorsiflexion. With the patient supine, the tibia is stabilized on the table, and pressure is applied to the anterior aspect of the talus to glide it posteriorly.

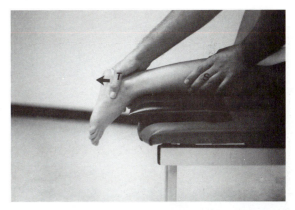

Figure 25-35 Subtalar joint traction reduces pain and increases inversion and eversion. The lower leg is stabilized on the table, and traction is applied by grasping the posterior aspect of the calcaneus.

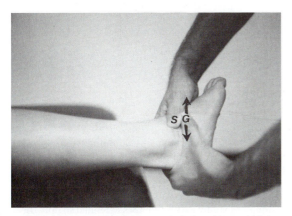

Figure 25-36 Subtalar joint medial and lateral glides increase eversion and inversion. The talus must be stabilized while the calcaneus is mobilized medially to increase inversion and laterally to increase eversion.

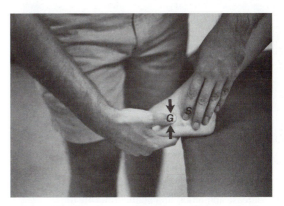

Figure 25-37 Anterior/posterior calcaneocuboid glides may be used for increasing adduction and abduction. The calcaneus should be stabilized while the cuboid is mobilized.

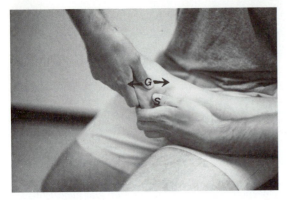

Figure 25-38 Anterior/posterior cuboidmetatarsal glides are done with one hand stabilizing the cuboid and the other gliding the base of the fifth metatarsal. They are used for increasing mobility of the fifth metatarsal.

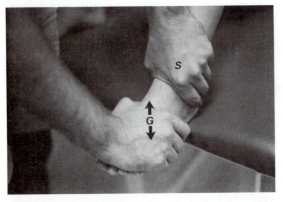

Figure 25-39 Anterior/posterior carpometacarpal glides decrease hypomobility of the metacarpals.

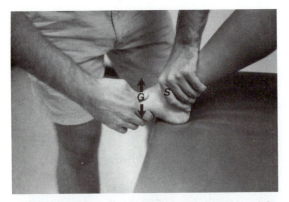

Figure 25-40 Anterior/posterior talonavicular glides also increase adduction and abduction. One hand stabilizes the talus while the other mobilizes the navicular bone.

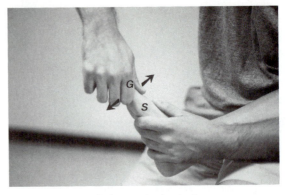

Figure 25-41 With anterior/posterior metacarpophalangeal glides, the anterior glides increase extension, and posterior glides increase flexion. Mobilizations are accomplished by isolating individual segments.

Exercises to Reestablish Neuromuscular Control.

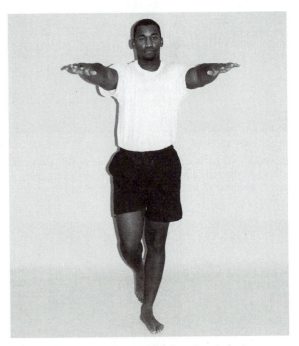

Figure 25-42 Static single-leg standing balance progression. Used to improve balance and proprioception of the lower extremity. This activity can be made more difficult with the following progression: (a) single-leg stand, eyes open; (b) single-leg stand, eyes closed; (c) single-leg stand, eyes open, toes extended so only the heel and metatarsal heads are in contact with the ground; (d) single-leg stand, eyes closed, toes extended.

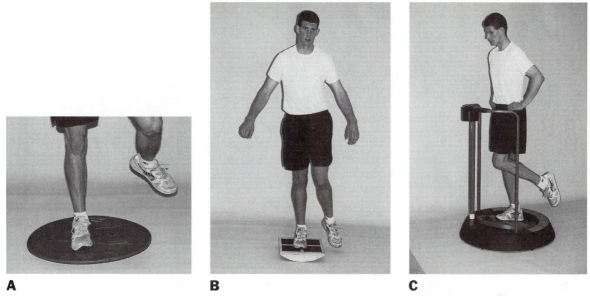

A **B** **C**

Figure 25-43 Standing single-leg balance board activity. Used to activate the lower-leg musculature and improve balance and proprioception of the involved extremity. **A,** BAPS board. **B,** Wedge board. **C,** KAT system.

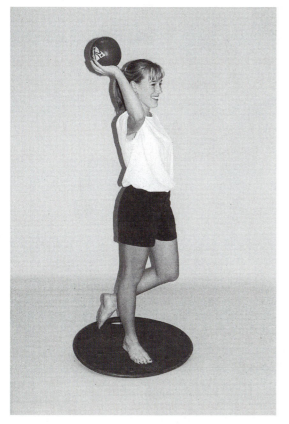

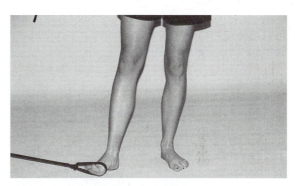

Figure 25-45 Single-leg standing rubber-tubing kicks. Using kicks resisted by surgical tubing of the uninvolved side while weight bearing on the uninvolved side may encourage neuromuscular control.

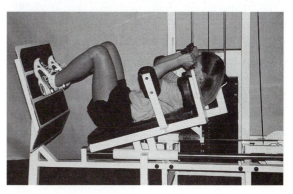

Figure 25-44 Single-leg stance on an unstable surface while performing functional activities.

Figure 25-46 Leg press.

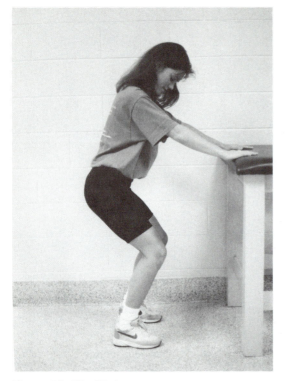

Figure 25-47 Minisquats.

Exercises to Improve Cardiorespiratory Endurance.

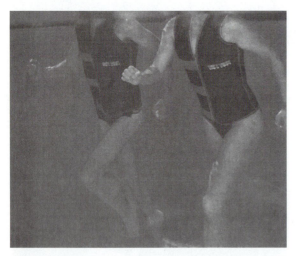

Figure 25-48 Pool running with flotation device. Used to reduce impact weight-bearing forces on the lower extremity while maintaining cardiovascular fitness level and running form.

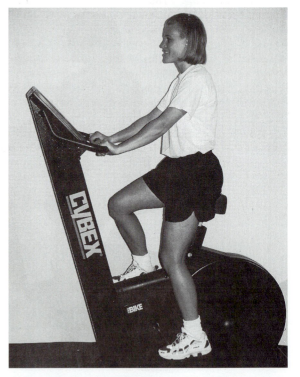

Figure 25-49 Upper-body ergometer. Used to maintain cardiovascular fitness when use of a lower-extremity ergometer is contraindicated or too difficult for the athlete to use.

Figure 25-50 Stationary exercise bike. Used to maintain cardiovascular fitness when lower-extremity weight bearing is difficult.

REHABILITATION TECHNIQUES FOR SPECIFIC INJURIES

Ankle Sprains

Pathomechanics and Injury Mechanism. Ankle sprains are among the more common injuries seen in sports medicine.[7,18,86] Injuries to the ligaments of the ankle may be classified according to either their location or the mechanism of injury.

Inversion sprains. An inversion ankle sprain that results in injury to the lateral ligaments is by far the most common. The anterior talofibular ligament is the weakest of the three lateral ligaments. Its major function is to stop forward subluxation of the talus. It is injured in an inverted, plantarflexed, and internally rotated position.[42,79] The calcaneofibular and posterior talofibular ligaments are also likely to be injured in inversion sprains as the force of inversion is increased. Increased inversion force is needed to tear the calcaneofibular ligament. Because the posterior talofibular ligament prevents posterior subluxation of the talus, its injuries are severe, such as is the case in complete dislocations.[8]

Eversion sprains. The eversion ankle sprain is less common than the inversion ankle sprain, largely because of the boney and ligamentous anatomy. As mention previously, the fibular malleolus extends further inferiorly than does the tibial malleolus. This, combined with the strength of the thick deltoid ligament, prevents excessive eversion. More often eversion injuries may involve an avulsion fracture of the tibia before the deltoid ligament tears.[13] The deltoid ligament may also be contused in inversion sprains due to impingement between the fibular malleolus and the calcaneous. Despite the fact that eversion sprains are less common, the severity is such that these sprains may take longer to heal than inversion sprains.[58]

Syndesmodic sprains. Isolated injuries to the distal tibiofemoral joint are referred to as syndesmodic sprains. The anterior and posterior tibiofibular ligaments are found between the distal tibia and fibula and extend up the lower leg as the interosseous ligament or syndesmodic ligament. Sprains of the ligaments are more common than has been realized in the past. These ligaments are torn with increased external rotational or forced dorsiflexion and are often injured in conjunction with a severe sprain of the medial and lateral ligament complexes.[77] Initial rupture of the ligaments occurs distally at the tibiofibular ligament above the ankle mortise. As the force of disruption is increased, the interosseous ligament is torn more proximally. Sprains of the syndesmodic ligaments are extremely hard to treat and often

take months to heal. Treatments for this problem are essentially the same as for medial or lateral sprains, with the difference being an extended period of immobilization. Functional activities and return to sport may be delayed for a longer period of time than for the inversion or eversion sprains.

Severity of the sprain. In a grade 1 sprain, there is some stretching or perhaps tearing of the ligamentous fibers with little or no joint instability. Mild pain, little swelling, and joint stiffness may be apparent. With a grade 2 sprain, there is some tearing and separation of the ligamentous fibers and moderate instability of the joint. Moderate to severe pain, swelling, and joint stiffness should be expected. Grade 3 sprains involve total rupture of the ligament, manifested primarily by gross instability of the joint. Severe pain may be present initially, followed by little or no pain due to total disruption of nerve fibers. Swelling may be profuse, and thus the joint tends to become very stiff some hours after the injury. A grade 3 sprain with marked instability usually requires some form of immobilization lasting several weeks. Frequently the force producing the ligament injury is so great that other ligaments or structures surrounding the joint may also be injured. With cases in which there is injury to multiple ligaments, surgical repair or reconstruction may be necessary to correct an instability.

Rehabilitation Concerns. During the initial phase of ankle rehabilitation, the major goals are reduction of postinjury swelling, bleeding, and pain and protection of the already healing ligament. As is the case in all acute musculoskeletal injuries, initial treatment efforts should be directed toward limiting the amount of swelling.[62] This is perhaps more true in the case of ankle sprains than with any other injury. Controlling initial swelling is the single most important treatment measure that can be taken during the entire rehabilitation process. There is no question that limiting the amount of acute swelling can significantly reduce the time required for rehabilitation. Initial management includes ice, compression, elevation, rest, and protection.

Compression. Immediately following injury and evaluation, a compression wrap should be applied to the sprained ankle. An elastic bandage should be firmly and evenly applied wrapping distal to proximal. It is also recommended that the elastic bandage be wet to facilitate the passage of cold. To add more compression, a horseshoe-shaped felt pad may be inserted under the wrap over the area of maximum swelling.

Following initial treatment, open Gibney taping may be applied under an elastic wrap to provide additional compression and support. Care should be taken not to compartmentalize this treatment by placing tape across

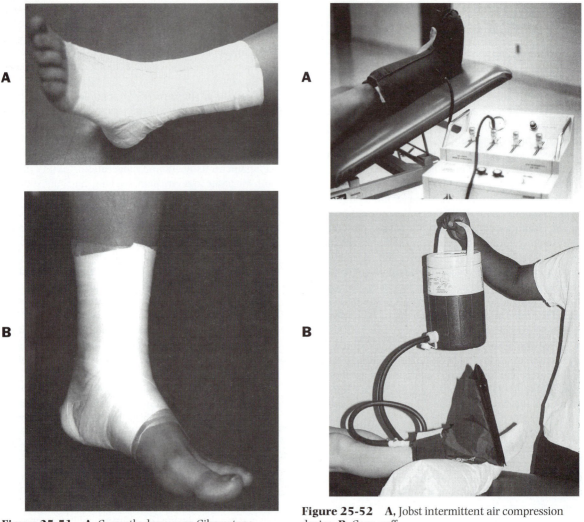

Figure 25-51 **A,** Correctly done open Gibney tape. **B,** Closed Basketweave tape.

Figure 25-52 **A,** Jobst intermittent air compression device. **B,** Cryo-cuff.

the top and bottom of the open area of the open Gibney (Figure 25-51). Uneven pressure or uncovered areas over any part of the extremity may allow the swelling to accumulate.

Other devices are available that apply external compression to the ankle to control or reduce swelling. This can be used both initially throughout the rehabilitative process. Most of these use either air or cold water within an enclosed bag to provide pressure to reduce swelling. Among these are intermittent compression devices such as a Josbt Pump or a Cryo-cuff (Figure 25-52).

Ice. The use of ice on acute injuries has been well documented in the literature. Ice must initially be used with compression, because ice used alone is not as effec-

tive as ice used in conjunction with compression.[72] The initial use of ice has its basis in constricting superficial blood flow to prevent hemorrhage as well as in reducing the hypoxic response to injury by decreasing cellular metabolism. Long-term benefits may be from reduction of pain and guarding.[2] Garrick suggests the use of ice for a minimum of 20 minutes once every 4 waking hours.[27] Ice should not be used longer than 30 minutes, especially over superficial nerves such as the peroneal and ulnar nerves; prolonged use of ice in such areas can produce transient nerve palsy.[22]

Current literature suggests that ice can be used during all phases of rehabilitation,[45] but is most effective if used immediately after injury.[62] Ice can certainly do no

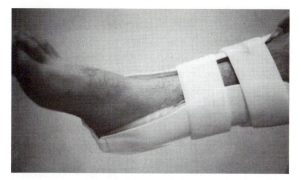

Figure 25-53 Commercially available Aircast ankle stirrup.

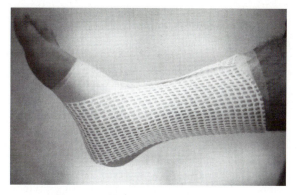

Figure 25-54 Molded Hexalite ankle stirrup.

harm if used properly, but heat, if applied too soon after injury, may lead to increased swelling. Often the switch from ice to heat cannot be made for weeks or months.

Elevation. Elevation is an essential part of edema control. Pressure in any vessel below the level of the heart is increased, which may lead to increased edema.[14] Elevation allows gravity to work with the lymphatic system rather than against it and decreases hydrostatic pressure to decrease fluid loss and also assists venous and lymphatic return through gravity.[62] Athletes with ankle sprains should be encouraged to maintain an elevated position as often as possible, particularly during the first 24 to 48 hours following injury. An attempt should be made to treat in the elevated position rather than the gravity dependent position. Any treatment done in the dependent position will allow edema to increase.[62,70]

Rest. It is important to allow the inflammatory process to have a chance to accomplish what it is supposed to during the first 24 to 48 hours before incorporating aggressive exercise techniques. However, rest does not mean that the injured athlete does nothing. Contralateral exercises may be performed to obtain cross-transfer effects on the muscles of the injured side.[44] Isometric exercises may be performed very early in dorsiflexion, plantarflexion, inversion, and eversion (Figures 25-5 through 25-8). These types of exercises may be performed to prevent atrophy without fear of further injury to the ligament. Active plantarflexion and dorsiflexion may be initiated early because they also do not endanger the healing ligament as long as they are done in a pain-free range. These active plantarflexion and dorsiflexion exercises can be done while the athlete is iced and elevated. Inversion and eversion are to be avoided, because they might initiate bleeding and further traumatize ligaments.

Protection. Several appliances are available to accomplish this early protected motion. Quillen[63] recommends the ankle stirrup, which allows motion in the

sagittal plane while limiting movement of the frontal plane and thus avoids stressing the ligaments through inversion and eversion (Figure 25-53). Several commercially available braces accomplish this goal and also apply cushioned pressure to help with edema.[73] When a commercially available product is not feasible, a similar protective device may be fashioned from thermoplastic materials such as Hexalite or Orthoplast (Figure 25-54).

The open Gibney taping technique also provides early medial and lateral protection while allowing plantarflexion and dorsiflexion, in addition to being an excellent mechanism of edema control (Figure 25-51).

Gross, Lapp, and Davis compared the effectiveness of a number of commercial ankle orthoses and taping in restricting eversion and inversion. All of these support systems significantly reduced inversion and eversion immediately after initial application and after exercise when compared to preapplication measures. Of the orthoses tested, taping provided the least support after exercise.[32] Early application of these devices allows early ambulation.

Rehabilitation Progression. In the early phase of rehabilitation, vigorous exercise is discouraged. The injured ligament must be maintained in a stable position so that healing can occur. Thus during the period of maximum protection following injury, the athlete should be either non-weight-bearing or perhaps partial-weight-bearing on crutches. Partial weight bearing with crutches helps control several complications to healing. Muscle atrophy, proprioceptive loss, and circulatory stasis are all reduced when even limited weight bearing is allowed. Weight bearing also inhibits contracture of the tendons, which can lead to tendinitis. For these reasons, early ambulation, even if only touchdown weight bearing, is essential.[48] It has been clearly demonstrated that a healing ligament needs a certain amount of stress to heal properly. Recent literature suggests that early limited stress following the initial period of inflammation might promote faster and stronger healing.[8,59] These studies found that protected motion facilitated proper collagen reorientation and thus increased the strength of the healing ligament.

As swelling is controlled and pain decreases, indicating that ligaments have reached that point in the healing process at which they are not in danger from minimal stress, rehabilitation can become more aggressive.

Range of motion. In the early stages of the rehabilitation, inversion and eversion should be minimized. Light joint mobilization concentrating on dorsiflexion and plantarflexion should be started first.[47] It can be accomplished by manual joint mobilization techniques (Figures 25-31 through 25-34) or through exercises such as towel stretching for the plantarflexors (Figure 25-27) and standing or kneeling stretches for the dorsiflexors (Figure 25-28). Athletes are encouraged to do these exercises slowly, without pain, and to use high repetitions (two sets of 40).

As tenderness over the ligament decreases, inversion-eversion exercises may be initiated in conjunction with plantarflexion and dorsiflexion exercises. Early exercises include pulling a towel from one side to the other by alternatively inverting and everting the foot (Figure 25-15*B*) and alphabet drawing in an ice bath, which should be done in capital letters to ensure that full range is used.

Exercises performed on a BAPS board, wedge board, or KAT (Figure 25-43) may be beneficial for range of motion, as well as a beginning exercise for regaining neuromuscular control.[80] These exercises should at first be done seated, progressing to standing (Figure 25-25). Initially the athlete should start in the seated position with a wedge board in the plantarflexion-dorsiflexion direction. As pain decreases and ligament healing progresses, the board may be turned in the inversion-eversion direction. As the athlete performs these movements easily, a seated BAPS board may be used for full range-of-motion exercises. When seated exercises are performed with ease, standing balance exercises should be initiated. They may be started on one leg standing without a board. The athlete then supports weight with the hands and maintains balance on a wedge board in either plantarflexion-dorsiflexion or inversion-eversion. Next, hand support may be eliminated while the athlete balances on the wedge board. The same sequence is then used on the BAPS board. The BAPS board is initially used with assistance from the hands. Then balance is practiced on the BAPS board unassisted.

Vigorous heelcord stretching should be initiated as soon as possible (Figure 25-26). McCluskey, Blackburn, and Lewis[50] found that the heelcord acts as a bowstring when tight and may increase the chance of ankle sprains.

Strengthening. Isometrics may be done in the four major ankle motion planes, frontal and sagittal (Figures 25-5 through 25-8). They may be accompanied early in the rehabilitative phase by plantarflexion and dorsiflexion isotonic exercises, which do not endanger the ligaments (Figures 25-11 and 25-12). As the ligaments heal further and range of motion increases, strengthening exercises may be begun in all planes of motion (Figures 25-9 and 25-10). Care must be taken when exercising the ankle in inversion and eversion to avoid tibial rotation as a substitute movement. Pain should be the basic guideline for deciding when to start inversion-eversion isotonic exercises. Light resistance with high repetitions has fewer detrimental effects on the ligaments (two to four sets of 10 repetitions). Resistive tubing exercises, ankle weights around the foot, or a multidirectional Elgin ankle exerciser (Figure 25-13) are excellent methods of strengthening inversion and eversion. Tubing has advantages in that it may be used both eccentrically and concentrically. Isokinetics have advantages in that more functional speeds may be obtained (Figures 25-19 and 25-20). PNF strengthening exercises that isolate the desired motions at the talocrural joint can also be used (Figures 25-21 through 25-24).

Proprioception and neuromuscular control. The role of proprioception in repeated ankle trauma has been questioned.[12,23,25,57] The literature suggests that proprioception is certainly a factor in recurrent ankle sprains. Rebman[64] reported that 83 percent of his patients experienced a reduction in chronic ankle sprains after a program of proprioceptive exercises. Glencross and Thornton[30] found that the greater the ligamentous disruption, the greater the proprioceptive loss. Early weight bearing has previously been mentioned as a method of reducing proprioceptive loss. During the rehabilitation phase, standing on both feet with closed eyes with progression to standing on one leg is an exercise to recoup proprioception (Figure 25-42). This exercise may be followed by standing and balancing on a BAPS board, which should be done initially with support from the hands. As a final-stage exercise, the athlete can progress to free standing and controlling the board through all ranges (Figure 25-43).

Other closed-kinetic-chain exercises may be beneficial. Leg presses (Figure 25-46) and minisquats (Figure 25-47) on the involved leg will encourage weight bearing and increase proprioceptive return. Single-leg standing kicks using abduction, adduction, extension, and flexion of the uninvolved side while weight bearing on the affected side will increase both strength and proprioception. This may be accomplished either free-standing (Figure 25-45) or on a machine.

Cardiorespiratory endurance. Cardiorespiratory conditioning should be maintained during the entire rehabilitation process. Pedaling a stationary bike (Figure 25-50) or an upper-extremity ergometer (Figure 25-49) with the hands provides excellent cardiovascular exercise without placing stress on the ankle. Pool running using a float vest and swimming are also good cardiovascular exercises (Figure 25-48).

Functional progressions. Functional progressions may be as complex or simple as needed. The more severe the injury, the more the need for a detailed functional progression. The typical progression begins early in the rehabilitation process as the athlete becomes partially weight bearing. Full weight bearing should be started when ambulation is performed without a limp. Running may be begun as soon as ambulation is pain free. Pain-free hopping on the affected side may also be a guideline to determine when running is appropriate. Exercising in a pool allows for early running. The athlete is placed in the pool in a swim vest that supports the body in water. The athlete then runs in place without touching the bottom of the pool. Proper running form should be stressed. Eventually the athlete is moved into shallow water so that more weight is placed on the ankle. Progression is then made to running on a smooth, flat surface, ideally a track. Initially the athlete should jog the straights and walk the curves and then progress to jogging the entire track. Speed may be increased to a sprint in a straight line. The cutting sequence should begin with circles of diminishing diameter. Cones may be set up for the athlete to run figure eights as the next cutting progression. The crossover or sidestep is next.[1] The athlete sprints to a predesignated spot and cuts or sidesteps abruptly. When this progression is accomplished, the cut should be done without warning on the command of another person. Jumping and hopping exercises should be started on both legs simultaneously and gradually reduced to only the injured side.

The athlete may perform at different levels for each of these functional sequences. One functional sequence may be done at half speed while another is done at full speed. An example of this is the athlete who is running full speed on straights of the track while doing figure eights at only half speed. Once the upper levels of all the sequences are reached, the athlete may return to limited practice, which may include early teaching and fundamental drills.

Criteria for Full Return. Estimates are that 30 to 40 percent of all inversion injuries result in reinjury.[23,37,38,49,68] In the past, athletes were simply returned to sports once the pain was low enough to tolerate the activity. Returning to full activity should include a gradual progression of functional activities that slowly

increase the stress on the ligament.[43] The specific demands of each individual sport dictate the individual drills of this progression.

It is most desirable to have the athlete return to sport without the aid of ankle support. However, it is common practice that some type of ankle support be worn initially. It appears that ankle taping does have a stabilizing effect on unstable ankles,[26,81] without interfering with motor performance.[24,50] McCluskey and others[50] suggest taping the ankle and also taping the shoe onto the foot to make the shoe and ankle function as one unit. High-topped footwear may further stabilize the ankle.[33] If cleated shoes are worn, cleats should be outset along the periphery of the shoe to provide stability.[50] An Aircast or some other supportive ankle brace can also be worn for support as a substitute for taping (Figure 25-54).

The athlete should have complete range of motion and at least 80 to 90 percent of preinjury strength before considering a return to the sport.[69] Finally, if full practice is tolerated without insult to the injured part, the athlete may return to competition.

Ankle Fractures and Dislocation

Pathomechanics and Injury Mechanism. When dealing with injuries to the ankle joint, the sports therapist must always be cautious about suspecting an ankle sprain when a fracture might actually exist. A fracture of the malleoli will generally result in immediate swelling. Ankle fractures can occur from several mechanisms that are similar to those for ankle sprains. In an inversion injury, medial malleolar fractures are often accompanied by a sprain of the lateral ligaments of the ankle. A fracture of the lateral malleolus is often more likely to occur than a sprain if an eversion force is applied to the ankle. This is due to the fact that the lateral malleolus extends as far as the distal aspect of the talus. With a fracture of the lateral malleolus, however, there may also be a sprain of the deltoid ligament. Fractures result from either avulsion or compression forces. With avulsion injuries it is often the injured ligaments that prolong the rehabilitation period.[31]

Osteochondral fractures are sometimes seen in the talus. These fractures may also be referred to as dome fractures of the talus. Generally they will be either undisplaced fractures or compression fractures.[31]

While sprains and fractures are very common, dislocations in the ankle and foot are rare. They most often occur in conjunction with fractures and require open reduction and internal fixation.[69]

Rehabilitation Concerns. Generally, undisplaced ankle fractures should be managed with rest and

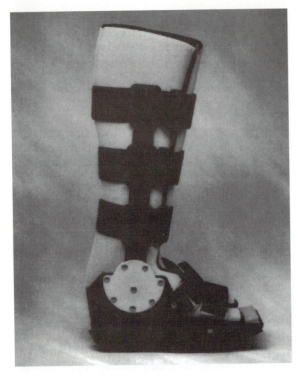

Figure 25-55 Short leg walking brace.

protection until the fracture has healed, whereas displaced fractures are treated with open reduction and internal fixation. Undisplaced fractures are treated by casting in a short leg walking cast for 6 weeks with early weight bearing. The course of rehabilitation following this period of immobilization is generally the same as for ankle sprains. Following surgery for displaced or unstable fractures, the athlete may be placed in a removable walking cast. However, it is essential to closely monitor the rehabilitative process to make certain that the patient is compliant.[31]

If an osteochondral fracture is displaced and there is a fragment, surgery is required to remove the fragment. In other cases, if the fragment has not healed within a year, surgery may be considered to remove the fragment.[31]

Rehabilitation Progression. Following open reduction and internal fixation, a posterior splint with the ankle in neutral should be applied and the athlete should be non-weight-bearing for about 2 weeks. During this period efforts should be directed at controlling swelling and wound management.

At 2 to 3 weeks the athlete may be placed in a short leg walking brace (Figure 25-55) which allows for partial weight bearing that should continue for 6 weeks. Active ROM plantarflexion and dorsiflexion exercises can begin

and should be done 2 to 3 times a day, along with general strengthening exercises for the rest of the lower extremity.

At 6 weeks, the athlete can be weight bearing in the walking brace, and this should continue for 2 to 4 weeks more. Isometric exercises (Figures 25-5 through 25-8) can be performed initially without the brace, progressing to isotonic strengthening exercises (Figures 25-9 through 25-12) that concentrate on eccentrics. Stretching exercises can also be incorporated (Figures 25-25 through 25-28). Joint mobilization exercises should be used to reduce capsular tightness (Figures 25-30 through 25-36). Exercises to regain proprioception and neuromuscular control can progress from sitting to standing as tolerated (Figures 25-42 through 25-47). As strength and neuromuscular control continue to increase, more functional closed-kinetic-chain strengthening activities can begin (Figures 25-16 through 25-18).

Criteria for Full Return. Once near-normal levels of strength, flexibility, and neuromuscular control have been regained and the injured athlete has progressed through an appropriate functional progression, full activity may be resumed.

Subluxation and Dislocation of the Peroneal Tendons

Pathomechanics. The peroneus brevis and longus tendons pass posterior to the fibula in the peroneal groove under the superior peroneal retinaculum. Peroneal tendon dislocation may occur because of rupture of the superior retinaculum or because the retinaculum strips the periosteum away from the lateral malleolus, creating laxity in the retinaculum. It appears that there is no anatomic correlation between peroneal groove size or shape and instability of the peroneal tendons.[41] An avulsion fracture of the lateral ridge of the distal fibula may also occur with a subluxation or dislocation of the peroneal tendons.

Injury Mechanism. Subluxation of peroneal tendons can occur from any mechanism causing sudden and forceful contraction of the peroneal muscles that involves dorsiflexion and eversion of the foot.[41] This forces the tendons anteriorly, rupturing the retinaculum and potentially causing an avulsion fracture of the lateral malleolus. The athlete will often hear or feel a "pop." And differentiating peroneal subluxation from a lateral ligament sprain or tear, there will be tenderness over the peroneal tendons and swelling and ecchymosis in the retromalleolar area. During active eversion the foot subluxation of the peroneal tendons may be observed and palpated. This is easier to observe when acute symptoms have subsided. The athlete will typically complain of chronic "giving way" or popping. If the tendon is dislocated on initial evaluation, it should be reduced using gentle inversion and plantarflexion with pressure on the peroneal tendon.[41]

Rehabilitation Concerns and Progression. Following reduction the athlete should be initially placed in a compression dressing with a felt pad cut in the shape of a keyhole strapped over the lateral malleolus, placing gentle pressure on the peroneal tendons. Once the acute symptoms abate, the athlete should be placed in a short leg cast in slight plantarflexion and non-weight-bearing for 5 to 6 weeks (Figure 25-55). Aggressive ankle rehabilitation, as previously described, is initiated after cast removal.

In the case of an avulsion injury or when this becomes a chronic problem, conservative treatment is unlikely to be successful and surgery is needed to prevent the problem from recurring. A number of surgical procedures have been recommended, including repair or reconstruction of the superior peroneal retinaculum, deepening of the peroneal groove, or rerouting the tendon. Following surgery, the athlete should be placed in a non-weight-bearing short leg cast for about 4 weeks. The course of rehabilitation is similar to that described for ankle fractures with increased emphasis on strengthening of the peroneal tendons in eversion.[41]

Criteria for Full Return. The athlete may return to full activity at approximately 10 to 12 weeks as tolerated, when normal strength, ROM, and neuromuscular control in the ankle joint are demonstrated.

Tendinitis

Pathomechanics and Injury Mechanism. Inflammation of the tendons surrounding the ankle joint is a common problem in athletes. The tendons most often involved are the posterior tibialis tendon behind the medial malleolus, the anterior tibialis under the extensor retinaculum on the dorsal surface of the ankle, and the peroneal tendons both behind the lateral malleolus and at the base of the fifth metatarsal.[77]

Tendinitis in these tendons may result from one specific cause or from a collection of mechanisms including faulty foot mechanics, which will be discussed later in this chapter; inappropriate or poor footwear that can create faulty foot mechanics; acute trauma to the tendon; tightness in the heel chord complex; or training errors. Training errors would include training at intensities that are too high or too often; changing training surfaces; or changes in activities within the training program.[77]

Athletes who develop tendinitis are likely to complain of pain with both active movement and passive stretching; swelling around the area of the tendon due to inflammation of the tendon and the tendon sheath; crepi-

tus on movement; and stiffness and pain following periods of inactivity but particularly in the morning.

Rehabilitation Concerns and Progression. In the early stages of rehabilitation, exercises are used to produce increased circulation. The increased lymphatic flow facilitates removal of fluid and the by-products of the inflammatory process, and increases nutrition to the healing tendon. Exercise should also be used to limit atrophy, which can occur with disuse, and to minimize loss of strength, proprioception, and neuromuscular control.

Rehabilitation should incorporate techniques that reduce or eliminate inflammation. These include rest, therapeutic modalities (ice, ultrasound, diathermy), and anti-inflammatory medications.

If faulty foot mechanics are a cause of tendinitis, it may be helpful to construct an appropriate orthotic devise to correct the biomechanics. Taping of the foot may also help reduce stress on the tendons (Figure 25-87).

In many instances, if the mechanism that is causing the irritation and inflammation of the tendon is removed, and the inflammatory process is allowed to accomplish what it is supposed to, the tendinitis will often resolve within 10 days to 2 weeks. This is particularly true if rest and treatment are begun as soon as the symptoms begin. Unfortunately, if treatment does not begin until the symptoms have been present for several weeks or even months, as is most often the case, the tendinitis will take much longer to resolve. Long-standing inflammation causes the tendon to thicken and significantly increases the period of time required for that tendon to remodel.

Criteria for Full Return. In our experience, it is better to allow the athlete sufficient rest so that tendon healing can take place. The rehabilitation philosophy in sports medicine is usually aggressive, but with tendinitis an aggressive approach that does not allow the tendon to first of all eliminate the inflammatory response and then to begin tissue realignment and remodeling will not allow the tendon to heal and can exacerbate the existing inflammation. The rehabilitation progression must be slow and controlled, with full return only when the athlete seems to be free of pain.

Excessive Pronation and Supination

Pathomechanics and Injury Mechanism. Often, when we hear the terms *pronation* or *supination,* we automatically think of some pathological condition related to gait. It must be reemphasized that pronation and supination of the foot and subtalar joint are normal movements that occur during the support phase of gait. However, if pronation or supination is excessive or prolonged, overuse injuries may develop. Excessive or prolonged

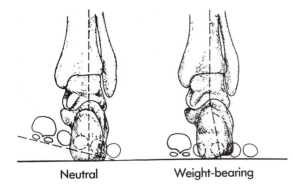

Figure 25-56   Forefoot varus. Comparing neutral and weight-bearing positions.

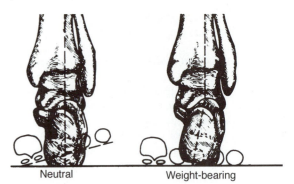

Figure 25-57   Forefoot valgus. Comparing neutral and weight-bearing positions.

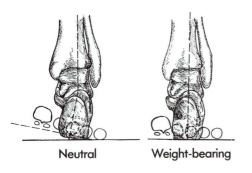

Figure 25-58   Rearfoot varus. Comparing neutral and weight-bearing positions.

supination or pronation at the subtalar joint is likely to result from some structural or functional deformity in the foot or leg. The structural deformity forces the subtalar joint to compensate in a manner that will allow the weight-bearing surfaces of the foot to make stable contact with the ground and get into a weight-bearing position. Thus, excessive pronation or supination is a compensation for an existing structural deformity. Three of the most common structural deformities of the foot are a forefoot varus (Figure 25-56), a forefoot valgus (Figure 25-57), and a rearfoot varus (Figure 25-58).

Structural forefoot varus and structural rearfoot varus deformities are usually associated with excessive pronation. A structural forefoot valgus causes excessive supination. The deformities usually exist in one plane, but the subtalar joint will interfere with the normal functions of the foot and make it more difficult for it to act as a shock absorber, adapt to uneven surfaces, and act as a rigid lever for push-off. The compensation, rather than the deformity itself, usually causes overuse injuries.

Excessive or prolonged pronation of the subtalar joint during the support phase of running is one of the major causes of stress injuries. Overload of specific structures re-

sults when excessive pronation is produced in the support phase or when pronation is prolonged into the propulsive phase of running. Excessive pronation during the support phase will cause compensatory subtalar joint motion such that the midtarsal joint remains unlocked, resulting in an excessively loose foot. There is also an increase in tibial rotation, which forces the knee joint to absorb more transverse rotation motion. Prolonged pronation of the subtalar joint will not allow the foot to resupinate in time to provide a rigid lever for push-off, resulting in a less powerful and less efficient force. Thus various foot and leg problems occur with excessive or prolonged pronation during the support phase. These include callus formation under the second metatarsal, stress fractures of the second metatarsal, bunions due to hypermobility of the first ray, plantar fascitis, posterior tibial tendinitis, Achilles tendinitis, tibial stress syndrome, and medial knee pain.

Several extrinsic keys may be observed that indicate pronation.[67] Excessive eversion of the calcaneus during the stance phase indicates pronation (Figure 25-59). Excessive or prolonged internal rotation of the tibia is another sign of pronation. This internal rotation can cause increased symptoms in the shin or knee, especially in repetitive sports such as running. A lowering of the medial arch accompanies pronation. It may be measured as the navicular differential,[54] the difference between the height of the navicular tuberosity from the floor in a non-weight-bearing position and its height in a weight-bearing position (Figure 25-60). As previously discussed, the talus plantarflexes and adducts with pronation. It may be seen as a medial bulging of the talar head (Figure 25-61). This same talar adduction causes increased concavity below the lateral malleolus in a posterior view while the calcaneus everts[52] (Figure 25-62).

At heel strike in prolonged or excessive supination, compensatory movement at the subtalar joint will not allow the midtarsal joint to unlock, causing the foot to re-

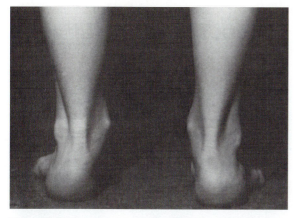

Figure 25-59   Eversion of the calcaneus indicating pronation.

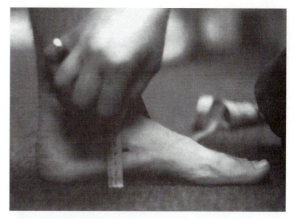

Figure 25-60   Measurement of the navicular differential.

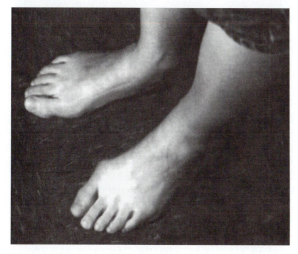

Figure 25-61   Medial bulge of the talar head indicating pronation.

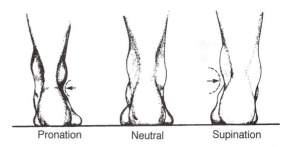

Pronation   Neutral   Supination

Figure 25-62   Concavity below the lateral malleolus indicating pronation.

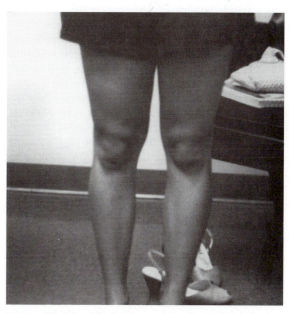

Figure 25-63   Tibial varum, or bowleg deformity.

main excessively rigid. The foot cannot absorb the ground reaction forces as efficiently. Excessive supination limits tibial internal rotation. Injuries typically associated with excessive supination include inversion ankle sprains, tibial stress syndrome, peroneal tendinitis, iliotibial band friction syndrome, and trochanteric bursitis.

Structural deformities originating outside the foot also require compensation by the foot for a proper weight-bearing position to be attained. Tibial varum is the common bowleg deformity.[52] The distal tibia is medial to the proximal tibia[21] (Figure 25-63). This measurement is taken weight-bearing with the foot in neutral position.[35] The angle of deviation of the distal tibia from a perpendicular line from the calcaneal midline is considered tibial varum.[28] Tibial varum increases pronation to

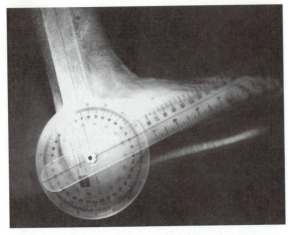

Figure 25-64 Ten degrees of dorsiflexion is necessary for normal gait.

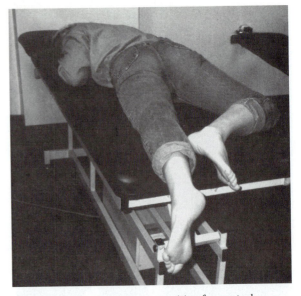

Figure 25-65 Examination position for neutral position.

allow proper foot function.[10] At heel strike the calcaneus must evert to attain a perpendicular position.[74]

Ankle joint equinus is another extrinsic deformity that may require abnormal compensation. It may be considered an extrinsic or intrinsic problem.

During normal gait, the tibia must move anterior to the talar dome.[52] Approximately 10 degrees of dorsiflexion are required for this movement[52] (Figure 25-64). Lack of dorsiflexion may cause compensatory pronation of the foot with resultant foot and lower-extremity pain. Often this lack of dorsiflexion results from tightness of the posterior leg muscles. Other causes include forefoot equinus, in which the plane of the forefoot is below the plane of the rearfoot.[52] It occurs in many high-arched feet. This deformity requires more ankle dorsiflexion. When enough dorsiflexion is not available at the ankle, the additional movement is required at other sites, such as dorsiflexion of the midtarsal joint and rotation of the leg.

Rehabilitation Concerns. In individuals who excessively pronate or supinate, the goal of treatment is quite simply to correct the faulty biomechanics that occur due to the existing structural deformity. An accurate biomechanical analysis of the foot and lower extremity should identify those deformities that require abnormal compensatory movements. In the majority of cases faulty biomechanics can be corrected by constructing an appropriate orthotic device.

Despite arguments in the literature, the author has found orthotic therapy to be of tremendous value in the treatment of many lower extremity problems. This view is supported in the literature by several clinical studies. Donatelli et al.[21] found that 96 percent of their patients reported pain relief from orthotics and that 52 percent

would not leave home without the devices in their shoes. McPoil, Adrian, and Pidcoe found that orthotics were an important treatment for valgus forefoot deformities only.[51] Riegler reported that 80 percent of his patients experienced at least a 50 percent improvement with orthotics.[65] This same study reported improvements in sport performance with orthotics. Hunt reported decreased muscular activity with orthotics.[35]

The process for evaluating the foot biomechanically, for constructing an orthotic device, and for selecting the appropriate footwear is detailed below.

Examination. The first step in the evaluation process is to establish a position of *subtalar neutral*. The athlete should be prone with the distal third of the leg hanging off the end of the table (Figure 25-65). A line should be drawn bisecting the leg from the start of the musculotendinous junction of the gastrocnemius to the distal portion of the calcaneus[78] (Figure 25-66). With the athlete still prone, the sports therapist palpates the talus while the forefoot is inverted and everted. One finger should palpate the talus at the anterior aspect of the fibula and another finger at the anterior portion of the medial malleolus (Figure 25-67). The position at which the talus is equally prominent on both sides is considered neutral subtalar position.[40] Root, Orien, and Weed[67] describe this as the position of the subtalar joint where it is neither pronated or supinated. It is the standard position in which the foot should be placed to examine deformities.[60] In this position, the lines on the lower leg and cal-

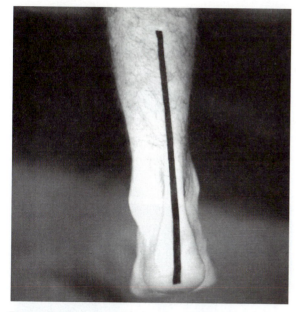

Figure 25-66 Line bisecting the gastrocnemius and posterior calcaneus.

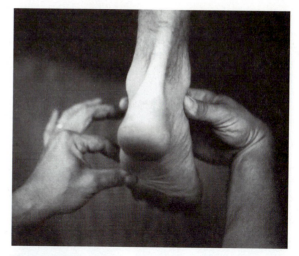

Figure 25-67 Palpation of the talus to determine neutral position.

caneus should form a straight line. Any variance is considered to be a rearfoot valgus or varus deformity. The most common deformity of the foot is a rearfoot varus deformity.[53] A deviation of 2 to 3 degrees is normal.[83]

Another method of determining subtalar neutral position involves the lines that were drawn previously on the leg and back of the heel. With the athlete prone, the heel is swung into full eversion and inversion, with measurements taken at each position. Angles of the two lines are taken at each extreme. Neutral position is considered two-thirds away from maximum inversion or one-third away from maximum eversion. The normal foot pronates 6 to 8 degrees from neutral.[67] For example, from neutral position a foot inverts 27 degrees and everts 3 degrees. The position at which this foot is neither pronated nor supinated is that point at which the calcaneus is inverted 7 degrees.

Once the subtalar joint is placed in a neutral position, mild dorsiflexion should be applied while observing the metatarsal heads in relation to the plantar surface of the calcaneous. Forefoot varus is an osseous deformity in which the medial metatarsal heads are inverted in relation to the plane of the calcaneus (Figure 25-56). Forefoot varus is the most common cause of excessive pronation, according to Subotnick.[75] Forefoot valgus is a position in which the lateral metatarsals are everted in relation to the rearfoot (Figure 25-57). These forefoot deformities are benign in a non-weight-bearing position,

but in stance the foot or metatarsal heads must somehow get to the floor to bear weight. This movement is accomplished by the talus rolling down and in and the calcaneus everting for a forefoot varus. For the forefoot valgus, the calcaneus inverts and the talus abducts and dorsiflexes. McPoil, Knecht, and Schmit[53] report that forefoot valgus is the most common forefoot deformity in their sample group.

In a rearfoot varus deformity, when the foot is in subtalar neutral position non-weight-bearing, the medial metatarsal heads are inverted as in a forefoot varus, and the calcaneous is also in an inverted position. To get to footflat in weight bearing, the subtalar joint must pronate (Figure 25-58). Minimal osseous deformities of the forefoot have little effect on the function of the foot. When either forefoot varus or valgus is too large, the foot compensates through abnormal movements to bear weight.

Constructing orthotics. Almost any problem of the lower extremity appears at one time to have been treated by orthotic therapy. The use of orthotics in control of foot deformities has been argued for many years.[4,15,17,29,40,66,74,75,84] The normal foot functions most efficiently when no deformities are present that predispose it to injury or exacerbate existing injuries. Orthotics are used to control abnormal compensatory movements of the foot by "bringing the floor to the foot."[36]

The foot functions most efficiently in neutral position. By providing support so that the foot does not have to move abnormally, an orthotic should help prevent compensatory problems. For problems that have already occurred, the orthotic provides a platform of support so that soft tissues can heal properly without undue stress.

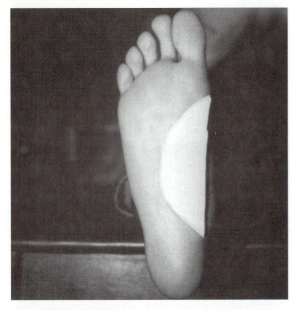

Figure 25-68 Felt pads.

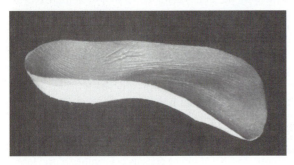

Figure 25-69 Semirigid orthotics.

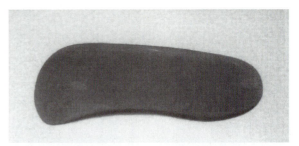

Figure 25-70 Hard orthotic.

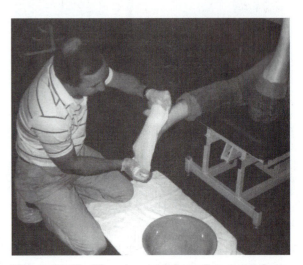

Figure 25-71 Three layers of plaster form neutral mold.

Basically there are three types of orthotics:[36,46,74]

1. Pads and soft flexible felt supports (Figure 25-68). These soft inserts are readily fabricated and are advocated for mild overuse syndromes. Pads are particularly useful in shoes, such as spikes and ski boots, that are too narrow to hold orthotics.

2. Semirigid orthotics made of flexible thermoplastics, rubber, or leather (Figure 26-69). These orthotics are prescribed for athletes who have increased symptoms. These orthotics are molded from a neutral cast. They are well tolerated by athletes whose sports require speed or jumping.

3. Functional or rigid orthotics are made from hard plastic and also require neutral casting (Figure 25-70). These orthotics allow control for most overuse symptoms.

Many sports therapists make a neutral mold, put it in a box, mail it to an orthotic laboratory, and several weeks later receive an orthotic back in the mail. Others like to complete the entire orthotic from start to finish, which requires a much more skilled technician than the mail-in method, as well as approximately $1,000 in equipment and supplies. The obvious advantage is cost if many orthotics are to be made.

No matter which method is chosen, the first step is the fabrication of the neutral mold, done with the patient in the same position used to determine subtalar neutral position. Once subtalar neutral is found, three layers of plaster splints are applied to the plantar surface and sides of the foot (Figure 25-71). Subtalar neutral position is maintained as pressure is applied on the fifth metatarsal area in a dorsiflexion direction until the midtarsal joint is locked (Figure 25-72). This position is held until the plaster dries. At this point the plaster cast may be sent out to have the orthotic made or it may be finished

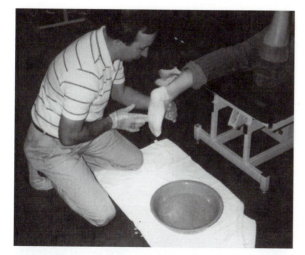

Figure 25-72 Mild pressure over the fifth metatarsal to lock the midtarsal joint.

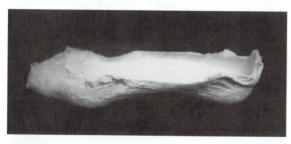

Figure 25-73 Neutral mold.

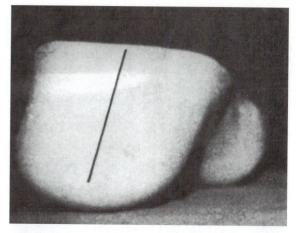

Figure 25-74 Positive mold.

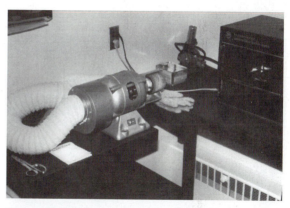

Figure 25-75 Convection oven and grinder.

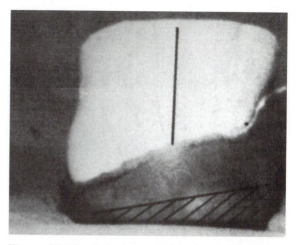

Figure 25-76 Orthotic material on the positive mold.

(Figure 25-73). If it is mailed out, the appropriate measurements of forefoot and rearfoot positions should be sent, along with any extrinsic measurements. If the orthotic is to be fabricated in-house, the plaster cast should be liberally lined interiorly with talc or powder. Plaster of paris should then be poured into the cast to form a positive mold of the foot (Figure 25-74).

Many different materials may be used to fabricate an orthotic from the positive mold. The author uses ⅛-inch Aliplast (Alimed Inc., Boston) covering with a ¼-inch Plastazote underneath. A rectangular piece of each material large enough to completely encompass the lower third of the mold is cut. These two pieces are placed in a convection oven (Figure 25-75) at approximately 275°F. At this temperature the two materials bond together and become moldable in about 5 to 7 minutes. At this time the orthotic materials are removed from the oven and placed on the positive mold (Figure 25-76). Ideally a form or vacuum press should be used to form the orthotic to the mold.[36]

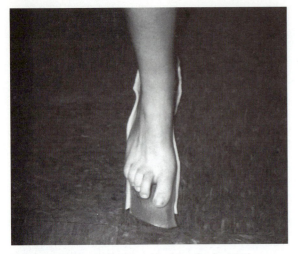

Figure 25-77 Orthotic mold under the foot with patient sitting.

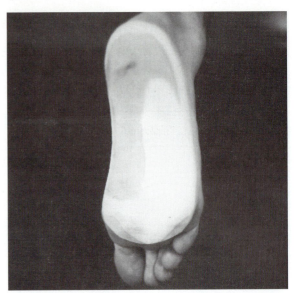

Figure 25-79 The length of the orthotic should bisect the metatarsal heads.

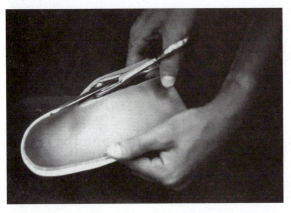

Figure 25-78 Trim excess material from orthotic.

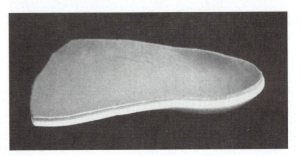

Figure 25-80 Sides of the orthotic should be leveled inward.

Once cooled, the uncut orthotic is placed under the foot while the athlete sits in a chair (Figure 25-77). Excess material is then trimmed from the sides of the orthotic with scissors. Any material that can be seen protruding from either side of the foot should be trimmed (Figure 25-78) to provide the proper width of the orthotic. The length should be trimmed so that the end of the orthotic bisects the metatarsal heads (Figure 25-79). This style is slightly longer than most orthotics are made, but the author has found that this length provides better comfort.[36]

Next a third layer of medial Plastazote may be glued to the arch to fill that area to the floor. Grinding begins with the sides of the orthotic, which should be ground so that the sides are slightly beveled inward (Figure 25-80) to allow better shoe fit. The bottom of the orthotic is leveled so that the surface is perpendicular to the bisection of the calcaneus. Grinding is continued until very little Plastazote remains under the Aliplast at the heel. The forefoot is posted by selectively grinding Plastazote just proximal to the metatarsal heads. Forefoot varus is posted by grinding more laterally than medially. Forefoot valgus requires grinding more medially than laterally. The final step is to grind the distal portion of the orthotic so that only a very thin piece of Aliplast is under the area where the orthotic ends. This prevents discomfort under the forefoot where the orthotic stops. If the athlete feels that this area is a problem, a full insole of Spenco or other material may be used to cover the orthotic to the end of the shoe to eliminate the drop off sometimes felt as the orthotic ends. Time must be allowed for proper break-in. The athlete should wear the orthotic for 3 to 4 hours the first day, 6 to 8 hours the next day, and then all day on the third day.

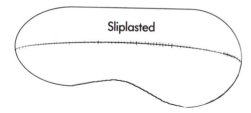

Figure 25-81 Slip-lasted shoe.

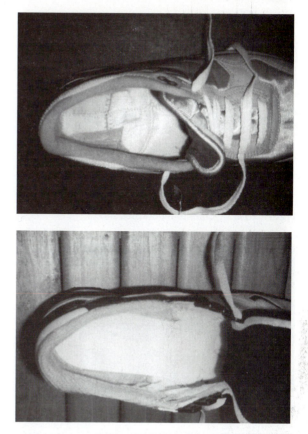

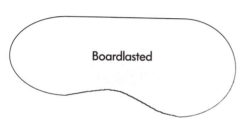

Figure 25-82 Board-lasted shoe.

Sports activities should be started with the orthotic only after it has been worn all day for several days.[36]

Shoe selection. The shoe is one of the biggest considerations in treating a foot problem.[76] Even a properly made orthotic is less effective if placed in a poorly constructed shoe.

As noted, pronation is a problem of hypermobility. Pronated feet need stability and firmness to reduce this excess movement. Research indicates that shoe compression may actually increase pronation, compared to barefoot.[3] The ideal shoe for a pronated foot is less flexible and has good rearfoot control.

Conversely, supinated feet are usually very rigid. Increased cushion and flexibility benefit this type of foot. Several construction factors may influence the firmness and stability of a shoe. The basic form upon which a shoe is built is called the *last*.[3] The upper is fitted onto a last in several ways. Each method has its own flexibility and control characteristics. A slip-lasted shoe is sewn together like a moccasin (Figure 25-81) and is very flexible. Board-lasting provides a piece of fiberboard upon which the upper is attached (Figure 25-82), which pro-

vides a very firm, inflexible base for the shoe. A combination-lasted shoe is boarded in the back half of the shoe and slip-lasted in the front (Figure 25-83), which provides rearfoot stability with forefoot mobility. The shape of the last may also be used in shoe selection. Most athletes with excessive pronation perform better in a straight-lasted shoe,[3] that is, a shoe in which the forefoot does not curve inward in relation to the rearfoot. Midsole design also affects the stability of a shoe. The midsole separates the upper from the outsole.[11] Ethylene vinyl acetate (EVA) is one of the most commonly used materials in the midsole.[61] Often denser EVA, which is colored differently to show that it is denser, is placed under the medial aspect of the foot to control pronation (Figure 25-84).

In an effort to control rearfoot movement, many shoe manufacturers have reinforced the heel counter both internally and externally, often in the form of extra plastic along the outside of the heel counter[54] (Figure 25-85). Other factors that may affect the performance of a shoe are the outsole contour and composition, lacing systems, and forefoot wedges.

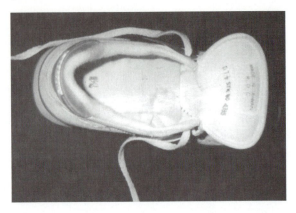

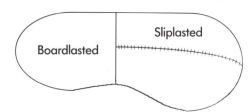

Figure 25-83 Combination-lasted shoe.

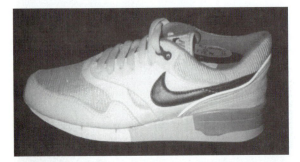

Figure 25-84 EVA in a midsole.

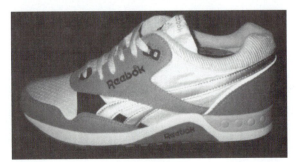

Figure 25-85 External heel counter.

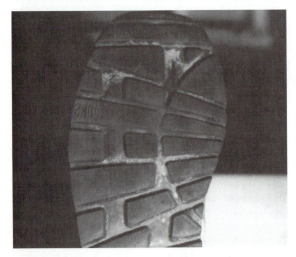

Figure 25-86 Front forefoot of a running shoe showing the typical wear pattern of a pronator.

Shoe wear patterns. Athletes with excessive pronation often wear out the front of the running shoe under the second metatarsal (Figure 25-86). Shoe wear patterns are commonly misinterpreted by athletes who think they must be pronators because they wear out the back

outside edges of their heels. Actually, most people wear out the back outside edges of their shoes. Just before heel-strike, the anterior tibial muscle fires to prevent the foot from slapping forward. The anterior tibial muscle not only dorsiflexes the foot but also slightly inverts it, hence the wear pattern on the back edge of the shoe. The key to inspection of wear patterns on shoes is observation of the heel counter and the forefoot.

Stress Fractures in the Foot

Pathomechanics and Injury Mechanism. The most common stress fractures in the foot involve the navicular, the second metatarsal (March fracture), and the diaphysis of the fifth metatarsal (Jones fracture). Navicular and second metatarsal stress fractures are likely to occur with excessive foot pronation, while fifth metatarsal stress fractures tend to occur in a more rigid pes cavus foot.

Navicular stress fractures. Individuals who excessively pronate during running gait are likely to develop a stress fracture of the navicular. Of the tarsal bones it is the most likely to have a stress fracture.

Second metatarsal fractures. Second metatarsal stress fractures occur most often in running and jumping

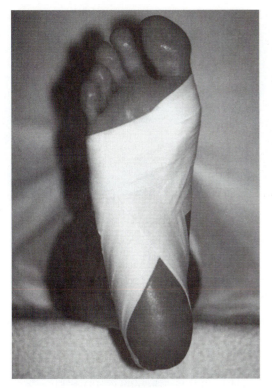

Figure 25-87   Low-dye taping for arch support.

Rehabilitation Concerns.   Rehabilitation efforts for stress fractures should focus on determining and alleviating the precipitating cause or causes. Second metatarsal stress fractures tend to do well with modified rest and non-weight-bearing exercises such as pool running (Figure 25-48), upper-body ergometer (Figure 25-49), or stationary bike (Figure 25-50) to maintain the athlete's cardiorespiratory fitness for 2 to 4 weeks. This is followed by a progressive return to running and jumping sports over a 2 or 3 week period using appropriately constructed orthotics and appropriate shoes.

Stress fractures of both the navicular of the proximal shaft of the fifth metatarsal usually require more aggressive treatment, requiring non-weight-bearing short leg casts for 6 to 8 weeks for nondisplaced fractures. With cases of delayed union, nonunion, or especially displaced fractures, both the Jones and navicular fractures require internal fixation, with or without bone grafting. In the highly competitive athlete, immediate internal fixation should be recommended.

Plantar Fasciitis

Pathomechanics.   Heel pain is a very common problem in the athletic and nonathletic population. This phenomenon has been attributed to several etiologies, including heel spurs, plantar fascia irritation, and bursitis. *Plantar fasciitis* is a catchall term that is commonly used to describe pain in the proximal arch and heel.

The plantar fascia (plantar aponeurosis) runs the length of the sole of the foot. It is a broad band of dense connective tissue that is attached proximally to the medial surface of the calcaneus. It fans out distally, with fibers and their various small branches attaching to the metatarsophalangeal articulations and merging into the capsular ligaments. Other fibers, arising from well within the aponeurosis, pass between the intrinsic muscles of the foot and the long flexor tendons of the sole and attach themselves to the deep fascia below the bones. The function of the plantar aponeurosis is to assist in maintaining the stability of the foot and in securing or bracing the longitudinal arch.[77]

Tension develops in the plantar fascia both during extension of the toes and during depression of the longitudinal arch as the result of weight bearing. When the weight is principally on the heel, as in ordinary standing, the tension exerted on the fascia is negligible. However, when the weight is shifted to the ball of the foot (on the heads of the metatarsals), fascial tension is increased. In running, because the push-off phase involves both a forceful extension of the toes and a powerful thrust by the ball of the foot (on the heads of the metatarsals), fascial tension is increased to approximately twice the body weight.

sports. As is the case with other injuries in the foot associated with overuse, the most common causes include rearfoot varus and forefoot varus structural deformities in the foot that result in excessive pronation, training errors, changes in training surfaces, and wearing inappropriate shoes. The base of the second metatarsal extends proximally into the distal row of tarsal bones and is held rigid and stable by the bony architecture and ligament support. In addition, the second metatarsal is particularly subjected to increased stress with excessive pronation, which causes a hypermobile foot. In addition, if the second metatarsal is longer than the first, as seen with a Morton's toe, it is theoretically subjected to greater bone stress during running. A bone scan, as opposed to a standard radiograph, is frequently necessary for diagnosis.

Fifth metatarsal stress fractures.   Fifth metatarsal stress fractures can occur from overuse, acute inversion, or high-velocity rotational forces. A Jones fracture occurs at the diaphysis of the fifth metatarsal most often as a sequela of a stress fracture.[69] The athlete will complain of a sharp pain on the lateral border of the foot and will usually report hearing a "pop." Because of a history of poor blood supply and delayed healing, a Jones fracture may result in nonunion requiring an extended period of rehabilitation.

Athletes who have a mild pes cavus are particularly prone to fascial strain. Modern street shoes, by the nature of their design, take on the characteristics of splints and tend to restrict foot action to such an extent that the arch may become somewhat rigid because of shortening of the ligaments and other mild abnormalities. The athlete, when changing from such footwear into a flexible gymnastic slipper or soft track shoe, often experiences trauma when the foot is subjected to stress. Trauma may also result from running, either from poor technique or because of lordosis, a condition in which the increased forward tilt of the pelvis produces an unfavorable angle of foot-strike when there is considerable force exerted on the ball of the foot.

Injury Mechanism. A number of anatomical and biomechanical conditions have been studied as possible causes of plantar fasciitis. They include leg length discrepancy, excessive pronation of the subtalar joint, inflexibility of the longitudinal arch, and tightness of the gastrocnemius-soleus unit. Wearing shoes without sufficient arch support, a lengthened stride during running, and running on soft surfaces are also potential causes of plantar fasciitis.

The athlete complains of pain in the anterior medial heel, usually at the attachment of the plantar fascia to the calcaneus that eventually moves more centrally into the central portion of the plantar fascia. This pain is particularly troublesome upon arising in the morning or upon bearing weight after sitting for a long period. However, the pain lessens after a few steps. Pain also will be intensified when the toes and forefoot are forcibly dorsiflexed.

Rehabilitation Concerns. Orthotic therapy is very useful in the treatment of this problem. The authors have found that soft orthotics in combination with exercises can significantly reduce the pain level of these patients. A soft orthotic works better than a hard orthotic. An extra-deep heel cup should be built into the orthotic. The orthotic should be worn at all times, especially upon arising from bed in the morning. Always have the athlete step into the orthotic rather than ambulating barefooted.[9]

Use of a heel cup compresses the fat pad under the calcaneous, providing a cushion under the area of irritation.

When soft orthotics are not feasible, taping may reduce the symptoms. A simple arch taping or alternative taping often allows pain-free ambulation.[87]

The use of a night splint to maintain a position of static stretch has also been recommended (Figure 25-88). In some cases it may be necessary to use a short leg walking cast for 4 to 6 weeks.

Vigorous heelcord stretching should be used, along with an exercise to stretch the plantar fascia in the arch. Exercises that increase dorsiflexion of the great toe also may be of benefit to this problem (Figures 25-26 and 25-29). Stretching should be done at least three times a day.

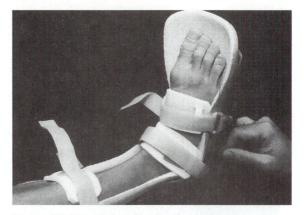

Figure 25-88 Night splint for plantar fasciitis.

Anti-inflammatory medications are recommended. Steroidal injection may be warranted at some point if symptoms fail to resolve.

Criteria for Full Return. Management of plantar fasciitis will generally require an extended period of treatment. It is not uncommon for symptoms to persist for as long as 8 to 12 weeks. The athlete's persistence in doing the recommended stretching exercises is critical. In some cases, particularly during a competitive season, the athlete may continue to train and compete if symptoms and associated pain are not prohibitive.

Cuboid Subluxation

Pathomechanics. A condition that often mimics plantar fasciitis is cuboid subluxation. Pronation and trauma have been reported to be prominent causes of this syndrome.[85] This displacement of the cuboid causes pain along the fourth and fifth metatarsals, as well as over the cuboid. The primary reason for pain is the stress placed on the long peroneal muscle when the foot is in pronation. In this position, the long peroneal muscle allows the cuboid bone to move downward medially. This problem often refers pain to the heel area as well. Many times this pain is increased upon arising after a prolonged non-weight-bearing period.

Rehabilitation Considerations. Dramatic treatment results may be obtained by manipulating to restore the cuboid to its natural position. The manipulation is done with the athlete prone (Figure 25-89). The plantar aspect of the forefoot is grasped by the thumbs with the fingers supporting the dorsum of the foot. The thumbs should be over the cuboid. The manipulation should be a thrust downward to move the cuboid into its more dorsal position. Often a pop is felt as the cuboid moves back into place. Once the cuboid is manipulated, an orthotic often helps to support it in its proper position.

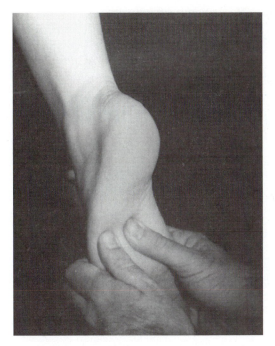

Figure 25-89   Prone position for cuboid manipulation.

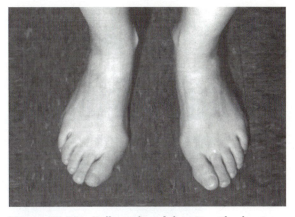

Figure 25-90   Hallux valgus deformity with a bunion.

Criteria for Full Return.   If manipulation is successful, quite often the athlete can return to play immediately with little or no pain. It should be recommended that the athlete wear an appropriately constructed orthotic when practicing or competing to reduce the chances of recurrence.

Hallux Valgus Deformity (Bunions)

Pathomechanics and Injury Mechanism.   A bunion is a deformity of the head of the first metatarsal in which the large toe assumes a valgus position[1] (Figure 25-90). Commonly it is associated with a structural forefoot varus in which the first ray tends to splay outward, putting pressure on the first metatarsal head. The bursa over the first metatarsophalangeal joint becomes inflamed and eventually thickens. The joint becomes enlarged and the great toe becomes malaligned, moving laterally toward the second toe, sometimes to such an extent that it eventually overlaps the second toe. This type of bunion may also be associated with a depressed or flattened transverse arch. Often the bunion occurs from wearing shoes that are pointed, too narrow, too short, or have high heels.

A bunion is one of the most frequent painful deformities of the great toe. As the bunion is developing there is tenderness, swelling, and enlargement with calcification

of the head of the first metatarsal. Poorly fitting shoes increase the irritation and pain.

Rehabilitation Concerns.   If the condition progresses, a special orthotic device may help normalize foot mechanics. Often an orthotic designed to correct a structural forefoot varus that can help increase stability of the first ray significantly reduces the symptoms and progression of a bunion. Shoe selection may also play an important role in the treatment of bunions. Shoes of the proper width cause less irritation to the bunion. Local therapy, including moist heat, soaks, and ultrasound, may alleviate some of the acute symptoms of a bunion. Protective devices such as wedges, pads, and tape can also be used. Surgery to correct the hallux valgus deformity is very common during the later stages of this condition.

Criteria for Full Return.   It is likely that an athlete with this condition can continue to compete while wearing an appropriately constructed orthotic, shoes with a wide toe box, and some type of donut pad over the bunion to disperse pressure.

Morton's Neuroma

Pathomechanics.   A neuroma is a mass occurring about the nerve sheath of the common plantar nerve where it divides into the two digital branches to adjacent toes. It occurs most commonly between the metatarsal heads and is the most common nerve problem of the lower extremity. A Morton's neuroma is located between the third and fourth metatarsal heads where the nerve is the thickest, receiving both branches from the medial and lateral plantar nerves. The athlete complains of severe intermittent pain radiating from the distal metatarsal heads to the tips of the toes and is often relieved when non-weight-bearing. Irritation increases with the collapse of the transverse arch of the foot, putting the transverse

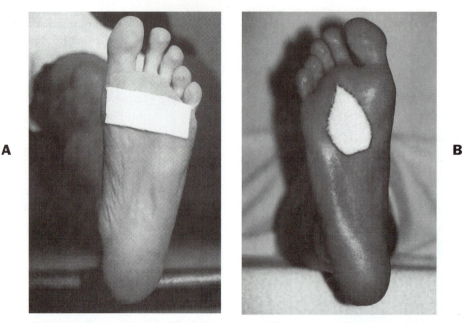

Figure 25-91 **A,** Metatarsal bar. **B,** Teardrop pad.

metatarsal ligaments under stretch and thus compressing the common digital nerve and vessels. Excessive foot pronation can also be a predisposing factor, with more metatarsal shearing forces occurring with the prolonged forefoot abduction.

The athlete complains of a burning paresthesia in the forefoot that is often localized to the third web space and radiating to the toes.[74] Hyperextension of the toes on weight bearing, as in squatting, stair climbing, or running, can increase the symptoms. Wearing shoes with a narrow toe box or high heels can increase the symptoms. If there is prolonged nerve irritation, the pain can become constant. A bone scan is often necessary to rule out a metatarsal stress fracture.

Rehabilitation Concerns. Orthotic therapy is essential to reduce the shearing movements of the metatarsal heads. To increase this effect, often either a metatarsal bar is placed just proximal to the metatarsal heads or a teardrop shaped pad is placed between the heads of the third and fourth metatarsals in an attempt to have these splay apart with weight bearing (Figure 25-91). It may decrease pressure on the affected area.

Therapeutic modalities can be used to help reduce inflammation. The author has used phonophoresis with hydrocortisone with some success in symptom reduction.

Shoe selection also plays an important role in treatment of neuromas. Narrow shoes, particularly women's shoes that are pointed in the toe area and certain men's

boots, may squeeze the metatarsal heads together and exacerbate the problem. A shoe that is wide in the toe box area should be selected. A straight-laced shoe often provides increased space in the toe box.[71] On a rare occasion surgical excision may be required.

Criteria for Full Return. Appropriate soft orthotic padding often will markedly reduce pain and allow the athlete to continue to play despite this condition.

Turf Toe

Pathomechanics and Injury Mechanism. Turf toe is a hyperextension injury resulting in a sprain of the metatarsophalangeal joint of the great toe, from either repetitive overuse or trauma.[82] Typically these injuries occur on unyielding synthetic turf, although it can occur on grass also. Many of these injuries occur because many artificial turf shoes are more flexible and allow more dorsiflexion of the great toe.

Rehabilitation Concerns. Some shoe companies have addressed this problem by adding steel or other materials to the forefoot of their turf shoes to stiffen them. Flat insoles that have thin sheets of steel under the forefoot are also available. When commercially made products are not available, a thin, flat piece of Orthoplast may be placed under the shoe insole or may be molded to the foot.[82] Taping the toe to prevent dorsiflexion may be done separately or with one of the shoe-stiffening suggestions (Figure 25-92).

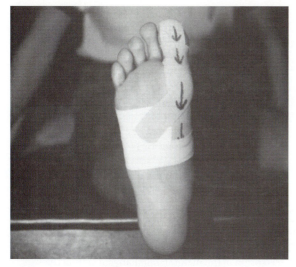

Figure 25-92   Turf toe taping.

Modalities of choice include ice and ultrasound. One of the major ingredients in any treatment for turf toe is rest. The athlete should be discouraged from returning to activity until the toe is pain-free.

Criteria for Full Return.   The athlete with turf toe can return to activity when the swelling in the metatarsophalangeal joint has resolved and full pain-free ROM from 0 to 90 degrees has been regained. In less severe cases the athlete can continue to play with the addition of a rigid insole. With more severe sprains, 3 to 4 weeks may be required for pain to reduce to the point where the athlete can push off on the great toe.

Tarsal Tunnel Syndrome

Pathomechanics and Injury Mechanism.   The tarsal tunnel is a loosely defined area about the medial malleolus that is bordered by the retinaculum, which binds the tibial nerve.[29] Pronation, overuse problems such as tendinitis, and trauma may cause neurovascular problems in the ankle and foot. Symptoms may vary, with pain, numbness, and paresthesia reported along the medial ankle and into the sole of the foot.[6] Tenderness may be present over the tibial nerve area behind the medial malleolus.

Rehabilitation Concerns.   Neutral foot control may alleviate symptoms in less involved cases. Surgery is often performed if symptoms do not respond to conservative treatment or if weakness occurs in the flexors of the toes.[6]

Summary

1. The movements that take place at the talocrural joint are ankle plantarflexion and dorsiflexion. Inversion and eversion occur at the subtalar joint.

2. The position of the subtalar joint determines whether the midtarsal joints will be hypermobile or hypomobile. Dysfunction at either joint can profoundly affect the foot and lower extremity.

3. Ankle sprains are very common. Inversion sprains usually involve the lateral ligaments of the ankle, and eversion sprains frequently involve the medial ligaments of the ankle. Rotational injuries often involve the tibiofibular and syndesmodic ligaments and can be very severe.

4. The early phase of treatment uses ice, compression, elevation, rest, and protection, all of which are critical components in preventing swelling.

5. Early weight bearing following ankle sprain is beneficial to the healing process. Rehabilitation may become more aggressive following the acute inflammatory response phase of healing.

6. Undisplaced ankle fractures should be managed with rest and protection until the fracture has healed. Displaced fractures are treated with open reduction and internal fixation.

7. Neutral casting is essential for the production of an orthotic, whether it is to be produced in-house or by someone else.

8. Subluxation of peroneal tendons can occur from any mechanism causing sudden and forceful contraction of the peroneal muscles that involves dorsiflexion and eversion of the foot. In the case of an avulsion injury or when this becomes a chronic problem, conservative treatment is unlikely to be successful and surgery is needed to prevent the problem from recurring.

9. Tendinitis in the posterior tibialis, anterior tibialis, and the peroneal tendons can result from one specific cause or from a collection of mechanisms. Rehabilitation should incorporate techniques that reduce or eliminate inflammation, including rest, therapeutic modalities (ice, ultrasound, diathermy), and anti-inflammatory medications.

10. Excessive or prolonged supination or pronation at the subtalar joint is likely to result from some structural or functional deformity, including forefoot varus, a forefoot valgus, or a rearfoot varus, which forces the subtalar joint to compensate in a manner that will allow the weight-bearing surfaces of the foot to make stable contact with the ground and get into a weight-bearing position.

11. Orthotics are used to control abnormal compensatory movements of the foot by "bringing the floor to the foot." By providing support so that the foot does not have to move abnormally, an orthotic should help prevent compensatory problems.

12. Shoe selection is an important parameter in the treatment of foot problems. The type of foot will dictate specific shoe features.

13. The most common stress fractures in the foot involve the navicular, the second metatarsal (March fracture), and the diaphysis of the fifth metatarsal (Jones fracture). Navicular and second metatarsal stress fractures are likely to occur with excessive foot pronation. Fifth metatarsal stress fractures tend to occur in a more rigid pes cavus foot.

14. A number of anatomical and biomechanical conditions have been studied as possible causes of plantar fasciitis. There is pain in the anterior medial heel, usually at the attachment of the plantar fascia to the calcaneus. Orthotics in combination with stretching exercises can significantly reduce pain.

15. Subluxation of the cuboid will create symptoms similar to those of plantar fasciitis and can be corrected with manipulation.

16. A bunion is a deformity of the head of the first metatarsal in which the large toe assumes a valgus position that is commonly associated with a structural forefoot varus in which the first ray tends to splay outward, putting pressure on the first metatarsal head.

17. In treating a Morton's neuroma, a metatarsal bar is placed just proximal to the metatarsal heads or a teardrop shaped pad is placed between the heads of the third and fourth metatarsals in an attempt to have these splay apart with weight bearing.

18. Turf toe is a hyperextension injury resulting in a sprain of the metatarsophalangeal joint of the great toe.

References

1. Andrews, J. R., W. McClod, T. Ward, et al. 1977. The cutting mechanism. *American Journal of Sports Medicine* 5:111–21.

2. Arnheim, D., and W. Prentice. 1997. *Principles of athletic training.* Madison, WI: Brown & Benchmark.

3. Baer, T. 1984. Designing for the long run. *Mechanical Engineering* (Sept.): 67–75.

4. Bates, B. T., L. Osternig, B. Mason, et al. 1979. Foot orthotic devices to modify selected aspects of lower extremity mechanics. *American Journal of Sports Medicine* 7:338.

5. Baxter, D. 1995. *The foot and ankle in sport.* St. Louis: Mosby.

6. Birnham, J. S. 1986. *The musculoskeletal manual.* Orlando: Grune and Stratton.

7. Bosien, W. R., O. S. Staples, and R. W. Russell. 1955. Residual disability following acute ankle sprains. *Journal of Bone and Joint Surgery* 37[A]:1237.

8. Bostrum, L. 1966. Treatment and prognosis in recent ligament ruptures. *Acta Chir Scand* 132:537–50.

9. Brotzman, B., and J. Brasel. 1996. Foot and ankle rehabilitation. In *Clinical orthopaedic rehabilitation,* edited by B. Brotzman. St. Louis: Mosby.

10. Brody, D. M. 1982. Techniques in the evaluation and treatment of the injured runner. *Orthop Clin North Am* 13:541.

11. Brunwich, T., and B. Wischnia. 1987. Battle of the midsoles. *Runners World,* April, p. 47.

12. Burgess, P. R., and J. Wei. 1982. Signalling of kinesthetic information by peripheral sensory receptors. *Ann Rev Neurosci* 5:171–87.

13. Calliet, R. 1968. *Foot and ankle pain.* Philadelphia: F. A. Davis.

14. Canoy, W. F. 1975. *Review of medical physiology,* 7th ed., Los Altos, CA: Lange Medical.

15. Cavanaugh, P. R. 1978. *An evaluation of the effects of orthotics force distribution and rearfoot movement during running.* Paper presented at the meeting of the American Orthopedic Society for Sports Medicine, Lake Placid, NY.

16. Choi, J. 1978. Acute conditions: Incidence and associated disability. *Vital Health Statistics* 120:10.

17. Collona, P. 1989. Fabrication of a custom molded orthotic using an intrinsic posting technique for a forefoot varus deformity. *Phys Ther Forum* 8(5): 3.

18. Cutler, J. M. 1984. Lateral ligamentous injuries of the ankle. In *Lateral ligamentous injuries of the ankle,* edited by W. C. Hamilton. New York: Springer-Verlag.

19. Delacerda, F. G. 1980. A study of anatomical factors involved in shinsplints. *Journal of Orthopaedic and Sports Physical Therapy* 2:55–59.

20. Donatelli, R., C. Hurlbert, D. Conaway, et al. 1988. Biomechanical foot orthotics: A retrospective study. *Journal of Orthopaedic and Sports Physical Therapy* 10:205–12.

21. Donatelli, R. 1985. Normal biomechanics of the foot and ankle. *Journal of Orthopaedic and Sports Physical Therapy* 7:91–95.

22. Drez, D., D. Faust, and P. Evans. 1981. Cryotherapy and nerve palsy. *American Journal of Sports Medicine* 9:256–57.

23. Freeman, M., M. Dean, and I. Hanhan. 1965. The etiology and prevention of functional instability at the foot. *Journal of Bone and Joint Surgery* 47[Br]: 678–85.

24. Fumich, R. M,. A. Ellison, G. Guerin, et al. 1981. The measured effect of taping on combined foot and ankle motion before and after exercise. *American Journal of Sports Medicine* 9:165–69.

25. Garn, S. N., and R. A. Newton. 1988. Kinesthetic awareness in subjects with multiple ankle sprains. *Journal of the American Physical Therapy Association* 68:1667–71.

26. Garrick, J. G., and R. K. Requa. 1977. Role of external supports in the prevention of ankle sprains. *Medicine and Science in Sports and Exercise* 5:200.

27. Garrick, J. G. 1981. When can I . . . ? A practical approach to rehabilitation illustrated by treatment of an ankle injury. *American Journal of Sports Medicine* 9:67–68.

28. Giallonardo, L. M. 1988. Clinical evaluation of foot and ankle dysfunction. *Physical Therapy* 68:1850–56.

29. Gill, E. 1985. Orthotics. *Runners World*, February, pp. 55–57.

30. Glencross, D., and E. Thornton. 1981. Position sense following joint injury. *Journal of Sports Medicine and Physical Fitness* 21:23–27.

31. Glick, J., and T. Sampson. 1996. Ankle and foot fractures in athletics. In *The lower extremity and spine in sports medicine*, edited by J. Nicholas and E. Hershman. St. Louis: Mosby.

32. Gross, M., A. Lapp, and M. Davis. 1991. Comparison of Swed-O-Universal ankle support and Aircast Sport Stirrup orthoses and ankle tape in restricting eversion-inversion before and after exercise. *Journal of Orthopaedic and Sports Physical Therapy* 13(1): 11–19.

33. Hirata, I. 1974. Proper playing conditions. *Journal of Sports Medicine* 4:228–34.

34. Hoppenfield, S. 1976. *Physical examination of the spine and extremities.* New York: Appleton-Century-Crofts.

35. Hunt, G. 1985. Examination of lower extremity dysfunction. In *Orthopedic and sports physical therapy*, vol. 2, edited by J. Gould and G. Davies. St Louis: Mosby.

36. Hunter, S., M. Dolan, and M. Davis. 1996. *Foot orthotics in therapy and sport.* Champaign, IL: Human Kinetics.

37. Isakov, E., J. Mizrahi, P. Solzi, et al. 1986. Response of the peroneal muscles to sudden inversion of the ankle during standing. *International Journal of Sport Biomechanics* 2:100–109.

38. Itay, S. 1982. Clinical and functional status following lateral ankle sprains: Followup of 90 young adults treated conservatively. *Orthop Rev* 11:73–76.

39. James, S. L., B. T. Bates, and L. R. Osternig. 1978. Injuries to runners. *American Journal of Sports Medicine* 6:43.

40. James, S. L. 1979. Chondromalacia of the patella in the adolescent. In *The injured adolescent*, edited by S. C. Kennedy. Baltimore: Williams & Wilkins.

41. Jones, D., and K. Singer. 1996. Soft-tissue conditions of the foot and ankle. In *The lower extremity and spine in sports medicine*, edited by J. Nicholas and E. Hershman. St. Louis: Mosby.

42. Kelikian, H., and A. S. Kelikian. 1985. *Disorders of the ankle.* Philadelphia: W. B. Saunders.

43. Kergerris, S. 1983. The construction and implementation of functional progressions as a component of athletic rehabilitation. *Journal of Orthopaedic and Sports Physical Therapy* 5:14–19.

44. Klein, K. K. 1955. A study of cross transfer of muscular strength and endurance resulting from progressive resistive exercises following surgery. *J Assoc Phys Mental Rehab* 9:5.

45. Kowal, M. A. 1983. Review of physiologic effects of cryotherapy. *Journal of Orthopaedic and Sports Physical Therapy* 5:66–73.

46. Lockard, M. A. 1988. Foot orthoses. *Physical Therapy* 68:1866–73.

47. Loudin, J., and S. Bel. 1996. The foot and ankle: An overview of arthrokinematics and selected joint techniques. *Journal of Athletic Training* 31(2): 173–78.

48. Mandelbaum, B. R., G. Finerman, T. Grant, et al. 1987. Collegiate football players with recurrent ankle sprains. *Physician and Sports Medicine* 15(11): 57–61.

49. Mayhew, J. L., and W. F. Riner. 1974. Effects of ankle wrapping on motor performance. *Ath Train* 3:128–30.

50. McCluskey, G. M., T. A. Blackburn, and T. Lewis. 1976. Prevention of ankle sprains. *American Journal of Sports Medicine* 4:151–57.

51. McPoil, T. G., M. Adrian, and P. Pidcoe. 1989. Effects of foot orthoses on center of pressure patterns in women. *Physical Therapy* 69:149–54.

52. McPoil, T. G., and R. S. Brocato. 1985. The foot and ankle: Biomechanical evaluation and treatment. In *Orthopedic and sports physical therapy*, edited by J. Gould and G. Davies. St. Louis: Mosby.

53. McPoil, T. G., H. G. Knecht, and D. Schmit. 1988. A survey of foot types in normal females between the ages of 18 and 30 years. *Journal of Orthopaedic and Sports Physical Therapy* 9:406–9.

54. McPoil, T. G. 1988. Footwear. *Physical Therapy* 68:1857–65.

55. Morris, J. M. 1977. Biomechanics of the foot and ankle. *Clin Orthop* 122:10–17.

56. Morton, D. J. 1937. Foot disorders in general practice. *Journal of American Medical Association* 109:1112–19.

57. Nawoczenski, D. A., M. Owen, M. Ecker, et al. 1985. Objective evaluation of peroneal response to sudden inversion stress. *Journal of Orthopaedic and Sports Physical Therapy* 7:107–19.

58. Nicholas, J. A., and E. B. Hershman. 1990. *The lower extremity and spine in sports medicine.* St. Louis: Mosby.

59. Noyes, F. R. 1977. Functional properties of knee ligaments and alterations induced by immobilization: A correlative biomechanical and histological study in primates. *Clin Orthop* 123:210–43.

60. Oatis, C. A. 1998. Biomechanics of the foot and ankle under static conditions. *Physical Therapy* 68:1815–21.

61. Pagliano, J. N. 1988. Athletic footwear. *Sports Medicine Digest* 10:1–2.

62. Prentice, W. 1998. *Therapeutic modalities in sports medicine.* Dubuque, IA: WCB/McGraw-Hill.

63. Quillen, S. 1980. Alternative management protocol for lateral ankle sprains. *Journal of Orthopaedic and Sports Physical Therapy* 12:187–90.

64. Rebman, L. W. 1986. Ankle injuries: Clinical observations. *Journal of Orthopaedic and Sports Physical Therapy* 8:153–56.

65. Riegler, H. F. 1987. Orthotic devices for the foot. *Orthop Rev* 16:293–303.

66. Rogers, M. M., and B. F. LeVeau. 1982. Effectiveness of foot orthotic devices used to modify pronation in runners. *Journal of Orthopaedic and Sports Physical Therapy* 4:86–90.

67. Root, M. L., W. P. Orien, and J. H. Weed. 1977. Normal and abnormal functions of the foot. Los Angeles: Clinical Biomechanics.

68. Sammarco, J. G. 1975. Biomechanics of foot and ankle injuries. *Ath Train* 10:96.

69. Sammarco, J. 1995. *Rehabilitation of the foot and ankle.* St. Louis: Mosby.

70. Sims, D. 1986. Effects of positioning on ankle edema. *Journal of Orthopaedic and Sports Physical Therapy* 8:30–33.

71. Sims, D. S., P. R. Cavanaugh, and J. S. Ulbrecht. 1988. Risk factors in the diabetic foot. *Physical Therapy* 68:1887–1901.

72. Sloan, J. P., P. Guddings, and R. Hain. 1988. Effects of cold and compression on edema. *Physician and Sports Medicine* 16:116–20.

73. Stover, C. N., and J. M. York. 1980. Air stirrup management of ankle injuries in the athlete. *American Journal of Sports Medicine* 8:360–65.

74. Subotnick, S. I., and S. G. Newell. 1975. *Podiatric sports medicine.* Mt. Kisko, NY: Futura.

75. Subotnick, S. I. 1981. The flat foot. *Physician and Sports Medicine* 9:85–91.

76. Subotnick, S. I. 1977. The running foot doctor. Mt. Vias, CA: World.

77. Taunton, J., C. Smith, and D. Magee. 1996. Leg, foot, and ankle injuries. In *Athletic injuries and rehabilitation,* edited by J. Zachazewski, D. Magee, and W. Quillen. Philadelphia: W. B. Saunders.

78. Tiberio, D. 1988. Pathomechanics of structural foot deformities. *Physical Therapy* 68:1840–49.

79. Tippett, S. R. 1982. A case study: The need for evaluation and reevaluation of acute ankle sprains. *Journal of Orthopaedic and Sports Physical Therapy* 4:44.

80. Tropp, H., C. Askling, and J. Gillquist. 1985. Prevention of ankle sprains. *American Journal of Sports Medicine* 13:259–66.

81. Vaes, P., H. DeBoeck, F. Handleberg, et al. 1985. Comparative radiologic study of the influence of ankle joint bandages on ankle stability. *American Journal of Sports Medicine* 13:46–49.

82. Visnich, A. L. 1987. A playing orthoses for "turf toe." *Athletic Training* 22:215.

83. Vogelbach, W. D., and L. C. Combs. 1987. A biomechanical approach to the management of chronic lower extremity pathologies as they relate to excessive pronation. *Athletic Training* 22:6–16.

84. Williams, J. G. P. 1980. The foot and chondromalacia: A case of biomechanical uncertainty. *Journal of Orthopaedic and Sports Physical Therapy* 2:50–51.

85. Woods, A., and W. Smith. 1983. Cuboid syndrome and the techniques used for treatment. *Athletic Training* 18:64–65.

86. Yablon, I. G., D. Segal, and R. E. Leach. 1983. *Ankle injuries.* New York: Churchill Livingstone.

87. Zylks, D. R. 1987. Alternative taping for plantar fasciitis. *Athletic Training* 22:317.

CHAPTER 26

Rehabilitation of Injuries to the Spine

Dan Hooker
William E. Prentice

After completion of this chapter, the student should be able to do the following:

- Discuss the functional anatomy and biomechanics of the spine.

- Discuss the rationale for using the different positioning exercises for treating pain in the spine.

- Discuss the importance of a thorough evaluation of the back before developing a rehabilitation plan.

- Explain the importance of using either joint mobilization or dynamic stabilization exercises for treating spine patients.

- Describe the acute vs. reinjury vs. chronic stage model for treating low back pain.

- Explain the eclectic approach for rehabilitation of back pain in the athletic population.

- Discuss basic- and advanced-level training in the reinjury stage of treatment.

- Discuss the rehabilitation approach to specific conditions affecting the low back.

- Discuss the rehabilitation approach to conditions of the cervical spine.

FUNCTIONAL ANATOMY AND BIOMECHANICS

From a biomechanical perspective, the spine is one of the most complex regions of the body. with numerous bones, joints, ligaments, and muscles, all of which are collectively involved in spinal movement. The proximity to and relationship of the spinal cord, the nerve roots, and the peripheral nerves to the vertebral column adds to the complexity of this region. Injury to the cervical spine has potentially life-threatening implications, and low back pain is one of the most common ailments known to man.

The 33 vertebrae of the spine are divided into five regions: cervical, thoracic, lumbar, sacral, and coccygeal. Between each of the cervical, thoracic, and lumbar vertebrae lie fibrocartilaginous intervertebral disks that act as important shock absorbers for the spine.

The design of the spine allows a high degree of flexibility forward and laterally and limited mobility backward.

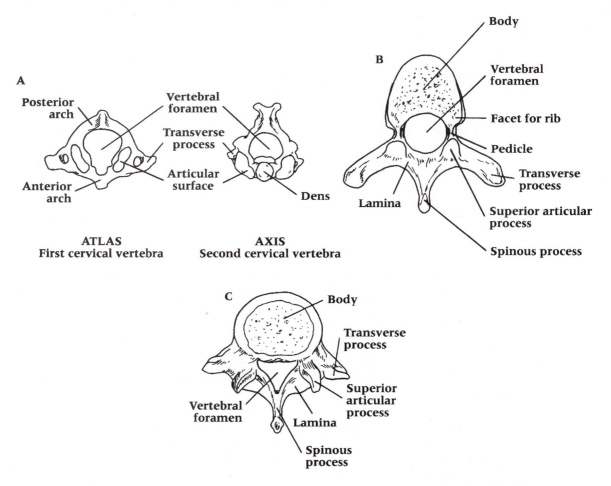

Figure 26-1 Anatomy of a vertebrae.

The movements of the vertebral column are flexion and extension, right and left lateral flexion, and rotation to the left and right. The degree of movement differs in the various regions of the vertebral column. The cervical and lumbar regions allow extension, flexion, and rotation around a central axis. Although the thoracic vertebrae have minimal movement, their combined movement between the first and twelfth thoracic vertebrae can account for 20 to 30 degrees of flexion and extension.

As the spinal vertebrae progress downward from the cervical region, they grow increasingly larger to accommodate the upright posture of the body, as well as to contribute to weight bearing. The shape of the vertebrae is irregular, but the vertebrae possess certain characteristics that are common to all. Each vertebra consists of a neural arch through which the spinal cord passes and several projecting processes that serve as attachments for muscles and ligaments. Each neural arch has two pedicles and two laminae. The pedicles are bony processes that project backward from the body of the vertebrae and connect with the laminae. The laminae are flat bony processes occurring on either side of the neural arch that project backward and inward from the pedicles. With the exception of the first and second cervical vertebrae, each vertebra has a spinous and transverse process for muscular and ligamentous attachment, and all vertebrae have an articular process (Figure 26-1).

Intervertebral articulations are between vertebral bodies and vertebral arches. Articulation between the bodies is of the symphysial type. Besides motion at articulations between the bodies of the vertebrae, movement takes place at four articular processes that derive from

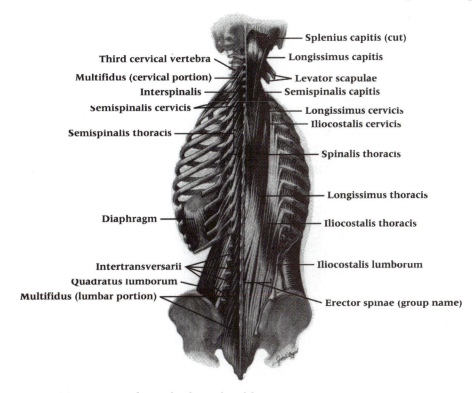

Third cervical vertebra

Multifidus (cervical portion)

Interspinalis

Semispinalis cervicis

Semispinalis thoracis

Diaphragm

Intertransversarii

Quadratus lumborum

Multifidus (lumbar portion)

Splenius capitis (cut)

Longissimus capitis

Levator scapulae

Semispinalis capitis

Longissimus cervicis

Iliocostalis cervicis

Spinalis thoracis

Longissimus thoracis

Iliocostalis thoracis

Iliocostalis lumborum

Erector spinae (group name)

Figure 26-2   Deep and superficial muscles of the spine.

the pedicles and laminae. The direction of movement of each vertebra is somewhat dependent on the direction in which the articular facets face. The sacrum articulates with the ilium to form the sacroiliac joint, which has a synovium and is lubricated by synovial fluid.

The major ligaments that join the various vertebral parts are the anterior longitudinal, the posterior longitudinal, and the supraspinous. The anterior longitudinal ligament is a wide, strong band that extends the full length of the anterior surface of the vertebral bodies. The posterior longitudinal ligament is contained within the vertebral canal and extends the full length of the posterior aspect of the bodies of the vertebrae. Ligaments connect one lamina to another. The interspinous, supraspinous, and intertransverse ligaments stabilize the transverse and spinous processes, extending between adjacent vertebrae. The sacroiliac joint is maintained by the extremely strong dorsal sacral ligaments. The sacrotuberous and the sacrospinous ligaments attach the sacrum to the ischium.

The muscles that extend the spine and rotate the vertebral column can be classified as either superficial or deep (Figure 26-2). The superficial muscles extend from the vertebrae to ribs. The erector spinae is a group of superficial paired muscles that is made up of three columns

or bands, the longissimus group, the iliocostalis group, and the spinalis group. Each of these groups is further divided into regions, the cervicis region in the neck, the thoracis region in the middle back, and the lumborum region in the low back. Generally the erector spinae muscles extend the spine. The deep muscles attach one vertebrae to another and function to extend and rotate the spine. The deep muscles include the interspinales, multifidus, rotatores, thoracis, and the semispinalis cervicis.

Flexion of the cervical region is produced primarily by the sternocleidomastoid muscles and the scalene muscle group on the anterior aspect of the neck. The scalenes flex the head and stabilize the cervical spine as the sternocleidomastoids flex the neck. The upper trapezius, semispinalis capitis, splenius capitus, and splenius cervicis muscles extend the neck. Lateral flexion of the neck is accomplished by all of the muscles on one side of the vertebral column contracting unilaterally. Rotation is produced when the sternocleidomastoid, the scalenes, the semispinalis cervicis, and the upper trapezius on the side opposite to the direction of rotation contract in addition to a contraction of the splenius capitus, splenius cervicis, and longissimus capitus on the same side of the direction of rotation.

Flexion of the trunk primarily involves lengthening of the deep and superficial back muscles and contraction of the abdominal muscles (rectus abdominus, internal oblique, external oblique) and hip flexors (rectus femoris, iliopsoas, tensor faciae lata, sartorius). Seventy-five percent of flexion occurs at the lumbosacral junction (L5-S1), whereas 15 to 70 percent occurs between L4 and L5. The rest of the lumbar vertebrae execute 5 to 10 percent of flexion.[5] Extension involves lengthening of the abdominal muscles and contraction of the erector spinae and the gluteus maximus, which extends the hip. Trunk rotation is produced by the external obliques and the internal obliques. Lateral flexion is produced primarily by the quadratus lumborum muscle, along with the obliques, latissimus dorsi, iliopsoas, and the rectus abdominus on the side of the direction of movement.

The spinal cord is that portion of the central nervous system that is contained within the vertebral canal of the spinal column. Thirty-one pairs of spinal nerves extend from the sides of the spinal cord, coursing downward and outward through the intervertebral foramen passing near the articular facets of the vertebrae. Any abnormal movement of these facets, such as in a dislocation or a fracture, may expose the spinal nerves to injury. Injuries that occur below the third lumbar vertebra usually result in nerve root damage but do not cause spinal cord damage.

The spinal nerve roots combine to form a network of nerves, or a plexus. There are five nerve plexuses: cervical, brachial, lumbar, sacral, and coccygeal.

THE IMPORTANCE OF EVALUATION IN TREATING BACK PAIN

In many instances after referral for medical evaluation, the athlete returns to the sports therapist with a diagnosis of low back pain. Even though this is a correct diagnosis, it does not offer the specificity needed to help direct the treatment planning. The sports therapist planning the treatment would be better served with a more specific diagnosis such as spondylolysis, disk herniation, quadratus lumborum strain, piriformis syndrome, or sacroiliac ligament sprain.

Regardless of the diagnosis or the specificity of the diagnosis, the importance of a thorough evaluation of the athlete's back pain is critical to good care. The sports therapist should become an expert on this individual athlete's back. Taking the time to perform a comprehensive evaluation will pay great rewards in the success of treatment and rehabilitation. The evaluation has six major purposes:

1. To clearly locate areas and tissues that might be part of the problem. The sports therapist should use this information to direct treatments and exercises.[21]

2. To establish the baseline measurements used to assess progress and guide the treatment progression and help the sports therapist make specific judgments on the progression of or changes in specific exercises. The improvement in these measurements also guides the return to practice and play and provides one measure of the success of the rehabilitation plan.[21]

3. To provide some provocative guidance to help the athlete probe the limits of their condition, help them better understand their problem, present limitations, and understand the management of their injury problem.[21]

4. To establish confidence in the sports therapist. This increases the placebo effect of the therapist-athlete interaction.[38,39]

5. To decrease the anxiety of the athlete. This increases the athlete's comfort, which will increase their compliance with the rehabilitation plan; a more positive environment is created, and the therapist and patient avoid the "no one knows what is wrong with me" trap.[8]

6. To provide information for making judgments on pads, braces, and corsets.

Table 26-1 provides a detailed scheme for evaluation of back pain.

REHABILITATION TECHNIQUES FOR THE LOW BACK

Positioning and Pain-Relieving Exercises

Most athletes with back pain have some fluctuation of their symptoms in response to certain postures and activities. The sports therapist logically treats this athlete by reinforcing pain-reducing postures and motions and by starting specific exercises aimed at specific muscle groups or specific ranges of motion. A general rule to follow in making these decisions is as follows: **Any movement that causes the back pain to radiate or spread over a larger area should not be included during this early phase of treatment.** Movements that centralize or diminish the pain are correct movements to include at this time.[3,24] Including some exercise during initial pain management generally has a positive effect on the athlete. The exercise encourages them to be active in the

■ **TABLE 26-1** Lumbar and Sacroiliac Joint Objective Examination

A. Observation
B. Standing Position
  1. Posture—alignment
  2. Gait
    a. Patient's trunk frequently bent laterally or hips shifted to one side
    b. Walks with difficulty and limps
  3. Alignment and symmetry
    a. Level of malleoli
    b. Level of popliteal crease
    c. Trochanteric levels
    d. PSIS and ASIS positioning
    e. Levels of iliac crests
      1. If there is sacroiliac dysfunction the iliac crests will be unlevel; the ASIS and the PSIS will also be unlevel but in the opposite direction. Slight changes in leg length are probably insignificant. With shortening of ½ inch or more, there is a tendency for the pelvis to try and right the upper sacral surface. In the long leg, the ilium tends to move posterior or the short leg ilium moves anterior
  4. Standing forward bending of trunk—(standing flexion test)
    a. Note extent of cranial movement of the PSIS
      1. If one PSIS moves further cranially, a motion restriction is possibly present on that side of the inominates
      2. If the PSISs move at different times, the side that moves first is usually the side with restriction
  5. Lumbar spine active movements
    a. With sacroiliac dysfunction, the athlete will experience exacerbation of pain with side bending toward painful side
    b. Often a lumbar lesion is present along with sacroiliac dysfunction. Side bending toward sacroiliac joints will often aggravate this
  6. Single leg standing backward bending is a provocation test to produce pain from spondylolysis or spondylolisthesis
C. Sitting Position
  1. Sitting forward bending trunk test (sitting forward flexion test)
    a. Note extent of cranial movement of PSIS
      1. Involved PSIS moves more cranially
        a. Blocked joint moves solidly as one, while the sacrum on the painless side is free to move through its small range with the lumbar spine

  2. Rotation—Check lumbar spine
  3. Hip internal rotation
    a. Leg on the involved side may reproduce pain. This is thought to be a piriformis irritation pain and is reproduced as the muscle is stretched
    b. Range of motion
  4. Hip external rotation
    a. Range of motion
D. Supine Position
  1. Hip external rotation—piriformis contracture may cause exaggerated external rotation posture of involved hip
  2. Palpation of symphysis pubis—for postural deviations and tenderness. Some sacroiliac joint problems create pain and tenderness in this area. Sometimes the presenting subjective symptoms mimic adductor or groin strain, but objective evaluation of muscle strength and tenderness are negative for strain of these groups
  3. Straight leg raising (SLR)
    a. Applies stress to sacroiliac joint— can indicate a unilateral torsional stress of the sacroiliac joint; however, could also be a coexisting lumbar problem
    b. Interpretation of SLR:
      1. 30 degrees—hip or very inflamed nerve
      2. 30 to 60 degrees—sciatic nerve involvement
      3. 70 to 90 degrees—sacroiliac joint
      4. Bilateral SLR—lumbar spine problem
      5. Neck flexion—exacerbates symptoms— disk or root irritation
      6. Ankle dorsiflexion or Lasègue sign— usually indicates sciatic nerve or root irritation
  4. Sacroiliac compression and distraction tests
    a. Tests useful in excluding joint irritability, hypermobility, and serious disease, usually negative unless classical pathology exists
  5. Patrick's test—flexion abduction external rotation (FABER)
    a. When pushed into extension may cause exacerbation of sacroiliac lesion—assess irritable motion
  6. Flexion adduction internal rotation (FADIR)— will give iliolumbar ligament stretch
  7. Bilateral knees to chest—will usually exacerbate lumbar spine symptoms as the sacroiliac joints move with the sacrum in this maneuver

Continued

■ **TABLE 26-1** Lumbar and Sacroiliac Joint Objective Examination—Cont'd.

8. Single knee to chest—if pain is reported to the posterolateral thigh—indicates sacrotuberous irritation
9. Single knee to opposite shoulder—if pain is reported in the PSIS area, this indicates sacroiliac ligament irritation

E. Sidelying—Each Side
1. Anterior and posterior pelvic tilt—pain on movement indicates irritation of sacroiliac joint. Also gives direction of movement clues used in treatment
2. Iliotibial band length—long standing sacroiliac joint problems sometimes create tightness of iliotibial band

F. Prone position
1. Palpation
   a. Tenderness medial to or around PSIS that is well localized indicates sacroiliac problem
   b. Gluteus maximus area—Sacrotuberous and sacrospinous ligaments are in this area, as well as piriformis and sciatic nerve. Changes in tension, tenderness, springiness can occur from positional changes of ilium
   c. Tenderness or alignment changes from S1 to T10 interspaces indicates lumbar problems

d. Anteroposterior or rotational stresses to lumbar spinous processes
e. Sacral provocation tests
   1. Do this series of tests only when applicable: If unable to reproduce signs and symptoms by now do not do if by previous tests the joint has been found to be hypermobile
      a. Anteroposterior pressure of sacrum at center of its base
      b. Anteroposterior pressure of sacrum on each side of sacrum just medial to PSIS
   2. Hip extension knee flexion stretch will provoke the L-3 nerve root. Pain similar to nerve pain down the anterolateral thigh would be a positive finding

G. Manual muscle test—if the lumbar spine or posterior hip muscle is strained, active movement against gravity or resistance should provoke the complaints of similar pain to pain under evaluation
1. Hip extension—isometric and isotonic
2. Hip internal rotation
3. Hip external rotation
4. Arm and shoulder extension
5. Arm, shoulder, and neck extension
6. Resisted trunk extension

---

rehabilitation plan and helps them to regain lumbar movement.[14,39]

When an athlete relieves pain through exercise and attention to proper postural control, he or she is much more likely to adopt these procedures into a daily routine. An athlete whose pain is relieved via some other passive procedure, and then is taught exercises, will not be able to readily see the connection between relief and exercise.[3]

The types of exercises that may be included in initial pain management include the following:
• Lateral shift corrections
• Extension exercises
• Flexion exercises

Lateral Shift Corrections. Lateral shift corrections and extension exercises probably should be discussed together because the indications for use are similar, and extension exercises will immediately follow the lateral shift corrections.

The indications for the use of lateral shift corrections are as follows:
• Subjectively, the athlete complains of unilateral pain reference in the lumbar or hip area.

• The typical posture is scoliotic with a hip shift and reduced lumbar lordosis.
• Walking and movements are very guarded and robotic.
• Forward bending is extremely limited and increases the pain.
• Backward bending is limited.
• Side bending toward the painful side is minimal to impossible.
• Side bending away from the painful side is usually reasonable to normal.
• A test correction of the hip shift either reduces the pain or causes the pain to centralize.
• The neurological examination may or may not elicit the following positive findings:
   1. Straight leg raising may be limited and painful, or it could be unaffected.
   2. Sensation may be dull, anesthetic, or unaffected.
   3. Manual muscle test may indicate unilateral weakness of specific movements, or the movements may be strong and painless.
   4. Reflexes may be diminished or unaffected.[3,24]

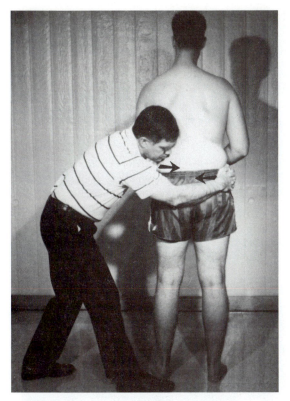

Figure 26-3 Lateral shift correction exercise.

The athlete will be assisted by the sports therapist with the initial lateral shift correction. The athlete is then instructed in the techniques of self-correction. The lateral shift correction is designed to guide the athlete back to a more symmetrical posture. The sports therapist's pressure should be firm and steady and more guiding than forcing. The use of a mirror to provide visual feedback is recommended for both the therapist-assisted and self-corrected maneuvers. The specific technique guide for sports-therapist-assisted lateral shift correction is as follows (Figure 26-3):

1. Preset the athlete by explaining the correction maneuver and the roles of the athlete and the sports therapist.
   a. The athlete is to keep the shoulders level and avoid the urge to side bend.
   b. The athlete should allow the hips to move under the trunk and should not resist the pressure from the sports therapist but allow the hips to shift with the pressure.
   c. The athlete should keep the sports therapist informed about the behavior of their back pain.
   d. The athlete should keep their feet stationary and not move after the hip shift correction until the standing extension part of the correction is completed.
   e. They should practice the standing extension exercise as part of this initial explanation.
2. The sports therapist should stand on the athlete's side that is opposite their hip shift. The athlete's feet should be a comfortable distance apart, and the sports therapist should have a comfortable stride stance aligned slightly behind the athlete.
3. Padding should be placed around the athlete's elbow, on the side next to the sports therapist, to provide comfortable contact between the athlete and the sports therapist.
4. The sports therapist should contact the athlete's elbow with their shoulder and chest with their head aligned along the athlete's back. Their arms should reach around the athlete's waist and apply pressure between the iliac crest and the greater trochanter.
5. The sports therapist should gradually pull the athlete's hips toward him or her. If the pain increases, the sports therapist should ease the pressure and maintain a more comfortable posture for 10 to 20 seconds, then again pull gently. If the pain increases again, the sports therapist should again lessen the pull and allow comfort, then instruct the athlete to actively extend gently, pushing their back into and matching the resistance supplied by the therapist. The goal for this maneuver is an overcorrection of the scoliosis, reversing its direction.
6. Once the corrected or overcorrected posture is achieved, the sports therapist should maintain this posture for 1 to 2 minutes. This procedure may take 2 to 3 minutes to complete, and the first attempt may be less than a total success. Repeated efforts 3 to 4 minutes apart should be attempted during the first treatment effort before the sports therapist stops the treatment for that episode.
7. The sports therapist gradually releases pressure on the hip while the athlete does a standing extension movement. The athlete should complete approximately six repetitions of the standing extension movement, holding each 15 to 20 seconds.
8. Once the athlete moves their feet and walks even a short distance, the lateral hip shift usually will recur, but to a lesser degree. The athlete then should be taught the self-correction maneuver. The athlete should stand in front of a mirror and place one hand on the hip where the sports

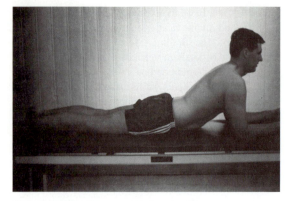

Figure 26-4   Prone extension on elbows.

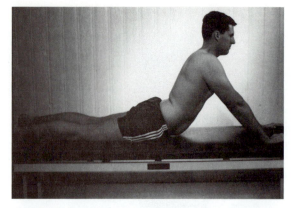

Figure 26-5   Prone extension on hands.

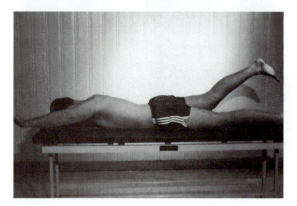

Figure 26-6   Alternate arm and leg extension.

therapist's hands were and the other hand on the lower ribs where the therapist's shoulder was.

9. The athlete then pushes their hip under their trunk, watching the mirror to keep their shoulders level and trying to achieve a corrected or overcorrected posture. They should hold this posture for 30 to 45 seconds and then follow with several standing extension movements as described in step 7.[3,24]

   Extension Exercises.   The indications for the use of extension exercise are as follows:

- Subjectively, back pain is diminished with lying down and increased with sitting. The location of the pain may be unilateral, bilateral, or central, and there may or may not be radiating pain into either or both legs.
- Forward bending is extremely limited and increases the pain, or the pain reference location enlarges as the athlete bends forward.
- Backward bending can be limited, but the movement centralizes or diminishes the pain.
- The neurological examination is the same as outlined for lateral shift correction.[3,25]

The efficacy of extension exercise is theorized to be from one or a combination of the following effects:

- A reduction in the neural tension
- A reduction of the load on the disk, which in turn decreases disk pressure
- Increases in the strength and endurance of the extensor muscles
- Proprioceptive interference with pain perception as the exercises allow self-mobilization of the spinal joints

Hip shift posture has previously been theoretically correlated to the anatomical location of the disk bulge or nucleus pulposus herniation. Creating a centralizing movement of the nucleus pulposus has been the theoreti-

cal emphasis of hip shift correction and extension exercise. This theory has good logic, but research on this phenomenon has not been supportive.[26] However, in explaining the exercises to the athlete, the use of this theory may help increase the athlete's motivation and compliance with the exercise plan.

End-range hyperextension exercise should be used cautiously when the athlete has facet joint degeneration or impingement of the vertebral foramen borders on neural structures. Also, spondylolysis and spondylolisthesis problems should be approached cautiously with any end-range movement exercise using either flexion or hyperextension.

Figures 26-4 through 26-11 are examples of extension exercises. These examples are not exhaustive but are representative of most of the exercises used clinically.

The order in which exercises are presented is not significant. Instead, each sports therapist should base the starting exercises on the evaluative findings. Jackson, in a review of back exercise, stated, "no support was found for the use of a preprogrammed flexion regimen that

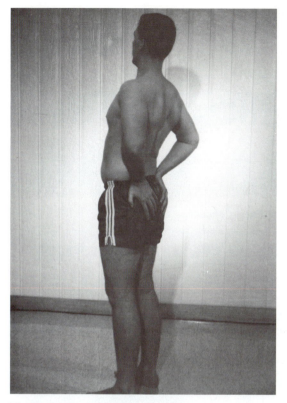

Figure 26-7 Standing extension.

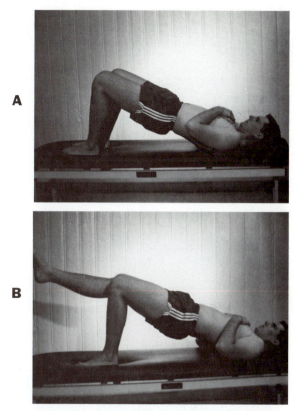

Figure 26-8 Supine hip extension—butt lift or bridge. **A,** Double-leg support. **B,** Single-leg support.

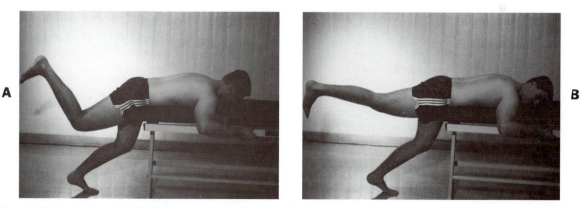

Figure 26-9 Prone single-leg hip extension. **A,** Knee flexed. **B,** Knee extended.

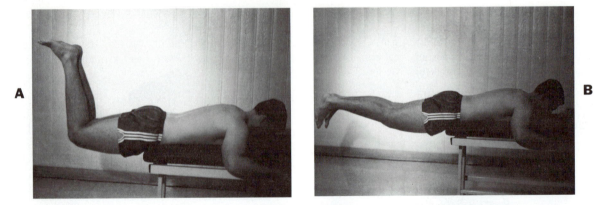

Figure 26-10 Prone double-leg hip extension. **A,** Knees flexed. **B,** Knees extended.

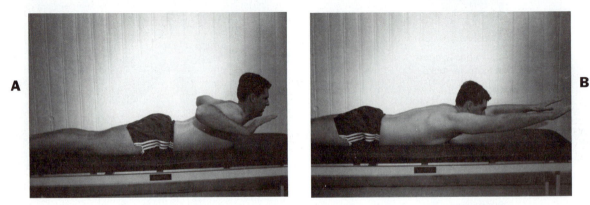

Figure 26-11 Trunk extension—prone. **A,** Hands near head. **B,** Arms extended—superman position.

includes exercises of little value or potential harm and is not specific to the current needs of the patient, as determined by a thorough back evaluation." The review also included a report of Kendall and Jenkins's study, which stated that one-third of the patients for whom hyperextension exercises had been prescribed worsened.[17]

Flexion Exercises.   The indications for the use of flexion exercises are as follows:

- Subjectively, back pain is diminished with sitting and increased with lying down or standing. Pain is also increased with walking.
- Repeated or sustained forward bending eases the pain.
- The athlete's lordotic curve does not reverse as they forward bend.
- The end range of sustained backward bending is painful or increases the pain.
- Abdominal tone and strength are poor.

In his approach, Saal elaborates on the thought that "No one should continue with one particular type of exercise regimen during the entire treatment program."[27] We concur with this and believe that starting with one type

of exercise should not preclude rapidly adding other exercises as the athlete's pain resolves and other movements become more comfortable.

The efficacy of flexion exercise is theorized to derive from one or a combination of the following effects:

- A reduction in the articular stresses on the facet joints
- Stretching to the dorsolumbar fascia and musculature
- Opening of the intervertebral foramen
- Relief of the stenosis of the spinal canal
- Improvement of the stabilizing effect of the abdominal musculature
- Increasing the intraabdominal pressure because of increased abdominal muscle strength and tone
- Proprioceptive interference with pain perception as the exercises allow self-mobilization of the spinal joints[17]

Flexion exercises should be used cautiously or avoided in most cases of acute disk prolapse and when a laterally shifted posture is present. In patients recovering from disk-related back pain, flexion exercise should not be commenced immediately after a flat-lying rest interval longer than 30 minutes. The disk can become more hydrated in this amount of time, and the athlete would be more susceptible to pain with postures that increase disk pressures. Other, less stressful exercises should be initi-

ated first and flexion exercise done later in the exercise program.[3,25]

Figures 26-12 through 26-20 show examples of flexion exercises. Again these examples are not exhaustive but are representative of the exercises used clinically.

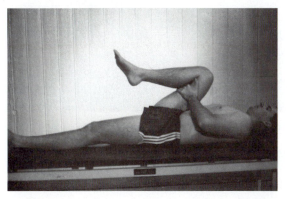

Figure 26-12   Single knee to chest. **A,** Stretch holding 15 to 20 seconds. **B,** Same as step 2.

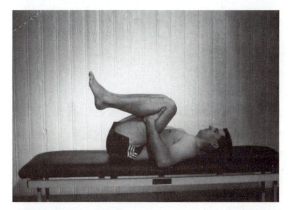

Figure 26-13   Double knee to chest. **A,** Stretching—holding posture 15 to 20 seconds. **B,** Mobilizing—using a rhythmic rocking motion within a pain-free range of motion.

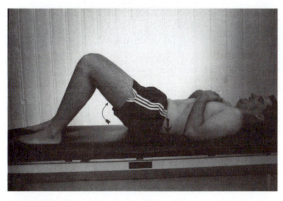

Figure 26-14   Posterior pelvic tilt.

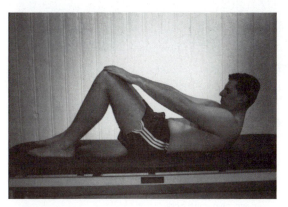

Figure 26-15   Partial sit-up.

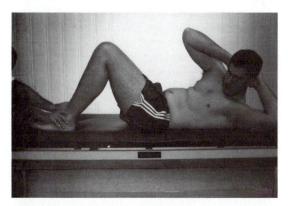

Figure 26-16   Rotation partial sit-up.

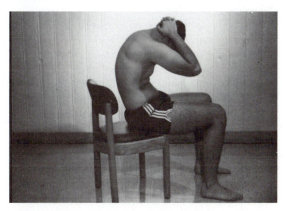

Figure 26-17   Slump sit stretch position.

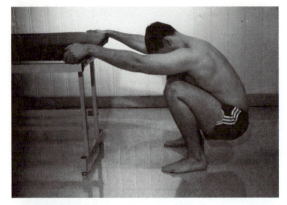

Figure 26-18 Flat-footed squat stretch.

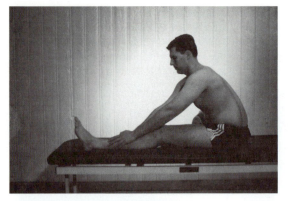

Figure 26-19 Hamstring stretch.

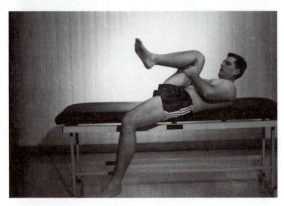

Figure 26-20 Hip flexor stretch.

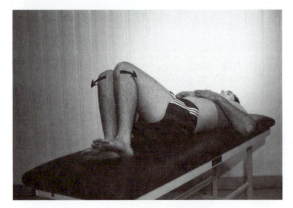

Figure 26-21 Knee rocking side to side.

Joint Mobilizations

The indications for the use of joint mobilizations are as follows:

- Subjectively, the athlete's pain is centered around a specific joint area and increases with activity and decreases with rest.
- The accessory motion available at individual spinal segments is diminished.
- Passive range of motion is diminished.
- Active range of motion is diminished.
- There may be muscular tightness or increased fascial tension in the area of the pain.
- Back movements are asymmetrical when comparing right and left rotation or sidebending.
- Forward and backward bending may steer away from the midline.

The efficacy of mobilization is theorized to be from one or a combination of the following effects:

- Tight structures can be stretched to increase the range of motion.
- The joint involved is stimulated by the movement to more normal mechanics, and irritation is reduced because of better nutrient waste exchange.
- Proprioceptive interference occurs with pain perception as the joint movement stimulates normal neural firing whose perception supercedes nociceptive perception.

Mobilization techniques are multidimensional and are easily adapted to any back pain problem. The mobilizations can be active or passive or assisted by the sports therapist. All ranges (flexion, extension, side-bending, rotation, and accessory) can be incorporated within the exercise plan. The mobilizations can be carried out according to Maitland's grades of oscillation as discussed in Chapter 12. The magnitude of the forces applied can range from grade 1 to grade 4 depending on levels of pain. The theory, technique, and application of the sports-therapist-assisted mobilizations are best gained through guided study with an expert practitioner.[21]

Figures 26-21 through 26-30 show the various self-mobilization exercises.

Figures 26-31 through 26-40 show joint mobilizations that can be used by the sports therapist.

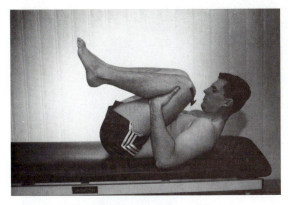

Figure 26-22   Knees toward chest rock.

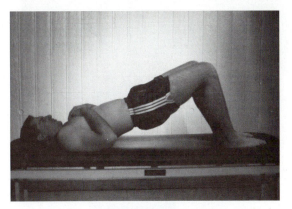

Figure 26-23   Supine hip lift-bridge-rock.

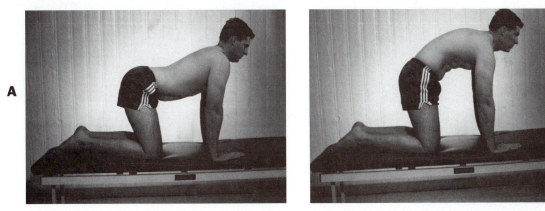

Figure 26-24   Pelvic tilt or pelvic rock. **A,** Butt out. **B,** Tail tuck.

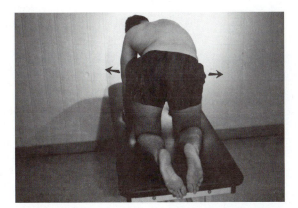

Figure 26-25   Kneeling—dog-tail wags.

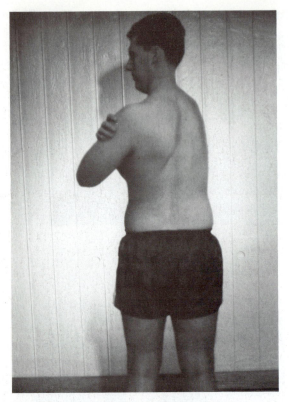

Figure 26-26   Sitting or standing rotation.

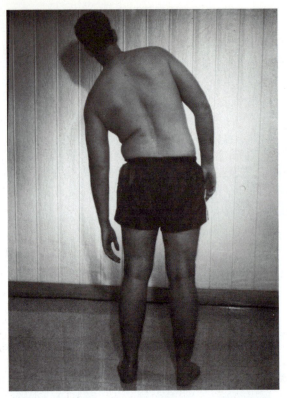

Figure 26-27   Sitting or standing side bending.

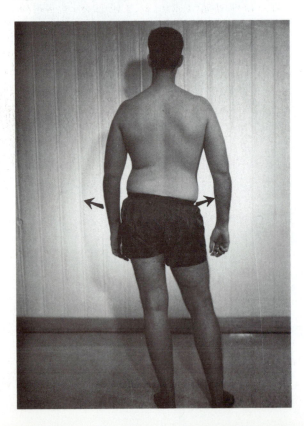

Figure 26-28   Standing hip shift side to side.

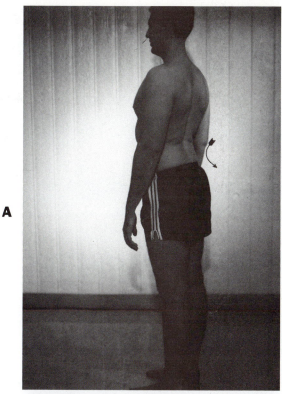

A

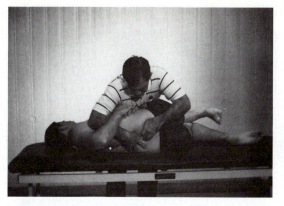

Figure 26-30 Various side-lying and back-lying positions can be used to both stretch and mobilize specific joint areas.

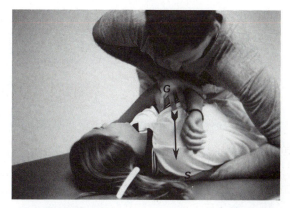

Figure 26-31 Thoracic vertebral facet rotations are accomplished with one hand underneath the patient providing stabilization and the weight of the body pressing downward through the rib cage to rotate an individual thoracic vertebra. Rotation of the thoracic vertebrae is minimal, and most of the movement with this mobilization involves the rib facet joint.

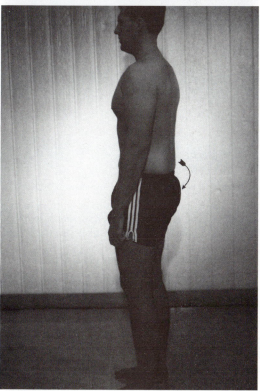

B

Figure 26-29 Standing pelvic rock. **A,** Butt out. **B,** Tail tuck.

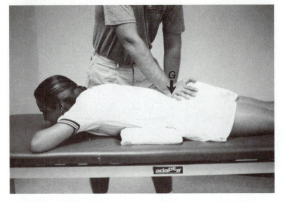

Figure 26-32 Anterior/posterior lumbar vertebral glides. In the lumbar region, anterior/posterior lumbar vertebral glides may be accomplished at individual segments using pressure on the spinous process through the pisiform in the hand. These decrease pain or increase mobility of individual lumbar vertebrae.

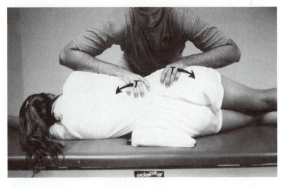

Figure 26-33 Lumbar lateral distraction increases the space between transverse process and increases the opening of the intervertebral foramen. This position is achieved by lying over a support, flexing the patient's upper knee to a point where there is gapping in the appropriate spinal segment, then rotating the upper trunk to place the segment in a close-packed position. Then finger and forearm pressure are used to separate individual spaces. This pressure is used for reducing pain in the lumbar vertebrae associated with some compression of a spinal nerve.

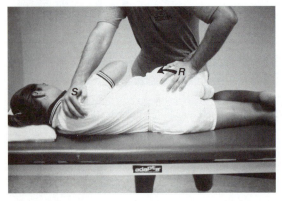

Figure 26-34 Lumbar vertebral rotations decrease pain and increase mobility in lumbar vertebrae. These rotations should be done in a side-lying position.

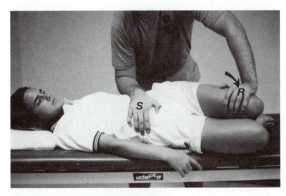

Figure 26-35 Lateral lumbar rotations may be done with the patient in supine position. In this position, one hand must stabilize the upper trunk, while the other produces rotation.

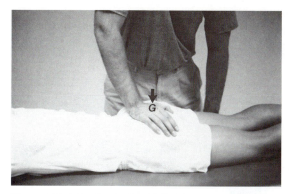

Figure 26-36   Anterior sacral glides decrease pain and reduce muscle guarding around the sacroiliac joint.

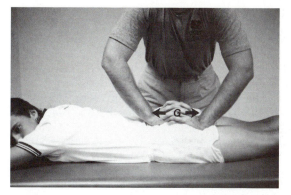

Figure 26-37   Superior/inferior sacral glides decrease pain and reduce muscle guarding around the sacroiliac joint.

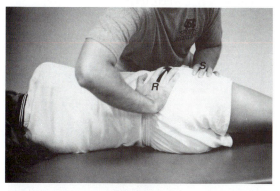

Figure 26-38   An anterior innominate rotation in a side-lying position is accomplished by extending the leg on the affected side, then stabilizing with one hand on the front of the thigh while the other hand applies pressure anteriorly over the posterosuperior iliac spine to produce an anterior rotation. This technique will correct a unilateral posterior rotation.

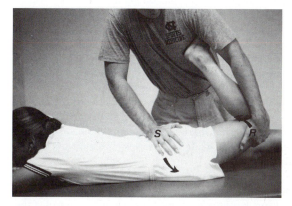

Figure 26-39   An anterior innominate rotation may also be accomplished by extending the hip, applying upward force on the upper thigh, and stabilizing over the posterosuperior iliac spine. This technique is once again used to correct a posterior unilateral innominate rotation.

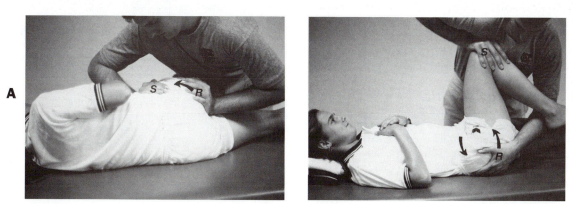

Figure 26-40   Posterior innominate rotations. **A,** A posterior innominate rotation with the patient in side-lying position is done by flexing the hip, stabilizing the anterosuperior iliac spine, and applying pressure to the ischium in an anterior direction. **B,** Another posterior innominate rotation with the hip flexed at 90 degrees stabilizes the knee and rotates the innominate anteriorly through upward pressure on the ischium.

Core Stabilization Exercises

Despite the fact that the athlete may have adequate strength and flexibility, there may be difficulty controlling the spine if the athlete does not learn to contract the appropriate muscles in a desired sequence. Stabilization, especially during complex functional movements, relies heavily on a learned response by the athlete to control the movement. Core stabilization exercises for the trunk and spine may help to minimize the cumulative effects of repetitive microtrauma to the spine. Spinal stabilization does not mean maintaining a static position. **Core stabilization** involves maintaining a controlled range of motion that varies with the position and the activity being performed. Core stabilization is achieved by conscious repetitive training, which over time eventually becomes an unconscious natural response. Core stabilization techniques are widely used in rehabilitation programs for the low back.[17]

The first step in core stabilization training involves learning to maintain the pelvis in a neutral position. A posterior tilt of the pelvis causes the lumbar curve to flatten and is caused by a simultaneous co-contraction of the abdominal and gluteal muscles (Figure 26-14). Once the athlete has learned to control pelvic tilt, progressively more advanced movement activities should be incorporated that involve movements of both the spine and extremities while the pelvis is maintained in a neutral position.[17]

Abdominal muscle control is another key to stabilization of the low back (Figures 26-15, 26-16). Abdominal bracing exercises focus attention on motor control of the external oblique muscles in different positions. There should also be co-contraction of the abdominal muscles and lumbar extensors to maintain a "corset" control of the lumbar spine.[13]

The progression of stabilization exercises should go from a supine activities (Figure 26-8), to prone activities (Figures 26-5, 26-9 to 26-11), to kneeling activities (quadriped to triped to biped), and eventually to weight-bearing activities, all performed while actively stabilizing the trunk. The athlete should be taught to perform a stabilization contraction before starting any movement. As the movement begins, the athlete will become less aware of the stabilization contraction. The athlete may begin by incorporating stabilization into every movement performed in their strengthening exercises. Stabilization contractions can also be used in aerobic conditioning activities. The exercises should include those activities that replicate the demands of the athlete's individual sport. The various components of a sport activity should be broken down into separate activities or skills that allow the athlete to consciously practice the stabilization technique

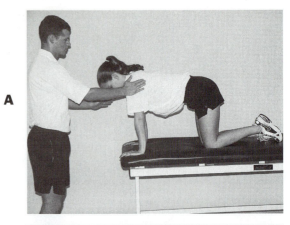

A

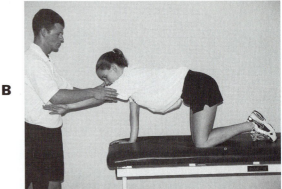

B

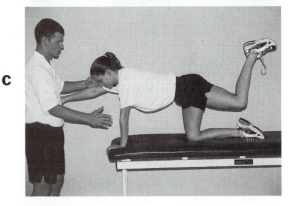

C

Figure 26-41 Weight shifting and stabilization exercises should progress from **A,** quadriped, to **B,** triped, to **C,** biped.

with each drill. Individual athletes differ in their degree of control and in the speed at which they can acquire the skills of core trunk stabilization.[13]

Figures 26-41 through 26-45 show additional examples of core stabilization exercises.

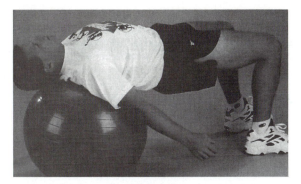

Figure 26-42   Bridging exercises on a Swiss ball.

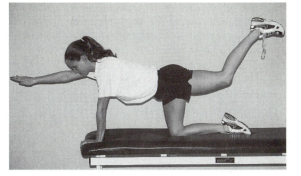

Figure 26-43   Alternate arm/leg extension.

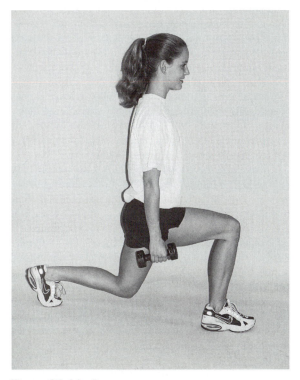

Figure 26-44   Lunges.

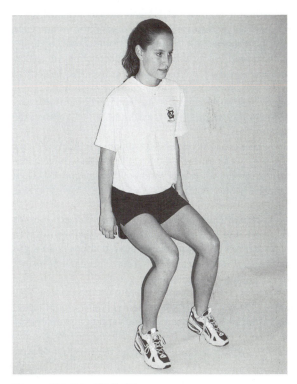

Figure 26-45   Wall slides.

REHABILITATION TECHNIQUES FOR LOW BACK PAIN

Low Back Pain

Pathomechanics.   In most cases, low back pain in athletes does not have serious or long-lasting pathology. It is generally accepted that the soft tissues (ligament, fascia, and muscle) can be the initial pain source. The ath-lete's response to the injury and to the provocative stresses of evaluation is usually proportional to the time since the injury and the magnitude of the physical trauma of the injury. The soft tissues of the lumbar region should react according to the biological process of healing, and the time lines for healing should be like those for other body parts. There is no substantiation that athletic injury to the low back should cause a pain syndrome that lasts longer than 6 to 8 weeks.[8,27]

Injury Mechanism. Back pain can result from one or a combination of the following problems: muscle strain, piriformis muscle or quadratus lumborum myofascial pain or strain, myofascial trigger points, lumbar facet joint sprains, hypermobility syndromes, disk-related back problems, or sacroiliac joint dysfunction.

Rehabilitation Concerns.

Acute versus chronic low back pain. The low back pain that athletes most often experience is an acute, painful experience rarely lasting longer than 3 weeks. The athlete rarely misses a practice and even more rarely misses a game because of this type of back pain. As with many athletic injuries, sports therapists often go through exercise or treatment fads in trying to rehabilitate the athlete with low back pain. The latest fad might involve flexion exercise, extension exercise, joint mobilization, dynamic muscular stabilization, abdominal bracing, myofascial release, electrical stimulation protocols, and so on. To keep perspective, as sports therapists select exercise and modalities, they should keep in mind that 90 percent of people with back pain get resolution of the symptoms in 6 weeks, regardless of the care administered.[27,39]

There are athletes who have pain persisting beyond 6 weeks. This group of athletes will generally have a history of reinjury or exacerbation of previous injury. They describe a low back pain that is similar to their previous back pain experience.

These athletes are experiencing an exacerbation or reinjury of previously injured tissues by continuing to apply stresses that may have created their original injury. This group of athletes needs a more specific and formal treatment and rehabilitation program.[8,27]

There are also people who have chronic low back pain. This is a very small percentage of the population suffering from low back pain and an even smaller percentage of the athletic low back pain subgroup. The difference between the athlete with an acute injury or reinjury and a person with chronic pain has been defined by Waddell. He states, "Chronic pain becomes a completely different clinical syndrome from acute pain."[39] Acute and chronic pain not only are different in time scale but are fundamentally different in kind. Acute and experimental pains bear a relatively straightforward relationship to peripheral stimulus, nociception, and tissue damage.

There may be some understandable anxiety about the meaning and consequences of the pain, but acute pain, disability, and illness behavior are generally proportionate to the physical findings. Pharmacological, physical, and even surgical treatments directed to the underlying physical disorder are generally highly effective in relieving acute pain. Chronic pain, disability, and illness behavior,

in contrast, become increasingly dissociated from their original physical basis, and there may be little objective evidence of any remaining nociceptive stimulus. Instead, chronic pain and disability become increasingly associated with emotional distress, depression, failed treatment, and adoption of a sick role. Chronic pain progressively becomes a self-sustaining condition that is resistant to traditional medical management. Physical treatment directed to a supposed but unidentified and possibly nonexistent nociceptive source is not only understandably unsuccessful but may cause additional physical damage. Failed treatment may both reinforce and aggravate pain, distress, disability, and illness behavior.[39]

Rehabilitation Progression. A discussion of the rehabilitation progression for the athlete with low back pain can be much more specific and meaningful if treatment plans are lumped into two stages. Stage I (acute stage) treatment consists mainly of the modality treatment and pain-relieving exercises. Stage II treatment involves treating athletes with a reinjury or exacerbation of a previous problem. The treatment plan in stage II goes beyond pain relief, strengthening, stretching, and mobilization to include trunk stabilization and movement training sequences and to provide a specific, guided program to return the athlete to the chosen sport.[27]

Stage I (acute stage) treatment. Modulating pain should be the initial focus of the sports therapist. Progressing rapidly from pain management to specific rehabilitation should be a primary goal of the acute stage of the rehabilitation plan. The most common treatment for pain relief in the acute stage is to use ice for analgesia. Rest, but not total bed rest, is used to allow the injured tissues to begin the healing process without the stresses that created the injury.[9]

Along with rest, during the initial treatment stage, the athlete should be taught to increase comfort by using the *appropriate* body positioning techniques, described previously, which may involve (1) lateral shift corrections (Figure 26-3), (2) extension exercises (Figures 26-4 through 26-11), (3) flexion exercises (Figures 26-12 through 26-20), or (4) self-mobilization exercises (Figures 26-21 through 26-30). Outside support, in the form of corsets and the use of props or pillows to enhance comfortable positions, also needs to be included in the initial pain management phase of treatment.[27,39] The athlete should also be taught to avoid positions and movements that increase any sharp, painful episodes. The limits of these movements and positions that provide comfort should be the initial focus of any exercises.

The athlete should be encouraged to move through this stage quickly and return to practice and play as soon as range, strength, and comfort will allow. The addition of a supportive corset for practice and play during this stage should be based mostly on athlete comfort. We suggest using an eclectic approach to the selection of the exercises, mixing the various protocols described according to the findings of the athlete's evaluation. Rarely will an athlete present with classic signs and symptoms that will dictate using one variety of exercise.

Stage II (reinjury stage) treatment. In the reinjury or chronic stage of back rehabilitation, the goals of the treatment and training should again be based on a thorough evaluation of the athlete. Identifying the causes of the athlete's back problem and recurrences is very important in the management of their rehabilitation and prevention of reinjury. A goal for this stage of care is to make the athlete responsible for the management of their back problem. The sports therapist should identify specific problems and corrections that will help the athlete better understand the mechanisms and management of their problem.[27]

Specific goals and exercises should be identified about the following:

- Which structures to stretch
- Which structures to strengthen
- Incorporating dynamic stabilization into the athlete's daily life and exercise routine
- Which movements need a motor learning approach to control faulty mechanics[27]

Stretching. The sports therapist and the athlete need to plan specific exercises to stretch restricted groups, maintain flexibility in normal muscle groups, and identify hypermobility that may be a part of the problem. In planning, instructing, and monitoring each exercise, adequate thought and good instruction must be used to ensure that the intended structures get stretched and areas of hypermobility are protected from overstretching.[10,16] Inadequate stabilization will lead to exercise movements that are so general that the exercise will encourage hyperflexibility at already hypermobile areas. Lack of proper stabilization during stretching may help perpetuate a structural problem that will continue to add to the athlete's back pain.

In the sports therapist's evaluation of the athlete with back pain, the following muscle groups should be assessed for flexibility:[10]

- Hip flexors
- Hamstrings
- Low back extensors
- Lumbar rotators
- Lumbar lateral flexors
- Hip adductors
- Hip abductors
- Hip rotators

Strengthening. There are numerous techniques for strengthening the muscles of the trunk and hip. Muscles are perhaps best strengthened by using techniques of progressive overload to achieve specific adaptation to imposed demands (SAID principle). The overload can take the form of increased weight load, increased repetition load, or increased stretch load to accomplish physiological changes in muscle strength, muscle endurance, or flexibility of a body part.[10]

The treatment plan should call for an exercise that the athlete can easily accomplish successfully. Rapidly but gradually, the overload should push the athlete to challenge the muscle group needing strengthening. The sports therapist and the athlete should monitor continuously for increases in the athlete's pain or recurrences of previous symptoms. If those changes occur, the exercises should be modified, delayed, or eliminated from the rehabilitation plan.[17,27]

Core stabilization. Core stabilization training, dynamic abdominal bracing, and finding neutral position all describe a technique used to increase the stability of the trunk. This increased stability will enable the athlete to maintain the spine and pelvis in the most comfortable and acceptable mechanical position that will control the forces of repetitive microtrauma and protect the structures of the back from further damage. Abdominal muscular control is one key to giving the athlete the ability to stabilize their trunk and control their posture. Abdominal strengthening routines are rigorous, and the athlete must complete them with vigor. However, in their functional activities, the athlete does not take advantage of abdominal strength to stabilize the trunk and protect the back.[16,22,29]

Kennedy's dynamic abdominal bracing exercises focus attention on the motor control of the external oblique muscles in various positions. Once this control is established, different positions and movements are added.[22] Saal describes this type of exercise as finding and maintaining the neutral position with muscle fusion. He specifically singles out the external oblique muscles as a major factor but describes a co-contraction of the abdominal and lumbar extensors, including the gluteus maximus, to maintain a corseting action on the lumbar spine. Adequate flexibility of hip muscles and other structures is also necessary to accomplish this muscle fusion concept.[27] The concept of increasing trunk stability with muscle contractions that support and limit the extremes of spinal movement is important, regardless of whether muscle fusion or dynamic abdominal bracing are the terms used to describe this action (Figures 26-40 through 26-45).

Basic functional training. The athlete must be constantly committed to improving body mechanics and trunk control in all postures in both sport-related activities and in their activities of daily living. The sports therapist needs to evaluate the athlete's daily patterns and give them instruction, practice, and monitoring on the best and least stressful body mechanics for them in as many activities as possible.

The basic program follows the developmental sequence of posture control, starting with supine and prone extremity movement while actively stabilizing the trunk. The athlete is then progressed to all fours, kneeling, and standing. Emphasis on trunk control and stability is maintained as the athlete works through this exercise sequence.[16,23,27]

The most critical aspect for developing motor control is repetition of exercise. However, variability in positioning, speed of movement, and changes in movement patterns must also be incorporated. The variability of the exercise will allow the athlete to generalize their newly learned trunk control to the constant changes necessary in their sport. The basic exercise, including a trunk stabilizing contraction, is the key. Incorporating this stabilization contraction into various activities helps reinforce trunk stabilization and makes trunk control a subconscious automatic response.

The use of augmented feedback (EMG, palpation) of the trunk stabilizing contraction may be needed early in the exercise plan to help maximize the results of this exercise. The sports therapist should have the athlete internalize this feedback as quickly as possible to make the athlete apparatus-free and more functional. With augmented feedback, it is recommended that the patient be rapidly and progressively weaned from dependency on external feedback.

Advanced functional training. Each activity that the athlete is involved in becomes part of the advanced exercise rehabilitation plan. The usual place to start is with the athlete's strength and conditioning program. Each step of the program is monitored and emphasis is placed on trunk stabilization for even the simple task of putting the weights on a bar or getting on and off of exercise equipment. Each exercise in their strength and conditioning program should be retaught, and the athlete is made aware of their best mechanical position and the proper stabilizing muscular contraction. The strength program is sport and athlete specific, attempting to strengthen weak areas and improve strength in muscle groups needed for better sports performance.[27]

Aerobic activities are also included in advanced programs. The same emphasis on technique and stabilization is used as the athlete begins aerobic conditioning activities. A functional progression should be used so that changes in symptoms can be controlled by working with lower-level exercises and then progressing to more difficult and stressful exercises.[27] Modification of normal aerobic conditioning for a particular sport may be an important part of eliminating some of the unnecessary stress from the athlete's overall program. Substituting an aquatic conditioning program for sprinting and running may keep the athlete participating effectively without increasing their back pain.

Using exercises designed to incorporate trunk control into specific skills is the next step in the exercise progression. Sport-specific skills should be tailored to the individual athlete. The sports therapist should work in concert with the coach and athlete to incorporate stabilization training with sport drills and postures. The sports therapist may not know the intricacies of pass blocking, but they can help the coach and athlete identify good alignment and stabilization as the athlete performs each drill.[27]

The athlete should be taught to start their stabilization contraction before starting any movement. This presets the athlete's posture and stabilization awareness before their movement takes place. As the movement occurs, they will become less aware of the stabilization contraction as they attempt to accomplish the drill.

They might revert to old postures and habits, so feedback is important. The next step is to incorporate a firmer stabilization contraction during the power phase of the drill. The athlete is instructed to contract more firmly during initiation of a jump or push during change in direction. The drills should be constructed to have several changes in contraction strength planned as the athlete moves through the drill. Expect that the athlete may experience paralysis by analysis as they try to think through stabilizing contraction plus drill execution. Adequate practice time will be necessary before the athlete is ready to reenter a team practice. The athlete should find this stabilization control comfortable, efficient, and powerful.

Each athlete is different, not only with their individual back problem but also with their abilities to gain motor skill. Athletes differ in degree of control and in the speed at which they acquire these new skills of trunk stabilization.

Reducing stress to the back by using braces, orthotics, shoes, or comfortable supportive furniture (beds, desks, or chairs) is essential to help the athlete minimize chronic or overload stresses to their back. The stabilization exercise should be incorporated into their activities of daily living and sport activities.[30]

The use of a low back corset or brace may also make the athlete more comfortable (Figure 26-62).

Criteria for Return. For most low back problems the stage I treatment and exercise programs will get the athlete back into their activities quickly. If the pain or dysfunction is pronounced or the problem becomes recurrent, an in-depth evaluation and treatment using stage I and stage II exercise protocols will be necessary. The team approach with athlete, doctor, sports therapist, and coach working together will provide the comprehensive approach needed to manage the athlete's back problem. Close attention to and emphasis on the athlete's progress will provide both the athlete and the sports therapist with the encouragement to continue this program.

Muscular Strains

Injury Mechanism. Evaluative findings include a history of sudden or chronic stress that initiates pain in a muscular area during the workout. There are three points on the physical examination that must be positive to indicate the muscle as the primary problem. There will be tenderness to palpation in the muscular area. The muscular pain will be provoked with contraction and with stretch of the involved muscle.

Rehabilitation Progression. The treatment should include the standard protection, ice, and compression. Ice may be applied in the form of ice massage or ice bags, depending on the area involved. An elastic wrap or corset would protect and compress the back musculature. Additional modalities would include pulsed ultrasound as a biostimulative and electrical stimulation for pain relief and muscle reeducation. The exercises used in rehabilitation should make the involved muscle contract and stretch, starting with very mild exercise and progressively increasing the intensity and repetition loads. In general this would include active extension exercises such as hip lifts (Figures 26-8 to 26-10), alternate arm and leg, hip extension (Figure 26-6), trunk extension (Figure 26-11), and quadratus hip shift exercises (Figures 26-55 to 26-57). A good series of abdominal strengthening and stabilization exercise would also be helpful (Figures 26-14 to 26-15). Stretching exercises might include the following: knee to chest (Figure 26-12, 26-13), side-lying leg hang to stretch the hip flexors (Figure 26-20), slump sitting (Figure 26-17), and knee rocking side to side (Figure 26-21).

Criteria for Return. When the athlete can perform functional activities on the same level as teammates, he or she may return to practice and competition. Initially, the athlete may wish to continue to use a brace or corset, but they should be encouraged to do away with the corset as their back strengthens and their performance returns to normal.[10,17]

Piriformis Muscle Strain

Pathomechanics. Piriformis syndrome was discussed in detail in Chapter 22. The piriformis muscle refers pain to the posterior sacroiliac region, to the buttocks, and sometimes down the posterior or posterolateral thigh. The pain is usually described as a deep ache that can get more intense with exercise and with sitting with the hips flexed, adducted, and medially rotated. The pain gets sharper and more intense with activities that require decelerating medial hip and leg rotation during weight bearing.

Tenderness to palpation has a characteristic pattern, with tenderness medial and proximal to the greater trochanter and just lateral to the posterosuperior iliac spine. Isometric abduction in the sitting position produces pain in the posterior hip buttock area, and the movement will be weak or hesitant. Passive hip internal rotation in the sitting position will also bring on posterior hip and buttock pain.

Rehabilitation Progression. Rehabilitation exercises should include both strengthening and stretching. Strengthening exercises should include prone-lying hip internal rotation with elastic resistance (Figure 26-48), hip-lift bridges (Figure 26-49), hand-knee position fire hydrant exercise (Figure 26-50), side-lying hip abduction straight leg raises (Figure 26-51), and prone hip extension exercise (Figure 26-52).

Stretching exercises for the piriformis include long-leg sitting with the involved hip and knee flexed and foot crossed over extended leg (Figure 26-53), back-lying legs-crossed hip adduction stretch (Figure 26-54), back-lying with the involved leg crossed over the uninvolved leg, ankle to knee position, pulling the uninvolved knee to the chest to create the stretch (Figure 26-55), contract-relax-stretch with elbow pressure to the muscle insertion during the relaxation phase (Figure 26-56).[18,32,35]

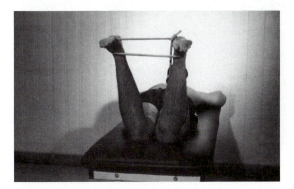

Figure 26-46 Prone-lying hip internal rotation with elastic resistance.

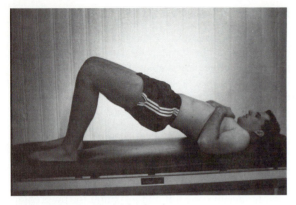

Figure 26-47 Hip-lift bridges.

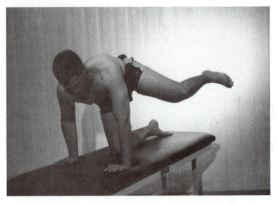

Figure 26-48 Hand-knee position—fire hydrant exercise.

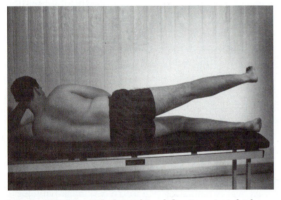

Figure 26-49 Side-lying hip abduction straight-leg raises.

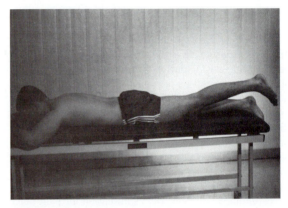

Figure 26-50 Prone hip extension exercise.

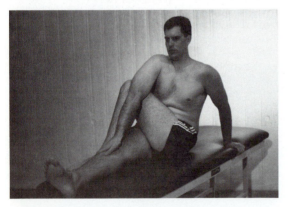

Figure 26-51 Long-leg sitting stretch.

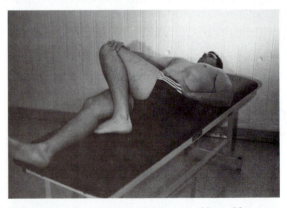

Figure 26-52 Back-lying legs-crossed hip adduction stretch.

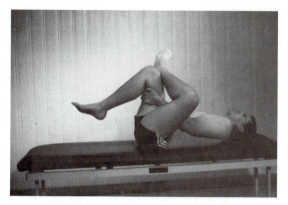

Figure 26-53 Back-lying legs-crossed pulling uninvolved knee.

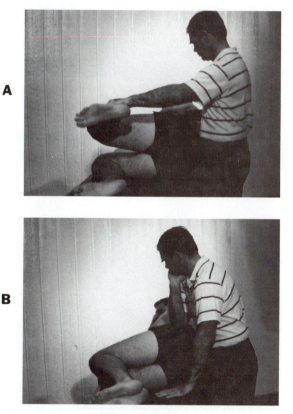

Figure 26-54 Piriformis stretch using elbow pressure. **A,** Start-contract. **B,** Relaxation-stretch.

Quadratus Lumborum Strain

Pathomechanics. Pain from the quadratus lumborum muscle is described as an aching, sharp pain located in the flank, in the lateral back area, and near the posterior sacroiliac region and upper buttocks. The athlete usually describes pain on moving from sitting to standing, standing for long periods, coughing, sneezing, and walking. Activities requiring trunk rotation or side bending aggravate the pain. The muscle is tender to palpation near the origin along the lower ribs and along the insertion on the iliac crest. Pain will be aggravated on side bending, and the pain will usually be localized to one side. For example, with a right quadratus problem, side bending right and left would provoke only right-side pain. Supine hip-hiking movements would also provoke the pain.

Rehabilitation Progression. Rehabilitation strengthening exercises should include back-lying hip-hike shifting (Figure 26-55), standing with one leg on elevated surface and the other free to move below that level, hip-hike on the free side (Figure 26-56), and back-lying hip-hike resisted by pulling on the involved leg (Figure 26-57).

Stretching exercises should include side-lying over a pillow roll leg-hand stretch (Figure 26-58), supine self-stretch with legs crossed (Figure 26-59), hip-hike exercise with hand pressure to increase stretch (Figure 26-60), and standing one leg on a small book stretch (Figure 26-61).[35]

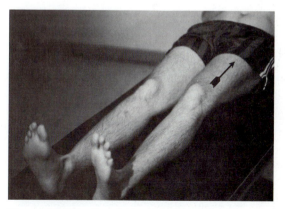

Figure 26-55 Back-lying—hip-hike shifting.

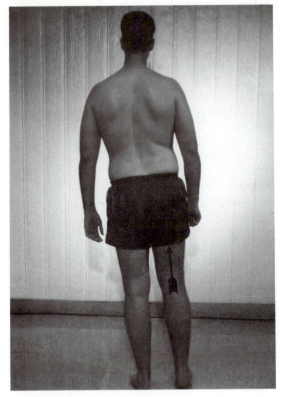

Figure 26-56 Standing hip hike.

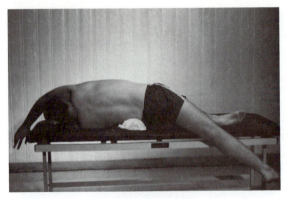

Figure 26-58 Sidelying stretch over pillow roll.

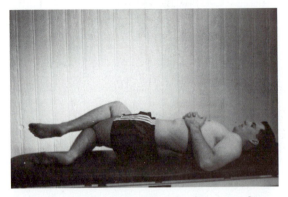

Figure 26-59 Supine self-stretch—legs crossed.

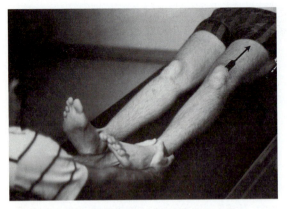

Figure 26-57 Back-lying—hip-hike resisted.

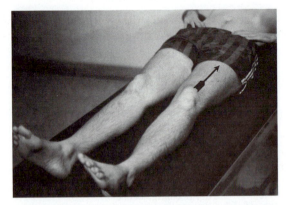

Figure 26-60 Hip-hike exercise with hand pressure.

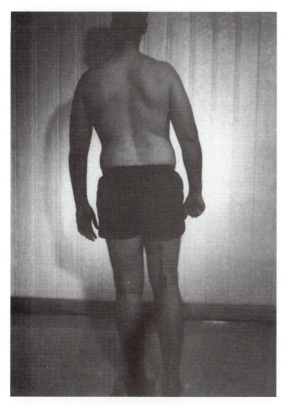

Figure 26-61   Standing one-leg-up stretch.

Myofascial Pain and Trigger Points

Pathomechanics and Injury Mechanism.   The above examples of muscle-oriented back pain in both the piriformis and quadratus lumborum could also have a myofascial origin. The major component in successfully changing myofascial pain is stretching the muscle back to a normal resting length. The muscle irritation and congestion that create the trigger points are relieved, and normal blood flow resumes, further reducing the irritants in the area. Stretching through a painful trigger point is difficult. A variety of comfort and counterirritant modalities can be used preliminary to, during, and after the stretching to enhance the effect of the exercise. Some of the methods used successfully are dry needling, local anesthetic injection, ice massage, friction massage, acupressure massage, ultrasound electrical stimulation, and cold sprays.

The indications for treating low back pain with myofascial stretching and treatment techniques are as follows:

1.   Subjectively, in athletes, early-season muscle soreness and fatigue from repetitive motions are common antecedent mechanisms. Athletes are also susceptible later in their season as fatigue and stress overload specific muscle groups. There may be a history of sudden onset during or shortly after an acute overload stress, or there may be a gradual onset with repetitive or postural overload of the affected muscle.

     The pain may be an incapacitating event in the case of acute onset, but it may also be a nagging, aggravating type of pain with an intensity that varies from an awareness of discomfort to a severe unrelenting type of pain. The pain location is usually a referred pain area remote from the actual myofascial trigger point. These trigger points can be present but quiescent until they are activated by overload, fatigue, trauma, or chilling. These points are called *latent trigger points.* This deep, aching pain can be specifically localized, but the athlete is not sensitive to palpation in these areas. This pain can often be reproduced by maintaining pressure on a hypersensitive myofascial trigger point.

2.   Passive or active stretching of the affected myofascial structure increases pain.

3.   The stretch range of muscle is restricted.

4.   The pain is increased when the muscle is contracted against a fixed resistance or the muscle is allowed to contract into a very shortened range. The pain in this case is described as a muscle cramping pain.

5.   The muscle may be slightly weak.

6.   Trigger points may be located within a taut band of the muscle. If taut bands are found during palpation, explore them for local hypersensitive areas.

7.   Pressure on the hypersensitive area will often cause a "jump sign"; as the sports therapist strums the sensitive area, the athlete's muscle involuntarily jumps in response.

8.   The primary muscle groups that create low back pain in athletes are the quadratus lumborum and the piriformis muscles.[18,32,35,36]

Travell and Simons have devoted two volumes to the causes and treatment of various myofascial pains.[35,36] They have done a very thorough job of describing the symptoms and signs of each area of the body, and they give very specific guidance on exercises and positioning in their treatment protocols.

Rehabilitation Technique. Myofascial trigger points may be treated using the following steps:

1. Position the athlete comfortably but in a position that will lend itself to stretching the involved muscle group.
2. Caution the athlete to use mild progressive stretches rather than sudden, sharp, hard stretches.
3. Hot pack the area for 10 minutes, and follow with an ultrasound and electrical stimulation treatment over the affected muscle.
4. Use an ice cup, and use 2 to 3 slow strokes starting at the trigger point and moving in one direction toward their pain reference area and over the full length of the muscle.
5. Begin stretching well within the athlete's comfort. A stretch should be maintained a minimum of 15 seconds. The stretch should be released until the athlete is comfortable again. The next stretch repetition should then be progressively more intense if tolerated, and the position of the stretch should also be varied slightly. Repeat the stretch 4 to 6 times.
6. Hot pack the area, and have the athlete go through some active stretches of the muscle.
7. Refer to Travell and Simons's manual for specific references on other muscle groups.[18,35,36]

Lumbar Facet Joint Sprains

Pathomechanics and Injury Mechanism. Sprains may occur in any of the ligaments in the lumbar spine. However, the most common sprain involves lumbar facet joints. Facet joint sprain typically occurs when bending forward and twisting while lifting or moving some object. The athlete will report a sudden acute episode that caused the problem, or they will give a history of a chronic repetitive stress that caused the gradual onset of a pain that got progressively worse with continuing activity. The pain is local to the structure that has been injured, and the athlete can clearly localize the area. The pain is described as a sore pain that gets sharper in response to certain movements or postures. The pain is located centrally or just lateral to the spinous process areas and is deep.

Local symptoms will occur in response to movements, and the athlete will usually limit the movement in those ranges that are painful. When the vertebra is moved passively with a posteroanterior or rotational pressure through the spinous process, the pain may be provoked.

Rehabilitation Progression. The treatment should include the standard protection, ice, and compres-

sion as mentioned previously. Both pulsed ultrasound and electrical stimulation could also be used similarly to the treatment of muscle strains but localized to the specific joint area.

Joint mobilization using anteroposterior (Figure 26-32) and rotational glides (Figures 26-34, 26-35) should help reduce pain and increase joint nutrition. The athlete should be instructed in trunk stabilization exercises using good postural control (Figures 26-41 to 26-45). Strengthening exercises for abdominals (Figures 26-14 to 26-16) and back extensors (Figures 26-8 to 26-11) should initially be limited to a pain-free range. Stretching in all ranges should start well within a comfort range and gradually increase until trunk movements reach normal ranges. Athletes should be supported with a corset or range limiting brace when they return to their competitive activity, which should be used only temporarily until normal strength, muscle control, and pain-free range are achieved.[10,20,21,34,37] It is important to guard against the development of postural changes that might occur in response to pain.

Hypermobility Syndromes (Spondylolysis/Spondylolisthesis)

Pathomechanics. Hypermobility of the low back may be attributed to spondylolysis or spondylolisthesis. Spondylolysis involves a degeneration of the vertebrae and, more commonly, a defect in the pars interarticularis of the articular processes of the vertebrae. It is often attributed to a congenital weakness, with the defect occurring as a stress fracture. Spondylolysis might produce no symptoms unless a disk herniation occurs or there is sudden trauma such as hyperextension. Commonly spondylolysis begins unilaterally. However, if it extends bilaterally, there may be some slipping of one vertebrae on the one below it.

A spondylolisthesis is considered to be a complication of spondylolysis often resulting in hypermobility of a vertebral segment.[11] Spondylolisthesis has the highest incidence with L5 slipping on S1.

Injury Mechanism. Sports movements that characteristically hyperextend the spine, such as the back arch in gymnastics, lifting weights, blocking in football, serving in tennis, spiking in volleyball, and the butterfly stroke in swimming, are most likely to cause this condition.

Rehabilitation Concerns. The athlete usually has a relatively long history of feeling "something go" in their back. They complain of a low back pain described as a persistent ache across the back (belt type). This pain does not usually interfere with their workout performance but is usually worse when fatigued or after sitting in a slumped posture for an extended time. The athlete

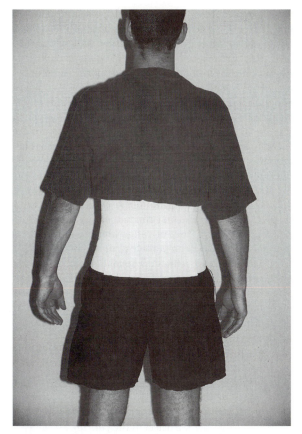

Figure 26-62 A lower-lumbar corset or brace.

may also complain of a tired feeling in the low back. They describe the need to move frequently and get temporary relief of pain through self-manipulation. They often describe self-manipulative behavior more than 20 times a day. Their pain is relieved by rest, and they do not usually feel the pain during exercise. On physical examination, the athlete usually will have full and painless trunk movements, but there will be a wiggle or hesitation at the midrange of forward bending. On backward bending their movement may appear to hinge at one spinal segment. When extremes of range are maintained for 15 to 30 seconds, the athlete feels a lumbosacral ache. On return from forward bending, the athlete will use thigh climbing to regain the neutral position. On palpation there may be tenderness localized to one spinal segment. Excessive movement may be noticed when applying posteroanterior pressure to the spinal segment.

Rehabilitation Progression. Athletes with this problem will fall into the reinjury stage of back pain and may require extensive treatment to regain stability of the trunk. The athlete's pain should be treated symptomati-

cally. Initially, bracing and occasionally bed rest for 1 to 3 days will help reduce pain. The major focus in rehabilitation should be on exercises that control or stabilize the hypermobile segment (Figures 26-41 to 26-45). Progressive trunk-strengthening exercises, especially through the midrange, should be incorporated. Core stabilization exercises that concentrate on abdominal muscles should also be used (Figures 26-14 to 26-16). The athlete should avoid manipulation and self-manipulation as well as stretching and flexibility exercises. Corsets and braces are beneficial if the athlete uses them only for support during higher-level activities and for short (1 to 2 hour) periods to help avoid fatigue[16,27] (Figure 26-62). Hypermobility of a lumbar vertebrae may make the athlete more susceptible to lumbar muscle strains and ligament sprains. Thus it may be necessary for the athlete to avoid vigorous activity. The use of a low back corset or brace might also make the athlete more comfortable (Figure 26-62).

Disk-Related Back Pain

Pathomechanics. The lumbar disks are subject to constant abnormal stresses stemming from faulty body mechanics, trauma, or both, which, over a period of time, can cause degeneration, tears, and cracks in the annulus fibrosus.[6] The disk most often injured lies between the L4 and L5 vertebrae. The L5-S1 disk is the second most commonly affected.

Injury Mechanism. In sports, the mechanism of a disk injury is the same as for the lumbosacral sprain—forward bending and twisting that places abnormal strain on the lumbar region. The movement that produces herniation or bulging of the nucleus pulposus may be minimal, and associated pain may be significant. Besides injuring soft tissues, such a stress may herniate an already degenerated disk by causing the nucleus pulposus to protrude into or through the annulus fibrosis. As the disk progressively degenerates, a prolapsed disk may develop in which the nucleus moves completely through the annulus. If the nucleus moves into the spinal canal and comes in contact with a nerve root, this is referred to as an extruded disk. This protrusion of the nucleus pulposus may place pressure on the cord of spinal nerves, causing radiating pains similar to those of sciatica, as occurs in piriformis syndrome. If the material of the nucleus separates from the disk and begins to migrate, a sequestrated disk exists.

Rehabilitation Concerns. The athlete will report a centrally located pain that radiates unilaterally or spreads across the back. They may describe a sudden or gradual onset after a workout that becomes particularly severe after they have rested and then tried to resume their activities. They may complain of tingling or numb feelings in a dermatomal pattern or sciatic radiation. Forward bending and sitting postures increase their pain. The athlete's symptoms are usually worse in the morning on first arising and get better through the day. Coughing and sneezing may increase their pain.

On physical examination, the athlete will have a hip shifted, forward bent posture. On active movements, side bending toward the hip shift is painful and limited. Side bending away from the shift is more mobile and does not provoke the pain. Forward bending is very limited and painful, and guarding is very apparent. On palpation there may be tenderness around the painful area. Posteroanterior pressure over the involved segment increases the pain. Passive straight-leg raising will increase the back or leg pain during the first 30 degrees of hip flexion. Bilateral knee-to-chest movement will increase the back pain. Neurological testing (strength, sensory reflex) may be positive for differences between right and left.

Rehabilitation Progression. The athlete should be treated with pain reducing modalities (ice, electrical stimulation) initially. The sports therapist should then use the lateral shift correction and extension exercise (Figure 26-3). This should be followed by self-correction instruction and gentle strengthening and mobilizing exercises. Manual traction combined with passive backward bending or extension makes the athlete more comfortable. The goal is to reduce the protrusion and restore normal posture.. When pain and posture return to normal, abdominal and back extensor strengthening should be emphasized. This athlete may recover easily from the first episode, but if repeated episodes occur, then they should also start on the reinjury stage of back rehabilitation.[7,10,12,14,17,29,30,33]

If the disk is extruded or sequestrated, about the only thing that can be done is to modulate pain with electrical stimulation. Flexion exercises and lying supine in a flexed position may help with comfort. The use of a low back corset or brace may also make the athlete more comfortable (Figure 26-62). Sometimes the symptoms will resolve with time. But if there are signs of nerve damage, surgery may be necessary.

Sacroiliac Joint Dysfunction

Pathomechanics and Injury Mechanism. A sprain of the sacroiliac joint may result from twisting with both feet on the ground, stumbling forward, falling backward, stepping too far down and landing heavily on one leg, or forward bending with the knees locked during lifting.[20] Athletic activities involving unilateral forceful movements, such as punting, hurdling, throwing, jumping, or trunk rotations with both feet fixed (swinging a club or bat), are the usual activities associated with the onset of pain. Any of these mechanisms can produce irritation and stretching of the sacrotuberous or sacrospinous ligaments. They may also cause either an anterior or posterior rotation of one side of the pelvis relative to the other. With rotation of the pelvis there is hypomobility. As healing occurs, the joint on the injured side may become hypermobile, allowing that joint to sublux in either an anteriorly or posteriorly rotated position.

Rehabilitation Concerns. On observation, the ASIS and/or PSIS may be asymmetrical when compared to the opposite side, due to either anterior or posterior rotation of one side of the pelvis relative to the other. There may appear to be a measurable leg length difference.

The athlete will relate a gradual onset of dull, achy back pain near or medial to the posterosuperior iliac spine (PSIS) with some associated muscle guarding. The pain may radiate into the buttocks and posterolateral thigh. The athlete may describe a heaviness, dullness, or deadness in the leg or referred pain to the groin, adductor, or hamstring on the same side. Doing a hip flexion activity with the affected leg may increase the pain. The pain may be more noticeable during the stance phase of walking.

On active movements in forward bending, there is a block to normal movement, and the PSIS on the affected side will move sooner than the normal side. Side-bending toward the painful side will increase the pain. Straight-leg raising will increase pain in the sacroiliac joint area after 45 degrees of motion. On palpation, there may be tenderness over the PSIS, medial to the PSIS, in the muscles of the buttocks, and anteriorly over the pubic symphysis. The back musculature will have increased tone on one side.

Rehabilitation Progression. To treat this problem, the sports therapist should mobilize the sacroiliac joint to correct the postural asymmetry (Figures 26-36 to 26-40). If the right side of the pelvis appears to be posteriorly rotated, it should be mobilized in an anterior direction. This should be followed by a contract-relax stretch of the hip, again aimed at correcting the postural asymmetry. Strengthening exercises should be used to help improve stability of a hypermobile joint. A bilateral hip-lifting bridge exercise may be used to help stabilize the pelvis (Figure 26-47). Corsets or belts may also help to stabilize the pelvis during activities (Figure 26-62). Self-stretching to correct the postural asymmetry should also be taught to the athlete.[4,5,11,15,40]

REHABILITATION TECHNIQUES FOR THE CERVICAL SPINE

Acute Facet Joint Lock

Pathomechanics.   Acute cervical joint lock is a very common condition, more frequently called wryneck or stiffneck. The athlete usually complains of pain on one side of the neck following a sudden backward bending, side bending, and/or rotation of the neck. Pain can also occur after holding the head in an unusual position over a period of time, as when awakening from sleep. This problem can also occasionally follow exposure to a cold draft of air. There is no report of other acute trauma that could have produced the pain. This usually occurs when a small piece of synovial membrane lining the joint capsule or a meniscoid body is impinged or trapped within a facet joint in the cervical vertebrae. During inspection, there is palpable point tenderness and marked muscle guarding. The athlete will report that the neck is "locked." Side bending and rotation are painful when moving in the direction opposite to the position in which there is locking. Other movements are relatively painless.[31]

Rehabilitation Progression.   Various therapeutic modalities may be used to modulate pain in an attempt to break a pain-spasm-pain cycle. Joint mobilizations involving gentle traction (Figure 26-63), rotation (Figure 26-64), and lateral bending (Figure 26-65), first in the pain-free direction and then in the direction of pain, can help reduce the guarding. Occasionally pain will be relieved almost immediately following mobilization. If not, it may be helpful to wear a soft cervical collar to provide for comfort (Figure 26-66). This muscle guarding will generally last for 2 or 3 days as the athlete progressively regains motion.

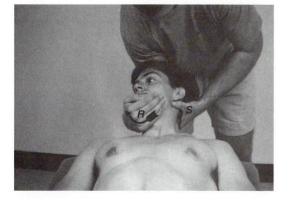

Figure 26-64   Cervical vertebrae rotation oscillations are done with one hand supporting the weight of the head and the other rotating the head in the direction of the restriction. These oscillations treat pain or stiffness when there is some resistance in the same direction as the rotation.

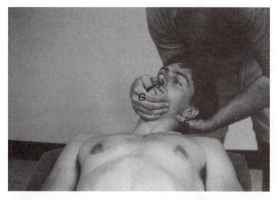

Figure 26-65   Cervical vertebrae side-bending may be used to treat pain or stiffness with resistance when side-bending the neck.

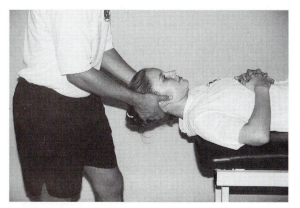

Figure 26-63   Cervical traction.

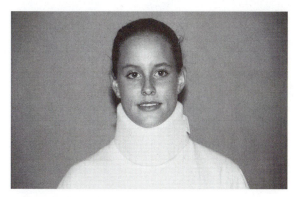

Figure 26-66   The use of a soft or hard collar can increase comfort.

Cervical Sprain

Pathomechanics and Injury Mechanism. A cervical sprain usually results from a moderate to severe trauma. More commonly the head snaps suddenly, such as when the athlete is tackled or blocked while unprepared. Frequently muscle strains occur with ligament sprains. A sprain of the neck can produce tears in the major supporting tissue of the anterior or posterior longitudinal ligaments, the interspinous ligament, and the supraspinous ligament. There may be palpable tenderness over the transverse and spinous processes that serve as sites of attachment for the ligaments.

The sprain displays all the signs of the facet joint lock, but the movement restriction is much greater and can potentially involve more than one vertebral segment. The main difference between the two is that acute joint lock can usually be dealt with in a very short period of time but a sprain will require a significantly longer period for rehabilitation. Pain may not be significant initially but always appears the day after the trauma. Pain stems from the inflammation of injured tissue and a protective muscle guarding that restricts motion.

Rehabilitation Progression. As soon as possible the athlete should have a physician evaluation to rule out the possibility of fracture, dislocation, disk injury, or injury to the spinal cord or nerve root. A soft cervical collar may be applied to reduce muscle guarding (Figure 26-66). Ice and electrical stimulation are used for 48 to 72 hours while the injury is in the acute stage of healing. In an athlete with a severe injury, the physician may prescribe 2 to 3 days of bed rest, along with analgesics and anti-inflammatory medication. Range-of-motion exercises through a pain-free range should begin as soon as possible, including flexion (Figure 26-67), extension (Figure 26-68), rotation (Figure 26-69), and side-bending (Figure 26-70). It has been demonstrated that using early ROM exercises, as opposed to long periods of immobility, tends to reduce the likelihood of neck hypomobility when the healing process is complete.[31] It is important to regain motion as soon as possible. However, it is critical to understand that a sprain, particularly one that involves a complete ligament tear, causes hypermobility. Thus strengthening exercises (Figures 26-71 to 26-74) along with stabilization exercises (Figures 26-75 to 26-76) should also be incorporated into the rehabilitation program.

Mechanical traction may also be prescribed to relieve pain and muscle guarding (Figure 26-65).

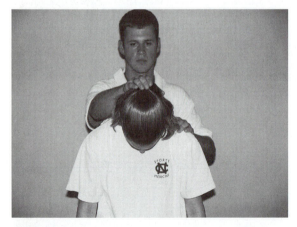

Figure 26-67   Manually assisted flexion stretching exercise.

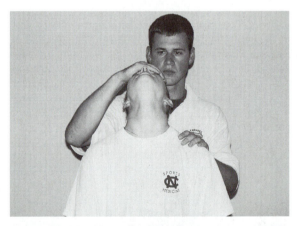

Figure 26-68   Manually assisted extension stretching exercise.

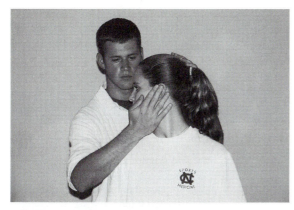

Figure 26-69 Manually assisted rotation stretching exercise.

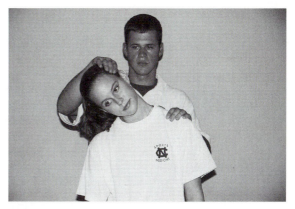

Figure 26-70 Manually assisted side-bending stretching exercise.

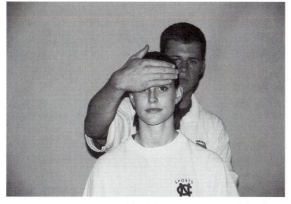

Figure 26-71 Manually resisted flexion strengthening exercise.

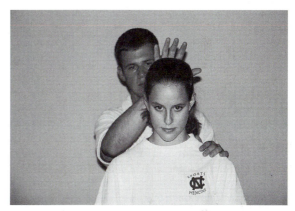

Figure 26-72 Manually resisted extension strengthening exercise.

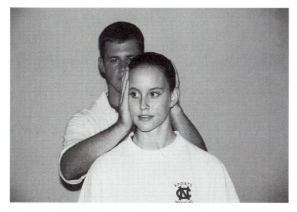

Figure 26-73 Manually resisted rotation strengthening exercise.

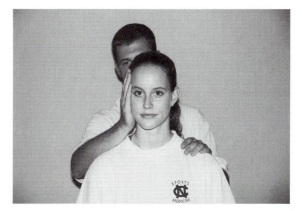

Figure 26-74 Manually resisted side-bending strengthening exercise.

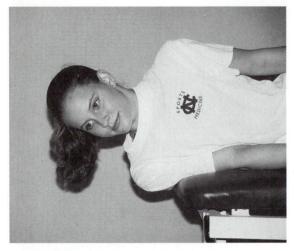

Figure 26-75 Gravity-assisted cervical stabilization exercise done on a treatment table with the head maintaining a static position. May be done side-lying(right and left), prone, supine.

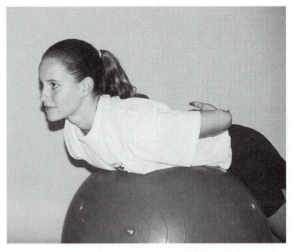

Figure 26-76 Cervical stabilization exercises done on a Swiss ball.

Summary

1. The low back pain that athletes most often experience is an acute, painful experience of relatively short duration that seldom causes significant time loss from practice or competition.
2. Regardless of the diagnosis or the specificity of the diagnosis, a thorough evaluation of the athlete's back pain is critical to good care.
3. Back rehabilitation may be classified as a two-stage approach. Stage I (acute stage) treatment consists mainly of the modality treatment and pain-relieving exercises. Stage II treatment involves treating athletes with a reinjury or exacerbation of a previous problem.
4. The types of exercises that may be included in the initial pain management phase include the following: lateral shift corrections, extension exercises, flexion exercises, mobilization exercises, and myofascial stretching exercises.
5. It is suggested that the sports therapist use an eclectic approach to the selection of exercises, mixing the various protocols described according to the findings of the athlete's evaluation.
6. Specific goals and exercises included in stage II should address which structures to stretch, which structures to strengthen, incorporating dynamic stabilization into the athlete's daily life and exercise routine, and which movements need a motor learning approach to control faulty mechanics.
7. The rehabilitation program should be based on functional training, which may be divided into basic and advanced phases.
8. Back pain can result from one or a combination of the following problems: muscle strain, piriformis muscle or quadratus lumborum myofascial pain or strain, myofascial trigger points, lumbar facet joint sprains, hypermobility syndromes, disk-related back problems, or sacroiliac joint dysfunction.
9. Cervical pain can result from muscle strains, acute cervical joint lock, ligament sprains, and various other problems.

References

1. Beattie, P. 1992. The use of an eclectic approach for the treatment of low back pain: A case study. *Physical Therapy* 72(12): 923–28.

2. Binkley, J., E. Finch, J. Hall, et al. 1993. Diagnostic classification of patients with low back pain: Report on a survey of physical therapy experts. *Physical Therapy* 73(3): 138–55.

3. Bittinger, J. 1980. *Management of the lumbar pain syndromes.* Course notes.

4. Cibulka, M. 1922. The treatment of the sacroiliac joint component to low back pain: A case report. *Physical Therapy* 72(12): 917–22.

5. Cibulka, M., A. Delitto, and R. Koldehoff. 1988. Changes in innominate tilt after manipulation of the sacroiliac joint in patients with low back pain: An experimental study. *Physical Therapy* 68(9): 1359–70.

6. Cibulka, M., S. Rose, A. Delitto, et al. 1986. Hamstring muscle strain treated by mobilizing the saroiliac joint. *Physical Therapy* 66(8): 1220–23.

7. Crock, H. 1986. Internal disk disruption: A challenge to disk-prolapse fifty years on: The Presidential address: ISSLS. *Spine* 11(6): 650–53.

8. DeRosa, C., and J. Porterfield. 1992. A physical therapy model for the treatment of low back pain. *Physical Therapy* 72(4): 261–72.

9. Deyo, R., A. Diehl, and M. Rosenthal. 1986. How many days of bed rest for acute low back pain? A randomized clinical trial. *New England Journal of Medicine* 315:1064–70.

10. Donley, P. 1977. Rehabilitation of low back pain in athletes: The 1976 Schering symposium on low back problems. *Athletic Training* 12(2).

11. Erhard, R., and R. Bowling. 1979. The recognition and management of the pelvic component of lowback and sciatic pain. *APTA* 2(3): 4–13.

12. Farfan, H. 1975. Muscular mechanism of the lumbar spine and the position of power and efficiency. *Orthop Clin North Am* 6(1): 135–44.

13. Friberg, O. 1983. Clinical symptoms and biomechanics of lumbar spine and hip joint in leg length inequality. *Spine* 8(6): 643–50.

14. Frymoyer, J. 1988. Back pain and sciatica: Medical progress. *New England Journal of Medicine* 318(5): 291–300.

15. Grieve, G. 1976. The sacro-iliac joint. *Physiotherapy* 62:384–400.

16. Grieve, G. 1982. Lumbar instability: Congress lecture. *Physiotherapy* 68(1): 2–9.

17. Jackson, C., and M. Brown. 1983. Analysis of current approaches and a practical guide to prescription of exercise. *Clin Orthop Rel Res* 179:46–54.

18. Lewit, K., and D. Simons. 1984. Myofascial pain: Relief by post-isometric relaxation. *Archives of Physical Medicine and Rehabilitation* 65(8): 452–56.

19. Lindstrom, I., C. Ohlund, C. Eek, et al. 1992. The effect of graded activity on patients with subacute low back pain: A randomized prospective clinical study with an operant-conditioning behavioral approach. *Physical Therapy* 72(4): 279–90.

20. Maigne, R. 1980. Low back pain of thoracolumbar origin. *Archives of Physical Medicine and Rehabilitation* 61(9): 391–95.

21. Maitland, G. 1990. *Vertebral manipulation.* 5th ed. London: Butterworth.

22. Mapa, B. 1980. An Australian programme for management of low back problems. *Physiotherapy* 66(4): 108–11.

23. McGraw, M. 1966. *The neuro-muscular maturation of the human infant.* New York: Hafner.

24. McKenzie, R. 1972. Manual correction of sciatic scoliosis. *New Zealand Medical Journal* 76(484): 194–99.

25. McKenzie, R. 1981. *The lumbar spine: Mechanical diagnosis and therapy, spinal publications.* New Zealand: Lower Hutt.

26. Porter, R., and C. Miller. 1986. Back pain and trunk list. *Spine* 11(6): 596–600.

27. Saal, J. 1988. I. Rehabilitation of football players with lumbar spine injury. *Physician and Sports Medicine* 16(9): 61–68.

28. Saal, J. 1988. Rehabilitation of football players with lumbar spine injury. *Physician and Sports Medicine* 16(10): 117–25.

29. Saal, J. 1990. Dynamic muscular stabilization in the non-operative treatment of lumbar pain syndromes. *Orthop Rev* 19(8): 691–700.

30. Saal, J., and J. Saal. 1989. Nonoperative treatment of herniated lumbar intervertebral disk with radiculopathy: An outcome study. *Spine* 14(4): 431–37.

31. Saunders, D. 1985. *Evaluation, treatment, and prevention of musculoskeletal disorders.* Bloomington, MN: Educational Opportunities.

32. Steiner, C., C. Staubs, M. Ganon, et al. 1987. Piriformis syndrome: Pathogenesis, diagnosis, and treatment. *J AOA* 87(4): 318–23.

33. Tenhula, J., S. Rose, and A. Delitto. 1990. Association between direction of lateral lumbar shift, movement tests, and side of symptoms in patients with low back pain syndrome. *Physical Therapy* 70(8): 480–86.

34. Threlkeld, A. 1992. The effects of manual therapy on connective tissue. *Physical Therapy* 72(12): 893–902.

35. Travell, J., and D. Simon. 1992. *Myofascial pain and dysfunction: The lower extremities.* Baltimore: Williams & Wilkins.

36. Travell, J., and D. Simons. 1992. *Myofascial pain and dysfunction: The trigger point manual.* Baltimore: Williams & Wilkins.

37. Twomey, L. 1992. A rationale for treatment of back pain and joint pain by manual therapy. *Physical Therapy* 72(12): 885–92.

38. Waddell, G. 1987. Clinical assessment of lumbar impairment. *Clin Orthop Rel Res* 221:110–20.

39. Waddell, G. 1987. A new clinical model for the treatment of low-back pain. *Spine* 12(7): 632–44.

40. Walker, J. 1992. The sacroiliac joint: A critical review. *Physical Therapy* 72(12): 903–16.

Glossary

A

abduction Movement of a body part away from the midline of the body.

accessory motion The movement of one articulating joint surface relative to another, involving spin, roll, glide.

active range of motion That portion of the total range of motion through which a joint can be moved by an active muscle contraction.

acute injury An injury with a sudden onset and short duration

adduction Movement of a body part toward the midline of the body.

adherence A term used in a behavior modification setting/program for what is usually a long-term commitment to a rehabilitation program.

aerobic activity An activity in which the intensity of the activity is low enough that a sufficient amount of oxygen can be delivered to continue activity for an indefinite period of time.

agonist muscle The muscle that contracts to produce a movement.

anaerobic activity An activity in which the intensity is so great that the demand for oxygen is greater than the body's ability to deliver oxygen.

analgesia A loss of sensitivity to pain.

anemia An iron deficiency.

antagonist muscle The muscle being stretched in response to contraction of the agonist muscle.

anteversion Tipping forward of a part as a whole, without bending.

antiemetics Drugs used to treat nausea and vomiting arising from any of a variety of causes.

antipyretic An agent that relieves or reduces fever.

antitussives Drugs that suppress coughing.

aponeurosis A thin, sheetlike tendon made of dense connective tissue.

apophysis Bony outgrowth to which muscles attach.

arthokinematics The physiology of joint movement. The manner in which two articulated joint surfaces move relative to one another.

arthroscopic Technique, using an arthroscope, which uses a small camera lens, to view the inside of a body part, such as a joint.

arthrosis A degenerative process involving destruction of cartilage, remodeling of bone, and possible secondary inflammation.

atrophy A decrease in muscle size due to inactivity.

attenuation A decrease in energy intensity as the ultrasound wave is transmitted through various tissues; caused by scattering and dispersion.

avulsion Forcible tearing away of a part or a structure of a tissue from its normal attachment.

B

Bad Ragaz technique Aquatic therapy technique where buoyancy is used for flotation purposes only.

ballistic stretching A stretching technique in which repetitive contractions of the agonist muscle are used to produce quick stretches of the antagonist muscle.

basal metabolic rate The rate at which calories are used for carrying on the body's vital functions and maintenance activities when the body is at rest.

biomechanics The mechanics of biological movement, regarding forces that arise either from within or outside of the body.

buffers Techniques that allay the symptoms of stress but do not address the problem that initially caused the stressor.

buoyant force A force that assists motion toward the water's surface and resists submersive motion.

bursitis Inflammation of a bursa, especially of a bursa located around a joint.

C

calisthenic exercises Exercises that use body weight as resistance.

capacitor electrodes Air space plates or pad electrodes that create a stronger electrical field than a magnetic field.

cardiac output The volume of blood the heart is capable of pumping in exactly 1 minute.

cardiorespiratory endurance The ability to persist in a physical activity requiring oxygen for physical exertion without experiencing undue fatigue.

cavitation The formation of gas-filled bubbles that expand and compress because of ultrasonically induced pressure changes in tissue fluids.

chronic injury A injury with long onset and long duration.

circuit training A series of exercise stations; typically consisting of various combinations of weight training, flexibility, calisthenics, and brief aerobic exercises.

closed fracture A fracture that involves little or no displacement of bones and thus little or no soft-tissue disruption.

closed kinetic chain A position in which at least one foot or one hand are in a weight-bearing position.

collagen The main organic constituent of connective tissue.

compliance A term used in the rehabilitation setting to describe a patient's attitude toward the caregiver's instructions. The patient is obedient to the physician or health caregiver's directions, the care giver is in an authoritative position, and the treatment is short-term and usually has been prescribed.

concentric contraction A contraction in which the muscle shortens.

continuous training A technique that uses exercises performed at the same level of intensity for long periods of time.

contractile tissue Tissue capable on contraction (i.e., muscles).

coping rehearsal A technique in which an individual visually rehearses a problem they feel may be an obstacle to reaching a goal, such as a return to competition, and envisions being successful.

core stability The ability to transfer the vertical projection of the center of gravity around a stationary supporting base.

crepitation A crackling sound heard and felt during the movement of broken bones or in a case of soft tissue inflammation.

cryotherapy Cold therapy.

cubital tunnel syndrome Entrapment of the ulnar nerve in the cubital tunnel.

cyanosis Slightly bluish, grayish, slatelike, or dark purple discoloration of the skin caused by a lack of sufficient oxygen.

D

degeneration Deterioration of tissue.

diapedesis A passage of blood cells via ameboid action through the intact capillary wall.

disassociation A technique that can be used in rehabilitation for temporary pain modulation. The individual thinks about something other than the pain, such as a sunny day at the beach or the game-winning shot at the buzzer.

distal Farthest from a center, from the midline, or from the trunk.

dorsiflexion Bending toward the dorsum or rear of the foot; opposite of plantarflexion.

E

eccentric contraction A contraction in which the muscle lengthens while contracting.

edema Swelling as a result of a collection of fluid in connective tissue.

energy Biologically, the ability to do work that is produced as body cells break down the chemical units of glucose, fats, or amino acids.

epiphysis A cartilaginous growth region of a bone.

etiology The science of dealing with causes of disease or trauma; or the chain of conditions that give rise to a disease or trauma.

eversion Turning the foot outward.

exudate An accumulation of fluid in an area.

F

fartlek A type of workout that involves jogging at varying speeds over varying terrain.

fascia A fibrous membrane that covers, supports, and separates muscles.

fasciotomy An incision into the fascia to release pressure within the compartment.

fast-twitch muscle fibers A type of muscle fiber responsible for speed or power activities such as sprinting or weight lifting.

fibrinogen A blood plasma protein that is converted into a fibrin clot.

fibroblast Any cell component from which fibers are developed.

fibrocartilage A type of cartilage (e.g., intervertebral disks) in which the matrix contains thick bundles of collaginous fibers.

fibroplasia The period of scar formation that occurs during the fibroblastic-repair phase.

flexibility The ability to move the arms, legs and trunk freely throughout a full, nonrestricted, pain-free range of motion.

foot pronation Combined foot movement of eversion and abduction.

foot supination Combined foot movement of inversion and abduction.

force A push or a pull produced by the action of one object or another; measured in pounds or newtons.

force couple Action of two forces in opposing direction about some axis of rotation.

force-velocity relationship The faster a muscle is loaded or lengthened eccentrically, the greater the resultant force output.

frequency With therapeutic modalities, the number of cycles per seconds that a specific exercise is performed during a training cycle.

functional progression A series of gradual progressive activities designed to prepare an individual for return to a specific sport.

G

genu recurvatum Hyperextension at the knee joint.

genu valgum Knock-knee.

genu varum Bowleg.

Golgi tendon organ (GTO) A mechanoreceptor sensitive to changes in tension of the musculotendinous unit.

H

hemorrhage A discharge or loss of blood.

herniation A bulging or enlargement of soft tissue.

hip pointer A subcutaneus contusion that can cause, in most cases, a separation or tearing of the origins or insertions of the muscles. The injury is usually caused by a direct blow to the iliac crest or anterosuperior iliac spine.

hyperextension Extreme stretching of a body part.

hypermobile Extreme mobility of a joint.

hypertonic Having a higher osmotic pressure than a compared solution.

hypertrophy An increase in muscle size in response to training.

hyperventilation Abnormally deep breathing that is prolonged, resulting in too much oxygen intake and too little carbon dioxide outtake.

hypoxia Oxygen deficiency.

I

idiopathic Cause of a condition is unknown.

imagery A technique in which the athlete vividly imagines a sensory experience in order to practice or prepare for a situation.

infrared The portion of the electromagnetic spectrum associated with thermal changes. Infrared wavelengths, located adjacent to the red portion of the visible light spectrum.

interosseous membrane Connective tissue membrane between bones.

interval training Alternating periods of relatively intense work followed by active recovery.

inversion Turning the foot inward.

iontophoresis A therapeutic technique that involves introducing ions into the body tissue by means of a continuous direct electrical current.

ischemia Local anemia.

isokinetic exercise An exercise in which the speed of movement is constant regardless of the strength of a contraction.

isometric exercise An exercise in which the muscle contracts against resistance but does not change in length.

isotonic exercise An exercise in which the muscle contracts against resistance and changes in length.

J

joint capsule A saclike structure that encloses the ends of bones in a diarthrodial joint.

K

kinesthesia, kinesthesis Sensation or feeling of movement; the awareness one has of the spatial orientation of his or her body and the relationships among its parts.

M

macrotears Tears usually caused by acute trauma, involving significant destruction of soft tissue and resulting in clinical symptoms and function alteration.

margination An accumulation of leukocytes on blood vessel walls at the site of an injury during early stages of inflammation.

maximal oxygen uptake (VO$_2$max) A measurement taken in a laboratory to determine how much oxygen an athlete can use during maximal exercise.

microstreaming The unidirectional movement of fluids along the boundaries of cell membranes, resulting from the mechanical pressure wave in an ultrasonic field.

microtears Soft-tissue tears that involve only minor damage and most often are associated with overuse.

muscle guarding A protective response in muscle that occurs because of pain or fear of movement.

muscle spindle Mechanoreceptors within skeletal muscle sensitive to changes in length and rate of length changes in muscle.

muscular endurance The ability to perform repetitive muscular contractions against some resistance for an extended period of time.

muscular strength The ability of a muscle to generate force against some resistance.

myofilaments Small protein structures that are the contractile elements in a muscle fiber.

myositis Inflammation or soreness of muscle tissue.

N

negative reinforcement A punishment (verbal or a stimulus) to elicit a certain behavior or inhibit a specific behavior.

nerve entrapment Compression of a nerve between bone or soft tissue.

neuroma A tumor consisting mostly of nerve cells and nerve fibers.

neuromuscular control The interaction of the nervous and muscular systems to create coordinated movement.

O

open fracture A fracture that involves enough displacement of the fracture ends that the bone actually disrupts the cutaneous layers and breaks through the skin.

open kinetic chain The foot and hand are not in contact with the floor or any other surfaces.

orthosis An appliance or apparatus used in sports to support, align, prevent, or correct deformities or to improve function of a movable body part.

orthotics Devices used to control abnormal compensatory movement of the foot.

osteochondritis dissecans Trauma in which fragments of cartilage and underlying bone are detached from the articular surface.

osteokinematic motion A physiological movement that results from either concentric or eccentric active muscle contraction that moves a bone or joint.

osteoporosis A decrease in bone density.

overload Exercising at a higher level than normal.

P

pain threshold The amount of noxious stimulus required before pain is perceived.

painful arc Pain that occurs at some point in the midrange but disappears as the limb passes this point in either direction.

par cours A technique for improving cardiorespiratory endurance that basically combines continuous training and circuit training.

passive range of motion That portion of the total range of motion through which a joint may be moved passively with no muscle contraction.

pathology Science of the structural and functional manifestation of disease; the manifestations of disease.

pathomechanics Mechanical forces applied to a living organism that adversely change the body's structure and function.

periosteum A highly vascularized and innervated membrane lining the surface of bone.

phagocytosis Destruction of injurious cells or particles by phagocytes (white blood cells).

phalanges Bones of the fingers and toes.

phalanx Any one of the bones of the fingers or toes.

phonophoresis A technique in which ultrasound is used to drive a topical application of a selected medication into the tissue.

plyometric training A technique of exercise that involves a rapid eccentric (lengthening) stretch of a muscle, followed immediately by a rapid concentric contraction of that muscle for the purpose of producing a forceful explosive movement.

positive reinforcement A reward (verbal or a stimulus) that elicits a desired behavior.

posterior interosseus nerve compression Compression of the posterior interosseus nerve within the radial tunnel, producing motor weakness with no pain.

power The ability to generate great amounts of force against a certain resistance in a short period of time.

progression Gradually increases in the level and intensity of exercise.

progressive resistance exercise A technique that progressively strengthens muscles through a muscle contraction that overcomes some fixed resistance.

prone To be positioned, lying down, on one's ventral surface.

proprioception The ability to determine the position of a joint in space.

proprioceptive neuromuscular facilitation (PNF) A group of manually resisted strengthening and stretching techniques.

prothrombin A substance that interacts with calcium to produce thrombin.

proximal Nearest to the point of reference.

R

radial tunnel syndrome Entrapment of the radial nerve within the radial tunnel, which produces pain with no motor weakness.

rating of perceived exertion (RPE) A technique used to subjectively rate exercise intensity on a numerical scale.

regeneration The repair, regrowth, or restoration of a part of a tissue.

retroversion Tilting or turning backward of a part.

S

SAID principle When the body is subjected to stresses and overloads of varying intensities, it will gradually adapt, over time, to overcome whatever demands are placed on it.

scapulohumeral rhythm The movement of the scapula relative to the movement of the humerus throughout a full range of abduction.

scoliosis Lateral rotary curve of the spine.

slow-twitch muscle fibers Muscle fibers that are resistant to fatigue and more useful in long-term, endurance activities.

somatosensation Specialized variation of the sensory modality of touch that encompasses the sensation of joint movement (kinesthesia) and joint position (joint position sense).

speed The ability to perform a particular movement very rapidly. It is a function of distance and time.

spondylolysis Degeneration of the vertebrae: most commonly it is a defect in the pars interarticularis of the articular processes of the vertebrae.

sprains Damage to a ligament that provides support to a joint.

static balance The ability to maintain a center of gravity over a fixed base of support (unilateral or bilateral) while standing on a stable surface.

static stretching Passively stretching a given antagonist muscle by placing it in a maximal position of stretch and holding it there for an extended time.

steadiness The ability to keep the body as motionless as possible; this is a measurement of postural sway.

strain The extent of deformation of tissue under loading.

stress A positive or negative forces that can disrupt the body's equilibrium.

stressor Anything that affects the body's physiological or psychological condition, upsetting the homeostatic balance.

stroke volume The volume of blood being pumped out of the heart with each beat.

subluxation A partial or incomplete dislocation of an articulation.

supine To be positioned, lying down, on one's dorsal surface.

symmetry A sliding or gliding of one joint surface relative to another.

T

target heart rate A specific heart rate to be achieved and maintained during exercise.

tendinitis Inflammation of a tendon.

tenosynovitis Inflammation of a tendon synovial sheath.

thermotherapy Heat therapy.

torque The moment of force applied during rotational motion (measured in foot pounds or newton meters).

traction A tension applied to a body segment which separates joint surfaces.

translation Equality of body parts on one side of the body when compared to the opposite side.

traumatic Pertaining to an injury or wound.

trigger point Localized deep tenderness in a palpable firm band of muscle. When stretched, palpating finger can snap the band like a taut string, which produces local pain, a local twitch of that portion of muscle, and a jump by the patient. Sustained pressure on a trigger point reproduces the pattern of referred pain for that site.

V

valgus Position of a body part that is bent outward.

varus Position of a body part that is bent inward.

vasoconstriction A decrease in the diameter of a blood vessel.

vasodilation An increase in the diameter of a blood vessel.

volar Referring to the palm or the sole.

volume Regarding exercise, the total amount of work that is performed in a single workout session.

W

Wolff's law A law that states that bone remodels itself and provides increased strength along the lines of the mechanical forces placed on it.

Index